Celiac Disease and Non-Celiac Gluten Sensitivity

Edited by:
Luis Rodrigo
Amado Salvador Peña

Celiac Disease and Non-Celiac Gluten Sensitivity

1st edition © 2014 OmniaScience (Omnia Publisher SL)

www.omniascience.com

DOI: http://dx.doi.org/10.3926/oms.223

ISBN: 978-84-942118-2-9

DL: B-23979-2014

English Translation: Carlos Beirute Lucke, Translator in Chief, CIEC. Translator and Interpreter, Ministry of Foreign Relations, Costa Rica

Cover design: OmniaScience

Cover image: © askaja – Fotolia.com

Sponsors

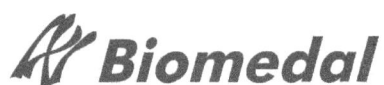 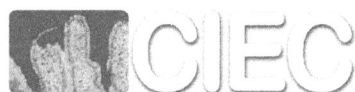

Applications for the detection of Gluten Immunogenic Peptides in celiac disease - Biomedal Diagnostics

Biomedal S.L. has developed tools for the management of celiac disease since 2003. The first collaborative research project with the Spanish National Research Council (CSIC), the Stanford University and the University of Seville was to obtain antibodies against the most immunogenic peptide found in prolamins, the gliadin 33-mer (1,2). In 2007, Biomedal Diagnostics division was created to commercialize Glutentox® product, the last generation tools for detection of the immunotoxic gluten proteins in food, based on the anti-gliadin33mer monoclonal antibodies A1 and G12. There is increasing evidence that these antibodies used in Glutentox® ELISAs and lateral flow tests correlate with the potential immunotoxicity found in food and beverages (2-9). Gliadin 33-mer structural related epitopes that react to either A1 or G12 antibodies are immunodominant for most of the patients with celiac disease. They therefore indicate the presence of Gluten Immunogenic Peptides (GIP).

Relevant research published in scientific journals of the use of these antibodies is shown under:

Generation of anti-gliadin 33-mer monoclonal antibodies

1. Sensitive detection of cereal fractions that are toxic to celiac disease patients by using monoclonal antibodies to a main immunogenic wheat peptide. Morón B et al., Am J Clin Nutr 2008, 87 405-14.

Monitoring gluten detoxification: reactivity to G12/A1 antibodies decreased in parallel to immunoactive gluten peptides in samples treated with glutenases.

2. Toward the assessment of food toxicity for celiac patients: characterization of monoclonal antibodies to a main immunogenic gluten peptide. Morón B et al., PLoS One 2008, 28 405-14

3. A food-grade enzyme preparation with modest gluten detoxification properties. Ehren J et al. PLoS One 2009, 4 e6313.

Analysis of the potential immunotoxicity of cereal varieties for celiac patients: reactivity of G12 antibody is proportional to the reactivity to different lines of oats, barley and engineered wheat.

4. Diversity in oat potential immunogenicity: basis for the selection of oat varieties with no toxicity in coeliac disease. Comino I, et al., Gut 2011, 60 915-22.

5. Molecular and immunological characterization of gluten proteins isolated from oat cultivars that differ in toxicity for celiac disease. Real A et al., Plos One 2012, 7 e48365.

6. Significant differences in potential immunotoxicity of barley varieties for celiac disease. Comino I et al. Mol. Nut. Food Res. 2012, 56 1697-707.

7. Reduced-Gliadin Wheat Bread: An Alternative to the Gluten-Free Diet for Consumers Suffering Gluten-Related Pathologies. Gil-Humanes J et al. Plos One, 2014, 9 e90898.

Analysis of the immunogenic peptides in hydrolyzed gluten (beers): Only HPLC fractions of beers reactive to a G12/A1 lateral flow test contained immunoactive peptides to celiac T Cells.

8. Immunological determination of gliadin 33-mer equivalent peptides in beers as a specific and practical analytical method to assess safety for celiac patients. Comino I, et al., J Sci Food Agric. 2013, 93 933-43

9. Identification and In Vitro Reactivity of Celiac Immunoactive Peptides in an Apparent Gluten-Free Beer. Real A et al. PLoS ONE 2014, 9 e100917.

iVYLISA GIP: an innovative tool for monitoring gluten-free diet compliance in patients with celiac disease by direct detection of gluten peptides in feces

Biomedal S.L. has introduced iVYLISA GIP an innovative application for the detection of gluten intake by using the highly specific monoclonal antibodies A1 and G12. The rationale of this new product is the detection of Gluten Immunogenic Peptides (GIP) in feces (10). The main application is the compliance of gluten-free diet (GFD) in celiac disease and other gluten-related pathologies (non-celiac gluten sensitivity or gluten allergy).

Why should the GFD adherence be monitored?

- Between 33 and 55% of celiac patients do not follow a completely GFD.

- More than 45% of patients still exhibit intestinal damage even after a year following a GFD. Within a week more than 90% of patients with celiac disease show symptoms indicating gluten intake.

- To reduce a long-term risk of complications such as nutritional deficiencies, low bone mineral density, etc.

- A non-treated celiac patient has a 4 fold increased risk of lymphoma (11).

- In the diagnosis of refractory celiac disease, it is necessary to ensure full adherence to GFD.

Conclusions of the method for the detection of GIP in stool

- A significant part of the ingested gluten peptides are excreted in feces. 98-100% of the people ingesting gluten show GIP in the feces as measured by the iVYLISA GIP.

- Transit of gluten peptides through the gastrointestinal track takes more than 24-48 hours.

- The time of GIP excretion in stools is between 2 and 4 days after ingestion of gluten.

- Despite a large variation between individuals, there is a correlation between the amount of gluten consumed and the amount of excreted GIPs as measured by the iVYLISA GIP.

- The iVYLISA GIP appears to be more reliable than serological marker to detect lack of strict adherence to GFD.

10. Monitoring of gluten-free diet compliance in celiac patients by assessment of gliadin 33-mer equivalent epitopes in feces. Comino I et al., Am J Clin Nutr 2012; 18: 670-77

11. Mucosal Healing and Risk for Lymphoproliferative Malignancy in Celiac Disease. Lebwohl et al. Annals Inter Med 2013; 159:169-176

Co-financed by MINECO and FEDER funds

::: iVYDAL ivydal@biomedal.com
In Vitro Diagnostics ivydal.biomedal.com

Developed by
Biomedal

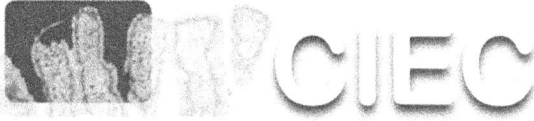

Centro de Información sobre la Enfermedad Celíaca

The *Celiac Disease Information Centre* is a non-profit, volunteer-staffed project aimed at disseminating, free of charge, up-to-date information on gluten-related disorders from scientific and academic sources.

This information is made available, through its different divisions, to patients and their close kin as well as to health care professionals of differing specialties, to restaurants and similar venues, as well as to the public, since a well-informed milieu contributes effectively to improve quality of life for those who suffer from such disorders. As part of its ongoing dissemination effort, CIEC gathers and translates relevant information from researchers from different regions of the world to make it available both in English and in Spanish.

On this occasion, CIEC is pleased to offer the English translation of this volume, whose original Spanish-language version, *Enfermedad Celiaca y Sensibilidad al Gluten no Celiaca*, from *Omniascience* Publishing, edited by Dr. Amado Salvador Peña and Dr. Luis Rodrigo, offers the work of renowned researchers in this field providing crucial perspectives on the management of these pathologies. This work has become an invaluable tool for patients and health care specialists in the Spanish-speaking world and we hope that this joint effort to render this work into English will likewise become a key contribution for a better understanding of this subject.

Amavilia Perez Villavicencio
Director
CIEC

Celiac Disease Information Centre

ciec.contacto@gmail.com   contactciec@gmail.com

Preface

This book which we have the honor and the pleasure to present to you, entitled *Celiac Disease and Non-Celiac Gluten Sensitivity*, has been written thanks to the efforts and collaboration of many authors, mostly from Spain and Latin America, all of whom are experts on the subjects of each one of its twenty-five chapters. We would like to acknowledge the great effort made by the "Centro de Información sobre la Enfermedad Celíaca" (CIEC) from Costa Rica, their support, and the organization of the English translation under the guidance of Carlos Beirute L. (translator in-chief) and the inspired dedication of Amavilia Perez V., its director. Since their main goal is to transmit and disseminate knowledge to patients with these ailments and Patient's Organizations they also realized that an English version of the book would bring original contributions of Spanish speaking experts to a wider audience.

The choice of its title is justified. Knowledge on celiac disease has deepened remarkably during recent decades. It is now firmly established, that is a common disorder, systemic in nature, genetically predetermined and triggered by gluten. However, the recent re-discovery of non-celiac gluten sensitivity has generated a new thrust in the quest for knowledge relating to these diseases, which have great social and public health repercussions. It is interesting that since the publication of the Spanish version of this book a year ago, studies mainly from Australia have demonstrated that improvement of symptoms with a gluten-free diet does not necessarily equate with an effect of withdrawing gluten and reintroducing gluten performing a gluten challenge. As Peter Gibson from Monash University, The Alfred Hospital, Melbourne, Vic, Australia has recently stated, "the story is only beginning".

There is a great amount of important scientific information, available through many informations, articles, revisions and monographs, which deals with a diversity of issues related to celiac disease, but there is a lack of books, particularly in the Spanish language, that gather its different aspects. This was one of the main objectives of the first book published in Spanish. The interdisciplinary approach that became clear with the different chapters is largely due to the *Sociedad Española de la Enfermedad Celíaca* (SEEC, "Spanish Celiac Disease Society"). In this preface, we warmly thank its present president, Professor Eduardo Arranz MD, PhD for his enthusiasm and we would like to acknowledge the contribution of the Society and its members for their approach to the study of celiac disease.

Our principal aim is the diffusion of knowledge, not only through its cost-free distribution by means of the internet, but also for those who may wish to purchase a printed copy. We intend to update current knowledge on celiac disease and we hope that this collective effort will help to improve the collaboration between the diverse groups in clinical and basic research. Knowledge on celiac disease has fully entered the field of biology and molecular genetics. It has become a model for the understanding of other autoimmune diseases. This book includes an important clinical component. We hope that it will be of use to those who carry on researches in basic disciplines in order to help them translate their findings for the benefit of people who suffer from celiac disease and other gluten-related disorders.

The book will be of use to physicians by helping them to identify a greater number of people who suffer from celiac disease and non-celiac gluten sensitivity and who have been not recognized as such throughout the world. These patients could benefit from a gluten-free diet, thus achieving an improvement of their ailments, as well as a complete recovery of their health and well-being.

We wish to thank all the authors who have selflessly collaborated in this project, providing all their knowledge and expertise and *OmniaScience Editorial* (Omnia Publisher S.L.), of Barcelona. Mrs. Irene Trullàs specially deserves our appreciation for the excellent and ongoing support she has provided us during the entire process in the preparation of the Spanish and English versions of the book.

We are also honored to dedicate this book to people who suffer from celiac disease or non-celiac gluten-related disorders. We agree with Ms. Karla Zaldívar, President of the *Asociación de Celíacos y Sensibles al Gluten de El Salvador* (ACELYSES) that it will be of help for people who suffer from these disorders and who wish to understand their condition beyond the explanations provided by their physician. These informed patients will make a better team with their physicians and specialists from related disciplines and may even, in some measure, contribute to generate a better approach to celiac disease and to non-celiac gluten sensitivity from a scientific perspective.

November 2014

Luis Rodrigo and Amado Salvador Peña

Authors' Index

AGÜERO LUENGO Carlos
Department of Gastroenterology, School of Medicine.
Pontificia Universidad Católica de Chile.
Santiago, Chile.

ARIAS RODRÍGUEZ Laura
Gastroenterology Service. University Hospital of León.
Biomedicine Institute. León University.
León, Spain.

ARRANZ SANZ Eduardo
Mucosal Immunology Laboratory, IBGM.
University of Valladolid.
Spanish National Research Council (CSIC), Consejo Superior de Investigaciones Científicas.
Valladolid, Spain.

BAI Julio César
Small Intestine Section, Clinical Unit. Department of Medicine.
 Bonorino Udaondo Gastroenterological Hospital.
Buenos Aires, Argentina.

BARRO LOSADA Francisco
Institute for Sustainable Agriculture.
Spanish National Research Council (CSIC), Consejo Superior de Investigaciones Científicas.
Córdoba, Spain.

BEIRUTE LUCKE Carlos
Anthropologist, University of Costa Rica.
M.Sci, Marketing and Communication Science.
Celiac Disease Information Centre.
San José, Costa Rica.

BILBAO José Ramón
Department of Genetics, Physical Anthropology and Animal Physiology.
Basque Country University (UPV-EHU).
BioCruces Research Institute.
Bizkaia, Spain.

BRENES Fernando
Laboratory of Pathology.
Hospital CIMA San José.
San José, Costa Rica.

CABRERA CHÁVEZ Francisco
Nutrition Sciences and Gastronomy Unit.
University of Sinaloa.
Culiacán, Sinaloa, Mexico.

CALDERÓN DE LA BARCA Ana María
Department of Nutrition.
Research Center for Food and Development (CIAD, A.C.)
Hermosillo, Sonora, Mexico.

CARRASCO Anna
Gastroenterology Service, Hospital Universitari Mutua de Terrassa.
University of Barcelona. CIBERehd
Terrassa, Barcelona, Spain.

CIMMINO Daniel
Endoscopy Service.
Hospital Alemán.
Buenos Aires, Argentina.

COMINO Isabel
Department of Microbiology and Parasitology.
Faculty of Pharmacy. University of Sevilla.
Sevilla, Spain.

COSTA Ana Florencia
Small Instestine Section, Clinical Unit. Department of Medicine.
Bonorino Udaondo Gastroenterological Hospital.
Buenos Aires, Argentina.

CROMEYER Mauricio
Diagnostic Hospital. Service of Pathology and Gastroenterology.
San Salvador, El Salvador.

CRUSIUS J. Bart A.
Laboratory of Immunogenetics, Department of Medical de Microbiology and Infection.
Control, VU University Medical Center (VUMC).
Amsterdam, The Netherlands.

CUETO-RÚA Eduardo A.
Pediatric Gastroenterology. Division of Gastroenterology, Hospital Sor MaríaLudovica.
La Plata, Argentina.

DOMÍNGUEZ CAJAL Manuel
San Jorge, Hospital.
Huesca, Spain.

ESTEVE Maria
Gastroenterology Service, Hospital Universitari Mutua de Terrassa.
University of Barcelona. CIBERehd
Terrassa, Barcelona, Spain.

FARRÉ MASIP Carme
Clinical Biochemistry Department, Sant Joan de Déu Pediatric University Hospital.
University of Barcelona.
Barcelona, Spain.

FERNÁNDEZ BAÑARES Fernando
Gastroenterology Service, Hospital Universitari Mutua de Terrassa.
University of Barcelona. CIBERehd
Terrassa, Barcelona, Spain.

FERNÁNDEZ JIMÉNEZ Nora
Department of Genetics, Physical Anthropology and Animal Physiology.
Basque Country University (UPV-EHU).
BioCruces Research Institute.
Bizkaia, Spain.

GARCÍA-MANZANARES Álvaro
Endocrinology and Nutrition.
La Mancha Centro Hospital
Alcázar de San Juan, Ciudad Real, Spain.

GARCÍA NIETO Víctor Manuel
History of Pediatrics Group Coordinator of the Spanish Pediatric Association.
Pediatrics Service of Nuestra Señora de Candelaria Hospital.
Santa Cruz de Tenerife, Spain.

GARROTE José Antonio
Genetics and Molecular Biology Laboratory.
Clinical Laboratory Service.
Rio Hortega University Hospital.
Valladolid, Spain.

GIL-HUMANES Javier
Department of Genetics, Cell Biology and Development and Center for Genome Engineering.
University of Minnesota.
Minneapolis, Minnesota, USA.

GIMÉNEZ María J.
Institute for Sustainable Agriculture.
Spanish National Research Council (CSIC), Consejo Superior de Investigaciones Científicas.
Córdoba, Spain.

GONZÁLEZ Nicolás
Department of Gastroenterology (Prof. Henry Cohen).
Faculty of Medicine, Hospital de Clínicas.
Montevideo, Uruguay.

GUTIÉRREZ Rafael A.
Diagnostic Hospital. Service of Pathology and Gastroenterology.
San Salvador, El Salvador.

GUZMÁN Luciana
Pediatric Gastroenterology. Division of Gastroenterology, Hospital Sor MaríaLudovica.
La Plata, Argentina.

HERRERA Adelita
Molecular Diagnosis Unit.
Sáenz Renauld Laboratories.
San José, Costa Rica.

IBÁÑEZ Patricio
Department of Gastroenterology, School of Medicine.
Pontificia Universidad Católica de Chile.
Santiago, Chile.

LAPARRA Moisés
Microbial Ecology, Nutrition and Health.
Institute of Agrochemistry and Food Technology. (IATA)
Spanish National Research Council (CSIC), Consejo Superior de Investigaciones Científicas.
Valencia, Spain.

LAURET BRAÑA Mª Eugenia
Gastroenterology Service.
Asturias Central University Hospital.
Oviedo, Spain.

LONGARINI Gabriela
Small Instestine Section, Clinical Unit. Department of Medicine.
Bonorino Udaondo Gastroenterological Hospital.
Buenos Aires, Argentina.

LUCENDO Alfredo J.
Gastroenterology Department.
Tomelloso General Hospital.
Tomelloso, Ciudad Real. Spain.

MANCINELLI Leopoldo
Clinical Psychology Gastroenterology Division, Hospital Sor María Ludovica.
La Plata, Argentina.

MARINÉ Meritxell
Gastroenterology Service, Hospital Universitari Mutua de Terrassa.
University of Barcelona. CIBERehd
Terrassa, Barcelona, Spain.

MAURIÑO Eduardo
Small Instestine Section, Clinical Unit. Department of Medicine.
Bonorino Udaondo Gastroenterological Hospital.
Buenos Aires, Argentina.

MONTALVILLO ÁLVAREZ Enrique
Mucosal Immunology Laboratory, IBGM.
University of Valladolid.
Spanish National Research Council (CSIC), Consejo Superior de Investigaciones Científicas.
Valladolid, Spain.

MONTORO HUGUET Miguel
Department of Medicine.
University of Zaragoza.
San Jorge Hospital.
Huesca, Spain.

MORENO Mª de Lourdes
Department of Microbiology and Parasitology.
Faculty of Pharmacy. University of Sevilla.
Sevilla, Spain.

NANFITO Gabriela Inés
Pediatric Gastroenterology. Division of Gastroenterology, Hospital Sor MaríaLudovica.
La Plata, Argentina.

OLIVARES Marta
Microbial Ecology, Nutrition and Health.
Institute of Agrochemistry and Food Technology. (IATA)
Spanish National Research Council (CSIC), Consejo Superior de Investigaciones Científicas.
Valencia, Spain.

OZUNA Carmen Victoria
Institute for Sustainable Agriculture.
Spanish National Research Council (CSIC), Consejo Superior de Investigaciones Científicas.
Córdoba, Spain.

PARRA BLANCO Adolfo
Department of Gastroenterology, School of Medicine.
Pontificia Universidad Católica de Chile.
Santiago, Chile.

PEDREIRA Silvia
Gastroenterology Service. Hospital Alemán.
Buenos Aires, Argentina.

PEÑA Amado Salvador
Professor Emeritus, Vrije Universiteit University Medical Center (VUmc), Laboratory of Immunogenetics, Department of Medical and Infection Control.
Amsterdam, The Netherlands.

PÉREZ MARTÍNEZ Isabel
Gastroenterology Service.
Asturias Central University Hospital.
Oviedo, Spain.

PEREZ VILLAVICENCIO Amavilia
Celiac Disease Expert, University of Sevilla, Spain.
M.Sci, Marketing and Communication Science.
Celiac Disease Information Centre.
San José, Costa Rica.

PLAZA IZURIETA Leticia
Department of Genetics, Physical Anthropology and Animal Physiology.
Basque Country University (UPV-EHU).
BioCruces Research Institute.
Bizkaia, Spain.

POLANCO Isabel
Full Professor of Pediatrics, School of Medicine, Autonomous University of Madrid.
Head of Gastroenterology and Pediatric Nutrition Service, La Paz University Children's Hospital.
Madrid, Spain.

RAMÓN Daniel
Biopolis S.L., Scientific Park of University of Valencia.
Valencia, Spain.

REAL Ana
Department of Microbiology and Parasitology.
Faculty of Pharmacy. University of Sevilla.
Sevilla, Spain.

RODRIGO Luis
Medicine Professor, University of Oviedo.
Gastroenterology Service. Asturias Central University Hospital (HUCA)
Oviedo, Spain.

ROSELL Cristina M.
Institute of Agrochemistry and Food Technology (IATA-CSIC).
Valencia, Spain.

ROSINACH Mercé
Gastroenterology Service, Hospital Universitari Mutua de Terrassa.
University of Barcelona. CIBERehd
Terrassa, Barcelona, Spain.

RUBIO TAPIA Alberto
Associated Consultant and Assistant Professor of Medicine.
Gastroenterology and Hepatology Division. Mayo Clinic.
Rochester, Minnesota, EE.UU.

SANTOLARIA PIEDRAFITA Santos
Gastroenterology and Hepatology Unit.
Hospital San Jorge.
Huesca, Spain.

SANZ Yolanda
Microbial Ecology, Nutrition and Health.
Institute of Agrochemistry and Food Technology. (IATA)
Spanish National Research Council (CSIC), Consejo Superior de Investigaciones Científicas.
Valencia, Spain.

SFOGGIA Cristina
Psychologist.
Small Instestine Section, Clinical Unit. Department of Medicine.
Bonorino Udaondo Gastroenterological Hospital.
Buenos Aires, Argentina.

SOUSA Carolina
Full Professor of Microbiology.
Department of Microbiology and Parasitology.
Faculty of Pharmacy. University of Sevilla.
Sevilla, Spain.

URRUTIA María Inés
Scientific Estimator, Licentiate in Computer Science.
Gastroenterology Division, Hospital Sor María Ludovica.
La Plata, Argentina.

VAQUERO AYALA Luis
Gastroenterology Service. University Hospital of León.
Biomedicine Institute. León University.
León, Spain.

VÁZQUEZ Horacio
Small Instestine Section, Clinical Unit. Department of Medicine.
Bonorino Udaondo Gastroenterological Hospital.
Buenos Aires, Argentina.

VIVAS ALEGRE Santiago
Gastroenterology Service. University Hospital of León.
Biomedicine Institute. León University.
León, Spain.

ZALDÍVAR Karla María
Asociación de Celíacos y Sensibles al Gluten de El Salvador.
San Salvador, El Salvador.

ZUBIRI Cecilia
Pediatric Gastroenterology. Division of Gastroenterology, Hospital Sor María Ludovica.
La Plata, Argentina.

Table of Contents

Foreword

On behalf of the *Sociedad Española de Enfermedad Celíaca* (SEEC, "Spanish Society for Celiac Disease"), it pleases me to welcome this book with which this Society shares a forward-looking vision that rests upon the pillars of education and the spreading of knowledge about this disease. As set down in its statutes, among SEEC's main objectives are to "Deepen the global knowledge on celiac disease, into its biological bases as well as into its clinical, diagnostic, and therapeutic aspects and its prevention", and also to "Promote the exchange of ideas among all professionals interested in the study of celiac disease".

The publishing of this volume is based on the amplitude and relevance of the subjects dealt with herein, which have been written by clinical specialists, researchers and teachers, many of whom are members of SEEC. Celiac disease has always been of interest for biomedical research as a model of the study of the interaction between factors that arise from the environment (specially the gluten from cereals) and genetics (HLA and genes that regulate the immune response), with the intestine as its main target organ and the immune system as mediator of inflammation and tissue damage. In recent years, significant breakthroughs in many of these aspects have been described, opening up new lines of enquiry and posing many questions to be solved.

The estimated prevalence data highlight the large number of undiagnosed cases along with the identification of cases on a scale that constantly grows worldwide. In the light of the acquired knowledge on its pathogenesis, its wide variety of clinical presentations still remain to be explained, not to mention the integration of the entire spectrum of pathological and immunological findings to the disease's definition and understanding the functional meaning of the new genetic variants. The development of serological and genetic markers has prompted the revision of the diagnostic criteria, leading to the establishment of practical protocols for each population under study, paying special attention to patients with atypical forms of expression.

I would like to acknowledge the outstanding work that Dr. Luis Rodrigo and Dr. Amado Salvador Peña have done as editors on starting and carrying out this project, which was first published in Spanish in 2013 and now is being brought forth in English thanks to the enthusiastic and disinterested translation skills of the group of Carlos Beirute L. and Amavilia Perez V. of the *Centro de Información de la Enfermedad Celíaca* (CIEC), "Celiac Disease Information Center".

PhD. Eduardo Arranz. President of SEEC

Chapter 1

Celiac Disease and Non-Celiac Gluten Sensitivity

A.S. Peña[1], L. Rodrigo[2]

[1] Emeritus Professor, Laboratory of Immunogenetics, Department of Medical Microbiology and Infection Control, Vrije Universiteit Medical Center (VUmc), Amsterdam, The Netherlands.

[2] Emeritus Professor of Medicine, Department of Gastroenterology and Medicine, University of Oviedo, Oviedo, Spain.

pena.as@gmail.com, lrodrigosaez@gmail.com

Doi: http://dx.doi.org/10.3926/oms.236

How to cite this chapter

Peña AS, Rodrigo L. *Celiac Disease and Non-Celiac Gluten Sensitivity.* In Rodrigo L and Peña AS, editors. *Celiac Disease and Non-Celiac Gluten Sensitivity.* Barcelona, Spain: OmniaScience; 2014. p. 25-44.

Abstract

This chapter explains the title of this volume and it highlights the importance of recognizing non-celiac gluten sensitivity. It briefly discusses the topics covered in all the chapters within the context of a new definition as well as recent developments in China, Mexico, El Salvador and Costa Rica. The immunological differences between celiac disease and non-celiac gluten sensitivity are reviewed as well as the clinical and pathological definition and the differences between celiac disease, gluten allergy, gluten sensitivity and non-celiac gluten intolerance.

The physiological and immunological effects that can be triggered by wheat products are also briefly summarized without mentioning somatization disorders that may apply to some patients with sensitivity or food intolerance. New concepts about placebo and nocebo are described. This new insight suggests the need to include protocols similar to those that can be applied to diets that include or exclude gluten. It is clear that the two opposing mechanisms of placebo and nocebo may come into play not only when administering drugs but also when specific diets are used as treatment. Subsequently, attention is drawn to the chapters on diagnostic techniques such as celiac disease serology, endoscopy and histopathology, as well as those that deal with the various clinical forms of CD in children and adults. Finally, there is a description of the topics relating to celiac disease on which the authors have expertise.

1. Introduction

This chapter sets out a great deal of the history of celiac disease from where Professor García Nieto leaves off in **chapter 2**: "History of celiac disease", that is to say, after Dicke's[1] discovery of the value of a gluten-free diet and the first description of morphological alterations of the proximal small intestine obtained in surgical resections by Paulley[2] as well as in Margot Shiner's[3,4] peroral biopsies. The chapters that follow explore the situation of celiac disease in countries like China and Costa Rica (**chapters 3 and 10**), El Salvador and Mexico (**chapters 4 and 5**, respectively). Knowledge in these countries is skimpy, but quite interesting since it pertains to very heterogeneous populations where celiac disease was thought to be inexistent. **Chapter 5** raises the possibility that other cereals, including maize, could affect some celiac patients. This last item is yet to be confirmed since it still must be rigorously proven that this is not due to cross contamination. These authors from Mexico argue that oats and maize, which belong to the same subfamily and family of gramineae as wheat[5] could stimulate an immune response. They also confirm that bovine milk caseins may exacerbate celiac disease. Previously, it had been observed that bovine caseins induce an inflammatory reaction in a contact test in the rectal mucosa of celiac patients.[6]

2. Non-Celiac Gluten Sensitivity (NCGS)

Before proceeding with a short description of this book, its title will be justified and the importance of recognizing non-celiac gluten sensitivity will be highlighted even though, for the time being, this syndrome is not fully understood.

This issue may have been the one with the greatest impact during the last decades, specially over the internet, in patients' associations and in the food industry. As discussed below, there is a lack of systematic studies which could enable an understanding and definition of this syndrome and, especially, an understanding of its possible impact on public health services. In this we fully agree with the view expressed by Corazza and his group, who emphasize the lack of a clear definition of non-celiac gluten sensitivity. This obstacle is of, course fundamentally related to the cause of this variegated disease, whose symptoms are presumably caused by different mechanisms.[7-10]

It is therefore unsurprising that, recently Dr. Spence of Glasgow, Scotland wrote: "Do you think non-celiac gluten sensitivity exists?" According to a recent poll undertaken by the general practitioners' magazine in England, the *British Journal of Medicine,* 66% of the 941 who were polled and who have had access to higher education, said they believe it does exist, despite lack of scientific evidence. Besides, about 20 % of the American population purchase gluten-free products and, by 2017, it is estimated that this market will be worth about 6.6 million dollars.[11]

The term *non-celiac gluten sensitivity* was first used in 1978, by Ellis and Linaker,[12,13] even though a few months before Hemmings[14] had reported two patients with satisfactory response to a gluten-free diet. In both cases, as in others later on, in Israel and England, those patients suffered from allergy to dietary wheat.[15,16] These isolated cases preceded the first double-blind study performed in six non-celiac patients who clearly showed the deleterious effects the ingestion of 20g of gluten per day.[17] Since then, a few randomized, placebo-controlled studies have shown that is increasingly clear that these patients suffer from non-celiac gluten sensitivity with heterogeneous etiology. Table 1 summarizes the systematic studies that have been published in medical literature until now. These are studies cannot be compared to each other since their patient selection is not uniform; besides, the protocols followed to establish the effects of gluten in each case are different. The first study group in Birmingham included seventeen patients with chronic diarrhea, of which nine responded to a GFD. Intestinal biopsy specimens revealed increased intraepithelial lymphocytes and plasma cells, not as high as in celiac patients, but returning to normal with a GFD. Three were HLA-B8+ (probably HLA-DQ2+). Several years later, the Peter R. Gibson's group[18] from Australian conducted a double-blind provocation, randomized, placebo-controlled trial in patients with irritable bowel syndrome, in which celiac disease was excluded; it was observed that participants who ingested gluten did not experience symptom improvement in their symptoms (13 of 19 patients) against those who received placebo, 6 of 15 (40%) while both groups followed a gluten-free diet. However, recently, the same Australian group,[19] in a double-blind crossover study of 37 subjects with non-celiac gluten sensitivity and irritable bowel syndrome, found no evidence of specific or dose-dependent gluten effects when patients consumed a diet low in FODMAPs (Fermentable Oligo-saccharides, Disaccharides, Mono-saccharides and Polyols). Even when given a high-gluten content diet (16g gluten/day) or a diet with low-gluten content (2g gluten/day supplemented with 14g whey protein) the patients had no more symptoms than with a control diet based on 6g whey protein per day for 1 week.

Ref.	Patients	Symptoms	Overload	Placebo or GFD
17	17 - patients with non-celiac chronic diarrhea	Diarrhea with positive response to GFD (9 females)	20 g. gluten/day Positive	Gluten-free flour
18	34 - Irritable Colon Syndrome Non-celiacs	Intestinal symptoms	16 g. gluten/day Positive	Gluten-free bread
20-22	276 - Irritable Colon Syndrome Non-celiacs	Intestinal symptoms 70 sensitivity only to wheat 206 sensitivity to several types of food	13 g. gluten capsules/day Positive	Xylose capsules
23-25	45 - Irritable colon Syndrome Non-celiacs	Diarrhea (Roma II)	22 NGFD (11 HLA-Q2/8 +) Altered intestinal barrier in HLA-DQ2/8+ patients	23 GFD (12 HLA-Q2/8 +)
19	59 - Irritable colon Syndrome Non-celiacs	Diarrhea (Roma III)	GFD, with FODMAP 16g gluten/day; 2g gluten/day 37 patients 7 days; 22 patients. 3 days Negative	GFD, without FODMAP 16g whey/day

GFD= gluten-free diet; NGFD= non-gluten-free diet; Ref.= Reference; FODMAP=Fermentable Oligo-saccharides, Disaccharides, Mono-saccharides and Polyols)

Table 1. Systematic randomized studies of patients with non-celiac gluten sensitivity.

Two different studies of patients with irritable bowel syndrome in whom celiac disease had been previously excluded (Table 1) have been published recently. In a study undertaken by Carroccio et al[20-22] wheat sensitivity also affected patients who do not have celiac disease and lack the specific HLA-DQ antigens associated with the disease. In these patients an increase of eosinophils and basophil activation in the lamina propria of the duodenum and colon were found. Therefore, in gluten sensitivity, wheat had multiple functions more consistent with food allergy. In a more recent study by Vazquez-Roque et al[25] it was shown that a diet containing gluten produces a reversible alteration of the intestinal barrier in patients with irritable bowel syndrome and diarrhea in those patients who carry HLA-DQ2/8.

Many of the described observations have helped to define non-celiac gluten sensitivity as a reaction to gluten in which allergic and autoimmune mechanisms are excluded. That is to say, anti-EMA and/or anti-tTG patients test are usually negative although antigliadin antibodies may be present; but their duodenal mucosa is normal. Symptoms disappear with a GFD and reappear with gluten overload. As Sapone et al. have written, so far, this is essentially an exclusion diagnosis.[26] his implies that this is an entity distinct from celiac disease although there is sufficient evidence that it is a syndrome since the alterations described in patients from Italy are not seen in similar patients in USA or Australia as it can be appreciated with immunological studies. In Germany it has been found that patients who have irritable bowel syndrome with a predominance of diarrhea with gliadin IgG antibodies and HLA-DQ2, but who have normal biopsies, usually respond to a GFD.[27, 28] These patients may be potentially celiac, since simple morphological studies may not be sensitive enough to exclude an immunological response. There patients are probably part of the heterogeneity of celiac disease. This does not apply to Carroccio's onservations[20, 21] since in their study wheat sensitivity also affected patients without HLA-DQ2 or HLA-DQ8 markers.

3. Immunological Differences between Celiac Disease and Non-Celiac Gluten Sensitivity

In many of Carroccio's[20, 21] patients, an increase of eosinophils in the duodenal and colon lamina propria was found, suggesting that basophil activation may be a useful marker for wheat sensitivity. In another group of non-celiac gluten sensitive patients, there was no increase in the expression of the IL-17 cytokine in comparison with a group of celiac patients who did show an increase of this same cytokine in the intestinal mucosa.[26, 29, 30] Subsequent studies by the same group have shown that non-celiac gluten sensitivity is not associated with an increased intestinal permeability and that, in these cases, the expression of T FOXP3 regulatory cell markers is decreased. Conversely, in these patients there is a significant increase in the expression of claudin 4 and of the innate immunity marker, the Toll-like receptor 2.[30] These studies suggest that the difference between these two groups is that, in celiac disease, both the innate and the acquired immunity are increased, whereas in gluten sensitivity patients only the innate immunity is activated by gluten. Recent Norwegian studies indicate that the immune response is more complicated and that more studies are needed to understand the symptoms. In one recent study, thirty HLA-DQ2+ celiac and fifteen with non-celiac gluten sensitivity patients were studied before and after a gluten-free diet , feeding them four slices of gluten-containing bread for three days. Duodenal biopsies were collected before and after exposure. In celiac patients the tumor necrosis factor alpha and interleukin-8 were increased after *in vivo* gluten challenge. The gamma interferon level in treated celiac patients was increased both before and after exposure to gluten and did not increase significantly. IFN-alpha was also found to be activated upon stimulation with gluten. By contrast, in patients with non-celiac gluten sensitivity, only IFN-gamma was significantly increased. The number of intra-epithelial lymphocytes CD3+ T was higher in patients compared with controls independently of gluten overload, although they were lower in the latter than in the former and there was an increase of IFN-gamma after gluten challenge.[31]

4. Celiac Disease: New Definitions

In the past 10 years it has become clear that, along with celiac disease, there are other conditions related to gluten consumption. a) Wheat allergy (the less common) b) Autoimmune disease, celiac disease, dermatitis herpetiformis and gluten ataxia, c) Sensitivity to gluten, which is possibly immune-mediated and now the most common.[26] and d) Gluten intolerance. Table 2 shows a classification system comprising four main types.

Celiac Disease	Allergy	Sensitivity	Intolerance
Intestinal and extraintestinal symptoms for days, weeks or years after ingesting gluten.	Intestinal and extraintestinal symptoms for minutes or hours after ingesting gluten.	Intestinal and extraintestinal symptoms for hours or days after ingesting gluten.	Intestinal and extraintestinal symptoms for hours or days after ingesting gluten.
No direct correlation with the amount, but enteropathy is still present. Reversibility feasible, but the mechanisms are unknown.	Small amounts provoke symptoms. Eosinophils in lamina propria. Wheat Anaphylaxis Desensitization is theoretically possible.	Variable response to different gluten amounts. Increased intraepitelial lymphocytes. Increased basophils in lamina propria.	The amount of gluten grams determines intensity and can be reversed. No enteropathy of any type.
Anti-Endomysium, anti-tTG, deamidated anti-gluten +.	Anti-IgE to wheat components including omega-5 gliadin and barley gamma3 hordein.	Anti-IgG-AGA+	Negative antibodies
HLA-DQ2 y/o HLA-DQ8	Unknown	No association	No association
Innate and acquired immunity activated	Allergy Anaphylaxis	Innate immunity	No immunological mechanisms
Associated and autoimmune diseases common.	Allergic diseases	Sensitivity to other kinds of food common.	Unknown.

Table 2. Clinical and pathophysiological differences between celiac disease, gluten allergy, non-celiac gluten sensitivity and gluten intolerance.

This classification does not include autoimmune enteropathy of unknown etiology. It is a fortunately rare and heterogeneous clinical condition, and few cases are described in adults.[32] It is characterized by malabsorption along with the presence of antibodies which react against intestinal epithelial cells; as opposed to celiac disease, the histopathology of the duodenal mucosa is characterized by hyperplastic crypts and villous atrophy, accompanied by lymphocytosis in deep crypts, an increase in the number of apoptotic bodies and very few intraepithelial lymphocytes. Most children described have associated autoimmune diseases.[33-35]

This proposed classification differs from the definitions recently accepted at Oslo Consensus meeting.[36] Celiac disease is defined as a genetically predisposed autoimmune enteropathy caused by the ingestion of some peptides derived from wheat (gliadins and glutenins), barley (hordeins), rye (secalins), oats (avenines) and hybrids of these grains, such as kalmut and triticale (**chapters 21 and 23**). These cereals contain epitopes for which deamidation is important for binding to HLA -DQ2 and/or HLA-DQ8 molecules and recognition of T cells contributing to produce the spectrum of the characteristic changes of the duodenal and jejunal mucosa. These changes lead to production of intestinal symptoms and autoimmune reactions that may affect extraintestinal organs. The immune response can remain inactive until unknown environmental elements trigger the disease and, as opposed to what was thought to be a lifelong disease, it may be transitory.[37-39]

Strict adherence to a gluten-free diet (GFD) leads, in a few months, to a rapid and complete recovery of small intestinal mucosa architecture and function, as well as to a remission of symptoms and normalization of serological tests.

In the second place, in Oslo it was recommended that the term "gluten-related disorders" be used as a general term for all diseases triggered by gluten and it was suggested that the term "gluten intolerance" should not be used.[36]

Peptides capable of stimulating T cells T	Components capable of stimulating dendritic cells	Alpha-amylase and trypsin Inhibitors	Opioid effect	Allergy and anaphylaxis	Placebo nocebo
Acquired immunity response	Innate immunity response	Increased IL-8 and TNF-alpha, through TLR4-MD2-CD14 stimulation	Increased intestinal transit	Intestinal and extraintestinal symptoms	
Gluten epitopes recognized by T-cells restricted by HLA-DQ molecules	Increase in Claudin		Response to Naloxone	Antibodies in response to Omega-5 gliadin	
40	30	41	7,8, 42-44	45,46,47	19

Table 3. Several components of wheat and related cereals with immunological and physiological effects.

5. A New View of Placebo and Nocebo

There are few observations on placebo/nocebo regarding GFD[19] but is appropriate to briefly review recent concepts about these mechanisms which doctors (due to their interest in patient response to GFD) as well as patients who respond to this diet ought to take into account. Until recently, the well-known therapeutic effect of placebo was based primarily on the fact that the patient did not know that what he was taking was an inert substance and that, without suggestion, the placebo's magic disappears. There is, however, evidence that the use of placebos as analgesics not only help alleviate pain, but also that they do so through the same humoral mechanisms and neuroendocrine pathways that many drugs use. It is therefore not surprising that placebos work even when patients know they are placebos.

It has been shown recently in patients who have irritable bowel syndrome the possibility of studying the placebo effect even when they know that the drug is an inert substance: "placebo without deception".[48,49] Patients taking placebos showed a far superior improvement of their condition than that of those who did not receive this treatment. In this study, 80 patients (70% female) randomized for a three-week treatment period, were divided into two branches in order to compare those who received no treatment compared to those who took a placebo. The latter were informed that what was being given to them was an inert substance (the bottle of pills was even labeled "placebo") but they were told that there was evidence that it had beneficial effects.

Therefore, placebos work even if the patient knows they are inert substances. This opens an interesting field in therapy and it makes the ethical issue of deceiving the patient disappear, since the fact that he or she is being given a placebo is not being hidden from the patient. From now on, conscious attempts to identify and exploit the characteristics of medical visits in order to increase the placebo's effects are an ethical way to use what is known about its mechanisms, to improve the clinical outcomes.

Regarding the nocebo effect, it generates negative expectations in the patient and, it exemplifies the old saying "fear makes you sick", it also explains why an analysis of placebo-controlled trials shows that almost 25% of patients taking placebo reported side effects that should not exist. Although there is less research on nocebo effects and therefore less documentation, the results of the studies are consistent with the fact that the placebo and nocebo effects are real. If, as argued before, a placebo can help the healing process or alleviate pain, a nocebo has the opposite effect – it makes patients feel worse. This is partly so because nocebo studies have been limited due to ethical restrictions, since a nocebo procedure is stressful and leads to anxiety. One theory that tries to explain the nocebo effect argues that just as placebo activates brain endorphins to relieve pain, nocebo activates other receptors that stimulate the production of hormones or other pathways that affect pain perception. In support of this view, it should be noted that drugs used to treat anxiety can mitigate the pain of the nocebo effect. Perhaps the chemical imbalances that contribute to anxiety can also be the basis of the nocebo response. The latest scientific evidence supports this theory; the placebo and nocebo effects arise from brain processes that triggered by psychological mechanisms such as expectation and conditioning.

Experimental tests have shown that negative verbal suggestions induce anticipatory anxiety about an impending increase in pain levels, this triggers the activation of the cholecystokinin which, in turn, facilitates pain transmission. It has been found that antagonists of this hormone block anxiety-induced hyperalgesia. These observations open up the possibility of new therapeutic strategies when pain has an important anxiety component.[50-53]

Psychological factors such as anxiety, depression and hypochondria increase the nocebo effect. Previous negative experiences and the words used to describe medical side effects may also increase the nocebo effect.

This new insight suggests the need to incorporate similar protocols to the effects that a gluten-free or non gluten-free diet may have. It is clear that these two opposing mechanisms, placebo and nocebo, are involved. Expectations can bias sensory evidence and therefore the patient and the physician must obtain an appropriate balance will result in the updating of expectations of a procedure, a drug or a product involved in the prescribed diet. The following chapters discuss relevant aspects of current understanding of celiac disease.

6. Genetics

As reviewed in the chapter by Dr. Bilbao's group (**chapter 6**), celiac disease has a genetic predisposition. Linkage in families and association studies have largely confirmed the importance of HLA-DQ although these genes account for approximately 50 % of inherited traits. Genome-wide association studies (GWAS) which analyzed thousands of single nucleotide polymorphisms (SNPs) have shown that celiac disease is not an exception among other autoimmune diseases in which multiple genes from different chromosomes contribute to modulating the immune response to gluten. However, epidemiological studies have shown that certain environmental factors also are important in the expression of the disease. In adults, a study from the Mayo Clinic in Rochester, Olmsted County , Minnesota, USA[54] found that between 2000 and 2010, the number of new cases of celiac disease has increased from 11 per 100,000 to 17 people 100,000. 63% of the new cases were women and specially until 2004. It is possible that this increased incidence of celiac disease may be due in part to improved diagnosis, as well as to a better understanding of the symptoms and signs of celiac disease along with knowledge of risk groups and changes in the environment, changes in diet and high consumption of foods containing gluten, use and abuse of antibiotics and infections. In Sweden, in two cohorts of children with different infant feeding, it was found that those born in 1997 (22 per 1000) have a significantly lower risk of developing celiac disease compared with those born in 1993 (29 per 1000). The 1997 cohort had a higher proportion of infants in which gluten was introduced into the diet in small amounts while still being breastfed.[55] Recent studies have clearly shown that neither breast feeding or the late introduction of gluten[56] nor introducing gluten to infants at 4 to 6 months of age 57 modified the risk for celiac disease in infants who had a first-degree relative with celiac disease. Since high-risk HLA–DQ genotypes are an important predictor of disease in these children[56, 57] further studies aimed at identifying environmental factors are important to understand the different prevalence of celiac disease.[42]

7. Immunology

Immunological theory explains the changes observed in the lamina propria of the intestinal mucosa invoking a response involving CD4+ T cells, HLA-DQ2/8 restricted and IFN- gamma release. However, innate immunity acts on the intraepithelial compartment and also contributes to this increase with a direct toxic effect of gluten on the epithelium (**chapter 7**).

Gluten-derived peptides, the insoluble protein fraction of wheat, barley or rye trigger an immune response in susceptible individuals. Some gluten peptides are relatively undigestible by human proteases. The 33-mer peptide, the 17-mer, and other gliadin oligopeptides contain epitopes that are toxic when deamidated by tissue transglutaminase. These may be presented to the immune system by HLA-DQ2/DQ8 molecules and induce a proinflammatory cytokines response, resulting in epithelial damage.

There are other additional peptide sequences which initiate innate immune cytotoxic responses in the epithelium and increase the intestinal permeability through the expression of zonulin which facilitates the passage of large peptide fragments to the lamina propria.[58-60]

8. Diagnostic Techniques in Celiac Disease

Chapter 8 describes the usefulness of several serological tests in screening, diagnosis and monitoring of patients with celiac disease. **Chapter 9** discusses the value of endoscopy and **chapter 10** discusses the difficulties and value of histopathological diagnosis. The advances in the sensitivity and specificity of serological tests and the difficult in assessing the histopathology of celiac disease are changing the view that the morphological spectrum of the intestinal biopsy specimens is not always the gold standard and particularly in children when the specific antibody titers are highly elevated the diagnosis can be reached without performing the biopsies.[61]

9. Clinical Presentation of Celiac Disease

Chapters 11 and 12 describe the variety and richness of this disease in children and adults. Both discuss new guidelines to facilitate diagnosis, risk groups and treatment, including emerging treatments.

Chapter 13 gives a thorough answer to such an important question in clinical practice as: When Marsh 1 type lesions can be considered indication of celiac disease? This histological finding is not produced exclusively by gluten, however, at present is thought to constitute one of the most common forms of presentation in adult celiac patients. Different anatomical and pathological classifications of celiac disease is discussed, along with its various application criteria and differential diagnoses in relation to other processes. A relevant issue to this kind of manifestation is that, despite having negative celiac serology in over 80% of the cases, the severity of the clinical symptoms can be very similar to the forms of celiac disease with clear villous atrophy.[62,63]

Chapter 14 reviews the diverse extra-intestinal manifestations of celiac disease. Some diseases are caused by chronic disorders associated with defects in intestinal absorption, others share the same genetic basis and some are rare. Celiac disease has been proposed as a model to understand the role of MHC class II molecules in human immunopathology, to analyze the mechanisms that link tolerance to food proteins and autoimmunity.[64,65] The importance of detection lies not only in its confirmation, but patients also benefit from dietary treatment since after the exclusion of gluten from the diet, some patients experience partial benefits while others experience a complete clinical remission. In a retrospective study of 924 celiac patients from 27 adult and pediatric centers in France it was found that those who were at greater risk of developing autoimmune diseases are those who were diagnosed early in life and who have a family history of autoimmune problems. The gluten-free diet has a clear protective effect.[66]

Chapter 15 tackles the interesting relationship between celiac disease and bone metabolism disorders, both in children and adults. There is high prevalence of osteoporosis and an increased risk of fractures, in all stages of life for CD patients, increasing after menopause and upon reaching an advanced age. It is advisable to attempt an early detection of these disorders, mainly osteoporosis by performing serial studies of metabolic bone density periodically. Its prevalence increases with the presence of atrophied villi.[67] The gluten-free diet improves the intestinal calcium absorption, but cases with advanced osteoporosis need not only supplementary calcium, but also vitamin D supplements and bisphosphonate intake.

Chapter 16 deals with the relationship between the so-called functional gastrointestinal disorders which are very common in clinical practice, and their possible relationship to celiac disease. Thus, patients diagnosed with a functional digestive disorder, such as functional dyspepsia and/or irritable bowel syndrome, may be misdiagnosed and actually have celiac disease. This happens more often if clinical diagnostic studies are not completed with celiac serology, genetic markers and duodenal biopsies. Many of them have Type-1 Marsh lymphocytic enteritis and clearly respond to a gluten-free diet. This consideration has important implications not only in terms of morbidity and mortality resulting from delayed diagnosis of celiac disease, but also leads to a prolonged decline in their quality of life which may be recovered following a gluten-free diet and also saving money by avoiding unnecessary pharmacological treatment.[68-71] The relationship between IBS and non-celiac gluten sensitivity has been amply discussed earlier in this chapter and in the recent medical literature including the role of FODMAPs in controlling the symptoms.[19,22,72]

Chapter 17 discusses the major intestinal complications of CD, such as refractoriness which fortunately is rare, since it occurs in fewer than 5% of celiac patients. There are two types of refractory celiac disease. Type I is less serious and can be treated more effectively with immunomodulators and therefore, has a better prognosis. Type 2, is more severe, it may lead to the development of intestinal T-cell lymphoma, which of course carries a worse prognosis. There is no consensus on the most effective treatment for this serious complication. For the differential diagnosis of both forms require immunophenotyping of intraepithelial lymphocyte populations by duodenal biopsies and studies of their characteristics using flow cytometry. Other possible causes of lack of response to GFD must be ruled out first.[73,74]

Chapter 18 discusses medical follow-up of celiac patients, which cannot be performed according to strict rules since there is no consensus about this subject. It describes the four most commonly used procedures: regular clinical follow-up, annual measurement of specific antibodies to celiac disease, regular duodenal biopsies (no clearly defined in time periods) and control of adherence to the GFD through structured questionnaires. All of these approaches are useful and necessary, as well as the detection and prevention of nutritional deficiencies and the periodical screening for the presence of associated diseases.[36,75,76]

Chapter 19 discusses the issue of quality of life and psychological distress in celiac patients. Undoubtedly the majority of patients with celiac disease have a marked worsening of their quality of life when diagnosed, secondary to multiple digestive and associated diseases that they have, together with the long diagnostic delay characteristic in most cases. This situation improves significantly with strict adherence to a gluten-free diet until a complete normalization is achieved.[77] Anxiety disorders are common at diagnosis and they are considered to be reactive forms due to lack of knowledge at the beginning or to difficulties in adhering to the diet. Depressive disorders have also negative effects and should be identified and, if necessary, treated properly, especially at the beginning of the GFD.[78-80] Recent studies at the Columbia University in New York indicate the frequent presence of chronic headaches in these patients and they found that up to 30% of their celiac patients, 56% of non-celiac gluten sensitivity, 23% in patients with inflammatory bowel disease and 14% of healthy controls. There was also a higher prevalence of migraine in these three groups of patients, being the female gender, depression and anxiety, the independent factors for migraine.[81]

Chapter 20 reviews the experiences of a large group of celiac patients, along with the results of various surveys on the acceptability of GFD, cultural aspects that influence adherence to GFD and the impact of a CD diagnosis, both personally and as a member of a family. It is a very interesting study which highlights the importance of the physician's attitude when diagnosing and explaining to the patient the disease characteristics as well as the cultural, personal and family variables determining compliance to GFD or the existence of various transgressions or even quitting GFD.[82-84] Recently in Norway, a comparative study was undertaken comparing 22 patients with celiac disease versus 31 patients with non-celiac gluten sensitivity during an overload of gluten for 3 days. A comparison group of 40 healthy controls was included. There were no significant differences between patients regarding personality traits, somatization level, quality of life, anxiety and depressive symptoms. Somatization was low in both groups. Patients with non-celiac gluten sensitivity had more symptoms than patients with celiac disease after exposure to gluten.[85]

Chapter 21 addresses the issue of detecting the immunotoxic gluten fractions in order to find applications in the food safety area. These researchers observed that there is a wide range of variability in the immunotoxic potential of different varieties of cereals, particularly barley and oats. They have shown that there is a strict correlation between the amount of gluten and immunotoxic potential due to the fact that some gluten epitopes may be less immunogenic than others and therefore require a higher concentration to cause an equivalent toxic effect. There are currently available specific monoclonal antibodies against various toxic gluten fractions, one of the most used methods in food analysis; these are very sensitive and specific and are determined by Elisa techniques. The authors study the toxic potential of oats, about which there is much discussion in the literature discussing whether they can be allowed as part of the GFD.[86, 87] They have analyzed three varieties of oats and found great variability in their gluten content, with different toxicity; this opens the future possibility to include the less toxic oats fractions in certain kinds of foods. A similar phenomenon occurs with several varieties of barley, demonstrating that the wild varieties are more toxic than the domestic ones. All this opens up exciting new possibilities for expanding a gluten-free diet, with the possible addition of oat flour and barley poor in toxic peptides and therefore well tolerated by celiac patients.[88,89]

Chapter 22 provides valuable information on the technological, nutritional and sensory characteristics of gluten-free cereal products and also discusses issues related to the design and development of these foods. Gluten-free diets can cause, in the long run, nutritional imbalances and due to specific nutrient deficiencies and it proposes the need to improve the nutritional composition of gluten-free food with the addition of nutrients such as omega-3 oils, specific proteins fiber, probiotics and prebiotics.[90-92] These recommendations are partially due to recent findings by Canadian researchers regarding the impact of long term gluten-free diets, highlighting the need for improved training and education of dietitians and other health care providers, as well as in workers in the gluten-free food industry, in order better help to the people for improving their adherence to a GFD and their quality of life.[93]

In **Chapter 23** contains clear and precise information regarding current possibilities of producing varieties of wheat gluten by the novel methods of silencing the genes involved in the generation of this peptide. This opens up numerous possibilities for future development of wheat flours which, prior to their modification and treatment, are practically free from gluten and therefore suitable for nutrition and treatment not only of celiac patients, but also for non-celiac gluten sensitives and people with anaphylactic reactions to the various components of wheat. In order to be marketed they will have to pass through numerous controls laid down by diverse national food agencies, as well as through the authorization of international health authorities, since they belong to the transgenic product category[94,95]

Chapter 24 discusses the issue of the relationship between intestinal microbiota and celiac disease. As it is well known, the intestinal flora of the colon is variegated and colonized by millions of bacteria. Its presence and characteristics are influenced by several variables, both in health as in illness. Nutrition is one of the important factors to consider and breastfeeding has a clear beneficial effect. Differences have been found in the characteristics of said flora between celiac and healthy individuals; there is as well a significant difference between untreated celiac patients and healthy adults, in celiac patients on GFD and in healthy adults, regarding acetic acid, propionic acid, butyric acid and all short-chained fatty acids.[96, 97] This raises an interesting and novel problem, since the use of probiotics can have a clearly beneficial effect in some of these patients, especially those with a partial response gluten-free diet or who have frequent relapses. Recent studies suggest that gut microbiota may play a role in some manifestations of celiac disease and these patients with gastrointestinal symptoms or anemia had lower microbial diversity than those with dermatitis herpetiformis.[98]

Chapter 25 describes the research design used in the preparation of a diary supplement with the addition of a probiotic (ES1) that has demonstrated to achieve a potent anti-inflammatory effect in in vitro studies and in experimental animals and being gluten-free, may be suitable for celiacs as nutritional support; it may also be used to improve and enhance the response to gluten-free diet, especially in patients with partial response or patients who have frequent relapses. There have been clinical trials in celiac and healthy controls, which have shown preliminary excellent results. This product is currently sold under the name of *Proceliac* by the *Central Lechera de Asturiana*.[99] Bakshi et al. discuss new treatments and include the use of probiotics with incorporated endopeptidases or transglutaminase inhibitors that could be used as GFD supplement and thus help patients to obtain a better quality of life.[100]

References

1. Dicke WK. *Treatment of celiac disease.* Ned Tijdschr Geneeskd. 1951; 95: 124-30.
2. De Re V, Caggiari L, Tabuso M, et al. *The versatile role of gliadin peptides in celiac disease.* Clin Biochem 2013; 46: 552-60.
    http://dx.doi.org/10.1016/j.clinbiochem.2012.10.038
3. Shiner M. *Jejunal-biopsy tube.* Lancet. 1956; 270: 85.
    http://dx.doi.org/10.1016/S0140-6736(56)92137-7
4. Shiner M. *Duodenal biopsy.* Lancet. 1956; 270: 17-9.
    http://dx.doi.org/10.1016/S0140-6736(56)91854-2
5. Kasarda DD, Okita TW, Bernardin JE et al. *Nucleic acid (cDNA) and amino acid sequences of alpha-type gliadins from wheat (Triticum aestivum).* Proc Natl Acad Sci USA. 1984; 81: 4712-6. http://dx.doi.org/10.1073/pnas.81.15.4712
6. Kristjansson G, Venge P, Hallgren R. *Mucosal reactivity to cow's milk protein in coeliac disease.* Clin Exp Immunol. 2007; 147: 449-55.
    http://dx.doi.org/10.1111/j.1365-2249.2007.03298.x
7. Di Sabatino A, Corazza GR. *Some clarification is necessary on the Oslo definitions for coceliac disease-related terms.* Gut 2013; 62: 182.
    http://dx.doi.org/10.1136/gutjnl-2012-302613
8. Di Sabatino A, Giuffrida P, Corazza GR. *Still Waiting for a Definition of Nonceliac Gluten Sensitivity.* J Clin Gastroenterol. 2013; febrero 18.
    http://dx.doi.org/10.1097/MCG.0b013e3182850dfe
9. Di Sabatino A, Corazza GR. *Nonceliac gluten sensitivity: sense or sensibility?* Ann Intern Med. 2012; 156: 309-11.
    http://dx.doi.org/10.7326/0003-4819-156-4-201202210-00010
10. Di Sabatino A, Vanoli A, Giufrrida P, et al. *The function of tissue transglutaminase in celiac disease.* Autoimmun Rev 2012; 11: 746:53.
11. Spence D. *Bad medicine: food intolerance.* BMJ. 2013; 346: f529.
    http://dx.doi.org/10.1136/bmj.f529
12. Ellis A, Linaker BD. *Non-coceliac gluten sensitivity?* Lancet 1978; 1: 1358-9.
    http://dx.doi.org/10.1016/S0140-6736(78)92427-3
13. Linaker BD, Calam J. *Is jejunal biopsy valuable in the elderly?* Age Ageing. 1978; 7: 244-5.
    http://dx.doi.org/10.1093/ageing/7.4.244
14. Hemmings WA. *Food allergy.* Lancet. 1978; 1: 608.
    http://dx.doi.org/10.1016/S0140-6736(78)91053-X
15. Jonas A. *Wheat-sensitive -but not coeliac.* Lancet. 1978; 2: 1047.
    http://dx.doi.org/10.1016/S0140-6736(78)92366-8
16. Dahl R. *Wheat sensitive - but not coeliac.* Lancet. 1979; 1: 43-4.
    http://dx.doi.org/10.1016/S0140-6736(79)90482-3
17. Cooper BT, Holmes GK, Ferguson R et al. *Gluten-sensitive diarrhea without evidence of celiac disease.* Gastroenterology. 1980; 79: 801-6.
18. Biesiekierski JR, Newnham ED, Irving PM et al. *Gluten causes gastrointestinal symptoms in subjects without celiac disease: a double-blind randomized placebo-controlled trial.* Am J Gastroenterol. 2011; 106: 508-14; quiz 515.
    http://dx.doi.org/10.1038/ajg.2010.487
19. Biesiekierski JRP, Peters SL, Newnham ED, Rosella O et al. *No Effects of Gluten in Patients with Self-Reported Non-Celiac Gluten Sensitivity Following Dietary Reduction of Low-Fermentable, Poorly-Absorbed, Short-Chain Carbohydrates.* Gastroenterology. 2013.
    http://dx.doi.org/10.1053/j.gastro.2013.04.051

20. Carroccio A, Brusca I, Mansueto P, It al. *A comparison between two different in vitro basophil activation tests for gluten- and cow's milk protein sensitivity in irritable bowel syndrome (IBS)-like patients.* Clin Chem Lab Med. 2012; 1-7.

21. Carroccio A, Mansueto P, Iacono G et al. *Non-celiac wheat sensitivity diagnosed by double-blind placebo-controlled challenge: exploring a new clinical entity.* Am J Gastroenterol. 2012; 107: 1898-906; quiz 1907.
http://dx.doi.org/10.1038/ajg.2012.236

22. Sanders DS, Aziz I. *Non-celiac wheat sensitivity: separating the wheat from the chat!* Am J Gastroenterol. 2012;107:1908-12. http://dx.doi.org/10.1038/ajg.2012.344

23. Camilleri M, Kolar GJ, Vazquez-Roque MI, et al. *Cannabinoid receptor 1 gene and irritable bowel syndrome: phenotype and quantitative traits.* Am J Physiol Gastrointest Liver Physiol 2013; 304: G553-60. Camilleri M, Kolar GJ, Vazquez-Roque MI, et al. Cannabinoid receptor 1 gene and irritable bowel syndrome: phenotype and quantitative traits. Am J Physiol Gastrointest Liver Physiol 2013; 304: G553-60.
http://dx.doi.org/10.1152/ajpgi.00376.2012

24. Vazquez-Roque MI, Bouras EP. *Linaclotide, novel therapy for the treatment of chronic idiopathic constipation and constipation-predominant irritable bowel syndrome.* Adv Ther. 2013; 30: 203-11. http://dx.doi.org/10.1007/s12325-013-0012-9

25. Vazquez-Roque MI, Camilleri M, Smyrk T et al. *A controlled trial of gluten-free diet in patients with irritable bowel syndrome-diarrhea: effects on bowel frequency and intestinal function.* Gastroenterology. 2013; 144: 903-11 e3.
http://dx.doi.org/10.1053/j.gastro.2013.01.049

26. Sapone A, Bai JC, Ciacci C et al. *Spectrum of gluten-related disorders: consensus on new nomenclature and classification.* BMC Med. 2012; 10: 13.
http://dx.doi.org/10.1186/1741-7015-10-13

27. Wahnschaffe U, Ignatius R, Loddenkemper C, et al. *Diagnostic value of endoscopy for the diagnosis of giardiasis and other intestinal diseases in patients with persistent diarrhea from tropical or subtropical areas.* Scand J Gastroenterol 2007; 42: 391-6.
http://dx.doi.org/10.1080/00365520600881193

28. Wahnschaffe U, Schulzke JD, Zeitz M et al. *Predictors of clinical response to gluten-free diet in patients diagnosed with diarrhea-predominant irritable bowel syndrome.* Clin Gastroenterol Hepatol. 2007; 5: 844-50; quiz 769.
http://dx.doi.org/10.1016/j.cgh.2007.03.021

29. Sapone A, Lammers KM, Mazzarella G et al. *Differential mucosal IL-17 expression in two gliadin-induced disorders: gluten sensitivity and the autoimmune enteropathy celiac disease.* Int Arch Allergy Immunol. 2010; 152: 75-80.
http://dx.doi.org/10.1159/000260087

30. Sapone A, Lammers KM, Casolaro V et al. *Divergence of gut permeability and mucosal immune gene expression in two gluten-associated conditions: celiac disease and gluten sensitivity.* BMC Med. 2011; 9: 23. http://dx.doi.org/10.1186/1741-7015-9-23

31. Brottveit M, Beitnes AC, Tollefsen S et al. *Mucosal Cytokine Response After Short-Term Gluten Challenge in Celiac Disease and Non-Celiac Gluten Sensitivity.* Am J Gastroen-terol. 2013; 108(5): 842-50. http://dx.doi.org/10.1038/ajg.2013.91

32. Akram S, Murray JA, Pardi DS et al. *Adult Autoimmune Enteropathy: Mayo Clinic Rochester Experience.* Clin Gastroenterol Hepatol. 2007; nov 5(11): 1282-90; quiz 1245.
http://dx.doi.org/10.1016/j.cgh.2007.05.013

33. Bernardos E, Solis-Herruzo JA. *Autoimmune enteropathy.* Rev Esp Enferm Dig. 2003; 95: 494-6, 490-3.

34. Colletti RB, Guillot AP, Rosen S et al. *Autoimmune enteropathy and nephropathy with circulating anti-epithelial cell antibodies.* J Pediatr. 1991; 118: 858-64.
http://dx.doi.org/10.1016/S0022-3476(05)82195-X

35. Murch SH, Fertleman CR, Rodrigues C et al. *Autoimmune enteropathy with distinct mucosal features in T-cell activation deficiency: the contribution of T cells to the mucosal lesion.* J Pediatr Gastroenterol Nutr. 1999; 28: 393-9.
http://dx.doi.org/10.1097/00005176-199904000-00009

36. Lebwohl B, Granath F, Ekbom A, et al. *Mucosal healing and mortality in coeliac disease.* Aliment Pharmacol Ther. 2013; 37: 332-9. http://dx.doi.org/10.1111/apt.12164

37. Cerf-Bensussan N, Matysiak-Budnik T, Cellier C, et al. *Oral proteases: a new approach to managing coeliac disease.* Gut 2007; 56: 157-60.
http://dx.doi.org/10.1136/gut.2005.090498

38. Marine M, Farre C, Alsina M et al. *The prevalence of coeliac disease is significantly higher in children compared with adults.* Aliment Pharmacol Ther. 2011; 33: 477-86.
http://dx.doi.org/10.1111/j.1365-2036.2010.04543.x

39. Monzon H, Forne M, Gonzalez C, et al. *Mild enteropathy as a cause of iron-deficiency anaemia of previously unknown origin.* Dig Liver Dis. 2011; 43: 448-53.
http://dx.doi.org/10.1016/j.dld.2010.12.003

40. Sollid LM, Qiao SW, Anderson RP et al. *Nomenclature and listing of celiac disease relevant gluten T-cell epitopes restricted by HLA-DQ molecules.* Immunogenetics. 2012; 64: 455-60. http://dx.doi.org/10.1007/s00251-012-0599-z

41. Junker Y, Zeissig S, Kim SJ et al. *Wheat amylase trypsin inhibitors drive intestinal inflammation via activation of toll-like receptor 4.* J Exp Med. 2012; 209: 2395-408.
http://dx.doi.org/10.1084/jem.20102660

42. Di Sabatino A, Brunetti L, Carnevale Maffe G, et al. *Is it worth investigating splenic function in patients with celiac disease?* World J Gastroenterol 2013; 19: 2313-8.
http://dx.doi.org/10.3748/wjg.v19.i15.2313

43. Di Sabatino A, Giuffrida P, Corazza GR. *From impending toxic megacolon to multiple organ failure in severe ulcerative colitis.* Intern Emerg Med. 2013; 8: 185-6.
http://dx.doi.org/10.1007/s11739-012-0849-y

44. Di Sabatino A, Rovedatti L, Vidali F, et al. *Recent advances in understanding Crohn's disease.* Intern Emerg Med. 2013; 8: 101-13.
http://dx.doi.org/10.1007/s11739-011-0599-2

45. Morita E, Chinuki Y, Takahashi H, et al. *Prevalence of wheat allergy in Japanese adults.* Allergol Int. 2012; 61: 101-5. http://dx.doi.org/10.2332/allergolint.11-OA-0345

46. Takahashi H, Matsuo H, Chinuki Y et al. *Recombinant high molecular weight-glutenin subunit-specific IgE detection is useful in identifying wheat-dependent exercise-induced anaphylaxis complementary to recombinant omega-5 gliadin-specific IgE test.* Clin Exp Allergy. 2012; 42: 1293-8. http://dx.doi.org/10.1111/j.1365-2222.2012.04039.x

47. Ebisawa M, Shibata R, Sato S et al. *Clinical utility of IgE antibodies to omega-5 gliadin in the diagnosis of wheat allergy: a pediatric multicenter challenge study.* Int Arch Allergy Immunol. 2012; 158: 71-6. http://dx.doi.org/10.1159/000330661

48. Kaptchuk TJ, Friedlander E, Kelley JM et al. *Placebos without deception: a randomized controlled trial in irritable bowel syndrome.* PLoS One. 2010; 5: e15591.
http://dx.doi.org/10.1371/journal.pone.0015591

49. Raicek JE, Stone BH, Kaptchuk TJ. *Placebos in 19th century medicine: a quantitative analysis of the BMJ.* BMJ. 2012; 345: e8326. http://dx.doi.org/10.1136/bmj.e8326

50. Sanderson C, Hardy J, Spruyt O et al. *Placebo and Nocebo Effects in Randomized Controlled Trials: The Implications for Research and Practice.* J Pain Symptom Manage. 2013; in-press. http://dx.doi.org/10.1016/j.jpainsymman.2012.12.005

51. Benedetti F. *Placebo-induced improvements: how therapeutic rituals affect the patient's brain.* J Acupunct Meridian Stud. 2012; 5: 97-103. http://dx.doi.org/10.1016/j.jams.2012.03.001

52. Enck P, Benedetti F, Schedlowski M. *New insights into the placebo and nocebo responses.* Neuron. 2008; 59: 195-206. http://dx.doi.org/10.1016/j.neuron.2008.06.030

53. Benedetti F, Lanotte M, Lopiano L et al. *When words are painful: unraveling the mechanisms of the nocebo effect.* Neuroscience. 2007; 147: 260-71. http://dx.doi.org/10.1016/j.neuroscience.2007.02.020

54. Ludvigsson JF, Rubio-Tapia A, van Dyke CT et al. *Increasing Incidence of Celiac Disease in a North American Population.* Am J Gastroenterol. 2013; 108(5): 818-24. http://dx.doi.org/10.1038/ajg.2013.60

55. Ivarsson A, Myleus A, Norstrom F et al. *Prevalence of childhood celiac disease and changes in infant feeding.* Pediatrics. 2013; 131: e687-94. http://dx.doi.org/10.1542/peds.2012-1015

56. Lionetti E, Castellaneta S, Francavilla R, et al. *Introduction of gluten, HLA status, and the risk of celiac disease in children.* N Engl J Med. 2014; 371: 1295-303. http://dx.doi.org/10.1056/NEJMoa1400697

57. Vriezinga SL, Auricchio R, Bravi E, et al. *Randomized feeding intervention in infants at high risk for celiac disease.* N Engl J Med. 2014; 371: 1304-15. http://dx.doi.org/10.1056/NEJMoa1404172

58. Drago S, El Asmar R, Di Pierro M, et al. *Gliadin, zonulin and gut permeability: Effects on celiac and non-celiac intestinal mucosa and intestinal cell lines.* Scand J Gastroenterol 2006; 41: 408-19. http://dx.doi.org/10.1080/00365520500235334

59. El Asmar R, Panigrahi P, Bamford P, et al. *Host-dependent zonulin secretion causes the impairment of the small intestine barrier function after bacterial exposure.* Gastroenterology 2002; 123: 1607-15. http://dx.doi.org/10.1053/gast.2002.36578

60. Smecuol E, Sugai E, Niveloni S, et al. *Permeability, zonulin production, and enteropathy in dermatitis herpetiformis.* Clinical gastroenterology and hepatology: the official clinical practice journal of the American Gastroenterological Association 2005; 3: 335-41. http://dx.doi.org/10.1016/S1542-3565(04)00778-5

61. Klapp G, Masip E, Bolonio M, et al. *Celiac disease: the new proposed ESPGHAN diagnostic criteria do work well in a selected population.* J Pediatr Gastroenterol Nutr 2013; 56: 251-6. http://dx.doi.org/10.1097/MPG.0b013e318279887b

62. Kurppa K, Collin P, Viljamaa M et al. *Diagnosing mild enteropathy celiac disease: a randomized, controlled clinical study.* Gastroenterology. 2009; 136: 816-23. http://dx.doi.org/10.1053/j.gastro.2008.11.040

63. Esteve M, Rosinach M, Fernandez-Banares F et al. *Spectrum of gluten-sensitive enteropathy in first-degree relatives of patients with coeliac disease: clinical relevance of lymphocytic enteritis.* Gut. 2006; 55: 1739-45. http://dx.doi.org/10.1136/gut.2006.095299

64. Meresse B, Malamut G, Cerf-Bensussan N. *Celiac disease: an immunological jigsaw.* Immunity. 2012; 36: 907-19. http://dx.doi.org/10.1016/j.immuni.2012.06.006

65. Sollid LM, Jabri B. *Triggers and drivers of autoimmunity: lessons from coeliac disease.* Nat Rev Immunol. 2013; 13: 294-302. http://dx.doi.org/10.1038/nri3407

66. Cosnes J, Cellier C, Viola S et al. *Incidence of autoimmune diseases in celiac disease: protective effect of the gluten-free diet.* Clin Gastroenterol Hepatol. 2008; 6: 753-8. http://dx.doi.org/10.1016/j.cgh.2007.12.022

67. Zanini B, Caselani F, Magni A et al. *Celiac disease with mild enteropathy is not mild disease.* Clin Gastroenterol Hepatol. 2013; 11: 253-8. http://dx.doi.org/10.1016/j.cgh.2012.09.027

68. Korkut E, Bektas M, Oztas E et al. *The prevalence of celiac disease in patients fulfilling Rome III criteria for irritable bowel syndrome.* Eur J Intern Med. 2010; 21: 389-92. http://dx.doi.org/10.1016/j.ejim.2010.06.004

69. Giangreco E, D'Agate C, Barbera C et al. *Prevalence of celiac disease in adult patients with refractory functional dyspepsia: value of routine duodenal biopsy.* World J Gastroenterol. 2008; 14: 6948-53. http://dx.doi.org/10.3748/wjg.14.6948

70. Santolaria Piedrafita S, Fernandez Banares F. *Gluten-sensitive enteropathy and functional dyspepsia.* Gastroenterol Hepatol. 2012; 35: 78-88. http://dx.doi.org/10.1016/j.gastrohep.2011.10.006

71. Sainsbury A, Sanders DS, Ford AC. *Prevalence of Irritable Bowel Syndrome-type Symptoms in Patients With Celiac Disease: A Meta-analysis.* Clin Gastroenterol Hepatol. 2013; 11: 359-65 e1. http://dx.doi.org/10.1016/j.cgh.2012.11.033

72. Aziz I, Sanders DS. *The irritable bowel syndrome-celiac disease connection.* Gastrointest Endosc Clin N Am. 2012; 22: 623-37. http://dx.doi.org/10.1016/j.giec.2012.07.009

73. Malamut G, Meresse B, Cellier C, et al. *Refractory celiac disease: from bench to bedside.* Semin Immunopathol 2012; 34: 601-13. http://dx.doi.org/10.1007/s00281-012-0322-z

74. Tack GJ, van Wanrooij RL, Langerak AW et al. *Origin and immunophenotype of aberrant IEL in RCDII patients.* Mol Immunol. 2012; 50: 262-70. http://dx.doi.org/10.1016/j.molimm.2012.01.014

75. Rubio-Tapia A, Hill ID, Kelly CP et al. *ACG Clinical Guidelines: Diagnosis and Management of Celiac Disease.* Am J Gastroenterol. 2013; 108(5): 656-76. http://dx.doi.org/10.1038/ajg.2013.79

76. Lebwohl B, Granath F, Ekbom A, et al. *Mucosal healing and risk for lymphoproliferative malignancy in celiac disease: a population-based cohort study.* Ann Intern Med. 2013; 159: 169-75. http://dx.doi.org/10.7326/0003-4819-159-3-201308060-00006

77. Nachman F, del Campo MP, Gonzalez A et al. *Long-term deterioration of quality of life in adult patients with celiac disease is associated with treatment noncompliance.* Dig Liver Dis. 2010; 42: 685-91. http://dx.doi.org/10.1016/j.dld.2010.03.004

78. Casellas F, Rodrigo L, Vivancos JL et al. *Factors that impact health-related quality of life in adults with celiac disease: a multicenter study.* World J Gastroenterol. 2008; 14: 46-52. http://dx.doi.org/10.3748/wjg.14.46

79. Pico M, Spirito MF, Roizen M. *Quality of life in children and adolescents with celiac disease: Argentinian version of the specific questionnaire CDDUX.* Acta Gastroenterol Latinoam. 2012; 42: 12-9.

80. Paarlahti P, Kurppa K, Ukkola A et al. *Predictors of persistent symptoms and reduced quality of life in treated coeliac disease patients: a large cross-sectional study.* BMC Gastroenterol. 2013; 13: 75. http://dx.doi.org/10.1186/1471-230X-13-75

81. Dimitrova AK, Ungaro RC, Lebwohl B et al. *Prevalence of migraine in patients with celiac disease and inflammatory bowel disease.* Headache. 2013; 53: 344-55. http://dx.doi.org/10.1111/j.1526-4610.2012.02260.x

82. Ukkola A, Maki M, Kurppa K et al. *Diet improves perception of health and well-being in symptomatic, but not asymptomatic, patients with celiac disease.* Clin Gastroenterol Hepatol. 2011; 9: 118-23. http://dx.doi.org/10.1016/j.cgh.2010.10.011

83. Lee AR, Hong SW, Ju SJ. *Development of a scale to measure life transition process in parents of children with autism.* J Korean Acad Nurs. 2012; 42: 861-9. http://dx.doi.org/10.4040/jkan.2012.42.6.861

84. Lee AR, Ng DL, Diamond B et al. *Living with coeliac disease: survey results from the USA.* J Hum Nutr Diet. 2012; 25: 233-8. http://dx.doi.org/10.1111/j.1365-277X.2012.01236.x

85. Brottveit M, Vandvik PO, Wojniusz S et al. *Absence of somatization in non-coeliac gluten sensitivity.* Scand J Gastroenterol. 2012; 47: 770-7. http://dx.doi.org/10.3109/00365521.2012.679685

86. Richman E. *The safety of oats in the dietary treatment of coeliac disease.* Proc Nutr Soc. 2012; 71: 534-7. http://dx.doi.org/10.1017/S0029665112000791

87. Cooper SE, Kennedy NP, Mohamed BM et al. *Immunological indicators of coeliac disease activity are not altered by long-term oats challenge.* Clin Exp Immunol. 2013; 171: 313-8. http://dx.doi.org/10.1111/cei.12014

88. Comino I, Real A, Gil-Humanes J et al. *Significant differences in coeliac immunotoxicity of barley varieties.* Mol Nutr Food Res. 2012; 56: 1697-707. http://dx.doi.org/10.1002/mnfr.201200358

89. Real A, Comino I, de Lorenzo L et al. *Molecular and immunological characterization of gluten proteins isolated from oat cultivars that differ in toxicity for celiac disease.* PLoS One. 2012; 7: e48365. http://dx.doi.org/10.1371/journal.pone.0048365

90. Ronda F, Rivero P, Caballero PA et al. *High insoluble fibre content increases in vitro starch digestibility in partially baked breads.* Int J Food Sci Nutr. 2012; 63: 971-7. http://dx.doi.org/10.3109/09637486.2012.690025

91. Gibert A, Kruizinga AG, Neuhold S et al. *Might gluten traces in wheat substitutes pose a risk in patients with celiac disease? A population-based probabilistic approach to risk estimation.* Am J Clin Nutr. 2013; 97: 109-16. http://dx.doi.org/10.3945/ajcn.112.047985

92. Bosmans GM, Lagrain B, Ooms N et al. *Biopolymer interactions, water dynamics, and bread crumb firming.* J Agric Food Chem. 2013; 61: 4646-54. http://dx.doi.org/10.1021/jf4010466

93. Zarkadas M, Dubois S, MacIsaac K et al. *Living with coeliac disease and a gluten-free diet: a Canadian perspective.* J Hum Nutr Diet. 2013; 26: 10-23. http://dx.doi.org/10.1111/j.1365-277X.2012.01288.x

94. Gil-Humanes J, Piston F, Gimenez MJ et al. *The introgression of RNAi silencing of gamma-gliadins into commercial lines of bread wheat changes the mixing and technological properties of the dough.* PLoS One. 2012; 7: e45937. http://dx.doi.org/10.1371/journal.pone.0045937

95. Beckles DM, Tananuwong K, Shoemaker CF. *Starch characteristics of transgenic wheat (Triticum aestivum L.) overexpressing the Dx5 high molecular weight glutenin subunit are substantially equivalent to those in nonmodified wheat.* J Food Sci. 2012; 77: C437-42. http://dx.doi.org/10.1111/j.1750-3841.2012.02648.x

96. Caminero A, Nistal E, Arias L, et al. *A gluten metabolism study in healthy individuals shows the presence of faecal glutenasic activity.* Eur J Nutr. 2012; 51: 293-9. http://dx.doi.org/10.1007/s00394-011-0214-3

97. Nistal E, Caminero A, Vivas S et al. *Differences in faecal bacteria populations and faecal bacteria metabolism in healthy adults and celiac disease patients.* Biochimie. 2012; 94: 1724-9. http://dx.doi.org/10.1016/j.biochi.2012.03.025

98. Wacklin P, Kaukinen K, Tuovinen E et al. *The duodenal microbiota composition of adult celiac disease patients is associated with the clinical manifestation of the disease.* Inflamm Bowel Dis. 2013; 19: 934-41.
http://dx.doi.org/10.1097/MIB.0b013e31828029a9

99. D'Arienzo R, Maurano F, Lavermicocca P et al. *Modulation of the immune response by probiotic strains in a mouse model of gluten sensitivity.* Cytokine. 2009; 48: 254-9.
http://dx.doi.org/10.1016/j.cyto.2009.08.003

100. Bakshi A, Stephen S, Borum ML et al. *Emerging Therapeutic Options for Celiac Disease: Potential Alternatives to a Gluten-Free Diet.* Gastroenterol Hepatol (NY). 2012; 8: 582-588.

Chapter 2

A History of Celiac Disease

Víctor M. García-Nieto

History of Pediatrics Group Coordinator of the Spanish Pediatric Association. Pediatrics Service of Nuestra Señora de Candelaria Hospital, Santa Cruz de Tenerife, Spain.
vgarcianieto@gmail.com

Doi: http://dx.doi.org/10.3926/oms.226

How to cite this chapter

García Nieto VM. *A History of Celiac Disease.* In Rodrigo L and Peña AS, editors. *Celiac Disease and Non-Celiac Gluten Sensitivity.* Barcelona, Spain: OmniaScience; 2014. p. 45-59.

Abstract

Celiac disease is known since ancient times. This chapter describes Aretaeus of Cappadocia's contribution, approximately 2,000 years ago and up until recent times when Marcelo Royer in Buenos Aires and Margot Shiner in London each independently designed a technique for peroral duodenal biopsy under fluoroscopic control. Over the centuries, doctors tried to treat this disease using different diets since the exact pathogenesis of CD was not clear. Special attention is given to the early history of celiac disease in Spain, highlighting the work of Santiago Cavengt and later writings by other Spanish doctors. The elucidation of the cause of celiac disease is due to Willem Karel Dicke. He published his first findings in 1941 in a Dutch Journal in an age when medical literature was based on the empirical knowledge that the diets by proposed by Fanconi and Haas were best for the treatment of the disease. The introduction of intestinal biopsy was the key in confirming the diagnosis of celiac disease since it revealed the characteristic flattening of the mucosa exposed to gluten and the response to a gluten-free diet. Afterwards came new, great advances in the knowledge of the pathophysiological mechanisms of the disease. But that is another history.

"Upon first sight the child appears to have a great pallor... he gives the impression of a balloon held up by two sticks"

(Recalde Cuestas JC, Travella EA.
La Medicina de los Niños. 1935; 36: 326-41)

Celiac disease is one of the nosological entities which has generated more writing in modern pediatric gastroenterology and in pediatrics in general.

Knowledge of the pathogenesis and treatment of the disease has progressed significantly since Willem Karel Dicke established the relationship between the consumption of gluten and the appearance of the disease's symptoms. However, celiac disease has been known for a long time. For centuries, doctors tried to treat it with different dietary regimes since they did not know its exact pathogenesis.

1. Aretaeus of Cappadocia and Gerónimo Soriano

Aretaeus of Cappadocia (85?-138 AD) was a physician, influenced by Greek culture, who flourished in Rome during the age of the Emperor Nero. He brought the clinical dimension of medical practice to the forefront, intensifying the return to the Hippocratic tradition.[1]

He hailed from Cappadocia (in what is now Central Turkey). Apparently, he studied at Alexandria in Egypt, where dissection was allowed. Aretaeus must have practiced it in order to acquire the profound and accurate knowledge about the internal structure of the human body he possessed. His work contains the best ancient descriptions of diseases like diabetes, tetanus, leprosy and pulmonary tuberculosis. He described the aura and hallucinations that precede epileptic seizures. His first description of diphtheric angina and croup are noted for their originality.[2]

His main work is a comprehensive treaty which has not been fully preserved. It consisted of four books which dealt with the causes and symptoms of acute and chronic diseases, plus four others on their treatment.[1] His work was printed in Venice in 1552. The first four books were published under the title *De Causis et Signis Acutorum et Diuturnorum Morborum*. They were regarded, together with the best Hippocratic texts, as classical antiquity's greatest contribution to clinical medicine and they exerted a significant influence on its development.[1] In Book IV, section VII, Aretaeus described the chronic disorder of *pepsis* and *anadosis*, terms which can be translated as "digestion" and "absorption", respectively. For contemporary physicians, *anadosis* included two phases, the passage of food from the intestines to the liver and, from there, to the tissues. According Aretaeus, the celiac condition consisted mainly in fecal elimination of undigested food and in a partially raw state. Being a chronic disease, it made the patient felt very weak "because of the body's hunger". The term "celiac" comes from the Greek word *koiliakos* (*koelia* means "belly" in Greek), which describes a characteristic symptom of the disease in children who begin exhibiting a classic clinical feature (i.e., bloating).

The explanation Aretaeus gives to this mixed disorder of digestion and assimilation was based on the then-current theory of digestive functions. It was based on the concept of "natural heat": as the heat of the sun is necessary for ripening fruit or as the heat used in cooking softens food, the "natural heat" of the stomach was thought to be necessary for the preparation (concoction) of ingested food as requirement for their subsequent absorption. To Aretaeus, the celiac state was thus caused by a cooling of the "natural heat" necessary for the *pepsis* and the *anadosis* of food. For this reason, celiac patients would be haggard, hungry, pale and devoid of the energy needed to perform their usual activities. The exclusion of "peptic" activity would lead to deterioration in the color, smell and consistency of their stools.

In Book VII, section VIII, Aretaeus explains the treatment for said disease. It was aimed at promoting *pepsis*, preventing cooling and restoring the "natural heat". The treatment included rest and fasting along with then current therapeutic measures to prevent flatulence and diarrhea. The prescribed diet was mentioned without excessive details, but it suggested that drinks should be taken before solid foods.

The first Spanish reference to celiac disease is found in a book written nearly three centuries before the work of Samuel Gee.[3]

Gerónimo Soriano, an aragonese physician born in Teruel, published, in 1600, one of the first Spanish language books on pediatrics, *Método y Orden de Curar las Enfermedades de los Niños* ("The Method and Order by which to Cure the Diseases of Children").[4] The book consists of 39 chapters, each referring to a pediatric disease, including topics as diverse as the treatment of fainting, cataracts and epilepsy. The second edition, which also appeared in Zaragoza in 1690, included a new chapter on the treatment of carbuncles.

In Chapter II, which dealt with the treatment of diarrhea, Soriano states that there are different types of diarrhea, one of which is characteristic of "those which are celiac" in which "that which is emptied is with little alteration or mutation". A few lines further on, he writes that "Regarding all these differences in diarrhea, we dwell long in the book on our medical experiments. Here you will find wonderful remedies".

2. Samuel Gee and Subsequent Works until the Late Nineteen Forties

London's St. Bartholomew's Hospital was founded in 1123. For centuries, numerous doctors and surgeons tried to alleviate the ills of their fellow citizens through the use of the methods, techniques and drugs current in the era in which they lived. Samuel Gee was one of the physicians who worked here (Figures 1 and 2).

He was born in London, on September 13, 1839. He died 72 years old, on August 3, 1911 in the English town of Keswick.[5] He began his medical studies at *University College Hospital* in London in 1857 and graduated from the University of London in 1861. Soon he began working at the prestigious *Hospital for Sick Children* in the same city and, in 1865, was appointed member of the Royal College of Physicians, the year in which he earned his doctorate. A year later, he began working at St. Bartholomew's Hospital.[5]

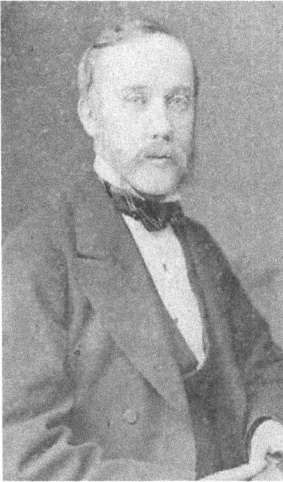

Figure 1. Samuel Jones Gee (1839-1911).

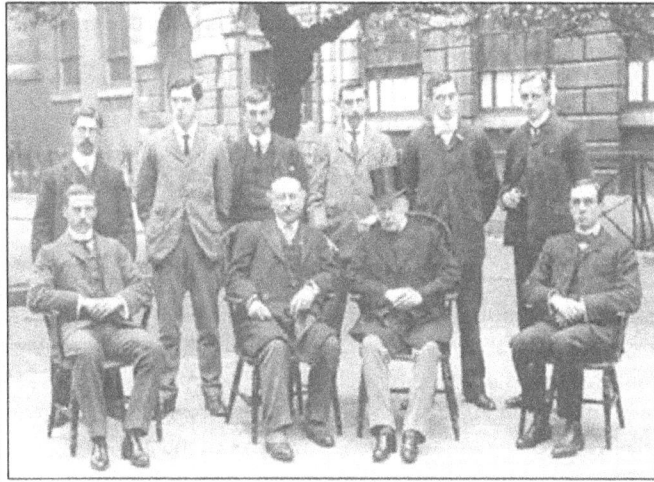

Figure 2. Samuel Gee in 1900. Picture taken in the yard of St. Bartholomew's Hospital, London. Dr. Gee is the second figure from the right, sitting, wearing top hat.

On October 5, 1887, Gee was invited to lecture at the *Hospital for Sick Children*. The contents of this lecture, published the following year in the journal *St. Bartholomew's Hospital Reports*, is the first recognizably modern description of celiac disease in children.[6] Gee describes a disease characterized as a kind of chronic indigestion which could be observed in all ages, although it mainly occurred in children aged between one and five years. This disease is characterized by the presence of soft, unformed stools, though not liquid, bulkier than the amount of food eaten, pale, as if devoid of bile, frothy and, sometimes, emitting a striking stench as if food had undergone putrefaction rather than *concoction* (digestion). Gee conducted autopsies on some of his patients and found no injuries to the stomach or intestines or other digestive organs, although he could not tell whether the atrophy which could be observed in the intestinal glandular crypts could be important to the pathogenesis of the disease. He thought that certain errors in the diet could be the cause of the disease, which led him to conclude that "if the patient can be cured at all, it must be by means of the diet".[6]

Indeed, he found that a patient who had been prescribed a daily "pint" of the "best" Dutch mussels thrived "wonderfully", even though he relapsed when the mussel season ended. The following season there was no way to repeat the experience.

In 1908, Christian Archibald Herter (1865-1910), who worked in New York, published his findings on new cases of the disease, which he called "intestinal infantilism". This author attributed this condition to an infection linked to abnormal persistence of acidic digestive flora (bifid bacilli) in the newly born; this theory was quite influential. Following the publication of his book[7] CD became known as the *Gee-Herter disease*.

In 1909, Johann Otto Leonhard Heubner (1843-1926), director of the Children's University Hospital at Berlin (Charité), described some cases of "serious digestive insufficiency" in which he supposed there might be a problem caused by starch fermentation, due to a faulty congenital disposition of the entire digestive tract.

In 1918, George Frederick Still (1868-1941), professor of pediatrics at King's College Hospital in London, considered the disease to be a serious digestive disorder and noted that bread particularly aggravated its symptoms, but was not aware of the importance of this observation.[8]

In 1924, Sydney Haas (1870-1964) reported success with eight children who were fed a diet based on bananas and which excluded bread, cereals and sugars, which ought to be maintained indefinitely. The author was right to recommend a gluten-free diet even though he did not understand the reason for his success, since he believed that what really mattered was the sugar content of the diet. It is possible that he may have based his recommendations on his observation that in Puerto Rico, "the inhabitants of the city suffer from sprue while farmers, who mostly live on bananas, never do".[9,10] (Figures 3 and 4)

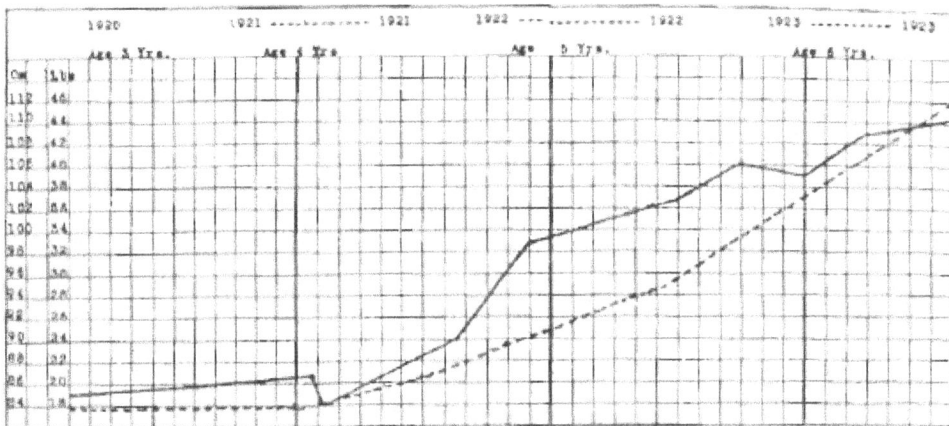

Figure 3. The effectiveness of Sydney Haas' banana diet. Case 2) . Progress S.D. The dashed line indicates height; the solid line, weight.[9]

In 1928 Guido Fanconi (1892-1979) suggested the possibility of the existence of profound metabolic changes in children suffering from this disease, such as hypocalcaemia, hypophosphatemia, vitamin C deficiency and, especially, metabolic acidosis. He therefore recommended that they be nourished with vitamin C-rich foods. The diet should be based on fruit and their juices, adding raw or pureed vegetables, crossing out flour, sucrose or baby food since they tend to be poorly tolerated by the small intestine and tend to produce acidosis.[11] This author, along Uehlinger and Knauer, published in 1936 a memorable article in which they revealed a new disease, mucoviscoidosis or cystic fibrosis.[12] Two years later, Dorothy Andersen (1901-1963) established the histopathological differences between this disease and celiac disease.[13] In 1947, Dr. Andersen defined celiac disease as "the disease which causes recurrent or chronic diarrhea in children between six months and six years, with no demonstrable pathological or bacteriological basis, showing intolerance to the food proper for their age and leading to a progressive increase in the volume of the stomach and halting of body weight gain".[14] In the late nineteen forties, Emery published some articles on carbohydrate[15] metabolism and on the tendency to hypoglycemia, with afebrile perspiration[16] in celiac children.

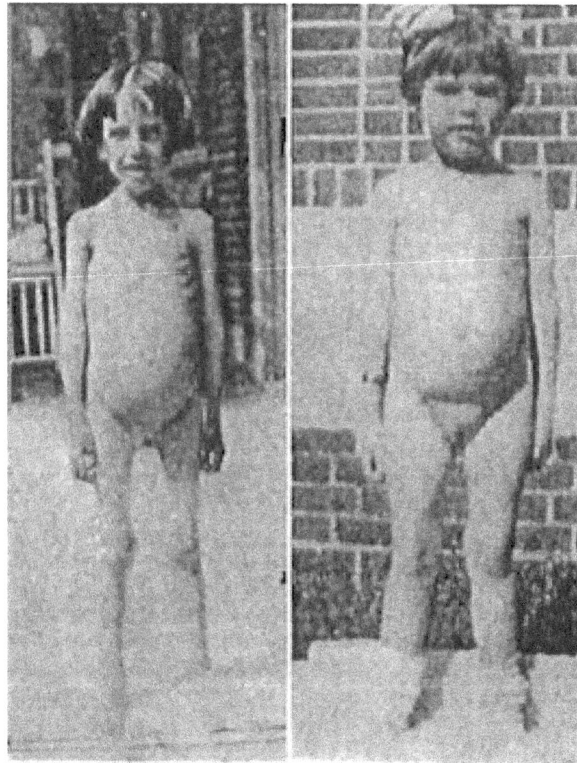

Figure 4. These pictures show the rate of change in celiac disease after the introduction of the gluten-free diet. The image on the left shows patient RB at age 7 years and 7 months, the right, at the age of 7 years, 10 months.[10]

3. Celiac Disease in Spain; Santiago Cavengt and the Later Writings of Spanish Physicians

In pediatrics textbooks as widely used in Spain as Apert's (1917) no reference is made to this entity, and the only thing that could be found approaching it was only a brief description of chronic dyspepsia, in which a distinction is made between "fatty dyspepsia" and "atrophic dyspepsia". Spanish pediatricians were aware of what was known as "serious digestive insufficiency" through the equally titled chapter in *Treatise of Children's Diseases*, edited by the German physician Bernardo Bendix and translated into Spanish in 1913. The author, who named to Heubner as his teacher, stated that this disease numbers among its symptoms "general depression, moodiness, loss of appetite, change in the appearance of the stool, bowel movements and halting of weight gain and growth. The abdomen may be distended". This text mentions a study by Herter which had shown an increase in the fecal excretion of calcium salts which might later help explain, at least in part, the osteomalacia and hyperoxaluria that can be seen in celiac children. Drawing from his experience in the treatment of the disease, which is defined as "faulty or weak congenital disposition of the entire digestive apparatus", Bendix recommended the exclusion of milk from the diet. Decades later, this decision would later be explained by the transient lactase deficiency that occurs in this disorder. The drugs that were recommended then were "occasionally, lactopepsin, acidolpepsin, pancreatin and pancreon tablets" a result of the fact that, by that date, celiac disease had not yet been differentiated from cystic fibrosis.

Santiago Cavengt Gutiérrez was one of the great Spanish pediatricians from the first half of the last century (Figure 5). He was a staff member at the of the *Hospital del Niño Jesús* at Madrid, where the *La Pediatría Española* ("Spanish Pediatrics") magazine was edited under the direction of Martin Aurelio Arquellada, a pediatric surgeon. Cavengt taught at the *Escuela Nacional de Puericultura* ("National Childcare School") and became Director of the *Dispensario Municipal de Puericultura* ("Municipal Childcare Dispensary"). In 1922 Santiago Cavengt wrote E*ndocrinología Infantil* ("Child Endocrinology") with a foreword by Gregorio Marañón. This was the first book written in Spain on the subject of pediatrics. Chapter 12 of said book is titled "Infantilism or *Patocativismo*" (this last Spanish-language term has fallen into disuse and it was used to denote a pathologically weak constitution).[17] The author recalls the different classifications made by contemporary writes on the different types of infantilism. Thus, he refers to Bauer's division of infantilism into two groups: thyroid infantilism or Brissaud's and "all the other types, that is to say (sic.) infantiles of the Lorain type, not regarding them as truly ill, but simply as constitutionally weak, physiologically miserable; he named them *chétivistes* (*chétivisme*), name which Marañón successfully rendered into Spanish as *cativistas* (*cativismo*)". Later that same chapter, Cavengt goes on to expound on "pluriglandular infant *patocativismo*" and one of them being "intestinal in origin". He quotes Herter, as the first author who studied this disease but he states that "Charrin and Le Play already in 1904 wrote about lack of intestinal development of toxic origin". He goes to say that "this *patocativismo* has also been described by Stoos, from Berne, who defines two varieties: one that begins during the second year of life (Herter type) and another one which features gastrointestinal disorders during the first year (Heubner type). The author goes on to relate the case of a child with a medical history absolutely typical for this disease, since it began with "vomiting since birth, without respite up until four years of age, sometimes not defecating for six or seven days, living in a state of athrepsia". Further on he adds "before, as an infant, he was very constipated, alternating between normality and ill-smelling diarrhea". At nine years old, the patient measured only 90 cm. The abdomen was distended and blood tests showed "decreased hemoglobin and red blood cells". This data suggest that the patient was affected by Hirschsprung's disease, rather than celiac disease. He closes the chapter admitting knowledge of the term "celiac infantilism" but points out that "the authors call it so, as they could name it otherwise, they are really cases of intestinal infantilism".[17]

Four years after the publication of his book, Santiago Cavengt publishes in *La Pediatría Española* reports on two new celiac disease cases, this time under the term *digestive infantilism*.[18] The author repeats concepts already mentioned. He admits knowledge of Gee's work: "thus, Samuel in 1888 speaks of the celiac affliction". He also mentions new concepts, such as the relationship of the disease with bone metabolism so that "along with Marfan, we admit that, among the root causes of rickets, the most common is chronic gastrointestinal toxicity; other authors such as Lehmann, Bluhdorn, Stollte and talk about osteoporosis". It is striking that these cases' symptoms began quite soon during lactation. Unless dietary cereals were introduced quite early, which is quite likely, it might be considered "that these children have actually suffered from diseases such as intolerance to the proteins in cow's milk or cystic fibrosis". Thus, the second patient acquired "pertussis one month after being born, which lasted a long time; the parents assure that he still coughs occasionally, catching cold quite easily".

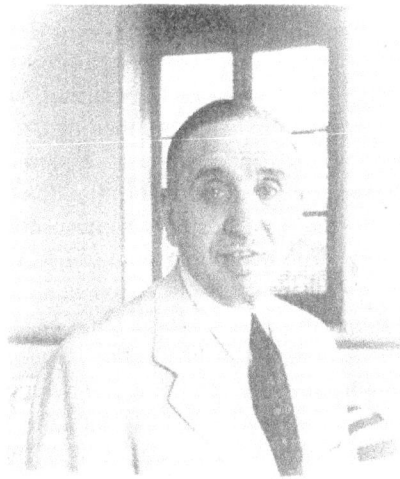

Figure 5. Santiago Cavengt Gutiérrez, the Spanish pediatrician who published the first cases of celiac disease in Spain. He was President of the Spanish Association of Pediatrics (1949-1952).

The nineteen thirties, especially near the end of the decade, were not conductive to promoting research and scientific development in Spain. In that span of time there are only two known papers written on the subject. In 1932, Tenerife pediatrician Isidoro González Hernández published the first known case described in the Canary Islands.[19] In 1935, Dr. Martinez Vargas, Professor of Pediatrics at the Faculty of Medicine, Barcelona, published in the journal *La Medicina de los Niños* ("The Children's Medicine") an article which now did use the term *celiac disease*. Actually, it was an article written by two argentine authors, Recalde Cuestas and Travella, who had already presented it at the V National Congress of Medicine at Rosario and in which they pointed out that "most of these children are neuropathic, capricious, and prone to anger, to lack of appetite and bulimia". Martinez Vargas, simply restricted himself to writing a few comments at the end of said text.[20]

The pediatric journals that were published in 1936, such as *La Medicina de los Niños* (Barcelona), *Archivos Españoles de Pediatría* ("Spanish Pediatrics Archives", Madrid), *La Pediatría Española* (Madrid) and *Pediatría y Puericultura* ("Pediatrics and Childcare, Granada) disappeared forever as a result of the civil war. Interestingly, in that decade, between 1934 and 1936, Dicke began his first experiments with wheat-free diets.

After the war, in 1943 Spanish pediatric journals reappeared with *Acta Pediátrica* ("Pediatric Act"), co-founded by Santiago Cavengt and which continues to this day. It was this author who would publish in the journal's first issue his *Contribución al Estudio Clínico del Síndrome Celíaco* ("Contribution to the Clinical Study of the Celiac Syndrome").[21] In this article, in which he already accepts celiac terminology, he also recognizes that it was Gee who gave the disease an "independent scientific personality"; he also reported the case histories of two new patients, the second of which was born with imperforate anus. The author, who no longer used the term *patocativismo*, summarized the three pathogenic theories at the time current at the time he wrote: "the one which defends the toxic influence of a bromo-infective origin, which would impinge upon the intestinal mucosa's function and absorption, the one that assigns the main role to altered adrenal glands and the one that posits the intervention of avitaminosis". This last hypothesis, then in vogue, was proposed by Dubois, who sought to explain the pathogenesis of celiac disease from a point of view essentially based on vitamins linked to lactoflavine, the vitamin B2 complex's thermostable factor. The author postulated that "it appears that vitamin B2 would be able to intervene in regulating the absorption process of the intestinal mucosa". Cavengt quoted data on mortality from various contemporary works and which ranged from 11% in the Shaap series up to 50% from Knofelmacher's. Discussing the issue of treatment, the author mentions renowned French pediatrician Marfan, who stated that "given the darkness that prevails about the aetiopathogenesis of this disease, treatment must depend on an empirical basis". Experience had already shown that a good way to start feeding the children again was based on rice flour and fruit juice. The author mentioned diets advocated by Haas and Fanconi, as well as those recommended by Marfan's, based modified milk compounds (albuminous milk, kefir) or more "exotic" ones, like Ribadeu-Dumas' comprising "heliotrope aleurone, vegetable protide, porridge made with water, sour milk or beef broth". In all these diets, experience had shown, in an empirical but effective way, to withdraw certain cereals and, in many cases, lactose from the diet of celiac children.

In 1945, Manuel Suárez Perdiguero, who then held the chair of Pediatrics at the University of Zaragoza, published the most comprehensive national study, consisting of 17 celiac children.[22]

From the point of view of the bodily functions, he mentioned that these patients had a flat glucose curve when the test was performed orally but a normal curve when checked intravenously. He mentioned as well radiological images obtained from the intestinal tract showing slow transit of pap in the small intestine, atonic dilated loops or "rainy" images. Dr. Suarez insisted on establishing differential diagnosis of celiac disease with pancreatic cystic fibrosis, lambliasis or B2 hypovitaminosis, rejecting the current pathogenic theories listed above, and thought, along with other authors like Stolte and Parssons, that the disease was due to functional impairment of the small intestine, which behaved like an infant's, able to accept only the "biological food of a woman's milk".

In 1948, Guillermo Arce, Chief of Pediatrics at the *Casa de Salud Valdecilla* ("Valdecilla House of Health"), at Santander, published a review summarizing current knowledge concerning chronic dyspepsia between three and six years of age.[3] The author reviewed contemporary etiologic systematizations including those of authors such as Nobécourt, Andersen, Hodges, Ramos and Fanconi, among others. The author explained his personal classification of the subject, in which distributed "chronic dyspepsias" into five subgroups, namely, simple chronic dyspepsia, chronic dyspepsia with accompanies genuine celiac disease, pseudoceliac chronic dyspepsia, chronic dyspepsia due to pancreatic insufficiency and dyspepsia with chronic enteritis or colitis.

In 1949 a work was published by one who would become one of the most internationally-minded Spanish pediatricians in the second half of the last century, Ángel Ballabriga Aguado. In this article, which had been awarded the Nestlé Prize by the *Sociedad Pediátrica de Madrid* ("Madrid Pediatric Society"), he mentioned that "it is more important to maximize the elimination or restriction of carbohydrates from the diet than the elimination or giving low-fat diet", and that this restriction "must be imposed on certain carbohydrates. Therefore, the administration of carbohydrates will take the form of disaccharides".[24] The reason for the removal of cereals is explained as done "in order to avoid or minimize hydrocarbon fermentation which causes bloating and diarrhea". The author advocated the effectiveness of a diet based on bananas, carob and buttermilk. The second part of this work mentioned the development of a new biochemical technique in Spain, referring to the determination of aminoacidemia levels following Krauel's micromethod. Ballabriga showed that the increase of these levels followed the administration of casein hydrolyzates, whose use he recommended.

Finally, in 1950, *Acta Pediátrica Española* published a reference to a meeting of the *Sociedad de Pediatría de Madrid* ("Madrid Pediatric Society"), which included a paper entitled *Consideraciones Clínicas sobre la Celiaquía* ("Clinical Considerations on Celiac Disease").[25] The author was none other than Santiago Cavengt, who, by then must have been 67 years old and yet still had enough enthusiasm to continue studying the disease he had made known in Spain. Little did he imagine that the question of its origins had already been solved.

4. The Elucidation of the Cause of Celiac Disease. The First Intestinal Biopsies

Willem Karel Dicke (1905-1962) (Figure 6) began his experiments in 1932 using wheat-free diets, inspired by Stheeman's report of the case of a child who experienced diarrhea after eating bread and biscuits. He published his first results in 1941 in a Dutch magazine, when literature had already empirically established that the Haas and Fanconi diets were the most suitable in the treatment of this disease.[26] At the International Congress of Pediatrics (New York, 1947) Dicke submitted comments about the bread or cookies aggravating celiac disease. He was not taken seriously.[27] With the help of colleagues from Utrecht, Weijers, a pediatrician and Van de Kamer, a biochemist who developed the fecal fat quantification technique, Dicke was able to show that the removal of wheat from the diet of celiac patients reduced fecal fat, while its reintroduction increased steatorrhea. These findings were presented at the International Congress of the International Pediatric Association (IPA) (Zurich, 1950).[27] The publication of the article which contained these results was delayed because it was rejected by a noted American magazine. It was later published in 1953 in *Acta Paediatrica Scandinavica*.[28] At the same time, Anderson et al. in Birmingham, noted that most of the fecal fat was of dietary origin and that it was due to a defect in intestinal absorption. This group concluded that improvement occurred only when a wheat flour component, gluten, was strictly removed.[29] This was what the Dutch group called the "wheat factor".[30]

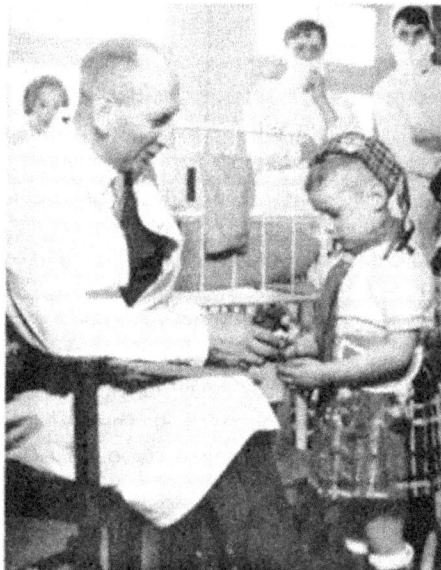

Figure 6. Willem Karel Dicke Stock (1905-1962) during the period in which he was Director of the Wilhelmina Children's Hospital at Utrecht.

The introduction of intestinal biopsy was instrumental in confirming the diagnosis of celiac disease, it highlighted the characteristic flattening of the mucosa when exposed to gluten. This finding was defined by Paulley in 1954, by means of laparotomy-obtained samples from adult individuals affected by idiopathic steatorrhea.[31] The difficulty in obtaining samples able to yield data suggested the need for a viable method to obtain intestinal biopsies from these patients. Wood et al. designed in Melbourne a simple biopsy tube which was flexible and could be used to perform gastric biopsies without the aid of a gastroscope or an X-ray screen; it was soon was used to establish the histological diagnosis of diffuse lesions such as chronic gastritis or atrophic gastritis.[32] Marcelo Royer et al. in Buenos Aires[33], and Margot Shiner, in London[34], each developed separately a technique for peroral duodenal biopsy under fluoroscopic control, based on a device designed by Wood (Figure 7).

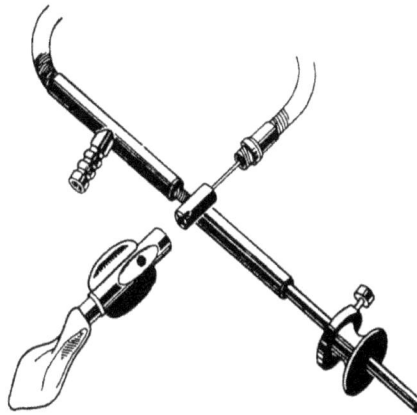

Figure 7. Margot Shiner's jejunal biopsy tube.[34]

Subsequently, other authors found flattening of the intestinal mucosa in celiac patients and that mucosal recovery followed the introduction of the gluten-free diet[35] (Figure 8).

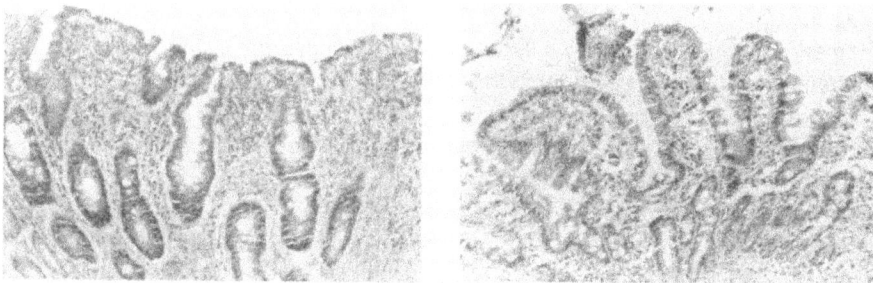

Figure 8. Left: initial biopsy. Right: Marked improvement in duodenal biopsy after 12 months of treatment with gluten-free diet.[35]

New and significant advances in the understanding of the pathophysiological mechanisms of the disease are yet to come. But that is another story.

References

1. López Piñero JM. *El helenismo romano. En: La Medicina en la Antigüedad.* Madrid: Cuadernos Historia. 1985; 16: 18-24.
2. Laín Entralgo P. *Historia de la Medicina.* Barcelona: Salvat Editores; 1978; 102.
3. García Nieto VM. *Cámaras celíacas y patocativismo o la historia de la enfermedad celíaca en España.* Granada: Editorial Comares; 1995.
4. Soriano G. Método y orden de curar las enfermedades de los niños. Madrid: Real Academia de Medicina; 1929.
5. Ortigosa del Castillo L. *Historia de la enfermedad celíaca (1), Samuel Gee.* Can Pediatr. 2008; 32: 57-9.
6. Gee S. *On the coeliac affection.* St. Bartholomew's Hospital Reports. 1888; 24: 17-20.
7. Herter CA. *On infantilism from chronic intestinal infection, characterized by the over growth and persistence of flora of the nursling period. A study of the clinical course, bacteriology, chemistry and therapeutics of arrested development in infancy.* New York: The Macmillan Company; 1908.
8. Still CF. *The Lumleian lectures on coeliac disease.* Lancet. 1918; 2: 163-6, 193-7, 227-9.
9. Haas SV. *Value of banane treatment in celiac disease.* Am J Dis Child. 1924; 28: 421-37.
10. Haas SV. *Celiac disease. Its specific treatment and cure without nutritional relapse.* JAMA. 1932; 99: 448-52. http://dx.doi.org/10.1001/jama.1932.02740580016004
11. Fanconi G. *Der intestinal infantilismus und ähnliche formen der chronischen verdauungstörung: Ihre behandlung mit früchten und gemüsen.* Berlin: S. Karger; 1928.
12. Fanconi G, Uehlinger E, Knauer C. *Das coeliakie-syndrom bei angeborener zystischer pankreasfibromatose und bronchiektasien.* Wien Med Wchnschr. 1936; 86: 753-6.
13. Andersen DH. *Cystic fibrosis of the pancreas and its relation to celiac disease: a clinical and pathological study.* Am J Dis Child. 1938; 56: 344-99.
14. Andersen DH. *Celiac síndrome VI. The relationship of celiac disease, starch intolerance, and steatorrhea.* J Pediatr. 1947; 30: 564-82. http://dx.doi.org/10.1016/S0022-3476(47)80050-2
15. Emery JL. *Carbohydrate metabolism in the coeliac syndrome.* Arch Dis Child. 1947; 22: 41-9. http://dx.doi.org/10.1136/adc.22.109.41
16. Emery JL. *Cold sweating, hypoglycaemia, and carbohydrate insufficiency; with particular reference to coeliac disease.* Arch Dis Child. 1947; 22: 34-40. http://dx.doi.org/10.1136/adc.22.109.34
17. Cavengt S. *Infantilismo o patocativismo.* En: Endocrinología infantil. Madrid: Ruiz Hermanos eds.; 1922. pp. 131-70.
18. Cavengt S. *Infantilismo digestivo.* La Pediatría Española. 1926; 15: 93-109.
19. Hernández González I. *Un caso de infantilismo digestivo.* Revista Médica de Canarias. 1932; 1: 215-16.
20. Recalde Cuestas JC, Travella EA, Martínez Vargas A. *Enfermedad celíaca.* La Medicina de los Niños. 1935; 36: 326-41.
21. Cavengt S. *Contribución al estudio clínico del síndrome celíaco.* Acta Ped. 1943; 1: 25-47.
22. Suárez Perdiguero M. *Enfermedad celíaca y síndrome celíaco. Concepto y patogénesis.* Rev Esp Pediatr. 1945; 1: 683-95.
23. Arce G. *Etiología y clasificación de las dispepsias crónicas en la segunda infancia.* Acta Ped Esp. 1948; 6: 837-41.

24. Ballabriga Aguado A. *Tratamiento de la enfermedad celíaca con especial consideración a sus aspectos dietéticos.* Acta Ped Esp. 1949; 7: 1519-41.

25. Cavengt S. *Consideraciones clínicas sobre la celiaquia.* Acta Ped Esp. 1950; 8: 199.

26. Dicke WK. *Simple dietary treatment for the syndrome of Gee-Herter.* Ned Tijdschr Geneeskd. 1941; 85: 1715-6.

27. Rossi E. *Pediatric Gastroenterology.* En: History of Pediatrics 1850-1950. Nichols Jr BL, Ballabriga A, Kretchmer N, eds. Nueva York: Raven Press; 1991; 105-12.

28. Dicke WK, Weijers HA, Van de Kamer JH. *Coeliac disease. II. The presence in wheat of a factor having a deleterious effect in cases of coeliac disease.* Acta Paediatr. 1953; 42: 34-42. http://dx.doi.org/10.1111/j.1651-2227.1953.tb05563.x

29. Anderson CM, French JM, Sammons HG, Frazer AC, Gerrard JW, Smellie JM. *Coeliac disease; gastrointestinal studies and the effect of dietary wheat flour.* Lancet. 1952; 1: 836-42. http://dx.doi.org/10.1016/S0140-6736(52)90795-2

30. Van de Kamer JH, Weijers HA, Dicke WK. *Coeliac disease IV. An investigation into the injurious constituents of wheat in connection with their action on patients with coeliac disease.* Acta Paediatr, 1953; 42: 223-31.
http://dx.doi.org/10.1111/j.1651-2227.1953.tb05586.x

31. Paulley JW. *Observation on the aetiology of idiopathic steatorrhoea. Jejunal and lymph-node biopsies.* Br Med J. 1954; 2: 1318-21. http://dx.doi.org/10.1136/bmj.2.4900.1318

32. Wood IJ, Doig RK, Motteram R, Hughes A. *Gastric biopsy.* Lancet. 1949; 2: 18-21. http://dx.doi.org/10.1016/S0140-6736(49)90344-X

33. Royer M, Croxatto 0, Biempica L, Morrison AJB. *Biopsia duodenal por aspiracion bajo control radioscopico.* Prensa Med Argentina. 1955; 42: 2515-9.

34. Shiner M. *Duodenal biopsy.* Lancet. 1956; 270: 17-9. http://dx.doi.org/10.1016/S0140-6736(56)91854-2

35. Anderson CM. *Histological changes in the duodenal mucosa in coeliac disease. Reversibility during treatment with a wheat gluten free diet.* Arch Dis Child. 1960; 35: 419-27. http://dx.doi.org/10.1136/adc.35.183.419

OmniaScience

Chapter 3

Perspectives to take into account when Studying Celiac Disease in China and Central America

Amavilia Perez Villavicencio[1], Carlos Beirute Lucke[2], Amado Salvador Peña[3]

[1]Celiac Disease Expert, University of Seville, Spain.

[2]Anthropologist, University of Costa Rica, *Centro de Información sobre la Enfermedad Celíaca*, San José, Costa Rica.

[1,2] MBA, Communication Science, Costa Rica.

[3]Professor Emeritus, University Medical Center, "VU" University, Amsterdam, The Netherlands.

cieccontacto@gmail.com, contactciec@gmail.com, pena.as@gmail.com

Doi: http://dx.doi.org/10.3926/oms.237

How to cite this chapter

Perez Villavicencio A, Beirute Lucke C, Peña AS. Perspectives to take into account when Studying Celiac Disease in China and Central America. In Rodrigo L and Peña AS, editors. *Celiac Disease and Non-Celiac Gluten Sensitivity*. Barcelona, Spain: OmniaScience; 2014. p. 61-74.

Abstract

Until quite recently, it was thought that celiac disease existed neither in China nor in Central America. The cultivation of rice in China and the cultivation of maize from the Mexican highlands have respectively been the basis of nourishment in China and Central America. Environmental, social and cultural changes in these regions allow foreseeing an increase of patients with celiac disease in both regions of the world. By way of example, we can point to the deworming of rural populations which contributes to a change in the TH2 to TH1 predominant intestinal immune response, changes in the intestinal microbiota, mainly in urban areas due to access to antibiotics, change in dietary habits due to the influence of "fast foods" and changes in traditional diets based on rice or maize due to the diffusion of diets with a higher gluten content. However, it is necessary to analyze difficulties in these countries regarding the identification of the disease as well as the techniques involved in its diagnosis. The main limitation of these studies lies in the absence of duodenal biopsy specimens. In fact, every population where celiac disease is thought to be emerging needs to adjust its array of detection procedures. Although it is true that sensitive and specific serologic tests for celiac disease have allowed greater confidence in establishing the prevalence of this disease in European and North American studies, the information from China and Central America is still scarce. The creation of interdisciplinary study groups is necessary to design specific protocols for each region.

1. Introduction

Until relatively recent times it was thought that celiac disease existed neither in China nor in Central America. Sporadic cases have been described in both continents and brief series of studies on the subject have been published in China, but not in the Central American countries, with the possible exception of Panama.

Rice cultivation in several regions of China and maize cultivation from the Mexican highlands have been the dominant staples in China and Central America, respectively, while potato cultivation was developed in the Peruvian Andes.

A Canadian university hospital in Vancouver[1] found in Asian-descended populations living in North America, from 1982 to 2002, that celiac disease was diagnosed in fourteen of these persons. Eleven were indo-Canadians, including ten with Punjabi ancestry and one Chinese patient.

Paleo-botanic evidence suggests that populations in north China could have been exposed to gluten-containing cereals for longer than it was recently thought. Findings made in August, 2010[2] suggest that the introduction of wheat in China could date from 2,500 B.C., but may have started to become significant about 2,000 B.C. Nowadays, China is a world-class center of wheat production, which encompasses its northern and southern regions. After the Han Dynasty (206 B.C.–A.D. 9), wheat became one of the main staples in northern China[3]. Since the Northern Song Dynasty (A.D. 960–1,127), wheat was also introduced in southern China.[4] In order to gain a better understanding of the impact of wheat in the presence of CD in China, it is necessary to compare it to rice and to frame both plants within the historical context of the nation. There are weighty reasons, relative to the nature of each of these grains, which made rice preferable in central and southern China: It can produce grains for up to three decades, grow on level land as well as on slopes and it has very high yields. Rice requires large quantities of water, especially due to the strategy of flooding the rice fields in the early stages of cultivation, which prevents the growth of other harmful plants and the arrival of certain pests (it is feasible to cultivate it without flooding the fields, but not doing so makes eventual plague control and fertilization more difficult). These requirements fit well with central and southern China's hydrography, regions that have the large Yangtze and Huanghe rivers and their enormous network of tributary streams, which provide enough water for widespread and intensive rice cultivation.

Chinese populations developed rice agriculture around 7,500 B.C. From this date onwards, this new means of subsistence slowly spread through Northern China until, around 2,100 B.C., the first Chinese state emerged, the Xia Dynasty, whose historicity is still being debated. With the next Dynasty, the Shang (1,800–1,027 B.C.) we stand on firm historical ground. This dynasty was an island of greater organization in the midst of a patchwork of other smaller-scale societies, whose influence and prestige, by means of a process of cultural diffusion, contributed to the spread of Shang culture (the basis of what today is known as China) among the diverse culture groups which, with the passing of millennia, were absorbed into the mainstream of Chinese culture.

The Shang collapse, still not fully understood, was probably brought about in part by the rise of another state, the Western Zhou Dynasty (1,027–771 B.C.), which assimilated the cultural and organizational achievements of their predecessors, consolidating and expanding their cultural influence.

The Zhou, however, were not able to keep direct control of the areas under their influence and, for the period spanning from 771 to 221 B.C., the Zhou sovereign was only the *de jure* ruler of the region. This could have arisen partly from what seems to have been a feudal system in which noblemen of diverse ranks were granted lands, which they ruled in the name of the king. With the passing of the centuries, these feudal lands acquired more and more power and independence up to the point where each one could have become an autonomous state in its own right.

Each one of these states, even when they initially paid nominal homage to the authority of the Zhou ruler, eventually came to develop its own political agenda. On the other hand, it is also likely that other states may have arisen by means of the diffusion of Zhou culture and achievements, which may not necessarily have been originally feudal vassals of the latter.

In any case, the second half of the Zhou period, known as the Warring States Period (as its name implies) was plagued by constant war. Towards the year 221 B.C., Shi Huangdi, ruler of the State of Qin, finally defeated all his opponents and became the first emperor of all of China, unifying for the first time writing, measurements and administration and finally managing to bring peace to the country.

However, the highly autocratic style of Qin administration generated great unrest and opposition and, by the year 207 B.C., this led to the collapse of the Dynasty.

The following dynasty, the Western Han (207 B.C.–A.D. 9), availed itself of the structure and administrative achievements of the Qin and it was the first which managed to impose a stable and relatively peaceful rule over almost the whole country, which laid the foundations for further growth. China's ethnic majority calls itself the "sons of Han" or simply the "Han". This stability generated the country's elevated demography,[5] which has been one of its defining features ever since. Within this historical context, possessing rice and enough water, China has been able to adequately satisfy its nutritional needs.[6]

North China, however, lacking a bountiful irrigation and having a less humid climate, was forced to depend more on grains adapted to drier climates, among which wheat stands out. Cultivation of this grain began to be given an emphasis since the nineteen thirties, midway through the short-lived Chinese Republic, an initiative that has been maintained and increased under the People's Republic of China.

Given rice's high water requirements, it would be reasonable to look for supplementary crops, which would require less water so as to be able to lessen the demand of this resource. China has had powerful reasons to become the world's foremost wheat producer and consumer. This country, in recent years has produced yearly some 115 million metric tons of wheat, about 40% more than India, the second biggest producer, and accounting for 17.06% of the world's total output.

This wheat, most of which is for internal consumption, must be having a widespread diffusion through massive consumer products. This is potentiated by China's insertion in the world market.

Wheat Production in China

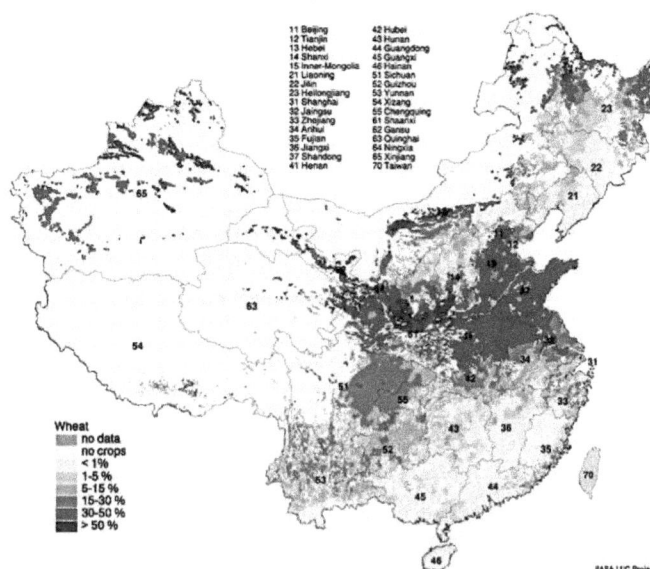

11 Beijing	42 Hubei
12 Tianjin	43 Hunan
13 Hebei	44 Guangdong
14 Shanxi	45 Guangxi
15 Inner-Mongolia	46 Hainan
21 Liaoning	51 Sichuan
22 Jilin	52 Guizhou
23 Heilongjiang	53 Yunnan
31 Shanghai	54 Xizang
32 Jiangsu	55 Chengquing
33 Zhejiang	61 Shaanxi
34 Anhui	62 Gansu
35 Fujian	63 Quinghai
36 Jiangxi	64 Ningxia
37 Shandong	65 Xinjiang
41 Henan	70 Taiwan

Wheat
no data
no crops
< 1%
1-5 %
5-15 %
15-30 %
30-50 %
> 50 %

IIASA LUC Project

http://webarchive.iiasa.ac.at/collections/IIASA_Research/SRD/ChinaFood/data/maps/crops/all_h.htm

Figure 1. Wheat Production in China

In spite of the lack of data on the subject, the prevalence of celiac disease in China and Japan is foreseeably low, due to a rice-based diet. However, with the traditional staple of rice slowly being replaced by western style food, which has a high wheat content,[7] celiac disease could become a health issue in China.

A similar situation is foreseen in Central America; however, in some small towns, which are distant from the capitals, a relatively gluten-free diet may still be widespread.

2. Current situation in China

Currently, the Chinese eat several kinds of wheat-derived products: noodles, steamed bread and cakes, to name a few. China has a long history of consuming *mianjin* or *kaofu*, which are basically gluten-based products. Wheat is the second leading cereal crop in China in terms of cultivated surface and production. More than 90% of this wheat grain is used to make steamed bread and noodles. Even though wheat is cultivated in twenty nine out of thirty Chinese provinces, more than 90% of it is produced in just thirteen provinces, five of which (Shandong, Henan, Jiangsu, Hebei and Anhui) contribute more than 60% of the total production.[8]

Dr. Luigi Greco, a pediatrician from Naples University, wrote in 1995:

> *"Over the last 200 years of our modern age active genetic selection, and actual genetic manipulation, have changed the aspect of the original* Triticacee *enormously: from few grains and little gluten to great wheat harvests very enriched in gluten (50% of the protein content), well adapted to cultivation practices and ready to be handled by monstrous machinery".*[9]

He considers enriched wheat gluten the reason behind the higher celiac disease frequency, especially in populations whose genetic inheritance stems from ancient groups, which did not successfully adapt to tolerate this protein.

Chinese agriculture is also advancing towards a new era, and wheat gluten content is also higher than before. Therefore, the "absence" of celiac disease in China cannot be predicted based on wheat consumption. Since China is a multiracial country, HLA-DQ distribution differs according to area. Currently there are fifty-five ethnic minorities in China, which are officially recognized by the government, even when there are other groups that are still waiting to receive official recognition. Historical and genetic evidence suggest that many of them have been intermixing with the Han for many centuries[10] so that the phenotypical and genotypical differences between these groups and the mainstream Chinese population do not seem to be, in any case, significant. Besides, these groups add up, all told, to less than 10% of the total population.

More interesting seems to be the genetic frontier that exists between North and South China, within the Han ethnic group, as revealed by an article published in 2008 in the *European Journal of Human Genetics*.[11]

This difference would be consistent with the historical division between these regions, which, as explained before, has been determined by their bio-geographical conditions of both. The frequency of haplotype HLA-DQ2, DR3-DQ2 (HLA-DRB1*0301-DQA1*05-DQB1*02) is high in North China along the Old Silk Road, where wheat consumption is higher than in the south. The risk of having celiac disease can be higher, too. In the Jiansu province, the province where Dr. Wu and colleagues undertook their first investigation[12,13] the frequency of allele HLA-DQB1*0201/02 was 17.8%, HLA-DQB1*0302 was 5.6%, the frequency of haplotype HLA-DQA1 0501-DQB1 0201/02 (HLA -DQ2) was 7.2% and the frequency of haplotypes HLA-DQA1 0301/02/03-HLA-DQB1 0302 (HLA-DQ8) was 4.7%.[14]

Only a small fraction of the Caucasoid population which has inherited the HLA-DQ2 and/or HLA-DQ8 genes suffers from celiac disease and the contribution of the HLA region to the development of celiac disease among brothers is of 36%.[15] However, only a small percentage of HLA-DQ2 and DQ8 positive individuals actually develop the disease. Recent investigations using wide field genome suggest that genes in the MHC and non-MHC loci jointly contribute to the likelihood of the disease. Thus, a meta-analysis of the full genome linking studies has pointed out a contribution from the genes in the telomeric region in chromosome 10 (10q26.12-qter) and in chromosome 8 (8q22.2-q24.21).[16]

However, as pointed out by Kumar and colleagues, the recent and sizable amount of information that already exists needs further research in order to clarify its importance. These authors discuss and sum up the results of genetic studies in celiac disease, centering on non-HLA genes besides introducing new perspectives to identify the causal variants of the susceptibility loci in complex diseases like celiac disease and other associated autoimmune diseases, as well as possible mechanisms which could explain the pathogenesis of these diseases.[17] It should not be forgotten that the allele variations found in patients from a Caucasoid background will probably be different in Asian populations and that we must wait for similar studies from these regions.

3. Situation in Central America

There is no doubt regarding the date when wheat began to have an impact on the Central American population. There has been, since the nineteenth century, a whole slew of attempts (with varying degrees of credibility) of vindicating the idea of strong pre-Columbian contacts with the Old World, but, so far (even when the possibility of said contacts cannot be discarded beforehand), there is no evidence at all that suggests a formative or even a perceptible influence, from Old World sources, on the development of native American cultures.

There is relatively certain evidence that, around 1,000 AD, there were small Scandinavian settlements from Greenland on some of the islands just off the coasts in Northern Canada. These lands were known by the Scandinavians as *Vinland* and *Markland* and there are records that the Norsemen had frequent contacts with those whom they called *skrælings*,[18] that is to say, Native Americans (Inuit, the people who until recent decades were known as "eskimos", or possibly members of other tribes).

However, to all intents and purposes, said contacts had no impact upon the ancestral cultural and subsistence patterns in the immediate region, much less on a continental scale.

In any case, the pre-Columbian diet was not only intrinsically gluten-free; it was also intrinsically free from any possibility of gluten cross-contamination, to boot. Additionally, the presence of human beings (*Homo sapiens*) in America dates from 13,000 years before the present and there is not, to date, evidence of any other kind of hominin in this continent. The most orthodox version regarding this fact argues that, near the end of the last ice age, the sea level was lower than it is today, so that there would have been a small strip of dry land where the Bering Strait is today.

Sometime during this period, according to this view, a small population or group of hunter-gatherers from Siberia would have migrated from the Old World towards what today is Alaska.

The members of this group, which is supposed to have been relatively homogenous genetically, would be the ultimate ancestors of all the native inhabitants of the New World.

This paradigm, however, known in archeology as "Clovis First" (based on the name of the eponymous paleoindian culture, the earliest and most archaic stage of American prehistory) is being strongly questioned since there is an ever-growing body of data which suggests the even earlier presence of humans in America, leading to the proposal of dates of 21,000 or even 40,000 years before the present for the peopling of the continent.[19]

Recent evidence, in fact, suggests a much more complex panorama than what was supposed before: A skeleton, known as the "Kennewick Man" (after the locale in Washington State, U.S.A., where it was found) was satisfactorily dated to a period between 7,300 and 7,600 B.C. Several anthropometric studies of its skull have yielded inconclusive results, but the evidence suggests that the cranial morphology of this individual has no exact parallels among known modern populations; in any case, he has more affinities with the Utari (the group formerly known as the Ainu) from North Japan or with the Polynesians than with typical native Americans.[20]

Something similar can be said of "Luzia", a female skeleton dating from about 9,500 B.C., found in the Vermelha cave near Belo Horizonte, Brazil. As with the Kennewick Man, cranial morphology analysis has yielded confusing results, of which the only thing that seems clear is that it differs substantially from the Siberian peoples who were the supposed sole ancestors of all Native Americans, up to the point where some have even classified its facial features as "negroid".[21]

This suggests that Native American populations have a much richer and complex genetic inheritance, and probably a much older one, than it had been supposed up until recent decades.

This panorama of phenotypical diversity is supported and made deeper by a study undertaken by a team headed by Dr. Antonio Torroni, from the University of Pavia, Italy[22,23] whose findings indicate that Native Americans descend from at least two genetically distinct groups. Another study recently published in *Nature* posits the existence of *three* very ancient migrations. These researchers, using a very high-resolution with 364,470 single-nucleotide polymorphisms have studied fifty-two Native American groups and seventeen Siberian groups.

They show that Native Americans descend from at least three Asian gene flows. Most descend from a single ancestral population, which they have named "First Americans", suggesting (according to some interpretations) that the initial population was followed by a southward expansion along the coast, with subsequent divisions but with little change in the gene flow after the divergence, above all in South America. The Chibchas seem to be an important exception on both sides of the Panama isthmus, since they possess ancestors from both North and South America.

To this panorama of inherent diversity in pre-Columbian Central America we can add the influx of European colonizers starting in the Sixteenth Century, who brought a very diverse genetic inheritance, the product of the complex history of their continent of origin.

The first wave of immigrants came mainly from the Iberian Peninsula and it includes a complex patchwork of peoples among which we can include (aside from the inheritance of the tribes that dwelt in it in pre-roman times, of uncertain relations) Iberians, Phoenicians, Romans, Basques, Greeks, Celts, Ostrogoths, Arabs, Berbers, etc.

To this, we must add the presence of large contingents of slaves forcibly brought from Africa, themselves, in turn, coming from various regions of this enormous continent, each of which possesses its own genetic diversity. Furthermore, to all this we must add the later arrival of groups, which hailed from other regions of Europe (Italy, Greece, etc.) or even Near Eastern groups, above all in the post-colonial period.

Clearly, it cannot be concluded that the mixing of peoples from the New World with peoples from the Old World could have easily foreseen genetic consequences, given the fact that we are talking about very large regions, each one of which, in turn, has a very complex genetic map.

When Spanish power collapsed in the New World, far from keeping any sort of cohesion, the diverse provinces of every Viceroyalty went, in a political and cultural sense, along their own separate ways, a fact that determined the way in which the descendants of recent immigrants and the descendants of Native Americans intermingled with each other. Due to this, neighboring Central American countries have clearly differentiated customs, habits, accents and even vocabulary.

Far from being a homogeneous region, Central America has a noteworthy genetic and cultural diversity that can affect the way CD manifests itself in each country and even within the different regions within each country, the social stratification imposed by Spanish administration and customs generated populations with different genetic compositions.

The Only Countries with a Significant Wheat Production in the Region are Mexico and Guatemala

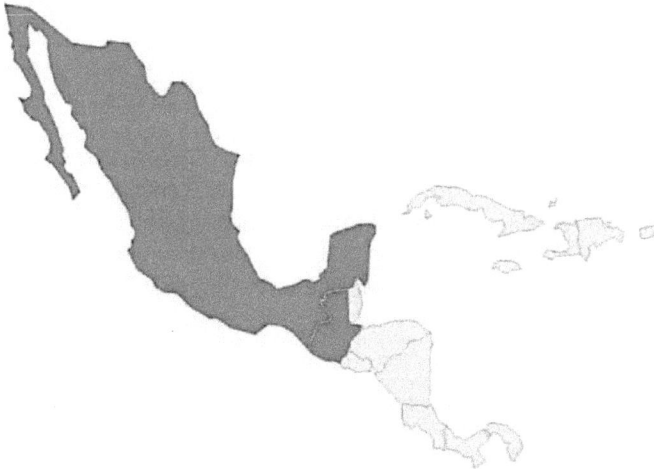

Mexico and Central America

Figure 2. México and Guatemala; the only countries with significant wheat production

Currently, commercial influence from consumer patterns from the United States of America and Europe are being intensified by modern telecommunications networks and by recent free trade treaties. This influence includes an influx of great quantities of gluten-bearing industrial products.

This tendency has been developing for decades, particularly after the end (in the middle of the nineteen-eighties) of the internal military conflicts formerly endemic to the region. For this reason, it should not be unlikely that gluten may have already reached even the inhabitants of areas that are distant or at the margins of the commercial centers by means of medicines or food provided by welfare services or humanitarian organizations, or else by the growing penetration of affordable products in rural areas.

Even making tentative generalizations about the prevalence of celiac disease in this region would be inherently risky. Given the elevated number of variables that have been acting on the region, it is imperative to undertake properly designed epidemiologic and genetic studies. The prevalence may vary from one country to another, even from one region within a country to another. For example, in the highlands of Guatemala the ethnic composition of the population is markedly different from that of the larger cities. This is due to the fact that colonial cities tended to act as administrative centers, so that European-descended people would gather there, relegating the original inhabitants to rural areas.

Studies of genetic markers in these countries are practically non-existent. Confirmed celiac patients have been found in El Salvador by Dr. Mauricio Cromeyer with the cooperation of Ms. Karla María Zaldívar, MBA, PMP, of the *Asociación de Celíacos y Sensibles al Gluten de El Salvador* ("Celiac and Gluten Sensitive Patients' Association of El Salvador) ACELYSES and preliminary results are presented in Chapter 4 of this book.

4. Present and Future

Several environmental changes point to an increase of celiac disease in these regions. We can mentioned the deworming of rural populations which contribute to a change in the TH2 to TH1 predominant intestinal immune response, changes in the intestinal microbiota (mainly in urban areas due to access to antibiotics), changes in dietary habits due to the influence of "fast foods" and changes in traditional diets based on rice or maize due to the diffusion of diets with a higher gluten content.

5. Diagnostic Difficulties

It is necessary to analyze the difficulties in these countries regarding the identification of the disease as well as the techniques involved in its diagnosis. It is possible that general practitioners, specialists and pediatricians may not be familiar with this disease due to clinical heterogeneity of the disease and the low prevalence of the disease.

The main limitations of these studies lie in the absence of duodenal biopsies specimens, the lack of experience in optimizing the quantity and location of the biopsy samples as well as in a lack of experience among the pathologists who analyze the samples. Every population where celiac disease is emerging needs to adjust its array of detection procedures to its particular conditions and needs.

Thus, in the aforementioned study by Wu and colleagues, seventy-three Han patients with irritable bowel syndrome with diarrhea (IBS-D) and five patients with insulin dependent diabetes mellitus were analyzed by serological tests. Six (7.7%) tested positive for antigliadin IgG antibodies (IgG AGA) and two (2.6%) tested positive for tissular transglutaminase IgA antibodies (tTG IgA)[12,13] in the Wuhan region. These initial data have been confirmed by a wider study in the region of Wuhan, which has only been published in abstract form. In this study, two hundred and eighty-two patients with irritable bowel syndrome with diarrhea and two hundred and ninety-six healthy controls underwent a combined serological test (QUANTA LiteTM h-tTG/DGP) which has, as antigen, human transglutaminase and deamidated peptides. Five patients with IBS tested positive for antibodies, as well as two healthy controls. The antibody levels were relatively low in comparison to what is reported from other countries.

6. Conclusion

Current sensitive and specific serological tests for celiac disease have allowed observing an increase of this disease's prevalence in several countries but the priority in emerging countries is the creation of interdisciplinary study groups, which will help to design specific protocols for each region.

6.1 Patients' Associations

Patients' associations in Central America are playing an important role in spreading knowledge about celiac disease. Besides ACELYSES, the *Asociación de Celíacos de Guatemala* ("Celiac Patients' Association of Guatemala") was founded in 2013 in that same country, by Dr.Estuardo Ligorría, who is deeply involved in the study of celiac disease and the treatment of local celiac patients. This association, which has just begun to hold meetings, has established communication with the relevant government institutions so as to secure a legal framework, which will benefit said patients.

In Panama, the *Fundación Celíacos de Panamá* ("Panama Celiac Patients' Foundation", FUCEPA) is also striving to help local celiac patients and their families by means of the dissemination of information, which will improve these patients' quality of life; it has also, among its aims, the improvement of medical criteria and diagnostic procedures, as well as the passing of laws regarding the labelling of products regarding their gluten content.

In Costa Rica, the *Asociación Pro-Personas Celíacas* ("Pro Celiac Persons' Association", APPCEL), founded in 2004, has worked towards the same ends, offering psychological support as well as useful information by means of an electronic newsletter and has been involved in changing this country's laws so that celiac patients may have access to safe food and properly labelled products.

The *Centro de Información sobre la Enfermedad Celíaca* ("Celiac Disease Information Center", CIEC), founded by Ms. Amavilia Pérez Villavicencio, MSc, has its headquarters also in Costa Rica. In Honduras and Nicaragua there is still very little information available to the general population, but in these countries efforts are being made, by some of their gastroenterologists, whose interest has been aroused by recent developments in the field, to better understand this disease and to lessen its impact on the population and on their countries' health care systems.

Acknowledgements

We would like to acknowledge the work of our colleagues in China, Dr. Wu Jing (Digestive Disease Department, *Jiangsu Provincial Hospital of Traditional Chinese Medicine*, Nanjing, Jiangsu Province, P.R. China) and Prof. Xia Bing (Director of Department of Gastroenterology, Chair of Department of Internal Medicine Zhongnan Hospital, Wuhan University School of Medicine, Wuhan, Hubei, P.R. China).

In Central America we are grateful to Dr. Mauricio Cromeyer (*Hospital de Diagnóstico Escalón*, Villavicencio Plaza, Paseo General Escalón, Colonia Escalón, San Salvador, El Salvador C.A.) and Ms. Karla María Zaldívar, MBA, PMP., (San Salvador, El Salvador, C.A.) for the enthusiasm with which they dedicate themselves to the study of celiac disease and provided interesting data.

References

1. Freeman HJ. Biopsy-defined adult celiac disease in Asian-Canadians. Can J Gastroenterol 2003; 17: 433-6.
2. Flad R, Shuicheng L, Xiaohong W, Zhijun Z. *Early Wheat in China: Results from New Studies at Donghuishan in the Hexi Corridor.* The Holocene. 2010; Sept 20(6): 955-65. http://hol.sagepub.com/content/20/6/955
3. Maoli H. *On wheat dissemination in regions south of the Changjiang river.* Studies in the History of Natural Sciences. 1992; 4: 010.
4. Zhonghu H, Rajaram S, Xin Z, Huang G. *A history of wheat breeding in China*: Cimmyt; 2001.
5. Issues and Trends in China's Demographic History. I http://afe.easia.columbia.edu/special/china_1950_population.htm
6. International Year of Rice 2004. Rice is life. Issues and Trends in China's Demographic History. http://www.fao.org/rice2004/en/f-sheet/factsheet3.pdf
7. Cummins AG, Roberts-Thomson IC. *Prevalence of celiac disease in the Asia-Pacific region.* J Gastroenterol Hepatol. 2009; 24(8): 1347-51. http://dx.doi.org/10.1111/j.1440-1746.2009.05932.x
8. Lee GA, Crawford GW, Liu L, Chen X. *Plants and people from the Early Neolithic to Shang periods in North China.* Proc Natl Acad Sci U S A. 2007; 104(3): 1087-92. http://dx.doi.org/10.1073/pnas.0609763104
9. Greco L. *From the neolithic revolution to gluten intolerance: benefits and problems associated with the cultivation of wheat.* J.Pediatr Gastroenterol Nutr. 1997; 24: S14-6; discussion S16-7. http://dx.doi.org/10.1097/00005176-199700001-00005
10. Lin H, Fan H, Zhang F, Huang X, Lin K, Shi L, et al. *Genetic relationships of ethnic minorities in Southwest China revealed by microsatellite markers.* PloS ONE. 2010; 5(3): e9895. http://www.plosone.org/article/info:doi/10.1371/journal.pone.0009895
11. Xue F, Wang Y, Xu S, Zhang F, Wen B, Wu X, et al. *A spatial analysis of genetic structure of human populations in China reveals distinct difference between maternal and paternal lineages.* European journal of human genetics : EJHG. 2008 Jun; 16(6): 705-17. http://www.nature.com/ejhg/journal/v16/n6/abs/5201998a.html
12. Wu J, Xia B, von Blomberg BM, Zhao C, Yang X,W Crusius J, et al. *Coeliac disease: emerging in China?* Gut. 2010; 59(3): 418-9. http://dx.doi.org/10.1136/gut.2009.197863
13. Wu J, Xia B, von Blomberg BM, Zhao C, Yang XW, Crusius J, et al. *Coeliac disease in China, a field waiting for exploration.* Revista Española de Enfermedades Digestivas. 2010; 102(8): 472. http://dx.doi.org/10.4321/S1130-01082010000800003
14. Yu RB, Hong X, Ding WL, Tan YF, Wu GL. *Polymorphism of the HLA-DQA1 and -DQB1 genes of Han population in Jiangsu Province, China.* Chin Med J (Engl). 2006; 119(22): 1930-3. http://www.cmj.org/Periodical/PDF/2006112040946940.pdf
15. Petronzelli F, Bonamico M, Ferrante P, Grillo R, Mora B, Mariani P, et al. *Genetic contribution of the HLA region to the familial clustering of coeliac disease.* Ann Hum Genet. 1997; 61(Pt 4): 307-17. http://www.ncbi.nlm.nih.gov/pubmed/9365784

16. Forabosco P, Neuhausen SL, Greco L, Naluai AT, Wijmenga C, Saavalainen P, et al. *Meta-analysis of genome-wide linkage studies in celiac disease*. Hum Hered. 2009; 68(4): 223-30. http://dx.doi.org/10.1159/000228920

17. Kumar V, Wijmenga C, Withoff S, editors. *From genome-wide association studies to disease mechanisms: celiac disease as a model for autoimmune diseases*. Seminars in immunopathology; 2012: Jul; 34(4): 567-80.
http://dx.doi.org/10.1007/s00281-012-0312-1
http://www.ncbi.nlm.nih.gov/pubmed/22580835

18. Jones G. *El Primer descubrimiento de América :establecimiento de los vikingos en Islandia, Groenlandia y América.* Traducción José A. Zabalbeascoa (Barcelona, Orbis: 1988)

19. Gruhn R. *The South American Twist: Clovis First Doesn't fit the Rich Prehistory of Southern Continent".* Discovering Archeology. 2000 January / February; 2(1). Scientific American, Inc. N.Y.

20. Chatters JC. Kennewick man. 1996 Copyright © 2004. Smithsonian Institution.
http://www.mnh.si.edu/arctic/html/kennewick_man.html

21. Rohter L. An Ancient Skull Challenges Long-Held Theories. 1999.
http://www.nytimes.com/1999/10/26/science/an-ancient-skull-challenges-long-held-theories.html

22. First Americans Arrived As Two Separate Migrations, According To New Genetic Evidence. Science News 2009.
 http://www.sciencedaily.com/releases/2009/01/090108121618.htm

23. Perego UA, Achilli A, Angerhofer N, Accetturo M, Pala M, Olivieri A, et al. *Distinctive Paleo-Indian migration routes from Beringia marked by two rare mtDNA haplogroups.* Current biology. 2009: Jan 13; 19(1): 1-8. http://eprints.hud.ac.uk/15489/

24. Reich D, Patterson N, Campbell D, et al. *Reconstructing Native American population history.* Nature 2012; 488: 370-4. http://dx.doi.org/10.1038/nature11258

Chapter 4

Celiac Disease in El Salvador

Mauricio Cromeyer[1], Rafael A. Gutiérrez [1], Karla Zaldívar[2], J. Bart A. Crusius[3], Amado Salvador Peña[3]

[1] Hospital de Diagnóstico, Service of Pathology and Gastroenterology, San Salvador, El Salvador.

[2] Asociación de Celíacos y Sensibles al Gluten, San Salvador, El Salvador.

[3] Laboratory of Immunogenetics, Department of Medical Microbiology and Infection Control, VU University Medical Center (VUMC), Amsterdam, The Netherlands.

mcromeyermd@yahoo.com, labguti@navegante.com.sv, celiac_sv@yahoo.com, b.crusius@gmail.com, pena.as@gmail.com

Doi: http://dx.doi.org/10.3926/oms.231

How to cite this chapter

Cromeyer M, Gutiérrez RA, Zaldívar K, Crusius JBA, Peña AS. *Celiac Disease in El Salvador.* In Rodrigo L and Peña AS, editors. *Celiac Disease and Non-Celiac Gluten Sensitivity.* Barcelona, Spain: OmniaScience; 2014. p. 75-88.

M. Cromeyer, R.A. Gutiérrez, K. Zaldívar, J.B.A. Crusius, A.S.Peña

Abstract

Celiac disease is insufficiently known in El Salvador. Between July and August 2012, 32 patients (23F, 9M) with ages between 19 and 77 diagnosed with celiac disease, 21 relatives (13F, 8M) of the celiac patients and 8 persons who were in undergoing the diagnostic process were studied. Genomic DNA was extracted from peripheral blood for HLA-DQA1 and HLA-DQB1 genotyping. Polymerase chain reaction-amplified exon 2 amplicons were generated for low-to-medium resolution typing in a combined, single-stranded conformation polymorphism heteroduplex assay by a semi-automated electrophoresis and gel-staining method on the PhastSystem. The biopsy specimens were revised and classified according to a modified Marsh classification of Oberhüber et al. All participants in this study reside in urban areas.

Of the 32 cases, 23 were celiac disease risk genotype carriers, with the following distribution: 14 HLA-DQ8 (12F and 2M), 7 HLA-DQ2.5 (3F and 4M), 2 HLA-DQ2.5 and DQ8 (1F,1M). A review was made of clinical history of 9 cases (7F, 2M) who were neither DQ2.5 nor DQ8. Three of them had a Marsh II and 4 Marsh IIIA of the modified histological classification. All patients have responded to a gluten-free diet. Of the seven families studied, the daughter of one patient was found to suffer from celiac disease, one daughter of another patient suffered from Sjogrën's syndrome, and the other of rheumatoid arthritis and the sister of another patient has thyroid disease, early menopause and suffered from attacks of migraine. The rest of the first- and second- degree relatives of the seven families have, so far, no clinical evidence of the disease in spite of the fact that 17 have HLA-DQ2.5 and/or DQ8 or DQ9.3/DQ2.2. Therefore, careful follow-up of these individuals is indicated. Eight other subjects mentioned above were not included in the final study because no reliable information could be gathered on their cases.

This is the first study using the modified Marsh classification and the full HLA-DQ tying in El Salvador.

1. Introduction

El Salvador is the smallest country in Central America, with an area of 20,742.66 km^2 and a population of 5,744,113, according to the 2007 census. It has a population density of 276 inhabitants per km^2. This population of which 53% are women and 47% men, is distributed so that 63% lives in urban areas and 37% in rural areas.[1]

In 2012 the budget allocated to the Ministry of Health was equivalent to 11.5% of the state budget[2], reaching 2.1 % of gross domestic product at prices estimated for 2012.[3]

Celiac disease is still a little-known entity in El Salvador, even among health care professionals. This limits the possibility of suspecting celiac disease and therefore also its diagnosis. Cases of confirmed celiac disease come mainly from people diagnosed in domestic and foreign private clinics. Only a few celiac patients are identified in national public health institutions. The tests used in this country for diagnosis focus on serological markers and biopsy since no local laboratories perform genetic analysis of HLA-DQ; the only way to obtain HLA-DQ typing results them is to send samples to laboratories abroad, specifically to the United States of America, which raises costs and reduces the number of people who have access to such tests. Given the widespread ignorance on celiac disease and therefore the lack of guidance, support and monitoring for gluten intolerant people, a group of celiac patients have united to form a self-help organization: "Asociación de Celíacos y Sensibles al Gluten de El Salvador"(ACELYSES) ("Celiac and Gluten Sensitive Association of El Salvador"), whose primary mission is the dissemination of information on gluten-related disorders as well as promoting education and awareness among celiac disease and gluten-sensitive patients, their families, public and private health institutions and other organizations which have an impact on the quality of life of celiac and gluten-sensitive people in El Salvador. ACELYSES facilitates access to and consumption of gluten-free products to people who need a lifelong gluten-free diet to improve their quality of life through actions such as early diagnosis, health services and the continuous quality control and labeling of products.

The early work aimed at creating a support group for patients with celiac disease in El Salvador began in June 2010 and its first public meeting took place on August 31, 2010. Meetings continued to take place monthly under the name "Celíacos de El Salvador" with the support of various health care professionals. On June 18, 2011, one year after taking its first steps, the association appointed its first Board of Directors and changed its name from "Asociación de Celíacos de El Salvador"(ACELES) ("Celiac Association of El Salvador") to "Asociación de Celíacos y Sensibles al Gluten de El Salvador (ACELYSES) ("Celiac and Gluten Sensitive Association of El Salvador").

The association's Advisory Committee is the consultative body which issues recommendations on health to achieve the association's goals; the committee is composed by Dr. Mauricio Cromeyer, Dr. Amado Salvador Peña, Dr. Roberto Zablah as well as Mrs. Gloria Durán de Renderos, a professional in Public Health and Nutrition. More recently, Dr Eduardo Ángel Cueto-Rúa from La Plata, Argentina has joined the Advisory Committee.

People with celiac disease and gluten-sensitivity share the vital goal to adhere to gluten-free diet, which implies a peculiar life style involving the rigorous monitoring of food, drugs, cosmetics and any product that may come into physical contact with the body, which forces the patient to read labels carefully, to consult the manufacturer when the labeling is unclear, to prevent cross-contamination, to promote certification of food and other measures and actions to improve their quality of life; that is why ACELES deemed it positive that gluten sensitive people also join the association. This proposal was consulted with Doctors Peña and Cromeyer, who gave it their endorsement.

2. Diagnosis of Celiac Disease and HLA-DQ Studies in El Salvador

In El Salvador intestinal biopsy is the gold standard regarding the diagnosis of celiac disease. Despite this, it is noteworthy, however, that although endoscopies are performed in public and private clinics and hospitals, only those doctors who have adequate knowledge of celiac disease apply the procedure for the proper sampling needed for their subsequent study and, unfortunately not all pathologists have the interest and knowledge to make an accurate diagnosis. It is not surprising that the patient is often misdiagnosed with other disorders and the diagnosis celiac disease remains hidden.

3. Intestinal biopsy Classification

In the present study the biopsy specimens were reviewed by one of us (R.A.G.) with special interest in the histopathology of celiac disease using the Marsh classification described in 1992[4] and modified in 1999 by Oberhüber, Granditsch and Vogelsang.[5]

4. Serological tests

The majority of the patients had as serological test, anti-Tissue Transglutaminase IgA ELISA, of DRG Diagnostics GmbH, Germany according to the instructions of the manufacturer and performed at the *Laboratorios Clínicos Max Bloch* in Colonia Escalón, San Salvador, El Salvador C.A. Few patients were tested abroad.

5. HLA-DQ Typing

Currently, there are few cases in which the patients had been genotyped outside of El Salvador. There is no information on the distribution of HLA-DQ genotypes in the Salvadoran population.

Between July and August 2012, the Laboratory of Immunogenetics at the Department of Microbiology and Infection Control of the VU University Medical Center, Amsterdam, provided an opportunity for a group of 69 Salvadoran patients with celiac disease and their relatives, as well as others, who were undergoing the process of being diagnosed for celiac disease, to also undergo genetic testing for HLA-DQ. The blood samples were taken at a local diagnostic laboratory, where they were packaged in accordance with the standards required to ensure their optimal preservation, transportation and receipt at their final destination. The typing process consisted of the extraction of genomic DNA from peripheral blood. For the HLA-DQA1* and DQB1* genotyping the method used was generating exons 2 amplicons by polymerase chain reaction for low- to medium- resolution typing in a combined, single-stranded conformation polymorphism heteroduplex assay by semiautomated electrophoresis and gel staining method on the PhastSystem (GE Healthcare/Amersham Pharmacia Biotech, Uppsala, Sweden). This method has been validated using a panel of reference DNA against DynallAllSet sequence specific primer high resolution typing kits (Dynal AS, Oslo, Norway).[6,7] The persons studied received full information about the study and gave oral consent to their physicians. Subjects who were recruited from ACELYSES informed their physicians and those who accepted signed informed consent forms afterwards. In the case of children younger than 18 years of age, consent was granted in writing by their parents/legal guardians.

6. Results

Table 1 shows 32 individuals diagnosed with celiac disease. The age at diagnosis ranges from 19 to 77 years; 23 are women and 9 are men, all are urban residents. Upon revision of the biopsy specimens and classification of the histological features, 28 showed the histological features that are compatible with celiac disease.

Of the 32 cases, 23 were celiac disease risk genotype carriers, with the following distribution: 14 HLA-DQ8 (DQA1*03/DQB1*0302; 12F and 2M), 7 HLA-DQ2.5 (DQA1*05/DQB1*02; 3F and 4M), 2 HLA-DQ2.5 and DQ8 (1F, 1M), and 9 cases (7F, 2M) who had neither DQ2.5 nor DQ8.

All nine non-DQ2.5/non-DQ8 cases reported an improvement of symptoms with a gluten-free diet (GFD); two had been diagnosed abroad. The clinical characteristics, the histological classification and the results of the HLA-DQ typing are summarized in Table 2. Seven out of nine non-DQ2.5/non-DQ8 celiac disease patients were heterozygous carriers of allele DQA1*05 only (No. 3, 14, 16, 20, 21, 27, 29) and one had HLA-DQ2.2 (DQA1*0201/DQB1*02) only (No. 13) and another (No. 19) did not possess an HLA-DQ genotype associated with celiac disease. Of note, one patient (No.20) also has dermatitis herpetiformis.[8]

#	Gender	Age	a-TTG	Biopsy	HLA-DQA1* genotype	HLA-DQB1* genotype	DQ2.5 and/or DQ8
1	F	19	P	Marsh IIIb	03/05	02/0302	DQ2.5 and DQ8 Heterozygous
2	F	21	P	Marsh II	03/03	0302/0402	DQ8 Heterozygous
3	F	21	P	Marsh IIIa	03/05	0301/0402	non DQ2.5 non DQ8
4	F	35	P	Marsh IIIa	03/03	0302/0302	DQ8 Homozygous
5	F	43	P	Marsh IIIb	05/05	02/0301	DQ2.5 Heterozygous
6	F	44	P	Marsh IIIa	03/05	0301/0302	DQ8 Heterozygous
7	F	44	P	Marsh IIIa	0102/03	0302/0604	DQ8 Heterozygous
8	F	45	P	NT	0102/03	0302/0602 or 0603	DQ8 Heterozygous
9	F	46	P	Marsh II	0102/03	0302/0604	DQ8 Heterozygous
10	F	48	P	Marsh IIIa	05/05	02/02	DQ2.5 Homozygous
11	F	51	NT	Marsh IIIb	03/03	0302/0302	DQ8 Homozygous
12	F	53	P	Marsh IIIa	0101 or 0102/0201	02/0501	non DQ2.5 non DQ8
13	F	54	NT	Marsh IIIb	0101/03	0302/0503	DQ8 Heterozygous
14	F	55	P	Marsh IIIa	0101 or 0102/05	0301/0602 or 0603	non DQ2.5 non DQ8
15	F	56	NT	Marsh IIIa	03/05	0301/0302	DQ8 Heterozygous
16	F	57	P	NA	0101 or 0102/05	0301/0501	non DQ2.5 non DQ8
17	F	60	P	Marsh IIIa	05/05	02/02	DQ2.5 Homozygous
18	F	61	P	Marsh IIIa	03/03	0302/0302	DQ8 Homozygous
19	F	63	P	Marsh II	0101/0103	0503/0602 or 0603	non DQ2.5 non DQ8
20	F	65	P	NA	0101 or 0102/05	0301/0502	non DQ2.5 non DQ8
21	F	66	P	Marsh II	0401 or 0601/05	0301/0402	non DQ2.5 non DQ8
22	F	75	P	Marsh IIIa	03/03	0302/0302	DQ8 Homozygous
23	F	77	P	Marsh II	03/03	0302/0302	DQ8 Homozygous
24	M	22	P	Marsh IIIb	0101 or 0102/05	02/0501	DQ2.5 Heterozygous
25	M	24	P	Marsh IIIa	0103/05	02/0602 or 0603	DQ2.5 Heterozygous
26	M	25	P	Marsh IIIb	03/05	02/0302	DQ2.5 and DQ8 Heterozygous
27	M	44	P	Marsh II	0101 or 0102/05	0301/0501	non DQ2.5 and non DQ8
28	M	47	P	Marsh IIIa	0101 or 0102/05	02/0501	DQ2.5 Heterozygous
29	M	50	P	Marsh IIIa	0103/05	0301/0601	non DQ2.5 and non DQ8
30	M	54	P	NT	0102/03	0302/0602 or 0603	DQ8 Heterozygous
31	M	64	P	Marsh IIIb	0102/03	0302/0602 or 0603	DQ8 Heterozygous
32	M	65	P	Marsh IIIa	0201/05	02/0301	DQ2.5 Heterozygous

Abbreviations: F=Female; M=Male; aTTG=anti-tissue transglutaminase; P=Positive; NT=Not Tested; NA=Not Available

Table 1. Patients with celiac disease, gender, age at diagnosis, serological, histological and HLA-DQ results.

#	Gender	Age in years	PCC	a-TTG	Biopsy	GFD	HLA-DQA1* genotype	HLA-DQB1* genotype
3	F	21	Chronic diarrhea, bloating	P	Marsh IIIa	R	03/05	0301/0402
13	F	52	Chronic diarrhea, depression	P	Marsh IIIa	R	0101 or 0102/0201	02/0501
14	F	55	Chronic diarrhea, lactose intolerance	P	Marsh IIIa	R	0101 or 0102/05	0301/0602 or 0603
16	F	57	Chronic diarrhea	P	NA	R	0101 or 0102/05	03/0501
19	F	63	Alternating evacuation	P	Marsh II	R	0101/0103	0503/0602 or 0603
20	F	66	Chronic diarrhea Dermatitis herpetiformis	P	Marsh II	R	0101 or 0102/05	0301/0502
21	F	66	Chronic diarrhea	P	NA*	R	0401 or 0601/05	0301/0402
27	M	44	Alternating evacuation	P	Marsh II	R	0101 or 0102/05	03/0501
29	M	50	Chronic diarrhea	P	Marsh IIIa	R	0103/05	0301/0601

Abbreviations: GFD=Gluten-free diet; R= Responding to diet. F= Female; M=Male; PCC= Predominant clinical conditions; aTTG=anti-tissue transglutaminase; P=Positive; *Not available for revision. Biopsy specimen originally characterized as compatible with celiac disease

Table 2. Clinical characteristics and HLA-DQ genotype of non-DQ2.5/non-DQ8 celiac disease patients.

Out of 23 HLA-DQ2.5 and/or DQ8 genotype carriers, direct access to complete medical records of 15 patients (9 women and 6 men) was obtained. The symptomatology is variable, with mild to moderate manifestations. The pattern of alternating evacuation, bloating and/or flatulence comprises 2/3 of the cases. In other cases the predominant symptoms are: 3 with chronic diarrhea and 2 with constipation.

Other conditions associated in the group are: 3 women diagnosed with osteopenia or osteoporosis,[9,10] 2 women with anemia, a man with chronic myelocytic leukemia (CML); another woman has moderate elevation of AST-ALT. One case with a lack of clinical records, reported suffering from autoimmune hepatitis[11], was excluded due to incomplete data and normal intestinal biopsy specimens. Another patient had antecedents of spontaneous abortion.

Distribution of HLA-DQ2.5 and/or HLA-DQ8 positives in homo- or heterozygotes is displayed in Table 3.

Risk Alleles	Homozygotes		Heterozygotes		Total
	(F)	(M)	(F)	(M)	
HLA-DQ2.5	2	0	1	4	7
HLA-DQ8	5	0	7	2	14
HLA-DQ2.5 and HLA-DQ8	0	0	1	1	2
Total	7	0	9	7	23

Table 3. Distribution of HLA-DQ2.5 and/or HLA-DQ8 positive patients with celiac disease in homo- or heterozygotes.

7. Family Study

Seven patients with confirmed celiac disease expressed the wish to type some of their relatives. Some of these relatives had symptoms compatible with celiac disease but so far only the daughter of one patient was found to suffer from the disease (Table 4). Seventeen out of 21 relatives are carriers of DQ2.5 and/or DQ8 risk alleles. Careful follow-up of these relatives is indicated.

Group No.	Relation	Age in years	Gender	aTTG	Biopsy	HLA-DQA1* genotype	HLA-DQB1* genotype	DQ2.5 and/or DQ8
1	patient	61	F	P	Marsh IIIa	05/05	02/02	HLA-DQ2.5 homozygous
	daughter	39	F	N	NT	0201/05	02/02	HLA-DQ2.5 heterozygous
	granddaughter	17	F	NT	NT	0103/0201	02/0601	Non-DQ2.5 and non-DQ8
	grandson	13	M	NT	NT	0103/0201	02/0601	Non-DQ2.5 and non-DQ8
	son	37	M	N	NT	0101 or 0102/05	02/0501	HLA-DQ2.5 heterozygous
	daughter	34	F	N	NT	0201/05	02/02	HLA-DQ2.5 heterozygous
	granddaughter	11	F	NT	NT	0101 or 0102/05	02/0602 or 0603	HLA-DQ2.5 heterozygous
	grandson	4	M	NT	NT	0201/05	02/0301	HLA-DQ2.5 heterozygous
2	patient	44	F	P	Marsh IIIa	03/05	0301/0302	HLA-DQ8 heterozygous
	father	67	M	NT	NT	03/0401 or 0601	0302/0402	HLA-DQ8 heterozygous
	mother	66	F	N	NT	0101 or 0102/05	0301/0501	Non-DQ2.5 and non-DQ8
	sister	39	F	N	NT	03/05	0301/0302	HLA-DQ8 heterozygous
3	patient	22	M	P	Marsh IIIb	0101 or 0102/05	02/0501	HLA-DQ2.5 heterozygous
	father	53	M	NT	NT	0101 or 0102/05	02/0502	HLA-DQ2.5 heterozygous
	mother	50	F	NT	NT	0101/0103	0501/0602 or 0603	Non-DQ2.5 and non-DQ8
	sister	20	F	NT	NT	0101 or 0102/05	02/0501	HLA-DQ2.5 heterozygous
4	patient	65	F	NA	NA	03/05	02/0303	HLA-DQ2.5 heterozygous (DQ9.3)
	daughter	30	F	NT	NT	0201/05	02/02	HLA-DQ2.5 heterozygous
	son	38	M	NT	NT	0201/03	02/0303	Non-DQ2.5 and non-DQ8 (DQ9.3)

Group No.	Relation	Age in years	Gender	aTTG	Biopsy	HLA-DQA1* genotype	HLA-DQB1* genotype	DQ2.5 and/or DQ8
5	patient	51	F	NT	Marsh II	03/03	0302/0302	HLA-DQ8 homozygous
	daughter	25	F	NT	NT	03/05	02/0302	DQ2.5 and DQ8 heterozygous
6	patient	46	F	P	Marsh II	0102/03	0302/0604	HLA-DQ8 heterozygous
	mother	83	F	NT	NT	0102/03	0302/0602 or 0603	HLA-DQ8 heterozygous
	sister	52	F	N	NT	0102/03	0302/0602 or 0603	HLA-DQ8 heterozygous
	son	14	M	N	NT	0102/03	0302/0604	HLA-DQ8 heterozygous
	son	10	M	N	NT	03/05	0301/0302	HLA-DQ8 heterozygous
7	patient	65	M	P	Marsh IIIa	0201/05	02/0301	HLA-DQ2.5 heterozygous
	daughter	34	F	P	Marsh IIIb	0201/05	02/02	HLA-DQ2.5 heterozygous

Abbreviations: F, Female; M, Male; aTTG, anti-tissue transglutaminase; P, Positive; NT, Not Tested. *NA= this patient was later withdrawn for lack of information

Table 4. Clinical characteristics of patients with celiac disease and family members and HLA-DQ genotype.

In the case of family group No. 1, two of its members who were not diagnosed as celiacs had other autoimmune diseases such as rheumatoid arthritis and Sjögren's syndrome. In this table it can be seen that the male patient of group 7 most likely carries the haplotypes DQA1*05-DQB1*0301 and DQA1*0201-DQB1*02 (ie. DQ2.5 trans) and therefore passed DQA1*0201-DQB1*02 (DQ2.2) to his daughter and that the mother of the daughter contributed HLA-DQA1*05-DQB1*02 (ie. DQ2.5).

8. Demographic Characterization of the Studied Cases

Ethnic admixture is characteristic of El Salvador; several factors influenced this outcome: a) in El Salvador's current territory there was no place where indigenous peoples could find refuge, so that they and the Spaniards had to coexist in the same space; b) a decrease in the indigenous population due to diseases and massacres; c) population break up due to its exploitation for the cultivation of indigo in the XVIIIth and XIXth centuries.[12] In the ethnic categories identified in colonial times, the predominance of *mestizos* (people of mixed native and European heritage) is evidenced in Tables 5 and 6.

Categories	Number	%
Native Americans	79,652	60.30
Mestizos	46,232	35.00
Peninsular Spaniards	1,321	1.00
American-born Spaniards	3,038	2.30
Sub-saharian African or mixed sub-saharian African and Caucasoid ancestry	1,849	1.40
Total	132,092	100

Source: Rivas, R. Persistencia Indígena en El Salvador, (p.31) Universidad Don Bosco. http://old.udb.edu.sv/editorial/científica/científica5/articulo2.pdf

Table 5. Population of the province of San Salvador, by ethnic group (1770).

Categories	Number	%
Native Americans	71,175	43.06
Mestizos	87,722	53.08
Peninsular Spaniards	1,422	0.86
American-born Spaniards	3,307	2.00
Sub-saharian African or mixed sub-saharian African and Caucasoid ancestry	1,652	1.00
Total	165,278	100.00

Source: Rivas, R. Persistencia Indígena en El Salvador, (p.31) Universidad Don Bosco. http://old.udb.edu.sv/editorial/científica/científica5/articulo2.pdf

Table 6. Population of the province of San Salvador, by ethnic group (1807, excluding Sonsonate and Ahuachapán).

The people who participated in the study are mostly of mixed native/European heritage which is predominant; thus, the results, albeit limited in number, are a representative sample of the ethnicity of El Salvador.

Population in the year 2007 is distributed according to the ethnic groups presented in Table 7.

Ethnic group	%
Caucasoid	12.74
Mestizos	86.34
Sub-saharian African	0.13
Others	0.56
Native Americans:	
Lenca	0.04
Kakawira	0.07
Nahua-pipil	0.06
Other	0.06
Total	100

Source: Dirección General de Estadística y Censos, Tomo I Características Generales de la Población. VI Censo de Población y V de Vivienda 2007, (p. 48). Ministerio de Economía, El Salvador. http://www.digestyc.gob.sv/index.php/temas/des/poblacion-y-estadisticas-demograficas/censo-de-poblacion-y-vivienda/publicaciones-censos.html

Table 7. Percentual Distribution of the population, by ethnic group.

According to the *Dirección General de Estadística y Censos de El Salvador* ("National Statistics and Census Directorate", DIGESTYC) in 2007 more men than women were born but there is also a higher mortality rate among men than women, as a result, there is a balance of population. However, census data show that there are additional factors operating, such as a higher percentage of men migrating abroad than women, leading to an increase in the female population (53%) compared to male (47%).[13] Despite this correlation, of the 23 confirmed HLA-DQ positive patients, 19 were women, which is consistent with the published literature.

In El Salvador the projected life expectancy for the 2010-2015 periods is of 67.45 years for men and 76.86 years for women.[14] This study shows that the age at which people are diagnosed with celiac disease is above 40, the category of people over 60 years prevails.

9. Celiac Disease in El Salvador

Despite not having prevalence studies in El Salvador, it can be stated that celiac disease is present in this country and that it may be considered to be a missed diagnosis due to lack of knowledge and the stubbornly held outdated concept of it not being a prevalent disease in the Americas.

The genetic predisposition of celiac disease is widely known and it is also known that, although it is a complex polygenic condition, approximately 95% of the patients that have the risk alleles that make up the HLA-DQ2.5, HLA-DQ8 or HLA-DQ9.3 heterodimers[15,16] and, furthermore, those celiac patients who are negative also have at least one risk allele (HLA-DQ2.2 or HLA-DQA1*05), being rare those in which these alleles are absent.[17,18]

Studies in Europe showed that the predominant heterodimer in celiac disease is HLA-DQ2.5: 83.8 % in Italy and France,[19] 91 % in Finland, 91.4 % in Norway and Sweden, 87.7 % in the UK and 92% in Spain.[20] A study from Argentina showed that 95% of celiac patients were HLA-DQ2.5 positive[21] and a Cuban study reported an 86.3% proportion.[22] There is no information on other genetic studies in the general population of the Caribbean or Central America, except for one from Costa Rica.[23]

The results obtained in patients with celiac disease from El Salvador differ from data from other regions of the Americas such as in the Chilean population.[24]

It must be remembered that in Latin America, populations with different origins came in contact with each other and became intertwined: natives and individuals from various regions of Europe and Africa. In El Salvador individuals of African ancestry are very few in number, unlike other Central American, Caribbean or some southern countries of the American continent (Colombia, Venezuela, Brazil, etc.), thus explaining the regional variability of the population of African origin.

In the southernmost countries of South America, predominantly in Uruguay and Argentina, the urban population is primarily descended from Europeans; from 65% in Mar del Plata to 90% in Montevideo,[25] this being representative of the high penetration of Caucasoid European genes. This ratio is different in other regions such as Bolivia, Peru, Chile, Mexico and Central America, whose genetic bases stem from the characteristics of their colonization process and the mixture between European and Native American genes, each of which had their own regional variables according to the origin of its European colonizers (Spaniards, Italians, Portuguese, etc.), as well as from the different social classes that arose, leading to a further opening up of the field of genetic epidemiology.

10. Conclusions

Celiac disease can be diagnosed at any age; however, in the study group it can be seen that most of the people studied are over 40.

It advisable to perform prevalence studies in El Salvador in order to have a more precise knowledge of the country's situation regarding celiac disease and non-celiac gluten sensitivity, which in turn may lead to the promotion of health policies, programs and plans to ensure timely diagnosis and the comprehensive care of celiac and gluten-sensitive patients as well as the taking of measures to facilitate access to gluten-free products.

As demonstrated by the experiences of countries like Spain, Argentina and the United Kingdom, ACELYSES, a vital support entity, is important as a source of much needed information and support to celiac and gluten-sensitive people in El Salvador.

The creation of cooperation of networks, including communities of practice, are a viable form of effort with high potential benefits for both physicians and scientists interested in celiac disease as well as for celiac patients. This first study of HLA-DQ typing in celiac Salvadorans is an incipient test of collaborative work. It stimulated the authors to critically review their diagnostic resources in El Salvador and to revise the histological classification according to the Marsh classification.

References

1. Dirección General de Estadística y Censos (DIGESTYC). Ministerio de Economía, El Salvador, *VI Censo de Población y V de Vivienda, 2007*.
2. División de Integración y Análisis Global, Dirección General del Presupuesto, Ministerio de Hacienda, El Salvador. *Guía del Presupuesto General del Estado para el Ciudadano. Ejercicio Fiscal 2012*.
   http://www.transparenciafiscal.gob.sv/portal/page/portal/PTF/Presupuestos_Publicos/ Guias_del_presupuesto_para_el_ciudadano/Guia_del_Presupuesto_para_el_Ciudadano _2012.pdf
3. Dirección General del Presupuesto, Ministerio de Hacienda, El Salvador. *Mensaje del Proyecto de Presupuesto 2012*.
   http://www.transparenciafiscal.gob.sv/portal/page/portal/PTF/Presupuestos_Publicos/ Presupuestos_votados/Anio2012/Mensaje_2012.pdf
4. Marsh MN. *Gluten, major histocompatibility complex, and the small intestine. A molecular and immunobiologic approach to the spectrum of gluten sensitivity ('celiac sprue')*. Gastroenterology. 1992; 102: 330-54.
5. Oberhüber G, Granditsch G, Vogelsang H. *The histopathology of coeliac disease: time for a standardized report scheme for pathologists*. Eur J Gastroenterol Hepatol. 1999; 11: 1185-94. http://dx.doi.org/10.1097/00042737-199910000-00019
6. Crusius JBA. *The immunogenetcs of chronic infammatory and autoimmune disease [PhD dissertaton]*. Amsterdam, the Netherlands, ISBN 90-9016411-1. VU; 2002.
7. Hadithi M, von Blomberg BME, Crusius JBA, Bloemena E, Kostense PJ, Meijer JW et al. *Accuracy of serologic tests and HLA-DQ typing for diagnosing celiac disease*. Ann Intern Med. 2007; 147: 294-302. http://dx.doi.org/10.1136/gut.25.2.151
8. Gawkrodger DJ, Blackwell JN, Gilmour HM, Rifkind EA, Heading RC, Barnetson RS. *Dermatitis herpetiformis: diagnosis, diet and demography*. Gut. 1984; 25: 151-7. PubMed PMID: 6693042. Pubmed Central PMCID: 1432259.
9. Ludvigsson JF, Michaelsson K, Ekbom A, Montgomery SM. *Coeliac disease and the risk of fractures – a general population-based cohort study*. Aliment Pharmacol & Ther. 2007; 25: 273-85. PubMed PMID: 17269989.
   http://dx.doi.org/10.1111/j.1365-2036.2006.03203.x
10. Buchman AL. *Population-based screening for celiac disease: improvement in morbidity and mortality from osteoporosis?* Arch Intern Med. 2005; 165: 370-2. PubMed PMID: 15738364. http://dx.doi.org/10.1001/archinte.165.4.370
11. Rashtak S, Marietta EV, Murray JA. *Celiac sprue: a unique autoimmune disorder*. Expert review of clinical immunology. 2009; 5: 593-604. PubMed PMID: 20477645. Pubmed Central PMCID: 3228242. http://dx.doi.org/10.1586/eci.09.30
12. Rivas, R. *Persistencia Indígena en El Salvador*. Universidad Don Bosco. http://old.udb.edu.sv/editorial/cientifica/cientifica5/articulo2.pdf
13. Dirección General de Estadística y Censos. *Tomo I Características Generales de la Población. VI Censo de Población y V de Vivienda 2007*. Ministerio de Economía, El Salvador. http://www.digestyc.gob.sv/index.php/temas/des/poblacion-y-estadisticas-demograficas/censo-de-poblacion-y-vivienda/publicaciones-censos.html
14. Ministerio de Economía, Dirección General de Estadística y Censos – DIGESTYC, Fondo de Población de las Naciones Unidas – UNFPA, Centro Latinoamericano y Caribeño de

Demografía – CELADE, *Estimaciones y Proyecciones Nacionales de Población 1950-2050*, Mayo 2010, El Salvador.

15. Wolters VM, Wijmenga C. *Genetic background of celiac disease and its clinical implications.* Amer J Gastroenterol. 2008; 103: 190-5. PubMed PMID: 18184122. http://dx.doi.org/10.1111/j.1572-0241.2007.01471.x

16. Bodd M, Tollefsen S, Bergseng E, Lundin KEA, Sollid LM. *Evidence that HLA-DQ9 confers risk to Celiac Disease by presence of DQ9-restricted gluten-specific T cells.* Hum Immunol. 2012; 73: 376-81. http://dx.doi.org/10.1016/j.humimm.2012.01.016

17. Polvi AS, Arranz E, Fernandez-Arquero M, Collin P, Maki M, Sanz A, et al. *HLA-DQ2-negative celiac disease in Finland and Spain.* Hum Immunol. 1998; 59: 169-75. http://dx.doi.org/10.1016/S0198-8859(98)00008-1

18. Louka AS, Sollid LM. *HLA in coeliac disease: unravelling the complex genetics of a complex disorder.* Tissue Antigens. 2003; 61: 105-17. PubMed PMID: 12694579. http://dx.doi.org/10.1034/j.1399-0039.2003.00017.x

19. Karell K, Louka AS, Moodie SJ, Ascher H, Clot F, Greco L et al. *HLA types in celiac disease patients not carrying the DQA1*05-DQB1*02 (DQ2) heterodimer: results from the European Genetics Cluster on Celiac Disease.* Hum Immunol. 2003; 64: 469-77. PubMed PMID: 12651074. http://dx.doi.org/10.1016/S0198-8859(03)00027-2

20. Arranz E, Telleria JJ, Sanz A, Martin JF, Alonso M, Calvo C et al. *HLA-DQA1*0501 and DQB1*02 homozygosity and disease susceptibility in Spanish coeliac patients.* Exp Clin Immunogen. 1997; 14: 286-90. PubMed PMID: 9523165.

21. Herrera M, Theiler G, Augustovski F, Chertkoff L, Fainboim L, DeRosa S et al. *Molecular characterization of HLA class II genes in celiac disease patients of Latin American Caucasian origin.* Tissue Antigens. 1994; 43: 83-7. PubMed PMID: 8016846. http://dx.doi.org/10.1111/j.1399-0039.1994.tb02305.x

22. Cintado A, Sorell L, Galvan JA, Martinez L, Castaneda C, Fragoso T et al. *HLA DQA1*0501 and DQB1*02 in Cuban celiac patients.* Hum Immunol. 2006; 67: 639-42. PubMed PMID: 16916661. http://dx.doi.org/10.1016/j.humimm.2006.04.009

23. Arrieta-Bolanos E, Maldonado-Torres H, Dimitriu O, Hoddinott MA, Fowles F, Shah A et al. *HLA-A, -B, -C, -DQB1, and -DRB1,3,4,5 allele and haplotype frequencies in the Costa Rica Central Valley Population and its relationship to worldwide populations.* Hum Immunol. 2011; 72: 80-6. PubMed PMID: 20937338. http://dx.doi.org/10.1016/j.humimm.2010.10.005

24. Araya M, Mondragon A, Perez-Bravo F, Roessler JL, Alarcon T, Rios G et al. *Celiac disease in a Chilean population carrying Amerindian traits.* J Ped Gastroenterol and Nutr. 2000; 31: 381-6. PubMed PMID: 11045834. http://dx.doi.org/10.1097/00005176-200010000-00010

25. Poggio Favotto R, Mimbacas A et al. *Alelos HLA DQB1 y DRB1 Asociados con la Enfermedad Celíaca en pacientes hospitalarios.* Rev Med. Uruguay; 2001; 17: 107-11.

Chapter 5

Other Dietary Proteins besides Gluten could Affect some Celiac Patients

A.M. Calderón de la Barca[1], F. Cabrera-Chávez[2]

[1]Department of Nutrition, Research Center for Food and Development (CIAD; A.C.) km 0.6 to Victoria, Hermosillo 83000, Sonora, Mexico.

[2]Nutrition Sciences and Gastronomy Unit. University of Sinaloa. Culiacán, Sinaloa, Mexico.

amc@ciad.mx, fcabrera@uas.edu.mx

Doi: http://dx.doi.org/10.3926/oms.212

How to cite this chapter

Calderón de la Barca AM, Cabrera-Chávez F. *Other Dietary Proteins besides Gluten could Affect some Celiac Patients.* In Rodrigo L and Peña AS, editors. *Celiac Disease and Non-Celiac Gluten Sensitivity.* Barcelona, Spain: OmniaScience; 2014. p. 89-101.

Abstract

Some patients with celiac disease do not improve even after following a gluten-free diet upon diagnosis; therefore, nutritionists and physicians might conclude that this is due to the fact that their dietary recommendations were not strictly obeyed. However, in some cases, this is because these patients suffer from refractory celiac disease; dietary treatment is not the solution for these cases. Some of the cases considered to be refractory improve if, besides gluten, other dietary proteins, such as prolamins from oats (avenins) or maize (zeins) and sometimes, caseins from bovine milk, are withdrawn. Although there are very few published papers about such cases, there are clinical and practical facts, as well as published *in vitro* and *in silico* experiments, supporting the idea that other proteins induce an immune response similar to that provoked by gluten in celiac patients. In this chapter, the clinical evidence of these special celiac disease cases is discussed, as well as the information about experimental models and their possible relationship to an immune response against dietary protein antigens other than wheat gluten.

1. Introduction

By definition, celiac disease (CD) is an immunologically mediated systemic disorder, induced by gluten (the wheat protein fraction insoluble in water) and related prolamins (alcohol-soluble protein fraction from any cereal) in genetically predisposed individuals.[1] Thus considered, prolamins from oats or maize, which could affect some celiac patients, would not be excluded from this definition, even though they are not usually considered "related prolamins". Those that are recognized as such, rye and barley, are taxonomically closer to wheat since they belong to the same group and subgroup, while oats and maize belong to the same family and subfamily to which wheat belongs.[2] What seems far stranger is that bovine milk caseins may exacerbate CD.

The issue here is that some CD patients continue experiencing symptoms and signs typical of the disease even after removing gluten from their diet, although effective adherence to this diet fails between 9 and 58% of the cases.[3-5] Another cause which may keep the disease active may be that celiac patients ingest gluten inadvertently. This is because the "gluten-free" or "no gluten" labels which indicate a maximum level of 20 ppm[6] are not always truthful. In fact, nearly half of the cases that do not respond to a gluten-free diet are due to the ingestion of improperly labeled foods[7] and one quarter of these patients are not aware of what they consume.[3] Although some of the symptoms improve with a reduced gluten intake, if its suppression is not strict, there is damage to the intestinal mucosa.

When symptoms of CD remain despite a strict adherence to the gluten-free diet, it could be due to other non-immune causes such as exocrine pancreatic insufficiency or intestinal bacterial overgrowth. Similarly, intolerance to fructose and lactose, resulting from damage to the intestinal mucosa while CD was active, can induce some of the symptoms of the disease.[8]

However, there are real CD cases in which there is no response to the gluten-free diet. Due to this, various studies and practical experiences lead to consider the possibility that other proteins, in addition to wheat, barley and rye, increase the CD immune response. Thus, it is clear that there are aspects of CD which have not been sufficiently studied. For instance, "Non-celiac gluten hypersensitivity"[9] is a new entity, and unresponsive CD or refractory celiac disease, has only recently been characterized. Both entities are two different health problems.

Refractory CD is defined by persistent or recurrent malabsorption symptoms and the presence of intestinal villous atrophy despite having followed strict gluten-free diet for 6-12 months.[10] Although there is no epidemiological data, it is considered that 5-10% of celiac patients do not recover through the gluten-free diet (GFD).[3] Patients with Type 1 refractory CD do not respond to the gluten-free diet, but their intraepithelial lymphocytes are normal. Type 2 is characterized by the presence of abnormal intraepithelial lymphocyte clones, which do not express CD3 and CD8 T-cell receptor markers, but express instead intracellular CD3; it is associated with a poor prognosis since it could evolve into a T-cell intestinal lymphoma.[11] Thus, continuous monitoring of both the immunophenotype as well as of lymphocytes clonality is recommended in these cases.[10]

In refractory CD, especially in Type 1, we should consider the possible influence of other dietary proteins besides gluten. The question is not whether there is a closely-related taxonomy, because this presumes a high prolamin homology with those from gluten, but to what extent they share the same immunogenic peptide sequences. This is the key to CD pathogenesis.

CD is triggered in genetically predisposed individuals, due to the properties of the gluten proteins which contain 15% proline and 35% glutamine. Proline, due to its cyclic structure, prevents intestinal proteolytic enzymes from breaking the peptide bond which forms it. Thus, some peptides comprising 10 to 50 amino acid residues with high immunogenic potential still remain and are able to cross the damaged intestinal barrier into the intestinal lamina propria. The lateral amino groups of the glutamines are removed by tissue transglutaminase, producing negatively charged peptides. The new-formed charged sequences (neoepitopes) have an increased affinity for class II human leukocyte antigens (HLA), specifically HLA-DQ2 and DQ8 in antigen-presenting cells. These cells present the neoepitopes to T cells which activate and proliferate to produce pro-inflammatory cytokines and stimulate to B cells to produce antibodies against gluten and the body's own tissular transglutaminase.[12]

Thus, any dietary protein which, once digested by the gastrointestinal tract, produces peptides with sequences and/or loads similarly arranged to those of gluten peptides could exacerbate an already developed CD. This chapter discusses some CD cases as well as complementary experiments dealing with a possible reaction to dietary proteins other than those of wheat.

2. Response to Proteins Generally Regarded as Safe

The persistence of symptoms in CD despite the gluten-free diet should lead to look for other causes of malabsorption. Among these, the most common is intolerance to food proteins other than gluten.[13] It would be interesting to test whether these proteins exacerbate a CD case which was previously triggered by gluten proteins or if they were the primary instigators.

Table 1 summarizes a series of tests with antibodies, cells or cell lines from CD patients, case reports, dietary and food protein contact challenges and *in silico* studies. These, along with some clinical experiences, have in common the analysis of the effects on CD of dietary protein different to prolamins from wheat, barley and rye. Overall, in refereed publications, three types of dietary proteins have been tested, generally unrecognized, which are suspected to have some effect on this disease: prolamins from oats (avenines) and maize (zeins), as well as bovine caseins.

Protein	Test performed	Outcome	Reference
Oat Proteins	Stimulus of lysosomal and K562 cells.	Positive response of lysosomal cells and agglutination of K562 cells as indicators of cytotoxic activity.	Silano et al.[14]
	Proliferation and activation of lymphocytes from CD patients.	Proteins from three oat varieties with proliferative and stimulant capacity of mononuclear peripheral blood cells, releasing IFN-γ.	Silano et al.[15]
	Two-year follow-up of CD children cases.	The children (4/9) exhibited symptoms due to oat ingestion. Oat peptides were identified in a HLA-DQ2 context.	Arentz-Hansen et al.[20]
Maize Proteins	Case report. Recording of symptoms and markers under maize stimulus.	No response to gluten removal but positive to maize in an oral challenge (double blind test, using maize and rice). CD remission on a gluten-free and maize-free diet.	Accomando et al.[13]
	Reactivity of anti-maize proteins' antibodies.	The competitive ELISA demonstrated that CD patient antibodies were specific for maize proteins; there was no cross-reactivity.	Skerritt et al.[28]
	Reactivity of CD patients' IgA and *in silico* analysis.	Positive titers of 5/24 CD patients for IgA anti-maize prolamins. Digested peptides with potentially immunogenic sequences were identified *in silico* for recognition and binding to HLA-DQ2/DQ8.	Cabrera-Chávez et al.[33]
	T-cell response.	IFN-γ production by intestinal cell line of 1/7 CD patients after stimulation using maize prolamins.	Bergamo et al.[32]
	Rectal mucosa challenge using maize prolamins and inflammation analysis.	CD patients (6/13) developed inflammatory reaction signs (nitric oxide production and granulocyte markers).	Kristjansson et al.[27]
	In silico analysis.	Presentation of peptide sequences from different maize proteins with homology to toxic wheat peptides.	Darewickz et al.[24]
Bovine caseins	Rectal mucosa challenge using bovine caseins and inflammation analysis.	Caseins induced an inflammatory response similar to that induced by gluten in CD patients in remission (nitric oxide, myeloperoxidase and eosinophil cationic protein production).	Kristjansson et al. [43]
	IgA reactivity of 150 CD patients (ELISA).	Inmunoreactivity was of 39% to hydrolyzed caseins, considering 100% inmunoreactivity to wheat gliadins.	Berti et al.[38]
	Identification of reactive proteins by IgA from CD patients.	IgA antibodies from some CD patients (9/14) recognize bovine but not human caseins by ELISA and immune-blotting.	Cabrera-Chávez, et al.[30]

Tabla I. Studies on the possible involvement of oat and maize prolamins as well as bovine casein in CD

3. Oat Prolamins and their Controversial Effect on CD

Oats, used in various foods for CD patients, may not be so safe, even if they are not contaminated with wheat gluten. Their proteins may affect the regeneration of the intestinal mucosa in recovering patients because they are able to promote T-cell response due to their immunogenicity, as well as that of lysosomal and K562 cells, which highlights their cytotoxic properties.[14,15] Oats contain a very special prolamin which, once digested, provides a peptide structurally rich in beta twists, soluble and quite immunoreactive, which the IgA antibodies of CD children recognize with high sensitivity and specificity.[16]

In contrast, other studies show that oats are safe for CD patients. According to Kilmartin et al[17], oat prolamins are not involved in the pathogenesis of CD because they do not induce a Th1 response in intestinal biopsies from a cohort of CD patients. It has also been published that these proteins do not trigger the characteristic CD autoimmunity, that is to say, they do not induce production of anti-tissue transglutaminase antibodies.[18] To reach common ground in this dispute, several authors recognize that while many CD patients can eat oats without any symptoms, some may not be able to tolerate it.[19-21] The behavior must be taken into account when considering the introduction of this cereal in the diet of CD patients. It is a fact that barley, rye and oats contain proteins with varying degrees of homology to wheat prolamins, due to their taxonomic relationship. The immune response to wheat, barley and rye prolamins is based on T-cell response to its homologous peptides.[22-23] The homology of avenins with gliadins is lesser than that of barley and rye[24], since is not so close. This gives rise to non-immunodominant peptides in oats, which would induce a response only in some CD patients.

As for the cellular immune response, there is knowledge of at least two avenin peptides which stimulate the T-cells of CD patients within the context of antigen presentation involving the HLA-DQ2.[20,25]

Finally, the manner in which oats are prepared as breakfast cereal makes them have a lower prolamin content than analogue products based on wheat, barley and rye. This results in a lower exposure to the immunogenic peptides of oat than to those of wheat.

4. The Intriguing Maize Prolamins and their Effect on CD

Maize is widely accepted as safe wheat substitute in foodstuffs for CD patients. Thus, to evaluate the effect in CD of microbial transglutaminase (mTG) in baking, we compared regular wheat bread with gluten-free bread made with rice and maize flours. In both cases, the bread was prepared with and without mTG treatment. Prolamins were then extracted from the four bread samples and tested as antigens for IgA from CD patients using ELISA. Unexpectedly, the IgA in one of the sera showed a much higher titer against prolamins in rice and maize bread treated with mTG than for wheat prolamins. In this case, it was the serum of a young CD patient who was unresponsive to the gluten-free diet. After performing a membrane immunodetection test with the isolated prolamins, it was inferred that this patient's CD was exacerbated by deamidated maize prolamins, as it happens with wheat gliadins in the pathogenesis of CD.[26]

In a case very similar to the one described in the previous paragraph, Accomando et al.[13] describe the follow-up of a young female CD patient who did not respond to the gluten-free diet. During follow-up, the patient had decreased levels of anti-gliadin IgA, but continuing symptoms of classic CD, including damage to the intestinal mucosa. When performing a double-blind provocation test with maize and rice, intolerance to maize was observed, but not to rice. After prescribing a gluten-free and maize-free diet, the symptoms gradually disappeared as well as the damage to the intestinal mucosa.

The two previously mentioned cases involved 16 year-old adolescents with atypical CD manifestations. The male was emaciated, had developmental delay, anemia, malabsorption, but mainly neurological problems. The female patient, in turn, had recurrent fatigue and loss of consciousness due to anemia. In both cases, anti-gliadin IgA and anti-transglutaminase levels decreased with gluten-free diet, but malabsorption, diarrhea and abdominal pain persisted. Symptoms remited only when maize was excluded from the diet. On neither case there are data on the age of CD onset; it is possible that it had been developing years before diagnosis and maybe maize prolamins induced a side effect to those of wheat.

In Table 1, in addition to clinical cases involving maize, a challenge with zeins in direct contact with the rectal mucosa of 13 adult CD patients is summarized. In this study, 6/13 of the patients showed signs of inflammatory reaction, although the response was lesser than that obtained in a gluten wheat challenge.[27] In this same study, a group of healthy individuals, showed response neither to gluten nor to wheat or maize proteins. Although the study by Kristjansson et al[27] evaluated the innate response involved in CD, their results demonstrated the activation of neutrophils and eosinophils in the early stages of inflammatory reaction in CD patients.

Regarding the humoral response, several authors have argued that some CD patients show high levels of antibodies against maize antigens.[28-31] Competitive ELISA immunoassays have shown that IgA from some CD patients recognizes specific maize protein sequences and that this is not a case of simple cross-reactivity. In the stage previous to antibody production, T helper cells must be activated, so that they, in turn will stimulate B cells.

Although there is not much information on the subject, in a study where the intestinal T cells of celiac patients were stimulated, a cell line from a patient (from a cohort of seven) with CD produced gamma interferon (IFN-γ) after stimulation with maize prolamins.[32]

In order to explain maize antigen presentation in CD, there have been diverse *in vitro* and *in silico* modelling studies. From their results it is inferred that some sequences in maize prolamins are good candidates for an efficient binding to HLA-DQ2 and HLA-DQ8 molecules[33]; it is a key step in the pathogenesis of CD. It has also been shown that certain sequences in maize remain immunoreactive for IgA from CD patients after a simulated gastrointestinal digestion with pepsin and trypsin. Furthermore, once thoroughly treated with proteases, there are still zein peptide sequences capable of binding to HLA class II molecules, involved in the pathogenesis of CD.[33]

The side chains of amino acids that bind to the HLA class II receptors make contact with specific sites in the molecule. For HLA-DQ8, the amino acid residue on the antigen required for binding is glutamine (converted into glutamic acid by tissular transglutaminase) in positions P1 and P9 on the peptide. For HLA-DQ2, glutamine is required on the P4, P6 and P7 positions on the peptide.[34]

Among the products of an exhaustive zein digestion, LQQAIAASNIPLSPLLFQQSPALSLVQSLVQTIR can be found, a peptide with glutamine residues at the appropriate positions to effectively bind to HLA-DQ8.[33]

According to Köning[35], in the early stages of CD development, a broad, gluten-specific T-cell response originates and may be directed towards any of the immunogenic peptides. On the other hand, IFN-γ secretion increases expression of HLA-DQ2 in the surface of the antigen-presenting cells, making peptide presentation more efficient. Eventually T-cell response will focus on the most immunogenic and stable peptides. It is likely that, among them, one of the maize prolamin peptides could be found.

The fact that few studies have been published on the adverse effect of maize gluten requires extensive review. An important consideration would be the weight of dietary maize, especially its intake before the development of CD. In the Mexican and Central American populations maize is a primary staple food; *atole* (a porridge made with maize flour mixed with water or milk) is introduced early into the infant diet. Thus, in a recent study, a total of 5 members of a cohort of 24 celiac patients showed positive reactivity of IgA class against zeins.[33]

In the Northwest Mexican population involved in our study, maize is used as much as wheat in the current diet.[36] In this way, the zein immunogenic sequences would be introduced at the same time that the immunogenic gliadin sequences, in individuals with a genetic predisposition to CD. However, not in all cases there is an immune response against zeins because, as with avenins, they possess less immunogenic sequences than gliadins.

5. Bovine Casein and its Surprising Effect on CD

Lactose intolerance is common in CD patients, especially when the intestinal mucosa has not completely recovered when starting a gluten-free diet. However, there are cases in which, even if they have recovered well, cow's milk is not tolerated and not because of lactose intolerance. A few years ago, it was suspected that some gluten peptides could pass through the wheat-containing pasture into the cow's milk. Dekking et al.[37] demonstrated, in a very convincing experiment, that there were no immunogenic peptides in cow's milk proteins, even if they had been fed pasture containing 100% wheat. Therefore, symptoms which were triggered in CD patients after ingesting cow milk were not due to gluten protein contamination but to the bovine milk proteins themselves.

IgA in some CD patients recognizes certain alpha and beta-casein sequences but not kappa caseins from cow milk, while it does not recognize any of the human milk caseins.[30] According to Berti et al.[38], IgA immunoreactivity is considerably reduced after casein digestion. However, the *in vitro* hydrolysis conditions used are quite different of the physiological conditions for the gastrointestinal digestion. Moreover, due to the processing of milk (heat treatment), bovine caseins form aggregates, which increases their resistance to digestion.[39]

On the other hand, beta casein contains sequences homologous to those of wheat gluten.[24] For example, in the 33-mer (LQLQPFPQPQLPYPQPQLPYPQPQLPYPQPQPF) which is widely recognized as an immunogenic gluten peptide for CD, the PYPQ sequence is repeated three times.[40] This sequence can be found in seven peptides of digested bovine beta casein, with pepsin and trypsin.[41] The reason why IgA from CD patients does not recognize human beta casein may be due to small differences in contrast with sequences found in bovine casein and gluten. While the digestion of wheat gluten and bovine casein yields peptides with PYPQ sequences, hydrolysis of human milk casein peptides yields sequences such as PIPQ or PVPQ.[42] Thus, the residues of branched chain amino acids with aliphatic groups from human casein peptides, provide considerably different properties compared to the aromatic group of tyrosine from bovine beta casein peptides.

In an analogous fashion to what has been described above for maize proteins, bovine caseins may induce an inflammatory reaction in a patch test on the rectal mucosa of CD patients.[43] However, even with such evidences from humoral and cellular response, tissular anti-transglutaminase antibodies, characteristic of the CD autoimmune response, may not appear. For their generation, the presentation of the enzyme and its substrate to the gluten peptides is necessary. Evidence shows that the humoral response is the same for untreated bovine caseins than for those previously treated with transglutaminase.[29] Thus, the hypothetically immunogenic peptides of bovine caseins do not require deamination for an efficient binding to the HLA-DQ2/DQ8 molecules. Thus, with the mere presence of bovine beta casein, transglutaminase would not be presented and an immune response against it would not be launched with the consequent lack of autoimmunity.

The low proportion of CD patients with symptoms after ingesting of cow's milk is surprising in the light of the hypothesis of its immunogenic peptides. In this case, the same assumptions cannot be made regarding the scant number of reactive sequences or amount ingested according to dietary habits, as it was done for oat and maize prolamins, because milk is a widely consumed food. Perhaps there would be differences in the degree in casein digestion; some CD patients would digest it less than others, especially if they have exocrine pancreatic insufficiency.[44]

6. Non-Refractory Celiac Patients who do not respond to the Gluten-Free Diet

When there is no good response to gluten-free diet, it becomes necessary to monitor possible responses against other dietary proteins. Regardless of the mechanism by which the immune system of these patients is being activated or not, simple and relatively non-invasive tests, such as ELISA immunoassays, can be used to obtain helpful information about treatment. According to published evidence, the three types of proteins discussed in this chapter may be related to persistent symptoms in CD patients. Thus, they would be the first subjects of ELISA immunoreactivity analysis, followed by a dietary challenge.

Acknowledgments

This chapter was prepared with support from the CB-2008-1/106227 project, funded by the *Consejo Nacional de Ciencia y Tecnología* ("National Council for Science and Technology", CONACyT, Mexico). We thank to M.Sci. Adriana V. Bolaños Villar, for her editorial support, to Dr. Veronica Mata Haro and to M.Sci. Rosa Olivia Mendez, for their enriching feedback on this manuscript.

References

1. Husby S, Koletzko S, Korponay-Szabo IR, Mearin ML, Phillips A, Shamir R et al. for the ESPGHAN Working Group on Coeliac Disease Diagnosis, on behalf of the ESPGHAN Gastroenterology Committee. *European Society for Pediatric Gastroenterology, Hepatology, and Nutrition Guidelines for the Diagnosis of Coeliac Disease.* J Pediatr Gastroenterol Nutr. 2012; 54: 136-60.
   http://dx.doi.org/10.1097/MPG.0b013e31821a23d0
2. Kasarda DD, Okita TW, Bernardin JE, Baecker PA, Nimmo CC, Lew EJ et al. *Nucleic acid (cDNA) and amino acid sequences of α-type gliadin from wheat* (Triticumaestivum). Proc Natl Acad Sci USA. 1984; 81: 4712-6. http://dx.doi.org/10.1073/pnas.81.15.4712
3. Dewar DH, Donnelly SC, McLaughlin SD, Johnson MW, Ellis HJ, Ciclitira PJ. *Celiac disease: Management of persistent symptoms in patients on a gluten-free diet.* World J Gastroenterol. 2012; 18: 1348-56. http://dx.doi.org/10.3748/wjg.v18.i12.1348
4. Leffler DA, Edwards-George J, Dennis M, Schuppan D, Cook F, Franko DL et al. *Factors that influence adherence to a gluten-free diet in adults with celiac disease.* Dig Dis Sci. 2008; 53: 1573-81. http://dx.doi.org/10.1007/s10620-007-0055-3
5. Hall NJ, Rubin G, Charnock A. *Systematic review: adherence to a gluten-free diet in adult patients with coeliac disease.* Aliment Pharmacol Ther. 2009; 30: 315-30.
   http://dx.doi.org/10.1111/j.1365-2036.2009.04053.x
6. Codex Alimentarius Commission. *Draft revised standard for gluten-free foods.* 2008. Disponible en: http://www.codexalimentarius.net.
7. Abdulkarim AS, Burgart LJ, See J, Murray JA. *Etiology of nonresponsive celiac disease: results of a systematic approach.* Am J Gastroenterol. 2002; 97: 2016-21.
   http://dx.doi.org/10.1111/j.1572-0241.2002.05917.x
8. Leffler DA, Edwards-George JB, Dennis M, Cook EF, Schuppan D, Kelly CP. *A prospective comparative study of five measures of gluten-free diet adherence in adults with coeliac disease.* Aliment Pharmacol Ther. 2007; 26: 1227-35.
   http://dx.doi.org/10.1111/j.1365-2036.2007.03501.x
9. Carroccio A, Mansueto P, Iacono G, Soresi M, D' Alcamo A, Cavataio F et al. *Non-celiac wheat sensitivity diagnosed by double-blind placebo-controlled challenge: exploring a new clinical entity.* Am J Gastroenterol. 2012; 107: 1898-906.
   http://dx.doi.org/10.1038/ajg.2012.236
10. Rubio-Tapia A, Murray JA. *Classification and management of refractory celiac disease.* Gut. 2010; 59: 547–57. http://dx.doi.org/10.1136/gut.2009.195131
11. Di Sabatino A, Biagi F, Gobbi PG, Corazza GR. *How I treat enteropathy-associated T-cell lymphoma.* Blood. 2012; 119: 2458-68.
    http://dx.doi.org/10.1182/blood-2011-10-385559
12. McAllister CS, Kagnoff MF. *The immunopathogenesis of celiac disease reveals posible therapies beyond the gluten-free diet.* SeminImmunopathol. 2012; 34: 581-600.
    http://dx.doi.org/10.1007/s00281-012-0318-8
13. Accomando S, Albino C, Montaperto D, Amato GM, Corsello G. *Multiple food intolerance or refractory celiac sprue?* Dig Liver Dis. 2006; 38: 784-5.
    http://dx.doi.org/10.1016/j.dld.2005.07.004
14. Silano M, Dessì M, De Vincenzi M, Cornell H. In vitro *tests indicate that certain varieties of oats may be harmful to patients with coeliac disease.* J Gastroenterol Hepatol. 2007; 22: 528-31. http://dx.doi.org/10.1111/j.1440-1746.2006.04512.x

15. Silano M, Di Benedetto R, Maialetti F, De Vincenzi A, Calcaterra R, Cornell HJ et al. *Avenins from different cultivars of oats elicit response by coeliac peripheral lymphocytes.* Scand J Gastroenterol. 2007; 42: 1302-5. http://dx.doi.org/10.1080/00365520701420750

16. Ribes-Koninckx C, Alfonso P, Ortigosa L, Escobar H, Suárez L, Arranz E et al. *A beta-turn rich oats peptide as an antigen in an ELISA method for the screening of coeliac disease in pediatric population.* Eur J Clin Invest. 2000; 30: 702-8. http://dx.doi.org/10.1046/j.1365-2362.2000.00684.x

17. Kilmartin C, Lynch S, Abuzakouk M, Wieser H, Feighery C. *Avenin fails to induce a Th1 response in coeliac tissue following in vitro culture.* Gut. 2003; 52: 47-52. http://dx.doi.org/10.1136/gut.52.1.47

18. Picarelli A, Di Tola M, Sabbatella L, Gabrielli F, Di Cello T, Anania MC et al. *Immunologic evidence of no harmful effect of oats in celiac disease.* Am J Clin Nutr. 2001; 74: 137-40.

19. Lundin KE, Nilsen EM, Scott HG, Løberg EM, Gjøen A, Bratlie J et al. *Oats induced villous atrophy in coeliac disease.* Gut. 2003; 52: 1649-52. http://dx.doi.org/10.1136/gut.52.11.1649

20. Arentz-Hansen H, Fleckenstein B, Molberg Ø, Scott H, Koning F, Jung G et al. *The molecular basis for oat intolerance in patients with celiac disease.* PLoS Med. 2004; 1: e1. http://dx.doi.org/10.1371/journal.pmed.0010001

21. Holm K, Mäki M, Vuolteenaho N, Mustalahti K, Ashorn M, Ruuska T et al. *Oats in the treatment of childhood coeliac disease: A 2-year controlled trial and a long-term clinical follow-up study.* Aliment Pharmacol Ther. 2006; 23: 1463-72. http://dx.doi.org/10.1111/j.1365-2036.2006.02908.x

22. Tye-Din JA, Stewart JA, Dromey JA, Beissbarth T, van Heel DA, Tatham A et al. *Comprehensive, quantitative mapping of T cell epitopes in gluten in celiac disease.* Sci Transl Med. 2010; 2: 41-51. http://dx.doi.org/10.1126/scitranslmed.3001012

23. Vader LW, Stepniak DT, Bunnik EM, Kooy YM, De HW, Drijfhout JW et al. *Characterization of cereal toxicity for celiac disease patients based on protein homology in grains.* Gastroenterology. 2003; 125: 1105-13. http://dx.doi.org/10.1016/S0016-5085(03)01204-6

24. Darewicz M, Dziuba J, Minkiewicz P. *Computational characterization and identification of peptides for in silico detection of potentially celiac-toxic proteins.* Food Sci Technol Int. 2007; 13: 125-33. http://dx.doi.org/10.1177/1082013207077954

25. Vader W, Stepniak D, Kooy Y, Mearin L, Thompson A, van Rood JJ et al. *The HLA-DQ2 gene dose effect in celiac disease is directly related to the magnitude and breadth of gluten-specific T cell responses.* Proc Natl Acad Sci USA. 2003; 100: 12390-5. http://dx.doi.org/10.1073/pnas.2135229100

26. Cabrera-Chávez F, Rouzaud-Sández O, Sotelo-Cruz N, Calderón de la Barca AM. *Transglutaminase treatment of wheat and maize prolamins of bread increases the serum IgA reactivity of celiac disease patients.* J Agric Food Chem. 2008; 56: 1387-91. http://dx.doi.org/10.1021/jf0724163

27. Kristjánsson G, Högman M, Venge P, Hällgren R. *Gut mucosal granulocyte activation precedes nitric oxide production: Studies in coeliac patients challenged with gluten and corn.* Gut. 2005; 54: 769-74. http://dx.doi.org/10.1136/gut.2004.057174

28. Skerritt JH, Devery JM, Penttila IA, La Brooy JT. *Cellular and humoral responses in coeliac disease. 2. Protein extracts from different cereals.* Clin Chim Acta. 1991; 204: 109-22. http://dx.doi.org/10.1016/0009-8981(91)90222-X

29. Cabrera-Chávez F, Rouzaud-Sández O, Sotelo-Cruz N, Calderón de la Barca AM. *Bovine milk caseins and transglutaminase-treated cereal prolamins are diferentially recognized by IgA of celiac disease patients according to their age.* J Agric Food Chem. 2009; 57: 3754-9. http://dx.doi.org/10.1021/jf802596g

30. Cabrera-Chávez F, Calderón de la Barca AM. *Bovine milk intolerance in celiac disease is related to IgA reactivity to α and β-caseins.* Nutrition. 2009; 25: 715-6. http://dx.doi.org/10.1016/j.nut.2009.01.006

31. Hurtado-Valenzuela JG, Sotelo-Cruz N, López-Cervantes G, de la Barca AM. *Tetany caused by chronic diarrhea in a child with celiac disease: A case report.* Cases J. 2008; 1: 176. http://dx.doi.org/10.1186/1757-1626-1-176

32. Bergamo P, Maurano F, Mazzarella G, Iaquinto G, Vocca I, Rivelli AR et al. *Immunological evaluation of the alcohol-soluble protein fraction from gluten-free grains in relation to celiac disease.* Mol Nutr Food Res. 2011; 55: 1266-70. http://dx.doi.org/10.1002/mnfr.201100132

33. Cabrera-Chávez F, Iametti S, Miriani M, Calderón de la Barca AM, Mamone G, Bonomi F. *Maize prolamins resistant to peptic-tryptic digestion maintain immune-recognition by IgA from some celiac disease patients.* Plant Foods Hum Nutr. 2012; 67: 24-30. http://dx.doi.org/10.1007/s11130-012-0274-4

34. Qiao SW, Sollid LM, Blumberg RS. *Antigen presentation in celiac disease.* Curr Opin Immunol. 2009; 21: 111-7. http://dx.doi.org/10.1016/j.coi.2009.03.004

35. Köning F. *Celiac disease: quantity matters.* Semin Immunopathol. 2012; 34: 541-9. http://dx.doi.org/10.1007/s00281-012-0321-0

36. Ortega MI, Valencia ME. *Measuring the intakes of foods and nutrients of marginal populations in North-West Mexico.* Public Health Nutr. 2002; 5: 907-10. http://dx.doi.org/10.1079/PHN2002379

37. Dekking L, Koning F, Hosek D, Ondrak TD, Taylor SL, Schroeder JW et al. *Intolerance of celiac disease patients to bovine milk is not due to the presence of T-cell stimulatory epitopes of gluten.* Nutrition. 2009; 25: 122-3. http://dx.doi.org/10.1016/j.nut.2008.07.009

38. Berti C, Trovato C, Bardella MT, Forlani, F. *IgA anti-gliadin antibody immunoreactivity to food proteins.* Food Agric Immunol. 2003; 15: 217-23. http://dx.doi.org/10.1080/09540100400003204

39. Dupont D, Mandalari G, Mollé D, Jardin J, Rolet-Répécaud O, Duboz G et al. *Food processing increases casein resistance to simulated infant digestion.* Mol Nutr Food Res. 2010; 54: 1677-89. http://dx.doi.org/10.1002/mnfr.200900582

40. Qiao SW, Bergseng E, Molberg Ø, Xia J, Fleckenstein B, Khosla C et al. *Antigen presentation to celiac lesion-derived T cells of a 33-mer gliadin peptide naturally formed by gastrointestinal digestion.* J Immunol. 2004; 173: 1757-62.

41. Deutsch SM, Molle D, Gagnaire V, Piot M, Atlan D, Lortal S. *Hydrolysis of sequenced beta-casein peptides provides new insight into peptidase activity from thermophilic lactic acid bacteria and highlights intrinsic resistance of phosphopeptides.* Appl Environ Microbiol. 2000; 66: 5360-7. http://dx.doi.org/10.1128/AEM.66.12.5360-5367.2000

42. Greenberg R, Groves ML, Dower HJ. *Human beta-casein. Amino acid sequence and identification of phosphorylation sites.* J Biol Chem. 1984; 259: 5132-8.

43. Kristjánsson G, Venge P, Hällgren R. *Mucosal reactivity to cow's milk protein in coeliac disease.* Clin Exp Immunol. 2007; 147: 449-55. http://dx.doi.org/10.1111/j.1365-2249.2007.03298.x

44. Malterre T. *Digestive and nutritional considerations in celiac disease: Could supplementation help?* Altern Med Rev. 2009; 14: 247-57.

OmniaScience

Chapter 6

Genetic Markers in Celiac Disease

Nora Fernández-Jiménez, Leticia Plaza-Izurieta, Jose Ramón Bilbao

Department of Genetics, Physical Anthropology and Animal Physiology, Basque Country University (UPV-EHU), BioCruces Research Institute, Bizkaia, Spain.

immunogenetics.let@gmail.com

Doi: http://dx.doi.org/10.3926/oms.232

How to cite this chapter

Fernandez-Jimenez N, Plaza-Izurieta L, Bilbao JR. *Genetic Markers in Celiac Disease.* In Rodrigo L and Peña AS, editors. *Celiac Disease and Non-Celiac Gluten Sensitivity.* Barcelona, Spain: OmniaScience; 2014. p. 103-121.

N. Fernandez-Jimenez, L. Plaza-Izurieta, J.R. Bilbao

Abstract

Although the mode of inheritance of celiac disease (CD) is not completely understood, there is abundant evidence supporting the implication of genetic factors in susceptibility to CD and its heritability has been estimated to be of about 87%.

It has been known for a long time that certain HLA alleles are the major contributors to CD risk. However, despite playing a determinant role in the pathogenesis of the disease, their contribution to inheritance is modest (<50%) and it is believed that there must exist several non-HLA susceptibility loci, each one of them with a very small effect on the overall risk.

Consequently, during the last years, a great amount of effort has been made to locate and identify those additional susceptibility genes that might explain the genetics of the disease. Linkage studies in families, candidate gene association studies and (more recently) genome-wide association studies (GWAS) analyzing hundreds of thousands of Single-Nucleotide Polymorphisms (SNPs) have been performed. These approaches have identified several genes that are associated with CD, but not all of them have been confirmed in subsequent studies. Besides, the contribution of the identified genes remains modest, and a large part of the genetics of CD still remains to be clarified.

1. Introduction

Although the pattern of inheritance of celiac disease (CD) is still unknown, it has long been known that heredity is involved in the predisposition to the disease. Prevalence studies in affected families, especially those based on comparing twins, have been useful to estimate the proportions in which genetic and environmental factors contribute to the risk of disease development. According to these studies, Genetics plays an important role in both the initiation and subsequent development of CD. It is generally accepted that the proportion of pairs of monozygotic or identical twins in which both siblings suffer from the disease is of 75-86%, while among dizygotic or fraternal twins (who, like all siblings, share an average of 50% of the genome) this match is reduced to 16-20%. This difference between mono- and dizygotic twins has been used to calculate the magnitude of the genetic component in CD, which is higher than in other complex diseases of immunological origin, such as type 1 diabetes (about 30% concordance between identical twins and 6% for fraternal twins).[1] Furthermore, in CD, the correlation between sibling pairs and non-identical twins is almost the same, so that the environmental component would have a minimal effect on the risk of developing the disease. All this supports the idea that there is a strong genetic component in the development of celiac disease. At present, it is estimated that the heritability of CD (ratio of risk for a disease attributable to genetic factors versus environmental factors) is close to 87%.[2]

It has long been known that a large part of the genetic risk of developing CD is due to the presence of certain human leukocyte antigen (HLA) alleles. Despite their crucial role in the pathogenesis of the disease, the contribution of HLA to CD heritability is modest, so there has been a great deal of speculation about the existence of numerous susceptibility *loci* not linked to HLA, each of which would have a very small effect on the overall risk.

2. The HLA region and Celiac Disease

2.1. HLA Region

The Human Leukocyte Antigen or HLA is the name given to the Major Histocompatibility Complex (MHC) in humans. It is a *superlocus* located on the short arm of chromosome 6 that contains a large number of genes related to the immune system. HLA genes are responsible for encoding antigen-presenting proteins expressed on the surface of most human cells and constitute a major component in the ability to discriminate between self and non-self.

HLA genes influence the development of numerous inflammatory and autoimmune disorders, as well as susceptibility to infectious diseases, such as malaria and AIDS. However, due to the complexity of this region, the genetic components and specific pathogenic mechanisms for most of these diseases are unknown. The HLA region is one of the genome regions with the highest gene density. One explanation for this phenomenon is that, in this region, a high level of expression is favored.[3]

2.2. Contribution to genetic risk and susceptibility genes

As mentioned above, the HLA region is the most important CD susceptibility *locus* and accounts for about 50% of the heritability of the disease. The first evidence of association between HLA and CD was published in 1972 and was found using serological methods. Due to the high degree of linkage disequilibrium in the area, early studies identified HLA-A1, HLA-B8 and HLA-DR3 as the etiologic variants in the region, but molecular studies have shown that the factors directly involved are the HLA class II genes that code for HLA-DQ2 and HLA-DQ8 molecules. The association of HLA-DQ2 with the disease is the strongest; around 90% of celiac patients have at least one copy of the HLA-DQ2.5 heterodimer (formed by the combination of DQA1*05 and DQB1*02 alleles, responsible for encoding α and β heterodimer chains, respectively). On the other hand, 20-30% of the general population also carries this risk variant, demonstrating that although crucial for the disease, HLA-DQ2 alone is insufficient to develop it. The vast majority of CD patients lacking HLA-DQ2 carry the DQ8 variant present in the haplotype consisting of alleles DQA1*03:01 and DQB1*03:02.[4] A very small proportion of the patients are negative for both DQ2 and DQ8, but it has been observed that in most cases, these individuals have at least one of the two alleles encoding DQ2 molecule, i.e., DQA1*05 and DQB1*02.[4,5]

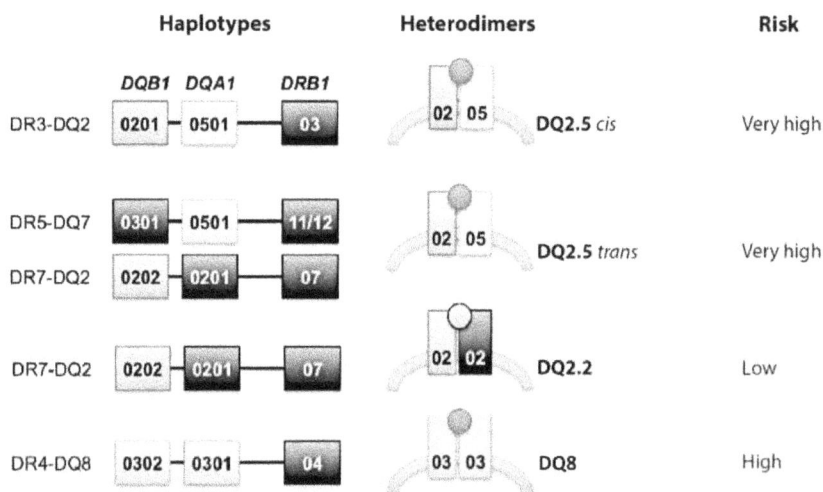

*Figure 1. Association of the HLA locus with CD. The HLA-DQ2 molecule is the major genetic risk factor for CD. Most celiac patients express the HLA-DQ2.5 heterodimer encoded by HLA-DQA1*05 (α chain) and HLA-DQB1*02 (β chain) alleles, which can be in cis in the haplotype DR3-DQ2 or in trans in DR5-DQ7 and DR7-DQ2.2 heterozygotes. The HLA-DQ2.2 dimer, an HLA-DQ2 variant (encoded by HLA-DQA1*02:01 and HLA-DQB1*02 alleles), confers a low risk of developing CD. Most DQ2-negative patients express HLA-DQ8 encoded by the haplotype DR4-DQ8.*

Risk variants DQ2 and DQ8 are in linkage disequilibrium (closely associated) with the HLA-DRB1 variants DR3 and DR4, respectively. Therefore, when referring to these risk variants, we might speak of haplotypes DR3-DQ2 and DR4-DQ8.[6] Haplotypes encoding the heterodimer HLA-DQ2.5

risk have been associated with CD in most populations (Figure 1). In certain haplotypes, such as DR3-DQ2, both alleles of the HLA-DQ2.5 heterodimer (DQA1*05:01 and DQB1*02:01) are located on the same chromosome and are encoded in cis. In heterozygous individuals with the DR5-DQ7 and DR7-DQ2 haplotypes, the two molecules are encoded in different chromosomes, or in *trans* (Figure 1). The differences between both HLA-DQ2.5 heterodimers affect an amino acid in the signal peptide of the DQα chains (DQA1*05:05 versus DQA1*05:01) and a residue in the membrane region of the DQβ chains (DQB1*02:01 versus DQB1*02:02) and seem not to have functional consequences, so they are attributed a similar risk. However, the risk conferred by another variant of the HLA DQ2 molecule, HLA-DQ2.2 dimer is very low (Figure 1).[7,8]

The degree of CD susceptibility is related to the number of DQ2.5 heterodimers. Individuals homozygous for DR3-DQ2 or DR3-DQ2/DR7-DQ2 heterozygotes express higher levels of DQ2.5 heterodimers and have maximum genetic risk of developing CD.[8-10] In this regard it is noteworthy that patients with refractory CD, unresponsive to the gluten-free diet, have a higher degree of DR3-DQ2 homozygosity (44-62%) compared to other celiac patients (20-24%). A similar allelic dose effect has been suggested for DQ8 molecules.

Together with the genes encoding DQ molecules, the HLA region contains other genes involved in the immune response that could also influence susceptibility to CD. Several studies have suggested that polymorphisms in genes such as *MICA*, *MICB* or *TNF* could contribute to the risk of developing the disease. However, most studies have not taken into account the high linkage disequilibrium between these genes and HLA-DQ and results are inconclusive. Sequencing and comprehensive mapping of the HLA region will help determine if it contains other susceptibility factors.

Despite the important contribution of HLA genes to the genetic risk, disease concordance for HLA identical siblings is only about 30%, so we can conclude that HLA genes are important but not sufficient to develop CD.[7]

2.3. Role in pathogenesis

The strong association of HLA class II genes with CD is explained by the fundamental role of CD4+ T lymphocytes in the pathogenesis of the disease. In fact, there are CD4+ T cells that recognize gluten peptides in the intestinal mucosa of celiac patients, but not in healthy individuals. These CD4+ cells present in the intestine of celiac patients are typically characterized by the HLA-DQ2 or -DQ8 molecules.[9]

When genetically susceptible individuals (expressing HLA-DQ2 or -DQ8 molecules) are exposed to certain gluten epitopes, these epitopes are presented by antigen presenting cells, stimulating the proliferation of gluten-specific CD4+ T cells.

An important milestone in the understanding of the molecular basis of the association of HLA with CD was the discovery that binding of HLA-DQ2 and -DQ8 molecules to gluten depends on enzymatic modifications of these peptides by the enzyme transglutaminase (TG2). This enzyme catalyzes a reaction that increases the negative charge of gluten epitopes, and enhances their binding to the HLA-DQ2 and -DQ8 molecules thus triggering the presentation of gluten peptides to T cells.

Given the importance of HLA molecules in the activation of autoreactive T cells against gluten, it makes sense that any distinct differences in their coding sequence may cause an alteration in any step of this process. Thus, polymorphisms in the sequence encoding the antigen-binding portion may cause changes in binding affinity, favoring the recognition of gluten peptides. Furthermore, certain polymorphisms located in regulatory regions may cause a sub-expression or over-expression of the HLA molecules, decreasing or increasing the immune response to gluten.

3. Search for genetic susceptibility genes in CD

In recent years, a great effort has been made to locate and identify susceptibility genes outside the HLA region and which may explain the Genetics of CD. For this purpose, two methods of analysis have been generally used: linkage studies in families and association studies. More recently, CD has been investigated by means of Genome-Wide Association Studies (GWAS) in which thousands of single nucleotide polymorphisms or SNPs have been analyzed. Through these studies, several genes associated with CD have been identified, but not all the observed associations have been subsequently confirmed.

3.1. Linkage regions and positional candidate genes

Linkage studies in families allow the identification of chromosomal regions repeatedly and consistently inherited by those family members affected by the disease through several generations. Through this type of analysis, the genome regions potentially involved in the pathogenesis of diseases can be further pinpointed. The genes located in these regions are positional candidate genes because their location confers upon them the suspicion of being involved in the pathogenesis of the disease.

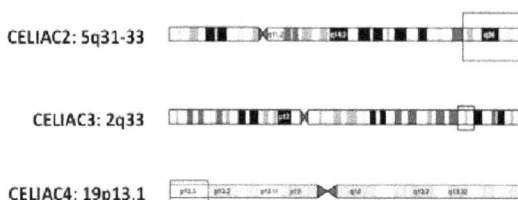

CELIAC2: 5q31-33

CELIAC3: 2q33

CELIAC4: 19p13.1

Fipure 2. Linkape repions replicated in different family studies.

To date, four candidate regions linked to CD have been identified: the first is the HLA region or CELIAC1, which is the most important genetic component in CD and which has already been discussed in depth previously. The other three regions are called CELIAC2, CELIAC3 and CELIAC4 (Figure 2), but analyses of these loci have not always been conclusive and consistent.

3.1.1. CELIAC2

The CELIAC2 region is located on chromosome 5q31-33 and was first identified by Greco et al. in 1998.[11] The replication of this *locus* has not been universal, and no gene functionally implicated in the disease has been identified. This region contains a set of genes coding for several cytokines, which may play a role in regulating the immune system and inflammation.[12] Anyway, specific genes associated with CD have not been identified yet.

Several studies have focused on specific candidates such as the *IL12B* genes or the *SPINK* family of genes, but no consistent associations have been found for any of them.[13] Thirteen potentially functional variants of *IL4, IL5, IL9, IL13, IL17B* genes and *NR3C1*, all in the CELIAC2 *locus*, were genotyped in the Irish population, but none of these variants or haplotypes showed association with the disease.[14]

On the other hand, in an association study of genes selected because they are differentially expressed in the disease and are located in linkage regions, evidence of association with the *YIPF5* gene, also located in this region, was observed.[15] In a subsequent study in the Finnish and Hungarian populations linkage of this region with CD was confirmed, and evidence of association with *YIPF5* was observed again, although not in a consistent fashion.[16]

Despite being a major risk *locus* described in several linkage studies, no gene has been found which may explain its association with disease.

3.1.2. CELIAC3

CELIAC3 was first identified in 1999 by Holopainen et al.[17] This region is located in the 2q33 chromosomal region and it contains, among others, genes that regulate the *CD28, CTLA4* and *ICOS* lymphocyte responses, which will be discussed further on.

In this first study, seven different genetic markers were analyzed in 100 families. The *D2S116* microsatellite presented the highest nonparametric linkage score in this study, a furthermore, significant association between the marker and the disease was detected. The linkage between CD and this *locus* has been replicated in several subsequent studies using different genetic markers (microsatellites and SNPs), in addition to the abovementioned microsatellite.

The CELIAC3 *locus* contains the *CD28, CTLA4* and *ICOS* genes, which are located in a block of around 300kb that controls various aspects of the T cell response. The binding of *CD28* and *ICOS* to their respective ligands creates a positive signal for cytokine proliferation and activation, while the binding of *CTLA4* creates a signal that negatively regulates T cell activation. The association of the *CTLA4* gene with CD has been described in several populations, but results have not always been positive. A study in which all SNPs in this gene were analyzed suggests that haplotypes rather than SNPs are more strongly associated with the disease. However, data for these variables and/or haplotypes in the disease are needed to determine whether the association is with the *CTLA4* gene or with another neighboring gene.[18]

In the study that analyzed differentially expressed genes in the disease located at the linkage regions (mentioned above)[13], the gene that showed the strongest association with the disease was *SERPINE2*. This gene is important in the initial stages of extracellular matrix formation, a process that is altered in CD. A subsequent study was unable to replicate the association of the disease with *SERPINE2* so, despite multiple attempts, the genetic factor that confers risk in the CELIAC3 region has not yet been identified.[19]

3.1.3. CELIAC4

The CELIAC4 *locus* is found on chromosome region 19p13.1 and was first identified by van Belzen et al in 2003.[20] This region contains more than 140 genes and some of them participate in the immune response and inflammation.

In the study, which identified CELIAC4, 82 families with affected members were analyzed. It was observed that the microsatellite D19S899 has a significant linkage peak with CD, with a LOD (*lop of likelihood ratio*) score of 4.31. Besides, this genetic marker was significantly associated with the disease when 216 CD patients and 216 controls were analyzed to confirm the results obtained in the linkage study. However, not all subsequent replication studies have achieved positive results on the linkage of this region and CD.[21]

The best CELIAC4 region candidate is the myosin *IXB* gene (*MYO9B*), since it encodes a myosin molecule probably involved in enterocyte actin remodeling. The specific function of *MYO9B* is unknown, but it is known to contain a protein domain similar to that of the genes involved in tight junctions, so that it has been hypothesized that variations in this gene may result in the disruption of the intestinal barrier, thus allowing immunogenic peptides to cross.[22] However, not all association studies conducted have found a positive association with *MYO9B*. There are about 140 additional genes in the region, some of which are involved in immunity and inflammation (*CYP4F3, HSH2D, IL12RB1, IFI30* and *KIR*, for example) and which might be good candidates. A study that analyzed ten genes from this region in a Dutch population found evidence of association with the *CYP4F3* and *CYP4F2* genes, both involved in the inhibition of leukotriene, a potent inflammatory mediator.[23] *ICAM-1*, a gene found in this region that is important for intercellular adhesion, also showed association in a French population.[24] These weak associations must be replicated in independent populations in order to determine the contribution of these genes to the development of the disease.

3.2. Functional candidate genes

3.2.1. Innate immune response penes

The involvement of the innate immune system in the development of CD is increasingly evident, therefore several of the innate response genes have been studied in search of risk polymorphisms. One study analyzed functional polymorphisms located in regulatory regions of different proinflammatory mediators (*IL-1α, IL-1β, IL-1RN, IL-18, RANTES* and *MCP-1*). None of the genes analyzed in this study, except *RANTES*, which has a dubious association, was connected with the risk of developing CD.[25]

The KIR (Killer Immunoglobulin-like receptors) gene family has also been studied in CD because it contains innate immune response candidate genes. These receptors are located in the 19q13.4 region, which has presented evidence for linkage with the disease and encode receptors for NK (Natural Killer) and certain T cells that modulate cytolytic activity through interaction with HLA class I ligands, participating in the innate immune response. The gene content, genotypes and haplotypes in the KIR genes from a Basque population were analyzed and it was observed that the frequency of the *KIR2DL5B*(+)/*KIR2DL5A*(-) combination was significantly higher in individuals with CD. This association was replicated in a Spanish population (odds ratio 3.63) suggesting the involvement of the KIR2DL5B gene with an increased risk of CD, probably due to the lack of an efficient inhibitory signal.[26] On the other hand, another study found that the *KIR3DL1* inhibitor gene was overexpressed in the intestinal mucosa in active disease, presumably due to increased subpopulations of lymphocytes with an NK phenotype.[27]

Toll-like receptors (TLR), which take part in pathogen recognition and immune response stimulation, have also been analyzed in search of association with CD. Although it has been shown that their expression is altered in patients, no association was found between polymorphisms in these genes and CD. Similarly, no association was found for copy number variation (CNV) of *TLR2* and *TLR4* with the disease.[28]

In turn, β-defensins form a cluster with variable number of copies in the population and are part of the innate immune response, acting as natural antibiotics. The genes that comprise this family have been previously associated with autoimmune and inflammatory diseases such as psoriasis or Crohn's disease. Although no association has been detected between SNPs in these genes and CD, there is an association between the copy number of the gene cluster and CD, since a lower presence of high copy numbers was observed (>4) among patients, suggesting a protective role of β-defensins in the disease.[28]

As mentioned previously, stress response genes *MICA* and *MICB* have also been studied in search of risk variants, but the location of these genes in the CELIAC1 *locus* has hindered conclusions about their independent contribution, due to high linkage disequilibrium in the HLA region.[29]

Although the innate immune system is activated in celiac patients, none of the candidate genes studied exhibited a strong association with the disease, so it may be assumed that many genes of the innate immune system, each with a weak effect, contribute to the development of disease activating the innate response.

3.2.2. Adaptive immune response penes

The Th1 response is one of the major inflammatory responses in CD and the characteristic cytokine of this type of response is IFN-γ. Production of this cytokine is significantly increased in active disease, reaching 240-fold higher levels in cases with total atrophy. The *IFNG* gene was studied in three Dutch and Finnish population cohorts, no differences between the allelic distributions of cases and controls were found. So far, there is no evidence that *IFNG* variants might predispose to the disease, despite its being highly overexpressed in the mucosa of celiac patients.[30]

Th17 cells have also been implicated in CD pathogenesis. Signaling by means of IL23 and its receptor (IL23R) is a key element in the differentiation of T cells towards Th17 cells. The *IL23R* gene has been associated with other autoimmune and/or inflammatory diseases such as psoriasis or ulcerative colitis. A coding variant in *IL23R* gene was analyzed in a Dutch population but was not associated with the disease.[31] However, the analysis of this same variant in a Spanish population showed an increase of the minor allele in patients, as opposed to what was observed in other diseases.[32] A later study found evidence of linkage in the *IL23R* gene region in Hungarian, Finnish and Italian populations, but no association was found with the studied polymorphisms.[33]

However, a recent study in Spanish populations in which the association of 101 SNPs in 16 genes related to the Th17 response (including *IL23R*) indicates that there is no association with the disease.[34]

On the other hand, the *CIITA* gene appears to be the major regulator of HLA class II genes. This gene has a complex expression pattern and two polymorphisms located in its promoter have been associated with other autoimmune diseases. These polymorphisms were analyzed in a Spanish CD cohort but no significant differences between patients and controls were detected.[9] On the contrary, the second GWAS does show an association between CD and the region containing the *CIITA* gene.

To date, no candidate gene from the adaptive immune response has been strongly associated with risk of developing CD.

3.2.3. Genes involved in intestinal epithelium remodelinp

It has been reported that the permeability of the intestinal epithelium is increased in CD patients in response to gliadin. This alteration of the intestinal barrier is associated with structural changes in intercellular junctions. Due to its possible role in intestinal epithelium remodeling, the *MYO9B* gene in the CELIAC4 linkage region has been scanned for disease-associated polymorphisms.[23] A 2008 study analyzed 197 SNPs from 41 genes associated with intercellular communication in Dutch and British populations. Two of the genes, *PARD3* (2 SNPs) and *MAGI2* (2 SNPs) showed weak association with the disease in the Dutch population. Replication in a British population confirmed association with one *PARD3* SNP. The combined analysis of both populations confirmed the association for both genes with Odds ratio values of 1.23 for *PARD3* and 1.19 for *MAGI2*. These genes also showed positive association with ulcerative colitis, suggesting a common causal defect in the intestinal barrier for both diseases.[36]

3.2.4. Cell sipnalinp pathways

Several signaling pathways are altered in CD, including the Jak-Stat signaling pathway, the kappa B (NFkB) transcription factor signaling pathway, the MAPK signaling pathway or the transforming growth factor beta (TGFB) signaling pathway.[15] Several genes of these pathways have been analyzed in search of an association with CD.

One of these genes is STAT1, whose expression is altered in the disease and is also a positional candidate since it is found in the CELIAC3 *locus*. An analysis was performed of five tag polymorphisms covering the entire gene in a Dutch population, but there was no evidence of association with CD.[37]

The *NFKB1* gene has also been studied in search of a genetic association with CD, but despite the fact that this transcription factor is constitutively active in the mucosa of celiac patients, no polymorphisms have been found to explain its increased activity in the disease. It has been suggested that the pathogenic effects attributed to this transcription factor may be caused by a regulatory defect instead of a polymorphism in the transcription factor itself. Genes located upstream in the biological cascade may be responsible for the increased genetic risk generating a higher NFkB-dependent transcriptional activity. Two of the genes identified in a GWAS follow-up study (*REL* and *TNFAIP3*) are located in this cascade and may be responsible for its deregulation. Recently, a regulatory polymorphism in *UBD*, a gene involved in NFkB activation has been associated with the disease in a Spanish population study. This gene is overexpressed in patients with active disease and the associated allelic polymorphism has a significant correlation with gene expression levels.[38]

The modifications observed in these complex biological pathways can alter the expression of genes located further downstream in the route, so that the analysis of individual genes can give rise to error. An exhaustive analysis of these routes may be crucial for the selection of association study candidates.

3.2.5. Extracellular Matrix

The extracellular matrix appears degraded in the intestinal epithelium of celiac patients. Metalloproteinases are enzymes that degrade matrix components, and it has been recorded that their expression is increased in the active stages of the disease, contributing to the morphological alterations of the intestinal mucosa. Therefore, these genes have been studied on several occasions in search of susceptibility variants. In any case, functional polymorphisms of the *MMP-1* gene have not been associated with CD.[39]

4. Genome-wide association studies in celiac disease

GWAS allow for fast scanning of markers in complete sets of DNA or genomes of several individuals, with the purpose of finding genetic variations associated with a particular disease. Having identified these genetic associations, researchers can use this information to develop new and improved technologies to detect, treat and prevent diseases. These studies are especially useful in finding genetic variations that contribute to the development of common and complex diseases, such as asthma, cancer, diabetes, and (in this case) CD.

In order to conduct a GWAS, researchers use two groups of participants: individuals with the disease under study and individuals with characteristics similar to those above but who do not have the disease. This is an association study on a genome-wide scale.

The full DNA or genome of each individual is purified from a blood sample. This DNA is placed on a chip and is automatically scanned in the laboratory. These devices strategically inspect the samples looking for genetic variation markers, in this case, SNPs.

If it is discovered that certain genetic variations turn out to be significantly more frequent in patients than in healthy individuals, it is said that these variations are associated with the disease. These associated genetic variations may be important markers since they could point to the region in the human genome wherein lies the variation responsible for the disease. The associated variant itself need not necessarily be the direct cause of the disease; it could simply be pointing to the region where for the true causal variant should be sought. Due to this, in most cases it may be necessary to continue with the investigation, for example, by sequencing this particular region so as to identify the exact genetic variant implicated in the disease, or by performing functional studies in order to find an association between specific variants and gene expression levels.

GWAS allow the definition of a new class of genetic variants associated with diseases. Association studies based on pedigrees use families in which clusters associated with the disease are useful to identify rare variants with great risk effect. On the other hand, GWAS depend on population-based samples and therefore require common variants with a more modest effect (since it will not be feasible to observe rare variants), which could not be observed using a traditional linkage-based approach.

4.1. Outcome of the first GWAS

In the first genome-wide study conducted on CD, 778 individuals with CD and 1,422 healthy controls were studied. Association analyses were performed on 310,605 SNPs with a minor allele frequency above 1%.[40]

As expected, the largest association was found around the HLA *locus*. The *rs2187668-A* allele was shown to be an efficient marker for HLA-DQ2.5cis, the most common HLA DQ2 haplotype associated with CD. In this first study, it was shown that 89.2 % of patients in the UK had one or two copies of HLA-DQ2.5cis, compared to 25.5 % in the control population.

Outside the HLA region a number of associated SNPs higher than what would be expected by chance alone was observed, 56 SNPs had an association with $p<10^{-4}$. Some of these SNPs are located close together, which suggests that the excess of SNPs with low p-values may be due to a true association of SNPs in linkage disequilibrium with the disease-causing variants.

The only SNP outside HLA that demonstrated significant association was *rs13119723*, in the 4q27 region, located in a linkage disequilibrium block containing the *IL2* and *IL21* genes. These results were repeated in collections of Dutch and Irish patients and controls.

It was estimated that the *IL2-IL21* alone could explain only 1% of the increased familial risk for CD, suggesting the existence of other susceptibility genes that had not yet been identified. For this reason, a study was undertaken to analyze the 1,164 most significant SNPs from the first study in a further 1,643 CD cases and 3,406 non-celiac controls from three independent European collections.[41] The associated regions identified in this new study were scrutinized for candidate genes that could play a role in the development of CD, especially those genes somehow implicated in the immune response (Figure 3).

It is important to be able to replicate the results of genetic discoveries in different populations when establishing a genetic effect in the predisposition to a disease. For this reason, efforts have been made to replicate, in several independent populations, the results obtained in the first GWAS, with different results, possibly due to population variations and the sample size of each one of these studies.

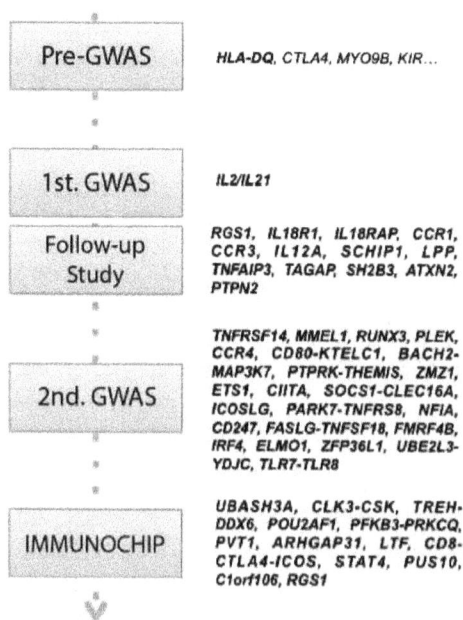

Pre-GWAS	*HLA-DQ, CTLA4, MYO9B, KIR...*
1st. GWAS	*IL2/IL21*
Follow-up Study	*RGS1, IL18R1, IL18RAP, CCR1, CCR3, IL12A, SCHIP1, LPP, TNFAIP3, TAGAP, SH2B3, ATXN2, PTPN2*
2nd. GWAS	*TNFRSF14, MMEL1, RUNX3, PLEK, CCR4, CD80-KTELC1, BACH2-MAP3K7, PTPRK-THEMIS, ZMZ1, ETS1, CIITA, SOCS1-CLEC16A, ICOSLG, PARK7-TNFRS8, NFIA, CD247, FASLG-TNFSF18, FMRF4B, IRF4, ELMO1, ZFP36L1, UBE2L3-YDJC, TLR7-TLR8*
IMMUNOCHIP	*UBASH3A, CLK3-CSK, TREH-DDX6, POU2AF1, PFKB3-PRKCQ, PVT1, ARHGAP31, LTF, CD8-CTLA4-ICOS, STAT4, PUS10, C1orf106, RGS1*

- Gene definition and etiological variants
- Functional analysis
- Studies on other types of genetic variability
- Creation of risk prediction algorithms

Figure 3. Advances in the Genetics of CD. After the Immunochip study, 40 loci that contribute to the risk of CD have been identified. Now is the time to perform functional studies in order to identify etiological variants and determine the practical applications of the association results (blue).

4.2. Outcome of the second GWAS

The second GWAS on CD was performed in 2009. To this end, an analysis was performed on 292,387 SNPs outside the HLA region in DNA samples from 4,533 individuals with celiac disease and 10,750 healthy controls of European origin. In addition, 231,362 non-HLA SNPs were also studied in 3,796 celiac patients and 8,154 controls.[42]

Thirteen new risk regions with significant evidence of association (Figure 3) were identified. There are several genes with immune functions in these regions: *BACH2, CCR4, CD80, CIITA-SOCS1-CLCD16A, ETS1, ICOSLG, RUNX3, THEMIS, TNFRSF14* and *ZMIZ1*. Another thirteen regions did not achieve significant association but did point to a trend and also contain genes with immune functions, including *CD247, FASLG-TNFSF18-TNFSF4, IRF4, TLR7-TLR8, TNFRSF9* and *YDJC*.

4.3. Immunochip

The most recent large-scale project performed to identify variants associated with CD and other autoimmune diseases is the *Immunochip Project*. Regarding CD, more than 200,000 variants from approximately 12,000 celiac patients and 12,000 controls from 7 geographical regions were analyzed.[43]

The analysis was performed on 183 loci related to the immune system that are outside the HLA region; 39 showed significant association with CD; the 26 regions identified in the GWAS plus 13 new *loci*. All associated variants have a minor allele frequency above 5%, that is, they are all common variants. Low frequency variants associated with the disease have only been detected in 4 loci. The advantage of the Immunochip over GWAS lies in the possibility of fine mapping the regions to locate and identify causal signals, due to the fact that in the Immunochip genotyping is much denser. One example of this is that out of 54 independent signals outside HLA that are found in high density in the 36 genotyped *loci*, 29 are located around a single gene (Figure 3).

After functional annotation of associated regions, one of the main conclusions that have been reached is that there are very few markers in the coding regions of genes, although some markers are close to transcription start sites and others in the 3 'UTR regions.

Some potentially causative genes proposed due to the existence of signals near the 5' or 3' regulatory regions are *THEMIS/PTPRK*, *TAGAP*, *ETS1*, *RUNX3* and *RGS1*. Some of them had already been proposed after the previous GWAS.

4.4. Replication of association studies and functional analysis of candidate genes

In 2011, the eight association peaks from the first CD GWAS were replicated in a Spanish population, identifying four genes (*IL12A*, *LPP*, *SCHIP1* and *SH2B3*) whose expression in the intestinal mucosa varied according to disease status and the genotype of the associated variant.[44] These results suggest that these genes may be constitutively altered in celiac patients, probably before the onset of observable symptoms of the disease, and therefore could have a primary role in its pathogenesis.

A second work takes a step forward and identifies two genes (*PTPRK* and *THEMIS*), located in the same associated region, which are co-expressed both in active disease and in response to *in vitro* stimulation by gliadin from intestinal biopsies of celiac patients with inactive disease who have adhered to the diet for at least two years.[45] Therefore, it seems that the variants associated in this region affect the expression of different genes, not constitutively from the time of birth of the future celiac patient, but after a toxic stimulus triggers an immune response.

The implications of this finding are of great importance because they highlight the existence of common regulatory mechanisms for different genes in the DNA sequence that only have an effect in the presence of a disease-provoking immunogenic stimulus.

These and other studies emphasize the need for functional studies and to avoid the selection of hypothetical susceptibility genes using arbitrary criteria. Similarly, this reveals that much about the immense complexity of the regulatory genome remains to be discovered and it opens the door to comprehensive analysis of the noncoding genome variants, the study of nonmessenger

RNA molecules and to the levels of expression of their trans targets at outermost positions of the genome.

4.5. Conclusions

Despite the enormous efforts of the past decades, genetic and molecular mechanisms underlying this disease have not yet been fully explained. GWAS and subsequent studies have begun to unravel the genetic contribution to the pathogenesis of CD. Although from the genetic standpoint, diseases of immune etiology show wide differences in the number of loci involved, the effect of each of these and the environmental factors involved, it is true that there is a strong overlap between this family of disorders. This overlap must involve the participation of common biological pathways and suggests that strategies for treatment may also be shared. However, the interpretation of association studies must be done with caution since it is true that each of the identified loci contains more than one gene. Strategies to identify potential etiological variants are indicated in Figure 3, and could, in the future, identify functional alterations underlying autoimmune diseases. Over time, these pathogenic variants may be included in risk prediction algorithms and allow for the diagnosis of individuals with a high genetic predisposition before the onset of symptoms, which could result in an improved quality of life and decreased healthcare costs. In addition, they could open the door to new therapeutic targets for CD itself and for other diseases of autoimmune etiology.

References

1. Sollid LM. Thorsby E. *HLA susceptibility penes in celiac disease: penetic mappinp and role in pathopenesis*. Gastroenterol. 1993; 105: 910-22.

2. Greco L. Romino R. Coto I. et al. *The first larpe population based twin study of coeliac disease*. Gut. 2002; 50: 624-8. http://dx.doi.org/10.1136/gut.50.5.624

3. Horton R. Wilming L. Rand V. Lovering RC. Bruford EA. Khodiyar VK. et al. *Gene map of the extended human MHC*. Nat Rev Genet. 2004; 5: 889-99. http://dx.doi.org/10.1038/nrg1489

4. Karell K. Louka AS. Moodie SJ. Ascher H. Clot F. Greco L. et al. *HLA types in celiac disease patients not carryinp the DQA1*05-DQB1*02 (DQ2) heterodimer: results from the European Genetics Cluster on Celiac Disease*. Hum Immunol. 2003; 64: 469-77. http://dx.doi.org/10.1016/S0198-8859(03)00027-2

5. Spurkland A. Sollid LM. Polanco I. Vartdal F. Thorsby E. *HLA-DR and -DQ penotypes of celiac disease patients serolopically typed to be non-DR3 or non-DR5/7*. Hum Immunol. 1992; 35: 188-92. http://dx.doi.org/10.1016/0198-8859(92)90104-U

6. Sollid LM. Thorsby E. *Evidence for a primary association of celiac disease to a particular HLA-DQ alpha/beta heterodimer*. J Exp Med. 1989; 169: 345–50. http://dx.doi.org/10.1084/jem.169.1.345

7. Sollid LM. *Coeliac disease: dissectinp a complex inflammatory disorder*. Nat Rev Immunol. 2002; 2: 647–55. http://dx.doi.org/10.1038/nri885

8. Van Belzen MJ. Koeleman BP. Crusius JB. et al. *Defininp the contribution of the HLA repion to cis DQ2-positive coeliac disease patients*. Genes Immun. 2004; 5: 215-20. http://dx.doi.org/10.1038/sj.gene.6364061

9. Ploski R. et al. *HLA-DQ (alpha 1*0501, beta 1*0201) associated susceptibility in celiac disease: a possible pene dosape effect of DQB1*0201*. Tissue Antigens 1993; 41: 173-7. http://dx.doi.org/10.1111/j.1399-0039.1993.tb01998.x

10. Lundin KE. Scott, H. Hansen T. Paulsen G. Halstensen TS. Fausa O. et al. *Gliadin-specific, HLA-DQ (alpha 1*0501, beta 1*0201) restricted T cells isolated from the small intestinal mucosa of celiac disease patients*. J Exp Med. 1993; 178: 187-96. http://dx.doi.org/10.1084/jem.178.1.187

11. Greco L. Corazza GR. Babron MC. Clot F. Fulchignoni-Lataud MCV. Percopo S. et al. *Genome search in celiac disease*. Am J Hum Genet. 1998; 62: 35-41. http://dx.doi.org/10.1086/301754

12. Greco L. Babron MC. Corazza GR. Percopo S. Sica R. Clot F. et al. *Existence of a penetic risk factor on chromosome 5q in Italian coeliac disease families*. Ann Hum Genet. 2001; 65: 35-41. http://dx.doi.org/10.1046/j.1469-1809.2001.6510035.x

13. Seegers D. Borm ME. Van Belzen MJ. et al. *IL12B and IRF1 pene polymorphisms and susceptibility to celiac disease*. Eur J Immunogenet. 2003; 30: 421-5. http://dx.doi.org/10.1111/j.1365-2370.2003.00428.x

14. Ryan AW. Thornton JM. Brophy K. Daly JS. McLoughlin RM. O'Morain C. et al. *Chromosome 5q candidate penes in coeliac disease: penetic variation at IL4, IL5, IL9, IL13, IL17B and NR3C1*. Tissue Antigens. 2005; 65: 150-5. http://dx.doi.org/10.1111/j.1399-0039.2005.00354.x

15. Castellanos-Rubio A. *Combined functional and positional pene information for the identification of susceptibility variants in celiac disease*. Gastroenterol. 2008; 134: 738-46. http://dx.doi.org/10.1053/j.gastro.2007.11.041

16. Koskinen LL. Einarsdottir E. Korponay-Szabo IR. et al. *Fine mappinp of the CELIAC2 locus on chromosome 5q31-q33 in the Finnish and Hunparian populations.* Tissue Antigens. 2009; 74: 408-16. http://dx.doi.org/10.1111/j.1399-0039.2009.01359.x

17. Holopainen P. Naluai AT. Moodie S. Percopo S. Coto I. Clot F. et al. *Candidate pene repion 2q33 in European families with coeliac disease.* Tissue Antigens. 2004; 63: 212-22. http://dx.doi.org/10.1111/j.1399-0039.2004.00189.x

18. Brophy K. Ryan AW. Thornton JM. et al. *Haplotypes in the CTLA4 repion are associated with coeliac disease in the Irish population.* Genes Immun. 2006; 7: 19-26. http://dx.doi.org/10.1038/sj.gene.6364265

19. Dema B. Martínez A. Fernández-Arquero M. Maluenda C. Polanco I. De la Concha EG. et al. *Lack of replication of celiac disease risk variants reported in a Spanish population usinp an independent Spanish sample.* Genes Immun. 2009; 10: 659-61. http://dx.doi.org/10.1038/gene.2009.54

20. Van Belzen MJ. Meijer JWR. Sandkuijl LA. Bardoel AFJ. Mulder CJJ. et al. *A major non-HLA locus in celiac disease maps to chromosome 19.* Gastroenterol. 2003; 125: 1032-41. http://dx.doi.org/10.1016/S0016-5085(03)01205-8

21. Capilla A. Donat E. Planelles D. Espinós C. Ribes-Koninckx C. Palau F. *Genetic analyses of celiac disease in a Spanish population confirm association with CELIAC3 but not with CELIAC4.* Tissue Antigens. 2007; 70: 324-9. http://dx.doi.org/10.1111/j.1399-0039.2007.00899.x

22. Monsuur AJ. De Bakker PIW. Alizadeh BZ. Xhernakova A. Bevova MR. Strengman E. et al. *Myosin IXB variant increases the risk of celiac disease and points toward a primary intestinal barrier defect.* Nat Genet. 2005; 37: 1341-4. http://dx.doi.org/10.1038/ng1680

23. Curley CR. Monsuur AJ. Wapenaar MC. Rioux JD. Wijmenga C. *A functional candidate screen for coeliac disease penes.* Eur J Hum Genet. 2006; 14: 1215-22. http://dx.doi.org/10.1038/sj.ejhg.5201687

24. Abel M. Cellier C. Kumar N. Cerf-Bensussan N. Schmitz J. Caillat-Zucman S. *Adulthood-onset celiac disease is associated with intercellular adhesion molecule-1 (ICAM-1) pene polymorphism.* Hum Immunol. 2006; 67: 612-7. http://dx.doi.org/10.1016/j.humimm.2006.04.011

25. Rueda B. Zhernakova A. López-Nevot MA. Martín J. Koeleman BPC. *Association study of functional penetic variants of innate immunity related penes in celiac disease.* BMC Med Genet. 2005; 3: 6-29. http://dx.doi.org/10.1186/1471-2350-6-29

26. Santin I. Castellanos-Rubio A. Perez de Nanclares G. Vitoria JC. Castaño L. Bilbao JR. *Association of KIR2DL5B pene with celiac disease supports the susceptibility locus on 19q13.4.* Genes Immun. 2007; 8: 171-6. http://dx.doi.org/10.1038/sj.gene.6364367

27. Fernandez-Jimenez N. et al. *Uprepulation of KIR3DL1 pene expression in intestinal mucosa in active celiac disease.* Hum Immunol. 2011; 72: 617-20. http://dx.doi.org/10.1016/j.humimm.2011.04.008

28. Fernandez-Jimenez N. Santín I. Irastorza I. Plaza-Izurieta L. Castellanos-Rubio A. Vitoria JC. Bilbao JR. *Analysis of beta-defensin and Toll-like receptor pene copy number variation in celiac disease.* Hum Immunol. 2010; 71: 833-6. http://dx.doi.org/10.1016/j.humimm.2010.05.012

29. Martín-Pagola A. Pérez-Nanclares G. Ortiz L. Vitoria JC. Hualde I. Zaballa R. et al. *MICA response to pliadin in intestinal mucosa from celiac patients.* Immunogenetics. 2004; 56: 549-54. http://dx.doi.org/10.1007/s00251-004-0724-8

30. Wapenaar MC. Van Belzen MJ. Fransen JH. Fariña Sarasqueta A. Houwen RHJ. Meijer JWR. et al. *The interferon pamma pene in celiac disease: aupmented expression correlates with tissue damape but no evidence for penetic susceptibility.* J. Autoimmun. 2004; 23: 183-90. http://dx.doi.org/10.1016/j.jaut.2004.05.004

31. Weersma RK. Zhernakova A. Nolte IM. Lefebvre C. Rioux JD. Mulder F. et al. *ATG16L1 and IL23R are associated with inflammatory bowel diseases but not with celiac disease in the Netherlands.* Am J Gastroenterol. 2008; 103: 621-7. http://dx.doi.org/10.1111/j.1572-0241.2007.01660.x

32. Núñez C. Dema B. Cénit MC. Polanco I. Maluenda C. Arroyo R. et al. *IL23R: a susceptibility locus for celiac disease and multiple sclerosis?* Genes Immun. 2008; 9: 289-93. http://dx.doi.org/10.1038/gene.2008.16

33. Einarsdottir E. Koskinen LLE. Dukes E. Kainu K. Suomela S. Lappalainen M. et al. *IL23R in the Swedish, Finnish, Hunparian and Italian populations: association with IBD and psoriasis, and linkape to celiac disease.* BMC Med Genet. 2009; 28: 10-8. http://dx.doi.org/10.1186/1471-2350-10-8

34. Medrano LM. García-Magariños M. Dema G. Espino L. Polanco I. Figueredo MA. et al. *Th17-related penes and celiac disease susceptibility.* PLoS One. 2012; 7: e31244. http://dx.doi.org/10.1371/journal.pone.0031244

35. Dema B. Martínez A. Fernández-Arquero M. Maluenda C. Polanco I. Figueredo MA. et al. *Autoimmune disease association sipnals in CIITA and KIAA0350 are not involved in celiac disease susceptibility.* Tissue Antigens. 2009; 73: 326-9. http://dx.doi.org/10.1111/j.1399-0039.2009.01216.x

36. Wapenaar MC. Monsuur AJ. Van Bodegraven AA. Weersma RK. Bevova MR. Linskens RK. et al. *Associations with tipht junction penes PARD3 and MAGI2 in Dutch patients point to a common barrier defect for coeliac disease and ulcerative colitis.* Gut. 2008; 57: 463-7. http://dx.doi.org/10.1136/gut.2007.133132

37. Diosdado B. Monsuur AJ. Mearin ML. Mulder C. Wijmenga C. *The downstream modulator of interferon-pamma, STAT1 is not penetically associated to the Dutch coeliac disease population.* Eur J Hum Genet. 2006; 14: 1120-4. http://dx.doi.org/10.1038/sj.ejhg.5201667

38. Castellanos-Rubio A. Santin I. Irastorza I. Sanchez-Valverde F. Castaño L. Vitoria JC. et al. *A repulatory sinple nucleotide polymorphism in the ubiquitin D pene associated with celiac disease.* Hum Immunol. 2010; 71: 96-9. http://dx.doi.org/10.1016/j.humimm.2009.09.359

39. Ciccocioppo R. Di Sabatino A. Bauer M. Della Riccia DN. Bizzini F. Biagi F. et al. *Matrix metalloproteinase pattern in celiac duodenal mucosa.* Lab. Invest. 2005; 85: 397-407. http://dx.doi.org/10.1038/labinvest.3700225

40. Van Heel DA. et al. *A penome-wide association study for celiac disease identifies risk variants in the repion harborinp IL2 and IL21.* Nat Genet. 2008; 39: 827-9. http://dx.doi.org/10.1038/ng2058

41. Hunt, KA. Zhernakova A. Turner G. Heap GAR. Franke L. Bruinenberg M. et al. *Newly identified penetic risk variants for celiac disease related to the immune response.* Nat Genet. 2008; 40: 395-402. http://dx.doi.org/10.1038/ng.102

42. Dubois PC. Trynka G. Franke L. Hunt KA. Romanos J. Curtotti A. et al. *Multiple common variants for celiac disease influencinp immune pene expression.* Nat Genet. 2010; 42: 295-302. http://dx.doi.org/10.1038/ng.543

43. Trynka G. Hunt KA. Bockett NA. Romanos J. Mistry V. Szperl A. et al. *Dense penotypinp identifies and localizes multiple common and rare variant association sipnals in celiac disease.* Nat Genet. 2011; 43: 1193-201. http://dx.doi.org/10.1038/ng.998

44. Plaza-Izurieta L. Castellanos-Rubio A, Irastorza I, Fernandez-Jimenez N, Gutierrez G, Bilbao JR. *Revisitinp penome wide association studies (GWAS) in coeliac disease: replication study in Spanish population and expression analysis of candidate penes.* J Med Genet. 2011; 48: 493-6. http://dx.doi.org/10.1136/jmg.2011.089714

45. Bondar C. Plaza-Izurieta L. Fernandez-Jimenez N. Irastorza I. Withoff S. CEGEC. Wijmenga C. Chirdo F. Bilbao JR. *THEMIS and PTPRK in celiac intestinal mucosa: coexpression in disease and after in vitro pliadin challenpe.* Eur J Hum Genet. 2013; 22: 358-62. http://dx.doi.org/10.1038/ejhg.2013.136

Chapter 7

Immunopathogenesis of Celiac Disease

E. Arranz[1], E. Montalvillo[1], J.A. Garrote[2]

[1]Mucosal Immunology Laboratory, IBGM, University of Valladolid-CSIC, Valladolid, Spain.

[2]Genetics and Molecular Biology Laboratory, Clinical Laboratory Service, Río Hortega University Hospital, Valladolid, Spain.

earranz@med.uva.es, enalmonn@hotmail.com, jagarrote@saludcastillayleon.es

Doi: http://dx.doi.org/10.3926/oms.213

How to cite this chapter

Arranz E, Montalvillo E, Garrote JA. *Immunopathogenesis of Celiac Disease.* In Rodrigo L and Peña AS, editors. *Celiac Disease and Non-Celiac Gluten Sensitivity.* Barcelona, Spain: OmniaScience; 2014. p. 123-149.

E Arranz, E. Montalvillo, J.A. Garrote

Abstract

Celiac disease is a chronic inflammatory process of the small intestine mediated by the immune system which affects genetically susceptible individuals following the ingestion of prolamins from wheat and other cereals. The interaction between genetic and environmental factors determines the loss of tolerance to gluten and the development of the intestinal lesion, with variable clinical and functional repercussions, characterized by an increased number of lymphocytes within the epithelium and the lamina propria, enterocyte apoptosis, the mucosal transformation, and the presence of anti-transglutaminase antibodies. The most accepted pathogenesis model for Celiac disease includes changes in digestion and in the transepithelial transport of gluten, and it is focused on the mechanisms of adaptive immunity triggered by the stimulation of CD4+ T lymphocytes after recognition of gluten peptides deaminated by the tissue transglutaminase (tTG) enzyme in the context of HLA-DQ2/DQ8 molecules, and the production of proinflammatory cytokines, specially IFNy. Furthermore, gluten has also a direct toxic effect on the epithelium, which depends on innate immunity with IL15 as the central mediator, manifested by the epithelial expression of stress molecules and the activation of cytotoxic functions by intraepithelial lymphocytes. The interaction between IL15 and its receptor, expressed by epithelial cells, may be also relevant for the induction of adaptive immunity to gluten. Further clarification is needed on several issues, like the passage of gluten into the lamina propria, the activation of free tTG, or the mechanisms regulating the activity of IL15, among others.

1. Introduction

Celiac disease (CD) is a chronic inflammatory disease of the small intestine caused by an improper immune response to wheat gluten and related proteins from other cereals[1-3] affecting genetically predisposed individuals at any stage of life. It is a common disorder with an estimated prevalence of nearly 1% in most of the populations studied[3-5], although only 1 of every 7-10 cases has been diagnosed.[6] Unfavorable interactions between susceptibility genes and environmental factors trigger this response against gluten in the intestinal mucosa, including an innate component responsible for epithelial injury and other adaptive mediated by CD4+ T lymphocytes specific to the lamina propria, and determines the remodeling of the mucosa. Along with the loss of oral tolerance to gluten, it generates other alterations which affect intraluminal digestion[7,8]; direct action of the gluten peptides on the epithelium and the transepithelial transport of lamina propria mucosa[9,10] have also been identified in CD.

The activation of CD4+ T lymphocytes from the mucosa on the lamina propria after the recognition of gliadin peptides modified by the transglutaminase 2 (TG2) enzyme, in the context of HLA-DQ2/DQ8 molecules, triggers an inflammatory response dominated by a Th1 cytokine profile, in which IFNγ predominates along with other proinflammatory cytokines (TNFα, IL 15 and IL 18), but with absence of IL 12 and a proportional decrease of immunoregulatory cytokine expression such as IL 10-14 and TGFβ.[11-14] Accordingly, a lesion of the small intestine mucosa occurs, which affects the absorption and utilization of nutrients and whose clinical and functional impact varies with the degree of atrophy or mucosal remodeling (Figure 1).

A   **B**

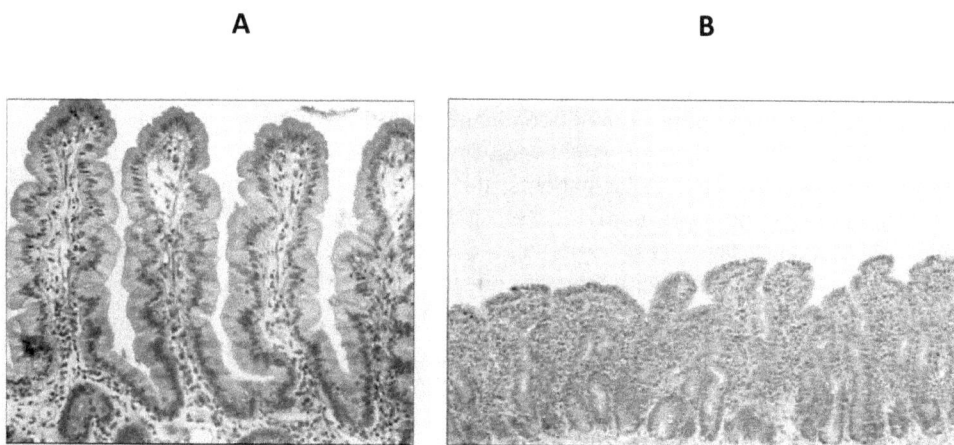

Figure 1. Duodenal mucosa from a non-celiac control patient (A) and from a celiac patient at the time of diagnosis (B) where the optic microscope reveals a lesion with villious atrophy and crypt hyperplasia.

In CD, the characteristic small intestine lesion can be recognized in several interrelated phases, described by Marsh.[15] Type 0, preinfiltrative, is characterized by mucosa with normal morphology, although local humoral immunity is altered; Type I, or infiltrative lesion, shows normal architecture in the mucosa, but with an increased IEL count (>25/100 enterocytes); Type II, hyperplastic lesion, is characterized by elongated or hyperplastic crypts with normal villious height and IEL infiltration; Type III, destructive lesion, may be partial (3a), subtotal (3b) or full (3c); this is the typical lesion diagnosis, with villi loss and tissue reorganization; Type IV, hypoplastic lesion is a true atrophic lesion with collagen deposits, observed in a small group of patients who do not respond to the gluten-free diet (Refractory CD).[16]

Gluten sensitization and activation of a specific response against gluten in the intestinal mucosa is an invariable feature of CD, however, the precipitant may be another factor which would be responsible for the full expression of the mucosal lesion; for example, in the form of a destructive lesion with loss of intestinal villi. According to the hypothesis proposed by Anne Ferguson[17] a few years ago, candidate factors may include an increase in intestinal permeability, nutritional defects, an increase in the amount of dietary gluten, alterations or defects in the intraluminal digestion of ingested gluten, adjuvant effects of a gastrointestinal infection, or some as yet unidentified gene not linked to HLA.

2. Pathogenic Theories of Celiac Disease

The metabolic theory held that CD was the result of an enzyme defect or some other mechanism that ultimately meant an incomplete gluten, or wheat gliadin digestion. Among the studies conducted to confirm this hypothesis, one in particular reported that homogenates from the small intestinal mucosa of untreated celiac patients were less efficient in degrading the product of gliadin digestion with pepsin and trypsin (PT), when compared with homogenates from non-celiac patients. These results led to propose that the incomplete digestion of gliadin was the trigger for the immune response, by means of the "lost peptidase hypothesis" or "metabolic hypothesis".[18]

This hypothesis, based on the incomplete digestion of gluten proteins in the intestinal mucosa of celiac patients, was subsequently confirmed using PT digests from alpha, beta, and gamma-gliadin, as well as many other immunodominant peptides.[19] It is striking that none of these studies found qualitative differences between the peptides generated in the mucosa of celiac patients and those from non-celiac patients; the only difference seemed to be their quantity, since in both cases the same peptides were generated, though in different amounts. Other studies did not find diferences[20]; instead, the enterocytic brush border enzymes in celiac patients, hydrolyzed PT-gliadin with the same effectiveness as those in non-celiacs.

Today, the enzyme-based hypothesis, formerly considered as a possible contributing factor in the pathogenesis of CD, has been virtually forgotten, due to a better molecular understanding of the pathophysiology of this disease. This has allowed the unraveling of many of the immunological mechanisms involved in the development of intestinal lesion, as well as to the discovery of the HLA-DQ2/DQ8 haplotype as a key factor in genetic predisposition.

3. The Immunological Theory of Celiac Disease

3.1. Immunity Against Dietary Antigens. Oral Tolerance

Under normal conditions, the response to the dietary proteins is oral tolerance, which is defined as the lack of a systemic immune response to certain antigens ingested after their systemic administration[21]. However, in CD there is a loss of tolerance to gluten and similar proteins. The capacity of the digestive tract's immune system to distinguish between dietary antigens and pathogenic microorganisms could be due to the fact that these furnish a persistent stimulus, associate other danger signals or else invade lymphoid tissues distant from the mucosa. Several mechanisms responsible for oral tolerance have been described: deletion (apoptosis), clonal anergy (functional inactivation of effector cells) and induction of regulatory T lymphocytes, which act through cytokines (IL 10 or TGF).[22,23]

The regulation of the response to dietary antigens, is determined by the way in which T lymphocytes recognize these antigens and the type and functional state of antigen-presenting cells (APCs) such as dendritic cells (DCs). Data from animal models and from observations in humans have led to explain oral tolerance as the result of immunoregulatory bowel conditions that lead to the differentiation of regulatory T lymphocytes (Treg)[24,25] and from other cells with a homeostatic function such as Tγδ+ cells and invariant NKT (iNKT). Another possibility is that the normal gut may respond with an IFNγ-dominated Th1 profile, even against dietary antigens, which would be the result of a balance between various factors (epithelial integrity, T lymphocytes development, immunoregulation, etc.). Th1 differentiation would not associate with tissue damage due to the control exerted by immature APCs upon effector lymphocytes, the former of which have a short half-life, and to the elimination induced by regulatory T lymphocytes.[25]

Dendritic cells (DCs) are the major APCs, especially for naive T lymphocytes and play a key role in intestinal homeostasis[26-28], as well as serving as a link between the innate and adaptive immune responses.[29,30] In the absence of other co-stimulatory signals, antigen presentation by these cells favors oral tolerance by decreasing its stimulatory capacity and/or promoting regulatory T lymphocyte differentiation[31], characterized by the CD4+ CD25high phenotype[24,32], and by the FoxP3 transcription factor, crucial for the functional development and maturation of these cells.[33] However, recent studies suggest that although FoxP3 is a transcription factor linked to the regulatory phenotype, it is not unique to a single cell type and would not be the best marker to identify regulatory T lymphocytes.[34] DCs also appear to have an important immunopathogenic role in CD due to their capacity to mature in response to danger signals from the innate immunity and to foster the induction of adaptive immune responses.[22,35]

Regulatory T lymphocytes (Treg) are the main homeostatic immune cells and have a key role in controlling of local inflammation. These cells perform their function by blocking T lymphocyte clonal expansion, both CD4+ and CD8+, as well as by inhibiting IL 2 production. By means of producing cytokines such as IL 10 and TGFß, Treg cells can modulate local inflammation by inhibiting Th1 responses and IFNγ production through cooperation with B cells in the IgA synthesis.[36,37] Other cells involved in gut homeostasis are CD4+ Th3, which perform their function through TGFβ production.[38] Recently, it has been determined that this cell population, at some point depends on the presence of FoxP3; it has been suggested, therefore, that Th3 and Treg cells could be the same cell population.[38]

There is another CD4+ population which expresses neither the FoxP3 transcription factor nor CD25 molecules on its surface and which has central role in controlling the inflammatory response to dietary antigens[39], such as the Tr1 lymphocytes, the leading IL 10 producers in the intestine. Under certain conditions, Th1, Th2 or Th17 lymphocytes can become IL10 producers, so Tr1 cells could not be other that CD4+ lymphocytes which have been chronically stimulated to reduce the production of pro-inflammatory cytokines and maintain IL 10 levels.[40] Within the gut, the activity of these non-Treg cells is more important than that of Treg in oral tolerance, since their number is far higher than that of CD4+CD25+FoxP3+ cells.

In addition to Treg cells, other cells that may be involved in the maintenance and regulation of intestinal homeostasis and oral tolerance are Tγδ+ intraepithelial lymphocytes (IEL), which significantly contribute to the circulating TCR+population[41], and their number is increased in the intestine of patients with CD.[42] Following their interaction with the antigen via TCR, these Tγδ+ cells quickly and transiently express the CCR7receptor, which allows their migration to the lymph nodes where they may act as APCs and induce specific Treg cell differentiation.[43]

Invariant NKT (iNKT) cells display NK cell markers such as CD161 (NK1.1), and an invariant Vα24β11 TCR that recognizes antigens along with CD1d molecules (MHC-1), highly expressed in the intestinal epithelium[44] and which represent 0.5-20% of the total cells.[45,46] A population with CD3-NK-like phenotype has also been described in the epithelium, which drastically decreases in CD patients.[47,48] Activated iNKT lymphocytes have a dual role, the iNKT CD4-CD8 subpopulation produces cytokines with a Th1 (IFNγ, TNFα) profile, while iNKTs CD4+ cells synthesize both Th1 and Th2 (IL 4, IL 13)cytokines.[32,49,50] The acquisition of a Th1 or Th2 profile depends on the strength of the interaction between the antigen and the CD1d molecule, the predominant cytokines in the local microenvironment and other co-stimulatory signals.[45] This ability to rapidly produce large amounts of Th1/Th2 cytokines, confers iNKT lymphocytes a significant role in oral tolerance, by modulating DC maturation towards the tolerogenic pathway, which is involved in the differentiation of Treg (IL 10 and TGFß) cells[44,51], as well as inducing clonal of antigen-specific T lymphocytes.[32]

The origin of immune cells in the duodenal mucosa is not clear at all. Under physiological conditions, during its activation, lymphocytes acquire recirculation properties which depend on the expression of adhesion molecules and chemokine receptors to direct their migration to specific tissues and microenvironments.[52,53] Activated lymphocytes in the intestinal lymphoid tissue tend to return to the intestine. This selective migration is directed by the α4β7 integrin, whose ligand is mucosal addressing (MAdCAM-1) from the high endothelial venules, Peyer's patches and mesenteric lymph nodes in the intestine.[53] The CCR9 chemokine receptor intervenes in the effector T lymphocyte recruitment for the intestine via interaction with its ligand CCL25 (TECK), selectively expressed in part of the intestine.[54] Conversely, selectin carbohydrate ligands P and E, are collectively referred to as human leukocyte antigens (CLA).[55] Other chemokine receptors such as CCR4, CCR8, and CCR10 have also been implicated in the selective migration to the skin.[55, 56]

Therefore, in diseases where the pathogenic involvement of immune response mediated by antigen-specific lymphocytes is known, as in the case of CD[2,57], an increase in the selective migration profile markers in the circulating cell populations in celiac patients is expected. However, little information is available on the expression of these cell markers not only in CD patients, but also in the general population. Preliminary results[31,58] from healthy adult volunteers without known autoimmune or malignant diseases, suggest that circulating blood CDs are double positive for migration markers to the intestine and skin while circulating monocytes preferably express intestinal markers and T lymphocytes express markers for bowels or skin. However, this information is yet to be confirmed in the case of CD patients.

3.2. The Two Signal Pathogenic Model

The immunological theory is the one that currently best explains the pathogenesis of CD. Formerly, it was thought that what happens in the lamina propria mucosa, in the context of a CD4+ T lymphocyte mediated response, with HLA-DQ2/8 restriction and IFNγ release, was fundamental in the development of this enteropathy. Recently, it has been observed that the innate immunity, which acts primarily in the intraepithelial compartment, is also critical to the immune response to gluten. The most accepted immunopathogenic model states that gluten has a double effect involving innate immunity (direct toxic effect of gluten on the epithelium) and adaptive or specific immunity (through T CD4+ lymphocytes of the lamina propria and underlying tissue).[59]

This immunopathogenic model integrates several necessary elements in the intestinal mucosa[1,60,61], such as the presence of gluten peptides (toxic and immunogenic), the effect of some of these peptides on the epithelium, TG2 enzyme activity, the presence APCs which express HLA-DQ molecules and CD4+ T lymphocytes reactive to gluten. Toxic peptides not recognized by T lymphocytes have a rapid and unspecific effect on the epithelium, while the response to immunogenic peptides is slower, after passing through the epithelium to reach the mucosal lamina propria there to undergo TG2 deamidation, after which to bind with high affinity to HLA DQ2 or DQ8 molecules. Gluten specific T lymphocytes recognize these T epitopes modified in the context of membrane DQ2 or DQ8 molecules in local APCs, such as DCs. These immune responses (innate and adaptive) trigger different mechanisms which cause damage through epithelial cytotoxicity and restructuring of the extracellular matrix (the so called mucosal transformation).

Wheat gluten contains two families of proteins, gliadin and glutenin (insoluble in alcohol), with fragments harmful for CD patients and which are also found in the proteins in rye (secalins), barley (hordeins) and oats (avenines). Gliadin proteins can be subdivided into α-, γ- and ω-gliadins and into subunits of high molecular weight (HMW), medium molecular weight (MMW) and low molecular weight (LMW) for glutenines.[62] All these proteins are designated by the generic name of prolamins since they share a very similar amino acid sequence and a high content of the hydrophobic amino acids glutamine and proline.[63,64] Peptides considered toxic induce damage in cultured intestinal duodenal biopsies[65], or after being administered in vivo on the proximal or distal intestine[66]; those which are immunogenic stimulate T lymphocyte lines with DQ2/DQ8 restriction, obtained from the intestine or peripheral blood from CD patients.[67]

3.3. Innate Immune Response to Gluten

Some gluten fragments, such as p31-49 or 31-43 from the α-gliadin, induce an immediate innate immune response, associated neither with T lymphocytes nor with HLA-DQ2/8 dependent antigen presentation, although these mechanisms are not yet fully understood.[68] In an *ex vivo* culture model from biopsies from CD patients, it has been observed that the immediate response induced by the 31-49 peptide is associated with IL 15 expression, cyclooxygenase (COX-2) and CD25 and CD83 activation markers by mononuclear cells from the lamina propria.[69] Furthermore, oxidative stress appears mediated by the formation of nitric oxide, which comes primarily from iNOS induction in enterocytes[70,71], which, in turn, induces the expression in these cells of ligands like MICA.[72] Gliadin is also able to weaken tight-junction type bonds located between intestinal epithelial cells.[9]

Intraepithelial lymphocytes (IELs) are found in the basolateral area of epithelial cells and have a crucial role in the immune surveillance of the intestinal epithelium. The population of IELs in the small intestine is a mixture of TCRαβ+ T lymphocytes, TCRγδ+ T lymphocytes and NK cells, although most of them are TCRαβ+CD8+ lymphocytes.[2] Furthermore, most TCR+ IELs express diverse NK receptors different from those expressed by T lymphocytes in the circulating peripheral blood.[73] These NK receptors act not only as costimulatory molecules, but also as T lymphocyte activators in stress situations.[74] In active CD, the number of CD8+ TCRαβ+ and TCRγδ+ IELs is very high. It is unclear whether this situation depends on epithelial homeostasis changes or if it is a consequence of the proinflammatory environment created by the CD4+ T lymphocyte mediated response in the lamina propria mucosa.

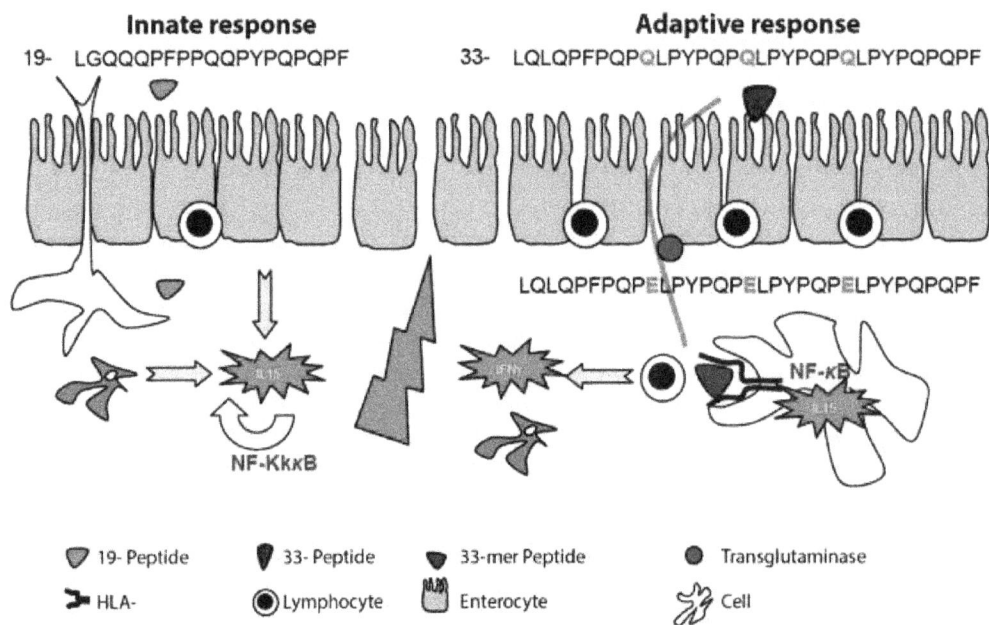

Innate response
19- LGQQQPFPPQQPYPQPQPF

Adaptive response
33- LQLQPFPQPQLPYPQPQPLPYPQPQPLPYPQPQPF

LQLQPFPQPELPYPQPELPYPQPELPYPQPQPF

NF-KB
NF-KkκB

▽ 19- Peptide   ▼ 33- Peptide   ◣ 33-mer Peptide   ● Transglutaminase
➤ HLA-   ◉ Lymphocyte   ⊔ Enterocyte   Cell

Figure 2. Gluten has a dual effect on the small intestine mucosa. Toxic peptides, such as the 19-mer, induce a nonspecific innate immune response characterized by the presence of IL 15, produced by enterocytes. IL 15, in turn, activates the NF-kB transcription factor in the adjacent cells, which enhances IL 15 production and iNOS induction, responsible for an oxidative stress and innate feedback situation. The expression of molecules such as MICA and/or HLA-E is increased in enterocytes and IL 15 triggers cytotoxicity (apoptosis) on these cells by inducing the expression of NKG2D and NKG2C molecules (ligands MICA and HLA-E respectively) in intraepithelial lymphocytes. Finally, IL 15 may weaken the tight-junctions between enterocytes. The adaptive response is facilitated by increased intestinal permeability allowing the passage of immunogenic peptides like 33-mer to the lamina propria, which are deaminated by the tissue transglutaminase (TG2) enzyme. Besides, IL 15 activates dendritic cells, which increases the surface expression of the costimulatory molecules necessary for an effective antigen presentation and restricted by HLA-DQ2/8, to T lymphocytes. These cells trigger an IFNγ predominant Th1 response with IL 10 absence, and the release by stromal cells of keratocinic growth factor and metalloproteinases. The Innate and Adaptive Immune Responses are responsible for the intestinal damage.

The principal mechanism that prompts the innate response depends on the release of IL 15 by enterocytes.[75] In CD, IL 15 expression is observed both in the epithelium surface enterocytes as well as on the mononuclear cells in the lamina propria mucosa.[76,77] IL 15 promotes the survival, activation and proliferation of IELs, independently of TCR interaction, besides controlling the clonal expansion TCRγδ IELs and of cells bearing NKG2D receptors[78,79], whose ligands are MICA molecules (MHC-I-non-classical) expressed by enterocytes.[76,77,80] In addition, IL 15 favors a NK-type reprogramming of IELs by activating intracellular perforin/granzyme signaling cascades as well as and Fas/FasL, which contribute to trigger inflammation and cytotoxicity on the enterocytes.[75,78,81] IL 15 favors immune response feedback by inducing the secretion of mediators of non-specific inflammation, such as arachidonic acid and leukotrienes, by the IEL. It also induces the formation of the inducible Nitric Oxide Synthase enzyme (iNOS)[67, 71] by stromal cells from the lamina propria by a means of a mechanism dependent on the NF-kB transcription factor, which favors the presence of oxygen-reactive species and oxidative stress. Finally, IL 15 contributes to the weakening of the tight junctions[9], with increased intestinal permeability and the passage of gluten the lamina propria mucosa. In CD pathogenesis, IL 15 acts as a mediator between the innate response and the epithelial lesion besides promoting the survival of specific T lymphocytes and the maintenance of the inflammatory response[82] (Figure 2).

In Refractory CD (RCD), the survival, expansion and acquisition of the NK phenotype by IELs is much more pronounced than in classical CD, possibly resulting from the presence of large amounts of IL 15. In type II RCD, patients have an aberrant clonal population of IELs that lose surface expression of TCR CD3. In studies using lines of aberrant IELs from patients with type II RCD, it has been observed that, under stimulation with IL 15, these cells express granzyme B and are capable of lysing the HT29 epithelial cell line, suggesting a role for aberrant IELs in the continuous epithelial damage in seen in RCD II.[83] Therefore, the NK transformation suffered by IELs via IL 15 is an essential step in the immunopathogenesis of RCD.

Gliadin might have a direct toxic effect on the intestine and the induction of a gliadin dependent innate immune response in the duodenum would not be unique to patients with CD. In Caco-2 cell lines, gliadin stimulation induces an apoptosis increase and transepithelial permeability.[84] Gliadin-induced CD maturation has been described in mice, as well as quimiocin release.[85] In enterocyte cell lines, gliadin and the derived peptides 13-and 33-mer increase zonulin dependent intestinal permeability[9] and also the expression of proinflammatory genes and cytokine secretion in macrophage lines.[86] Unlike other dietary proteins, gliadin can also induce expression of maturation markers and the release of cytokines and chemokines in DCs, through an NFkB-dependent mechanism.[85] In this context, it has been suggested that gliadin may be a nonspecific IL 15 inductor in the duodenum in both CD patients and non-CD individuals.[87] Recent studies indicate that the enterocyte apical membrane can recognize gluten fragments through the CXCR3 chemokine receptor.[88] Furthermore, some APCs such as monocytes, macrophages and DCs, can recognize gluten through the TLR4 pattern recognition receptor.[86,89] Remarkably, the intracellular signaling cascade in both mechanisms (CXCR3 and TLR4) converges on the myeloid differentiation factor (MyD88).[88] The role of these receptors in the context of the intestinal innate immune response and whether they are the only receptors involved in this response remain open questions.

3.4. Beyond the Innate Immune Response: IL 15/IL 15 Rα Interaction

Although the effects of IL 15 are traditionally considered to be associated with innate immunity, they are also important in the induction of adaptive immunity, which is particularly evident in CD, where, besides the innate effects like NK-like reprogramming of IELs[78,79,81] or stress molecule/MICA induction enterocytes[72], it can also act as a clear nexus between both types of immune responses being a potent DC activator[90,91], and so also to the specific CD4+ T lymphocytes. IL 15 thus becomes the initiator of the clonal expansion and the Th1-type immune response manifested by intraepithelial lymphocytosis, crypt hyperplasia and villous flattening.

The IL-15 receptor shares two subunits with the IL-2 receptor: the common γ chain and the IL 2Rβ subunit.[91,92] The former is also shared with other cytokines (IL 4, IL 7, IL 9 and IL 21) each of which have other specific sub-units responsible for the binding specificity and, thus for posterior signaling.[93] However, despite this similarity in the receptor, IL 15 and IL 2 have very different roles. Thus IL 2 appears to be a key modulator of the T lymphocyte dependent adaptive immune processes, while IL 15 has a much wider range of action, although focused primarily on the innate response.[90] The receptor's subunit, IL 15Rα, is responsible for bestowing ligand specificity. In fact, IL 15 has a high binding specificity to the IL 15Rα receptor, to type I transmembrane protein, even in the absence of IL 15Rβ and IL 15Rγ/γc subunits.[92] Messenger RNA levels from IL 15Rα have been detected on a wide variety of cellular systems, immunological as well as non-immunological[92,94], suggesting a complex regulatory mechanism as well as that IL 15/IL 15Rα signaling can interrelate various cell systems.[95] Furthermore, IL 15 is able to positively modulate IL 21, another cytokine involved in CD.[96]

Recent studies have found that the duodenum of CD patients exhibits increased levels of the IL 15 receptor (IL 15R) compared to the intestine of non-CD patients. The fact that higher levels of IL 15R are maintained even after complete normalization of mucosal histology in patients treated with GFD suggests that it is a pre-disposing factor in the development of this pathology. Such high levels of IL 15R confer CD patients a lower immune response threshold to IL 15.[97,98] This immune mechanism based on a lower threshold for IL 15 in CD patients may be key in the pathogenesis, as it facilitates the connection between the establishment of an innate immune response to gluten, and an adaptive immune response against this protein, which prevents the development of oral tolerance mechanisms.

3.5. Adaptive Immune response to gluten

Tissue transglutaminase (TG2) is a widely distributed enzyme in the body, whose main function is to catalyze the modification of proteins by transamination or deamination. In CD, TG2 has a fundamental role in the pathogenic mechanism through the enzymatic modification of immunodominant gliadin peptides, which increases their affinity for the HLA-DQ[99] molecule but is also the main (auto) antigen for specific serum antibodies, which are of great value for diagnosis.[100] In patients with active CD, TG2 is expressed in the epithelial brush border and in the subepithelial zone of the lamina propria area mucosa.[101] The main TG2 exogenous substrate is gliadin, which contains positively charged amino acids. TG2 induces ordered and specific glutamine residue substitution for negatively-charged glutamic acid residues[100], which promotes interaction with other basic amino acids located in anchoring positions to the HLA-DQ2 and DQ8 molecules, and increases their ability to stimulate CD4 T lymphocytes+.[101,102] The enzymatic modification which unmasks the most immunogenic epitopes to gliadin and other prolamins, or gives rise to new ones through interaction with extracellular matrix proteins, could be responsible for the loss of tolerance and the appearance of autoimmune diseases.[103,104]

Gliadins are a heterogeneous mixture of more than 40 components which contain multiple immunogenic peptides against which patients show different sensitivity and even a single patient may respond to more than one. Immunodominant peptides, such as those of from the α-gliadin region[57-75], induce specific immune responses in virtually all patients.[105-107] The major epitopes on α-and γ-gliadins, as well as on glutenins, have been identified; many bind to HLA-DQ2 and DQ8 others and, in most cases, TG2 deamidation shows an increased antigenicity, except for glutenin derivatives.[101,102,108] The richness of glutamine and proline, and their location in the primary structure influences peptide immunogenicity by determining the molecular structure and acting as preferential binding residue in the HLA-DQ molecule motifs as well as controlling TG2 specificity, which acts on glutamine residues at positions adjacent to those of proline in QXP-type sequences but not in QP or QXXP (Q=glutamine, P=proline, X=other).[1,107,108] By means of algorithms based on the separation these residues and through the presence/absence of other amino acids, it has been possible to predict more than the existence of more than 50 immunogenic peptides in wheat gluten, hordeins and secalins and which are nearly absent in avenins.[108]

In active CD, there has been an increase in the passage, through the epithelium, of both toxic as well as immunogenic fragments.[109] Incomplete intraluminal gluten digestion can generate residual fragments, such as the 33 amino acid peptide of α-gliadin[71,110], whose glutamine and proline content confers resistance to proteolysis by digestive enzymes, favoring the formation of large fragments with several immunodominant T epitopes, which are the preferred substrates of TG2.[111] The bacterial enzyme prolyl-endopeptidase (PEP) induces the rapid degradation of this fragment and prevents the formation of T epitopes able to activate the immune response harmful to the intestine.[110]

Adaptive immunity mediated by specific T lymphocytes requires that the antigen presentation to T lymphocytes of the lamina propria be performed by APCs bearing the HLA-DQ2/DQ8 restriction element. The HLA-DQ2 and DQ8 molecules confer susceptibility through their main function, that is to say, to present small gluten peptides to the intestinal CD4+ T lymphocytes in the APCs membrane, but which could also modulate the development of the repertoire of T lymphocytes in the thymus.[112] The CD4+ T lymphocytes recognize gliadin peptides in the DQ2/DQ8 molecule context that bind peptide fragments with negatively charged amino acids in certain positions of the structural binding motifs, located in the central position (4th, 6th, 7th) to HLA-DQ2 and outermost (1st, 4th, 9th) for HLA-DQ8.[104,112] The fact that, in each peptide, the residues are deaminated in different positions suggests that the specific immune response to gluten could be generated against various pathogenic causes.

The main APCs from the lamina propria mucosa are the macrophages (20%) and, especially, the DCs (80%). The DCs come mostly from extravasated monocytes recruited to the inflamed mucosa, where they differentiate *in situ*.[30,35] In active CD, there is an increase of APCs, mainly DCs expressing activation markers on the surface. These DCs, with a HLA-DQ2+ CD11c+ CD68-CD1c-BDCA3-phenotype play a central role in the activation of memory T lymphocytes reactive to gluten that accumulate in the small intestine of CD patients and which are ultimately responsible for tissular injury.[35,113] APCs can also be activated as a consequence of IL 15 released during the innate response induced by gluten.[114,115] In an animal model, digested wheat gluten was observed to induce maturation of DCs, along with the expression of costimulatory molecules and chemokine secretion.[85] In CD, a rapid accumulation of CD14+CD11c+ DCs can be seen preceding structural changes, indicating that this subtype is directly related to the immunopathology of the disease. The expression of CCR2 and CD14 in these cells may indicate that they are monocytes extravasated from peripheral blood.[116]

CD4+ T lymphocytes in the lamina propria mucosa recognize gliadin peptides such as the 33-mer (fragments 56-88 of α-gliadin), modified by TG2 and presented by HLA-DQ2 or DQ8 molecules by DCs[22,35,106,115,117], leading to response dominated by Th1 profile cytokines with IFNγ predominance and other pro-inflammatory cytokines (TNF, IL18, among others) and a proportional decrease of regulatory or anti-inflammatory cytokines (IL 10 and TGFβ).[118,119] This pro-inflammatory profile will be ultimately involved in the tissue remodeling mechanisms.

The presence of gluten specific CD4+ T lymphocytes has been confirmed in the lamina propria of the small intestine mucosa in CD patients, from which gluten specific cell clones were obtained.[118] These cells express the αβ T lymphocyte receptor (TCR) and a CD45RO+ memory cell phenotype and, after stimulation, they produce Th0/Th1 type cytokines, predominantly IFNγ but with absence of interleukin-12 (IL 12), a pattern which disappears under remission.[11,115,120] The increased production of Th1 cytokines is related to with delayed hypersensitivity reactions and autoimmune phenomena and, in functional studies, it has been shown that activation of these cells is associated with extracellular matrix alterations in the lamina propria and the epithelial proliferation.[120]

The differentiation of CD4+ T lymphocytes predominantly towards a Th1 or Th2 phenotype of cytokine production depends on the nature and concentration of the antigen, APC type and the local cytokine concentration.[26] An alteration in the cytokine balance could explain findings in the celiac intestine where an abnormal or uncontrolled Th response against gluten could lead to intestinal inflammation and damage. However, the absence of the main Th1-inducing factor (IL 12) suggests that the differentiation of Th1 effector cells could be related to other cytokines, among them, interferon-α (IFNα) or interleukin-18 (IL 18), which share some of their functions with it.[104] Additionally, other Th1-and IL 12-mediated enteropathies, such as Crohn's disease, show more severe damage with tissue loss and the degree of injury is related to the levels of Tumor Necrosis Factor-α (TNFα).

In the celiac intestine there could be an IFNγ increase along with an altered pro-and anti-inflammatory cytokine balance, such as the one between IFNγ and TGFß. The epithelium and the lamina propria in a healthy intestine express TGFβ, but in CD, it decreases in the epithelium surface and disappears from the crypts, increasing in the lamina propria around macrophages and activated T lymphocytes, where there is no tissue destruction. IFNα can intervene in the differentiation of Th1 cells, promoting the production of IFNγ, and it has been observed that administration of IFNα in susceptible individuals may promote Th1 responses associated with hyperplastic injuries.[115] Although yet to be confirmed, IFNα could be secreted by fibroblasts and activated macrophages or even by lamina propria DCs[75] after an intestinal infection episode, which would contribute to inflammation rescuing apoptosis activated T cells, maintaining memory T cells after stimulus disappearance and increasing the expression of costimulatory molecules in local APCs. In contrast to IL 12, IL 18, produced by macrophages, DCs and epithelial cells, does not act on naive cells but on memory and effector cells, enhancing the IL 12 or IFNα dependent IFNγ expression. Under normal conditions, the intestine expresses IL 18, however, it increases in CD at the expense of its mature form requiring intervention of the Converter Enzyme IL 1β (ICE) or local proteases.[12]

In active CD, there is an increase in plasma cells in the lamina propria, with a density two to three times higher in the celiac lesion[121], and CD is characterized by the presence of a variety of serum antibodies against self and foreign molecules.[122] In 1997, TG2 was identified as the main autoantigen to antiendomisium antibodies.[122] There have also been other different autoantibodies, including antibodies against actin-type proteins, different types of collagen and several members of the transglutaminase family: TG3, TG6, and Factor XII.[124] It ought to be mentioned that complexes formed by IgA/TG3 have been found in the skin of patients with dermatitis herpetiformes[57,123], and the presence of antibodies against the TG6 neuronal enzyme has been related to ataxia.[124] These findings could explain the development of extraintestinal manifestations in CD.

B lymphocytes are also professional APCs via BCR receptor. There are few virgin or memory B lymphocytes and most are plasma blasts or plasma cells from the lamina propria with low HLA class II expression.[125] It is likely that B lymphocytes have a more important role as a APCs in the mesenteric lymph nodes in order to amplify of the T cell response to the gluten. B lymphocytes specific for TG2 would preferentially stimulate reactive T lymphocytes against peptides specific to deaminated gliadin, which would explain why antibodies against these peptides are good CD predictors.

4. Interaction between Innate and Adaptive Immunity to Gluten

Induction of the adaptive response in CD is tightly controlled by innate immunity. DCs not only recognize invading pathogens but decide what kind of effector response must be deployed. Clearly, with no signals from intestinal DCs, the gluten specific T lymphocyte response could not be triggered. Recently, using the THP-1126 human macrophage cell line, it has been demonstrated that gliadin is able to stimulate cytokine production and induce monocyte derived DC maturation.[127] In other studies with *ex vivo* tissue cultures it was observed that gliadin and the p31-43 gliadin derived fragment can induce IL 15 secretion[67] and increase IEL cytotoxicity.[78,79] IL 15 is particularly produced by activated DCs and other APCs, in such a way that DCs simultaneously intervene in two effector responses: adaptive (mediated by gluten specific CD4+ T lymphocytes) and innate (mediated by IELs).[128, 129]

IL 15 production by DCs dependent on the specific T lymphocyte response may explain why the innate response to gliadin is produced only in the duodenum of celiac patients and not in other individuals. A pro-inflammatory state of the mucosa would be an essential prerequisite for gliadin triggering the innate immunity. It is still unknown by what means the mechanism by which gliadin, and especially the p31-43 fragment, is able to directly stimulate IL 15production, although recent studies suggest that TG2 may play an important role in this process.[68]

5. Gluten Transport across the Epithelium

Under normal conditions, protein peptides are hydrolyzed in the intestinal lumen leading to smaller peptides or isolated ones isolated aminoacids by means of gastric, pancreatic and intestinal peptidases and also from the brush border before transepithelial transport to the lamina propria mucosa. Incomplete intraluminal gluten digestion originates residual fragments such as the one at the 57-75 position of α-gliadin, resistant to enzymatic proteolysis due to its content of glutamine and proline, which includes several immunodominant T epitopes.[8] Due to their large size, gluten peptides like 33mer are not readily absorbed through the normal mechanisms followed by dietary proteins. The major theories state that gliadin could reach the lamina propria where the adaptive immune response takes place through two main routes: the transcellular route through enterocytes and the paracellular route through the *Tight-Junctions* (TJs) between enterocytes. A third possibility involves direct gluten access to the lamina propria gluten due to direct uptake by DCs. However, lack of studies that address this issue in model human biopsies make it difficult to elucidate the subject.

The great majority of dietary proteins are absorbed, as simple amino acids or small peptides, through the intestinal epithelium by transcellular transport. This process involves endocytosis mechanisms in the apical membrane and, in transit to the basal membrane, endosomes are generally conjugated with lysosomes carrying, in turn, more proteases, which facilitates complete peptide degradation.[130] However, the antigenic structure of gliadin favors differential transport within the enterocytes[10,109] which may associate lysosome evasion, reaching the lamina propria in an immunogenic context. Several studies support this possibility and it has been observed that, in CD patients, there is a high level of transport from the enterocyte apical membrane to the basal membrane by an IFNγ dependent mechanism.[131,132] IFNγ weakens the intestinal barrier, promoting the internalization of TJs, and in a Caco-2 cells model, it has been observed that stimulation with IFNγ is associated with increased translocation of the 33mer peptide.[10]

Recently, another transepithelial gliadin transport mechanism has been identified which would be mediated by the CD71 transferrin receptor.[109] This CD71 receptor is overexpressed on the apical surface of the enterocytes in active CD and it binds to the secreted IgA. Transcytosis experiments performed *ex vivo* suggest that CD71 can mediate the transport of IgA-gliadin complexes, and in patients with active CD, IgG-gliadin complexes have also been found. Given the fact that the neonatal Fc receptor (FcRn) is expressed in epithelial cells of the human intestine and that it can mediate apical to basolateral transcytosis of IgG-antigen immunocomplexes[109], FcRn could also transport antigens across the epithelial barrier by transcytosis of immunocomplexes formed by IgG anti-gliadin and gliadin.

The P31-43 peptide can produce two major effects on the alteration of intracellular vesicular traffic: it modifies recycling of the IL 15/IL 15Rα complex, which favors innate immunity overexpression and activation, it also increases enterocyte proliferation in the crypts through cooperation between the IL 15 receptor and the epidermal growth factor (EGFR), with consequent remodeling of the duodenal mucosa. Moreover, peptide accumulation in the enterocyte lysosomes activates the innate response via ROS-TG2, TG2 then acting as an activator of proteasomic ubiquitination of degradation leading to mucosal inflammation, decreasing the expression of the PPARγ molecule.[132]

The intestinal lumen proteins can pass inside by means of paracellular transport between enterocytes. Intestinal permeability is increased in celiac patients due to by alteration of TJs between enterocytes, compared to non-celiac control subjects. This finding appears to have a genetic component as also seen in non-affected relatives of celiac patients.[9] This, however, by itself does not explain the massive peptides traffic produced in active CD. Another possibility involves active gliadin effect on intestinal permeability favoring its weakening. Gluten is recognized in the apical membrane of enterocytes through the CXCR3 chemokine receptor, which promotes the paracrine secretion of the zonulin protein.[88] When it is recognized by adjacent enterocytes, zonulin triggers an intracellular signaling cascade which implies the reorganization of its cytoskeleton favoring TJ joints decoupling between enterocytes.[9,10,133] Therefore, gliadin, besides acting indirectly through IL 15, may also induce the opening the TJs, which destroys the integrity of the epithelial barrier and makes it possible that the larger peptides have easier access to the lamina propria.

6. Inflammatory Mechanisms in Celiac Disease

The presence of inflammatory mechanisms in the lamina propria is not enough to trigger tissue damage. None of the known cytokines involved in CD is ultimately responsible for the injury mechanisms, as mediator molecules are released as a consequence of the innate and adaptive responses, or as it seems likelier, as a result of the interaction between these two. Intestinal inflammation and damage are usually the result of the interaction between lymphoid and non-lymphoid cells that release different mediators, many of which are non-specific, able to interact and amplify signals culminating in intestinal mucosa tissue damage. Non-specific mechanisms are mediated by an innate immune response that does not require antigen presentation and therefore T lymphocyte intervention. Transcription factor NF-kβ[134,135] plays a major role in such responses, and among its many effects, enterocytic IL 15 secretion is included, as in the case of CD.[75] The IL 15 cytokine, the main innate immunological response, is itself a factor of positive feedback for the signal that induces the expression of NF-kβ in adjacent cells.[135] Another NFkβ effect is the induction of the iNOS (inducible nitric oxide synthase) enzyme[67,71], whose presence in the lamina propria is an oxidative stress factor that affects NF-kβ re-induction and the maintenance of an inflammatory response.

NF-kβ also has a key role in the connection between innate immunity and adaptive immunity. The DCs, which initiate adaptive immunity in the lamina propria by antigen presentation to gluten-reactive CD4+ T lymphocytes[136], need the activation of this transcription factor in order to increase the membrane expression of HLA (DQ2/8) molecules and of costimulatory ones (CD80/B7.1, CD86/B7.2, CD83) and thus, carrying out the antigen presentation function.[137] Furthermore, these cells can be activated by innate immunity cell populations, such as NK, iNKT and/or Tγδ, which in turn are activated by stress signals induced in an innate immunity context.[44,136] Thus, DCs act as a sensor capable of uniting both innate and adaptive responses which, once activated, would also stimulate growth and function of these innate immunity and the swift production of perforins and granzymes, besides being an IFNγ source.[44,45] Both feedback loops formed by the interaction between innate lymphocytes/DCs and the NFkB/IL 15-iNOS system activation, would help maintain the state of stress in the intestinal mucosa.

Stromal fibroblasts are also susceptible to the local stress microenvironment (presence of nitric oxide, IFNγ, IL 15, etc.). As a result, these cells secrete the keratinocyte growth factor (KGF) to the lamina propria[120], which seems to be involved in crypt hyperplasia, characteristic of a type II Marsh lesion. There is also an increase in the expression of adhesion molecules on the vascular endothelium and chemokines synthesis, which contribute to the recruitment of inflammatory cells, and the synthesis of metalloproteinases (MMPs) along with the blocking of their tissue inhibitors (TIMP-1). MMPs are an endopeptidase family whose primary role is the degradation of extracellular matrix components (such as proteoglycans and glycoproteins) and mucosal destruction[25,138], which is manifested, according to their of severity, as type III forms of destructive Marsh lesion. In the inflamed gut the expression of some MMPs increases, and in CD there has been described a correlation between non-specific inflammation mechanisms, as the levels of MMP-12 expression, and the presence of IFNγ, with the degree of mucosal injury.[139]

7. Celiac Disease and Intestinal Microbiota

In patients with CD-induced alterations in the intestinal microbiota have been detected, which are characterized by an increase of Gram-negative bacteria and reduced bifidobacteria.[140] Recent studies have found differences in the fecal microbiota of patients with untreated CD, which are partially restored after following the GFD.[141] Specific components of the intestinal microbiota can influence maturation of dendritic cells in terms of phenotype and function, as well as their interactions with epithelial cells. This would define the role of dendritic cells in the disease's progression.[142] However, further studies are required to explain how these changes in the intestinal flora may affect the pathogenesis and prognosis of CD.

Preliminary results from our group suggest the presence, in the intestinal protein extract, of 7 bands with specific gliadinase activity which are metalloproteasic in nature and can involve microbial activity. This could be a differentiating factor would allow to identify, with a confidence of more than 90%, whether the duodenal explant originated from a celiac patients (active or in remission), or from a non-EC control patient. Available data do not allow us to affirm that the different bacterial populations recently described in the duodenum of celiac patients are the carriers of these gliadinases.[143,144] However, the fact that this enzymatic activity has not been found virtually on no non-celiac individuals seems to indicate that the bacterial population and activity may participate in the pathogenesis of CD.[145]

8. Some Unresolved Issues

First, elucidation is still needed on how immunogenic gliadin peptides pass from the intestinal lumen to the lamina propria in the early stages of CD. It has been suggested that peptides can be transported over an increased intestinal permeability secondary to a viral intestinal infection[109,146], or by means of IgA-mediated retrotranscitosis.[147,148]

Second, the p31-49 peptide of the α-gliadin has a direct effect on the intestinal epithelium. However, although this seems clear, it is still unknown how it is produced and how it contributes to the development of CD.

Third, the TG2 is a crucial factor in antigen presentation of gluten derived peptides. In basal conditions, TG2 is expressed intracellularly in an inactive form or on the cell surface. It still not known how TG2 is activated and released in CD. It has been proposed that TG2 is released after tissue damage induced by the initial response of T lymphocytes to unprocessed gluten peptides. Another non-exclusive possibility is TLR3 activation by its ligands during an enteroviral infection which can result in TG2activation.[148]

Fourth, in active CD, the breakdown in IL 15 regulation leads to massive overexpression of IL 15, although it is unknown how this occurs. GFD has a direct effect on the decreased expression of IL 15 together with a decrease of the adaptive response mediated by CD4+ T lymphocytes, therefore, these cells may have a direct effect on IL 15 expression. Another possibility is that the signals derived from the innate immune response through TLRs may be responsible for the elevated IL 15 levels.[83]

References

1. Sollid LM. *Coeliac disease: dissecting a complex inflammatory disorder*. Nat Rev Immunol. 2002; 2(9): 647-55. http://dx.doi.org/10.1038/nri885

2. Jabri B, Sollid LM. *Tissue-mediated control of immunopathology in coeliac disease*. Nat Rev Immunol. 2009; 9(12): 858-70. http://dx.doi.org/10.1038/nri2670

3. Abadie V, Sollid LM, Barreiro LB, Jabri B. *Integration of genetic and immunological insights into a model of celiac disease pathogenesis*. Annu Rev Immunol. 2011; 29: 493-525. http://dx.doi.org/10.1146/annurev-immunol-040210-092915

4. Dube C, Rostom A, Sy R, Cranney A, Saloojee N, Garritty C, et al. *The prevalence of celiac disease in average-risk and at-risk Western European populations: a systematic review*. Gastroenterology. 2005; 128(4 Suppl 1): S57-67. http://dx.doi.org/10.1053/j.gastro.2005.02.014

5. Koning F. *Celiac disease: caught between a rock and a hard place*. Gastroenterology. 2005; 129(4): 1294-301. http://dx.doi.org/10.1053/j.gastro.2005.07.030

6. Catassi C, Ratsch IM, Fabiani E, Rossini M, Bordicchia F, Candela F, et al. *Coeliac disease in the year 2000: exploring the iceberg*. Lancet. 1994; 343(8891): 200-3. http://dx.doi.org/10.1016/S0140-6736(94)90989-X

7. Hausch F, Shan L, Santiago NA, Gray GM, Khosla C. *Intestinal digestive resistance of immunodominant gliadin peptides*. Am J Physiol Gastrointest Liver Physiol. 2002; 283(4): G996-G1003.

8. Shan L, Molberg O, Parrot I, Hausch F, Filiz F, Gray GM, et al. *Structural basis for gluten intolerance in celiac sprue*. Science. 2002; 297(5590): 2275-9. http://dx.doi.org/10.1126/science.1074129

9. Clemente MG, De Virgiliis S, Kang JS, Macatagney R, Musu MP, Di Pierro MR, et al. *Early effects of gliadin on enterocyte intracellular signalling involved in intestinal barrier function*. Gut. 2003; 52(2): 218-23. http://dx.doi.org/10.1136/gut.52.2.218

10. Menard S, Lebreton C, Schumann M, Matysiak-Budnik T, Dugave C, Bouhnik Y, et al. *Paracellular versus transcellular intestinal permeability to gliadin peptides in active celiac disease*. Am J Pathol. 2012; 180(2): 608-15. http://dx.doi.org/10.1016/j.ajpath.2011.10.019

11. Forsberg G, Hernell O, Melgar S, Israelsson A, Hammarstrom S, Hammarstrom ML. *Paradoxical coexpression of proinflammatory and down-regulatory cytokines in intestinal T cells in childhood celiac disease*. Gastroenterology. 2002; 123(3): 667-78. http://dx.doi.org/10.1053/gast.2002.35355

12. Salvati VM, MacDonald TT, Bajaj-Elliott M, Borrelli M, Staiano A, Auricchio S, et al. *Interleukin 18 and associated markers of T helper cell type 1 activity in coeliac disease*. Gut. 2002; 50(2): 186-90. http://dx.doi.org/10.1136/gut.50.2.186

13. Leon AJ, Garrote JA, Blanco-Quiros A, Calvo C, Fernandez-Salazar L, Del Villar A, et al. *Interleukin 18 maintains a long-standing inflammation in coeliac disease patients*. Clin Exp Immunol. 2006; 146(3): 479-85. http://dx.doi.org/10.1111/j.1365-2249.2006.03239.x

14. Leon AJ, Gomez E, Garrote JA, Arranz E. *The pattern of cytokine expression determines the degree of mucosal damage*. Gut. 2007; 56(3): 441-3. http://dx.doi.org/10.1136/gut.2006.110361

15. Marsh MN. *Gluten, major histocompatibility complex, and the small intestine. A molecular and immunobiologic approach to the spectrum of gluten sensitivity ('celiac sprue')*. Gastroenterology. 1992; 102(1): 330-54.

16. Malamut G, Meresse B, Cellier C, Cerf-Bensussan N. *Refractory celiac disease: from bench to bedside*. Semin Immunopathol. 2012; 34(4): 601-13. http://dx.doi.org/10.1007/s00281-012-0322-z

17. Ferguson A, Arranz E, O'Mahony S. *Clinical and pathological spectrum of coeliac disease--active, silent, latent, potential*. Gut. 1993; 34(2): 150-1. http://dx.doi.org/10.1136/gut.34.2.150

18. Carchon H, Serrus M, Eggermont E. *Digestion of gliadin peptides by intestinal mucosa from control or coeliac children*. Digestion. 1979; 19(1): 1-5. http://dx.doi.org/10.1159/000198315

19. Cornell HJ, Wills-Johnson G. *Structure-activity relationships in coeliac-toxic gliadin peptides*. Amino Acids. 2001; 21(3): 243-53. http://dx.doi.org/10.1007/s007260170010

20. Bruce G, Woodley JF, Swan CH. *Breakdown of gliadin peptides by intestinal brush borders from coeliac patients*. Gut. 1984; 25(9): 919-24. http://dx.doi.org/10.1136/gut.25.9.919

21. Chehade M, Mayer L. *Oral tolerance and its relation to food hypersensitivities*. J Allergy Clin Immunol. 2005; 115(1): 3-12; quiz 3. http://dx.doi.org/10.1016/j.jaci.2004.11.008

22. Mowat AM. *Anatomical basis of tolerance and immunity to intestinal antigens*. Nat Rev Immunol. 2003; 3(4): 331-41. http://dx.doi.org/10.1038/nri1057

23. Faria AM, Weiner HL. *Oral tolerance*. Immunol Rev. 2005;206:232-59. http://dx.doi.org/10.1111/j.0105-2896.2005.00280.x

24. Mills KH. *Regulatory T cells: friend or foe in immunity to infection?* Nat Rev Immunol. 2004; 4(11): 841-55. http://dx.doi.org/10.1038/nri1485

25. Macdonald TT, Monteleone G. *Immunity, inflammation, and allergy in the gut*. Science. 2005; 307(5717): 1920-5. http://dx.doi.org/10.1126/science.1106442

26. Mowat AM, Donachie AM, Parker LA, Robson NC, Beacock-Sharp H, McIntyre LJ, et al. *The role of dendritic cells in regulating mucosal immunity and tolerance*. Novartis Found Symp. 2003; 252: 291-302; discussion -5.

27. Rimoldi M, Chieppa M, Salucci V, Avogadri F, Sonzogni A, Sampietro GM, et al. *Intestinal immune homeostasis is regulated by the crosstalk between epithelial cells and dendritic cells*. Nat Immunol. 2005; 6(5): 507-14. http://dx.doi.org/10.1038/ni1192

28. Niess JH, Reinecker HC. *Dendritic cells: the commanders-in-chief of mucosal immune defenses*. Curr Opin Gastroenterol. 2006; 22(4): 354-60. http://dx.doi.org/10.1097/01.mog.0000231807.03149.54

29. Rossi M, Young JW. *Human dendritic cells: potent antigen-presenting cells at the crossroads of innate and adaptive immunity*. J Immunol. 2005; 175(3): 1373-81.

30. Beacock-Sharp H, Donachie AM, Robson NC, Mowat AM. *A role for dendritic cells in the priming of antigen-specific CD4+ and CD8+ T lymphocytes by immune-stimulating complexes in vivo*. Int Immunol. 2003; 15(6): 711-20. http://dx.doi.org/10.1093/intimm/dxg067

31. Mann ER, Bernardo D, Al-Hassi HO, English NR, Clark SK, McCarthy NE, et al. *Human gut-specific homeostatic dendritic cells are generated from blood precursors by the gut microenvironment*. Inflamm Bowel Dis. 2012; 18(7): 1275-86. http://dx.doi.org/10.1002/ibd.21893

32. La Cava A, Van Kaer L, Fu Dong S. *CD4+CD25+ Tregs and NKT cells: regulators regulating regulators*. Trends Immunol. 2006; 27(7): 322-7. http://dx.doi.org/10.1016/j.it.2006.05.003

33. Shevach EM, McHugh RS, Piccirillo CA, Thornton AM. *Control of T-cell activation by CD4+ CD25+ suppressor T cells*. Immunol Rev. 2001; 182: 58-67. http://dx.doi.org/10.1034/j.1600-065X.2001.1820104.x

34. Bernardo D, Al-Hassi HO, Mann ER, Tee CT, Murugananthan AU, Peake ST, et al. *T-cell proliferation and forkhead box P3 expression in human T cells are dependent on T-cell density: physics of a confined space?* Hum Immunol. 2011; 73(3): 223-31. http://dx.doi.org/10.1016/j.humimm.2011.12.017

35. Raki M, Tollefsen S, Molberg O, Lundin KE, Sollid LM, Jahnsen FL. *A unique dendritic cell subset accumulates in the celiac lesion and efficiently activates gluten-reactive T cells.* Gastroenterology. 2006; 131(2): 428-38. http://dx.doi.org/10.1053/j.gastro.2006.06.002

36. Mowat AM, Parker LA, Beacock-Sharp H, Millington OR, Chirdo F. *Oral tolerance: overview and historical perspectives.* Ann N Y Acad Sci. 2004; 1029: 1-8. http://dx.doi.org/10.1196/annals.1309.001

37. Hadis U, Wahl B, Schulz O, Hardtke-Wolenski M, Schippers A, Wagner N, et al. *Intestinal tolerance requires gut homing and expansion of FoxP3+ regulatory T cells in the lamina propria.* Immunity. 2012; 34(2): 237-46. http://dx.doi.org/10.1016/j.immuni.2011.01.016

38. Sun CM, Hall JA, Blank RB, Bouladoux N, Oukka M, Mora JR, et al. *Small intestine lamina propria dendritic cells promote de novo generation of Foxp3 T reg cells via retinoic acid.* J Exp Med. 2007; 204(8): 1775-85. http://dx.doi.org/10.1084/jem.20070602

39. Gianfrani C, Levings MK, Sartirana C, Mazzarella G, Barba G, Zanzi D, et al. *Gliadin-specific type 1 regulatory T cells from the intestinal mucosa of treated celiac patients inhibit pathogenic T cells.* J Immunol. 2006; 177(6): 4178-86.

40. O'Garra A, Vieira P. *T(H)1 cells control themselves by producing interleukin-10.* Nat Rev Immunol. 2007; 7(6): 425-8. http://dx.doi.org/10.1038/nri2097

41. Thielke KH, Hoffmann-Moujahid A, Weisser C, Waldkirch E, Pabst R, Holtmeier W, et al. *Proliferating intestinal gamma/delta T cells recirculate rapidly and are a major source of the gamma/delta T cell pool in the peripheral blood.* Eur J Immunol. 2003; 33(6): 1649-56. http://dx.doi.org/10.1002/eji.200323442

42. Arranz E, Bode J, Kingstone K, Ferguson A. *Intestinal antibody pattern of coeliac disease: association with gamma/delta T cell receptor expression by intraepithelial lymphocytes, and other indices of potential coeliac disease.* Gut. 1994; 35(4): 476-82. http://dx.doi.org/10.1136/gut.35.4.476

43. Locke NR, Stankovic S, Funda DP, Harrison LC. *TCR gamma delta intraepithelial lymphocytes are required for self-tolerance.* J Immunol. 2006; 176(11): 6553-9.

44. Yu KO, Porcelli SA. *The diverse functions of CD1d-restricted NKT cells and their potential for immunotherapy.* Immunol Lett. 2005; 100(1): 42-55. http://dx.doi.org/10.1016/j.imlet.2005.06.010

45. van der Vliet HJ, Molling JW, von Blomberg BM, Nishi N, Kolgen W, van den Eertwegh AJ, et al. *The immunoregulatory role of CD1d-restricted natural killer T cells in disease.* Clin Immunol. 2004; 112(1): 8-23. http://dx.doi.org/10.1016/j.clim.2004.03.003

46. Zeissig S, Kaser A, Dougan SK, Nieuwenhuis EE, Blumberg RS. *Role of NKT cells in the digestive system. III. Role of NKT cells in intestinal immunity.* Am J Physiol Gastrointest Liver Physiol. 2007; 293(6): G1101-5. http://dx.doi.org/10.1152/ajpgi.00342.2007

47. Eiras P, Leon F, Camarero C, Lombardia M, Roldan E, Bootello A, et al. *Intestinal intraepithelial lymphocytes contain a CD3- CD7+ subset expressing natural killer markers and a singular pattern of adhesion molecules.* Scand J Immunol. 2000; 52(1): 1-6. http://dx.doi.org/10.1046/j.1365-3083.2000.00761.x

48. Leon F, Roldan E, Sanchez L, Camarero C, Bootello A, Roy G. *Human small-intestinal epithelium contains functional natural killer lymphocytes.* Gastroenterology. 2003; 125(2): 345-56. http://dx.doi.org/10.1016/S0016-5085(03)00886-2

49. Cardell SL. *The natural killer T lymphocyte: a player in the complex regulation of autoimmune diabetes in non-obese diabetic mice*. Clin Exp Immunol. 2006; 143(2): 194-202. http://dx.doi.org/10.1111/j.1365-2249.2005.02942.x

50. Seino K, Taniguchi M. *Functionally distinct NKT cell subsets and subtypes*. J Exp Med. 2005; 202(12): 1623-6. http://dx.doi.org/10.1084/jem.20051600

51. Munz C, Dao T, Ferlazzo G, de Cos MA, Goodman K, Young JW. *Mature myeloid dendritic cell subsets have distinct roles for activation and viability of circulating human natural killer cells*. Blood. 2005; 105(1): 266-73. http://dx.doi.org/10.1182/blood-2004-06-2492

52. Johansson-Lindbom B, Agace WW. *Generation of gut-homing T cells and their localization to the small intestinal mucosa*. Immunol Rev. 2007; 215: 226-42. http://dx.doi.org/10.1111/j.1600-065X.2006.00482.x

53. Butcher EC, Williams M, Youngman K, Rott L, Briskin M. *Lymphocyte trafficking and regional immunity*. Adv Immunol. 1999; 72: 209-53. http://dx.doi.org/10.1016/S0065-2776(08)60022-X

54. Zabel BA, Agace WW, Campbell JJ, Heath HM, Parent D, Roberts AI, et al. *Human G protein-coupled receptor GPR-9-6/CC chemokine receptor 9 is selectively expressed on intestinal homing T lymphocytes, mucosal lymphocytes, and thymocytes and is required for thymus-expressed chemokine-mediated chemotaxis*. J Exp Med. 1999; 190(9): 1241-56. http://dx.doi.org/10.1084/jem.190.9.1241

55. Ohmori K, Fukui F, Kiso M, Imai T, Yoshie O, Hasegawa H, et al. *Identification of cutaneous lymphocyte-associated antigen as sialyl 6-sulfo Lewis X, a selectin ligand expressed on a subset of skin-homing helper memory T cells*. Blood. 2006; 107(8): 3197-204. http://dx.doi.org/10.1182/blood-2005-05-2185

56. Clark RA, Chong B, Mirchandani N, Brinster NK, Yamanaka K, Dowgiert RK, et al. *The vast majority of CLA+ T cells are resident in normal skin*. J Immunol. 2006; 176(7): 4431-9.

57. Qiao SW, Iversen R, Raki M, Sollid LM. *The adaptive immune response in celiac disease*. Semin Immunopathol. 2012; 34(4): 523-40. http://dx.doi.org/10.1007/s00281-012-0314-z

58. Ng SC, Benjamin JL, McCarthy NE, Hedin CR, Koutsoumpas A, Plamondon S, et al. *Relationship between human intestinal dendritic cells, gut microbiota, and disease activity in Crohn's disease*. Inflamm Bowel Dis. 2011; 17(10): 2027-37. http://dx.doi.org/10.1002/ibd.21590

59. Brandtzaeg P. *The changing immunological paradigm in coeliac disease*. Immunol Lett. 2006; 105(2): 127-39. http://dx.doi.org/10.1016/j.imlet.2006.03.004

60. Gianfrani C, Auricchio S, Troncone R. *Adaptive and innate immune responses in celiac disease*. Immunol Lett. 2005; 99(2): 141-5. http://dx.doi.org/10.1016/j.imlet.2005.02.017

61. Koning F, Gilissen L, Wijmenga C. *Gluten: a two-edged sword. Immunopathogenesis of celiac disease*. Springer Semin Immunopathol. 2005; 27(2): 217-32. http://dx.doi.org/10.1007/s00281-005-0203-9

62. Sollid LM, Qiao SW, Anderson RP, Gianfrani C, Koning F. *Nomenclature and listing of celiac disease relevant gluten T-cell epitopes restricted by HLA-DQ molecules*. Immunogenetics. 2012; 64(6): 455-60. http://dx.doi.org/10.1007/s00251-012-0599-z

63. Sturgess RP, Ellis HJ, Ciclitira PJ. *Cereal chemistry, molecular biology, and toxicity in coeliac disease*. Gut. 1991; 32(9): 1055-60. http://dx.doi.org/10.1136/gut.32.9.1055

64. Shewry PR, Halford NG, Tatham AS, Popineau Y, Lafiandra D, Belton PS. *The high molecular weight subunits of wheat glutenin and their role in determining wheat processing properties*. Adv Food Nutr Res. 2003; 45: 219-302.
http://dx.doi.org/10.1016/S1043-4526(03)45006-7

65. Howdle PD, Corazza GR, Bullen AW, Losowsky MS. *Gluten sensitivity of small intestinal mucosa in vitro: quantitative assessment of histologic change*. Gastroenterology. 1981; 80(3): 442-50.

66. Ellis HJ, Ciclitira PJ. *In vivo gluten challenge in celiac disease*. Can J Gastroenterol. 2001; 15(4): 243-7.

67. Maiuri L, Ciacci C, Ricciardelli I, Vacca L, Raia V, Auricchio S, et al. *Association between innate response to gliadin and activation of pathogenic T cells in coeliac disease*. Lancet. 2003; 362(9377): 30-7. http://dx.doi.org/10.1016/S0140-6736(03)13803-2

68. Maiuri L, Ciacci C, Ricciardelli I, Vacca L, Raia V, Rispo A, et al. *Unexpected role of surface transglutaminase type II in celiac disease*. Gastroenterology. 2005; 129(5): 1400-13.
http://dx.doi.org/10.1053/j.gastro.2005.07.054

69. Londei M, Ciacci C, Ricciardelli I, Vacca L, Quaratino S, Maiuri L. *Gliadin as a stimulator of innate responses in celiac disease*. Mol Immunol. 2005; 42(8): 913-8.
http://dx.doi.org/10.1016/j.molimm.2004.12.005

70. Beckett CG, Dell'Olio D, Shidrawi RG, Rosen-Bronson S, Ciclitira PJ. *Gluten-induced nitric oxide and pro-inflammatory cytokine release by cultured coeliac small intestinal biopsies*. Eur J Gastroenterol Hepatol. 1999; 11(5): 529-35.
http://dx.doi.org/10.1097/00042737-199905000-00011

71. De Stefano D, Maiuri MC, Iovine B, Ialenti A, Bevilacqua MA, Carnuccio R. *The role of NF-kappaB, IRF-1, and STAT-1alpha transcription factors in the iNOS gene induction by gliadin and IFN-gamma in RAW 264.7 macrophages*. J Mol Med (Berl). 2006; 84(1): 65-74. http://dx.doi.org/10.1007/s00109-005-0713-x

72. Martin-Pagola A, Perez-Nanclares G, Ortiz L, Vitoria JC, Hualde I, Zaballa R, et al. *MICA response to gliadin in intestinal mucosa from celiac patients*. Immunogenetics. 2004; 56(8): 549-54. http://dx.doi.org/10.1007/s00251-004-0724-8

73. Jabri B, de Serre NP, Cellier C, Evans K, Gache C, Carvalho C, et al. *Selective expansion of intraepithelial lymphocytes expressing the HLA-E-specific natural killer receptor CD94 in celiac disease*. Gastroenterology. 2000; 118(5): 867-79.
http://dx.doi.org/10.1016/S0016-5085(00)70173-9

74. Cheroutre H, Lambolez F, Mucida D. *The light and dark sides of intestinal intraepithelial lymphocytes*. Nat Rev Immunol. 2011; 11(7): 445-56.
http://dx.doi.org/10.1038/nri3007

75. Di Sabatino A, Ciccocioppo R, Cupelli F, Cinque B, Millimaggi D, Clarkson MM, et al. *Epithelium derived interleukin 15 regulates intraepithelial lymphocyte Th1 cytokine production, cytotoxicity, and survival in coeliac disease*. Gut. 2006; 55(4): 469-77.
http://dx.doi.org/10.1136/gut.2005.068684

76. Maiuri L, Ciacci C, Auricchio S, Brown V, Quaratino S, Londei M. *Interleukin 15 mediates epithelial changes in celiac disease*. Gastroenterology. 2000; 119(4): 996-1006.
http://dx.doi.org/10.1053/gast.2000.18149

77. Mention JJ, Ben Ahmed M, Begue B, Barbe U, Verkarre V, Asnafi V, et al. *Interleukin 15: a key to disrupted intraepithelial lymphocyte homeostasis and lymphomagenesis in celiac disease*. Gastroenterology. 2003; 125(3): 730-45.
http://dx.doi.org/10.1016/S0016-5085(03)01047-3

78. Meresse B, Chen Z, Ciszewski C, Tretiakova M, Bhagat G, Krausz TN, et al. *Coordinated induction by IL15 of a TCR-independent NKG2D signaling pathway converts CTL into*

lymphokine-activated killer cells in celiac disease. Immunity. 2004; 21(3): 357-66. http://dx.doi.org/10.1016/j.immuni.2004.06.020

79. Hue S, Mention JJ, Monteiro RC, Zhang S, Cellier C, Schmitz J, et al. *A direct role for NKG2D/MICA interaction in villous atrophy during celiac disease*. Immunity. 2004; 21(3): 367-77. http://dx.doi.org/10.1016/j.immuni.2004.06.018

80. Maiuri L, Ciacci C, Vacca L, Ricciardelli I, Auricchio S, Quaratino S, et al. *IL-15 drives the specific migration of CD94+ and TCR-gammadelta+ intraepithelial lymphocytes in organ cultures of treated celiac patients.* Am J Gastroenterol. 2001; 96(1): 150-6.

81. Ebert EC. *IL-15 converts human intestinal intraepithelial lymphocytes to CD94 producers of IFN-gamma and IL-10, the latter promoting Fas ligand-mediated cytotoxicity*. Immunology. 2005; 115(1): 118-26. http://dx.doi.org/10.1111/j.1365-2567.2005.02132.x

82. Fehniger TA, Caligiuri MA. *Interleukin 15: biology and relevance to human disease*. Blood. 2001; 97(1): 14-32. http://dx.doi.org/10.1182/blood.V97.1.14

83. Mention JJ, Ben Ahmed M, Begue B, Barbe U, Verkarre V, Asnafi V, et al. *Interleukin 15: a key to disrupted intraepithelial lymphocyte homeostasis and lymphomagenesis in celiac disease*. Gastroenterology. 2003; 125(3): 730-45. http://dx.doi.org/10.1016/S0016-5085(03)01047-3

84. Giovannini C, Sanchez M, Straface E, Scazzocchio B, Silano M, De Vincenzi M. *Induction of apoptosis in caco-2 cells by wheat gliadin peptides*. Toxicology. 2000; 145(1): 63-71. http://dx.doi.org/10.1016/S0300-483X(99)00223-1

85. Nikulina M, Habich C, Flohe SB, Scott FW, Kolb H. *Wheat gluten causes dendritic cell maturation and chemokine secretion*. J Immunol. 2004; 173(3): 1925-33.

86. Thomas KE, Sapone A, Fasano A, Vogel SN. *Gliadin stimulation of murine macrophage inflammatory gene expression and intestinal permeability are MyD88-dependent: role of the innate immune response in Celiac disease*. J Immunol. 2006; 176(4): 2512-21.

87. Bernardo D, Garrote JA, Fernandez-Salazar L, Riestra S, Arranz E. *Is gliadin really safe for non-coeliac individuals? Production of interleukin 15 in biopsy culture from non-coeliac individuals challenged with gliadin peptides*. Gut. 2007; 56(6): 889-90. http://dx.doi.org/10.1136/gut.2006.118265

88. Lammers KM, Lu R, Brownley J, Lu B, Gerard C, Thomas K, et al. *Gliadin induces an increase in intestinal permeability and zonulin release by binding to the chemokine receptor CXCR3*. Gastroenterology. 2008; 135(1): 194-204 e3. http://dx.doi.org/10.1053/j.gastro.2008.03.023

89. Freitag TL, Rietdijk S, Junker Y, Popov Y, Bhan AK, Kelly CP, et al. *Gliadin-primed CD4+CD45RBlowCD25- T cells drive gluten-dependent small intestinal damage after adoptive transfer into lymphopenic mice*. Gut. 2009; 58(12): 1597-605. http://dx.doi.org/10.1136/gut.2009.186361

90. Ohteki T, Suzue K, Maki C, Ota T, Koyasu S. *Critical role of IL-15-IL-15R for antigen-presenting cell functions in the innate immune response*. Nat Immunol. 2001; 2(12): 1138-43. http://dx.doi.org/10.1038/ni729

91. Mattei F, Schiavoni G, Belardelli F, Tough DF. *IL-15 is expressed by dendritic cells in response to type I IFN, double-stranded RNA, or lipopolysaccharide and promotes dendritic cell activation*. J Immunol. 2001; 167(3): 1179-87.

92. Abadie V, Discepolo V, Jabri B. *Intraepithelial lymphocytes in celiac disease immunopathology*. Semin Immunopathol. 2012; 34(4): 551-66. http://dx.doi.org/10.1007/s00281-012-0316-x

93. Anderson DM, Kumaki S, Ahdieh M, Bertles J, Tometsko M, Loomis A, et al. *Functional characterization of the human interleukin-15 receptor alpha chain and close linkage of IL15RA and IL2RA genes*. J Biol Chem. 1995; 270(50): 29862-9.
http://dx.doi.org/10.1074/jbc.270.50.29862

94. Waldmann TA, Tagaya Y. *The multifaceted regulation of interleukin-15 expression and the role of this cytokine in NK cell differentiation and host response to intracellular pathogens*. Annu Rev Immunol. 1999; 17: 19-49.
http://dx.doi.org/10.1146/annurev.immunol.17.1.19

95. Budagian V, Bulanova E, Paus R, Bulfone-Paus S. *IL-15/IL-15 receptor biology: a guided tour through an expanding universe*. Cytokine Growth Factor Rev. 2006; 17(4): 259-80.
http://dx.doi.org/10.1016/j.cytogfr.2006.05.001

96. Sarra M, Cupi ML, Monteleone I, Franze E, Ronchetti G, Di Sabatino A, et al. *IL-15 positively regulates IL-21 production in celiac disease mucosa*. Mucosal Immunol. 2013; 6(2): 244-55.

97. Bernardo D, Garrote JA, Allegretti Y, Leon A, Gomez E, Bermejo-Martin JF, et al. *Higher constitutive IL15R alpha expression and lower IL-15 response threshold in coeliac disease patients*. Clin Exp Immunol. 2008; 154(1): 64-73.
http://dx.doi.org/10.1111/j.1365-2249.2008.03743.x

98. Harris KM, Fasano A, Mann DL. *Monocytes differentiated with IL-15 support Th17 and Th1 responses to wheat gliadin: implications for celiac disease*. Clin Immunol. 2010; 135(3): 430-9. http://dx.doi.org/10.1016/j.clim.2010.01.003

99. Arentz-Hansen H, Korner R, Molberg O, Quarsten H, Vader W, Kooy YM, et al. *The intestinal T cell response to alpha-gliadin in adult celiac disease is focused on a single deamidated glutamine targeted by tissue transglutaminase*. J Exp Med. 2000; 191(4): 603-12. http://dx.doi.org/10.1084/jem.191.4.603

100. Dieterich W, Ehnis T, Bauer M, Donner P, Volta U, Riecken EO, et al. *Identification of tissue transglutaminase as the autoantigen of celiac disease*. Nat Med. 1997; 3(7): 797-801. http://dx.doi.org/10.1038/nm0797-797

101. Molberg O, McAdam SN, Korner R, Quarsten H, Kristiansen C, Madsen L, et al. *Tissue transglutaminase selectively modifies gliadin peptides that are recognized by gut-derived T cells in celiac disease*. Nat Med. 1998; 4(6): 713-7.
http://dx.doi.org/10.1038/nm0698-713

102. van de Wal Y, Kooy Y, van Veelen P, Pena S, Mearin L, Papadopoulos G, et al. *Selective deamidation by tissue transglutaminase strongly enhances gliadin-specific T cell reactivity*. J Immunol. 1998; 161(4): 1585-8.

103. Schuppan D. *Current concepts of celiac disease pathogenesis*. Gastroenterology. 2000; 119(1): 234-42. http://dx.doi.org/10.1053/gast.2000.8521

104. Sollid LM. *Coeliac disease: dissecting a complex inflammatory disorder*. Nat Rev Immunol. 2002; 2(9): 647-55. http://dx.doi.org/10.1038/nri885

105. Arentz-Hansen H, McAdam SN, Molberg O, Fleckenstein B, Lundin KE, Jorgensen TJ, et al. *Celiac lesion T cells recognize epitopes that cluster in regions of gliadins rich in proline residues*. Gastroenterology. 2002; 123(3): 803-9.
http://dx.doi.org/10.1053/gast.2002.35381

106. Anderson RP, Degano P, Godkin AJ, Jewell DP, Hill AV. *In vivo antigen challenge in celiac disease identifies a single transglutaminase-modified peptide as the dominant A-gliadin T-cell epitope*. Nat Med. 2000; 6(3): 337-42. http://dx.doi.org/10.1038/73200

107. Vader W, Kooy Y, Van Veelen P, De Ru A, Harris D, Benckhuijsen W, et al. *The gluten response in children with celiac disease is directed toward multiple gliadin and glutenin peptides*. Gastroenterology. 2002; 122(7): 1729-37.
http://dx.doi.org/10.1053/gast.2002.33606

108. Koning F, Vader W. *Gluten peptides and celiac disease*. Science. 2003; 299(5606): 513-5; author reply -5. http://dx.doi.org/10.1126/science.299.5606.513

109. Matysiak-Budnik T, Candalh C, Dugave C, Namane A, Cellier C, Cerf-Bensussan N, et al. *Alterations of the intestinal transport and processing of gliadin peptides in celiac disease*. Gastroenterology. 2003; 125(3): 696-707.
http://dx.doi.org/10.1016/S0016-5085(03)01049-7

110. Piper JL, Gray GM, Khosla C. *Effect of prolyl endopeptidase on digestive-resistant gliadin peptides in vivo*. J Pharmacol Exp Ther. 2004; 311(1): 213-9.
http://dx.doi.org/10.1124/jpet.104.068429

111. Shan L, Molberg O, Parrot I, Hausch F, Filiz F, Gray GM, et al. *Structural basis for gluten intolerance in celiac sprue*. Science. 2002; 297(5590): 2275-9.
http://dx.doi.org/10.1126/science.1074129

112. Sollid LM. *Molecular basis of celiac disease*. Annu Rev Immunol. 2000;18:53-81.
http://dx.doi.org/10.1146/annurev.immunol.18.1.53

113. Beitnes AC, Raki M, Lundin KE, Jahnsen J, Sollid LM, Jahnsen FL. *Density of CD163+ CD11c+ dendritic cells increases and CD103+ dendritic cells decreases in the coeliac lesion*. Scand J Immunol. 2011; 74(2): 186-94.
http://dx.doi.org/10.1111/j.1365-3083.2011.02549.x

114. Ouaaz F, Arron J, Zheng Y, Choi Y, Beg AA. *Dendritic cell development and survival require distinct NF-kappaB subunits*. Immunity. 2002; 16(2): 257-70.
http://dx.doi.org/10.1016/S1074-7613(02)00272-8

115. Monteleone G, Pender SL, Alstead E, Hauer AC, Lionetti P, McKenzie C, et al. *Role of interferon alpha in promoting T helper cell type 1 responses in the small intestine in coeliac disease*. Gut. 2001; 48(3): 425-9. http://dx.doi.org/10.1136/gut.48.3.425

116. Beitnes AC, Raki M, Brottveit M, Lundin KE, Jahnsen FL, Sollid LM. *Rapid accumulation of CD14+CD11c+ dendritic cells in gut mucosa of celiac disease after in vivo gluten challenge*. PLoS One. 7(3): e33556. http://dx.doi.org/10.1371/journal.pone.0033556

117. Arentz-Hansen H, McAdam SN, Molberg O, Fleckenstein B, Lundin KE, Jorgensen TJ, et al. *Celiac lesion T cells recognize epitopes that cluster in regions of gliadins rich in proline residues*. Gastroenterology. 2002; 123(3): 803-9.
http://dx.doi.org/10.1053/gast.2002.35381

118. Nilsen EM, Jahnsen FL, Lundin KE, Johansen FE, Fausa O, Sollid LM, et al. *Gluten induces an intestinal cytokine response strongly dominated by interferon gamma in patients with celiac disease*. Gastroenterology. 1998; 115(3): 551-63.
http://dx.doi.org/10.1016/S0016-5085(98)70134-9

119. Leon F, Sanchez L, Camarero C, Roy G. *Cytokine production by intestinal intraepithelial lymphocyte subsets in celiac disease*. Dig Dis Sci. 2005; 50(3): 593-600.
http://dx.doi.org/10.1007/s10620-005-2480-5

120. Salvati VM, Bajaj-Elliott M, Poulsom R, Mazzarella G, Lundin KE, Nilsen EM, et al. *Keratinocyte growth factor and coeliac disease*. Gut. 2001; 49(2): 176-81.
http://dx.doi.org/10.1136/gut.49.2.176

121. Farstad IN, Halstensen TS, Kvale D, Fausa O, Brandtzaeg P. *Topographic distribution of homing receptors on B and T cells in human gut-associated lymphoid tissue: relation of L-selectin and integrin alpha 4 beta 7 to naive and memory phenotypes*. Am J Pathol. 1997; 150(1): 187-99.

122. Dieterich W, Storch WB, Schuppan D. *Serum antibodies in celiac disease*. Clin Lab. 2000; 46(7-8): 361-4.

123. Sardy M, Karpati S, Merkl B, Paulsson M, Smyth N. *Epidermal transglutaminase (TGase 3) is the autoantigen of dermatitis herpetiformis*. J Exp Med. 2002; 195(6): 747-57. http://dx.doi.org/10.1084/jem.20011299

124. Hadjivassiliou M, Aeschlimann P, Strigun A, Sanders DS, Woodroofe N, Aeschlimann D. *Autoantibodies in gluten ataxia recognize a novel neuronal transglutaminase*. Ann Neurol. 2008; 64(3): 332-43. http://dx.doi.org/10.1002/ana.21450

125. Farstad IN, Carlsen H, Morton HC, Brandtzaeg P. *Immunoglobulin A cell distribution in the human small intestine: phenotypic and functional characteristics*. Immunology. 2000; 101(3): 354-63. http://dx.doi.org/10.1046/j.1365-2567.2000.00118.x

126. Jelinkova L, Tuckova L, Cinova J, Flegelova Z, Tlaskalova-Hogenova H. *Gliadin stimulates human monocytes to production of IL-8 and TNF-alpha through a mechanism involving NF-kappaB*. FEBS Lett. 2004; 571(1-3): 81-5. http://dx.doi.org/10.1016/j.febslet.2004.06.057

127. Palova-Jelinkova L, Rozkova D, Pecharova B, Bartova J, Sediva A, Tlaskalova-Hogenova H, et al. *Gliadin fragments induce phenotypic and functional maturation of human dendritic cells*. J Immunol. 2005; 175(10): 7038-45.

128. Stepniak D, Koning F. *Celiac disease--sandwiched between innate and adaptive immunity*. Hum Immunol. 2006; 67(6): 460-8. http://dx.doi.org/10.1016/j.humimm.2006.03.011

129. Meresse B, Malamut G, Cerf-Bensussan N. *Celiac disease: an immunological jigsaw*. Immunity. 2012; 36(6): 907-19. http://dx.doi.org/10.1016/j.immuni.2012.06.006

130. Visser J, Rozing J, Sapone A, Lammers K, Fasano A. *Tight junctions, intestinal permeability, and autoimmunity: celiac disease and type 1 diabetes paradigms*. Ann N Y Acad Sci. 2009; 1165: 195-205. http://dx.doi.org/10.1111/j.1749-6632.2009.04037.x

131. Zimmer KP, Fischer I, Mothes T, Weissen-Plenz G, Schmitz M, Wieser H, et al. *Endocytotic segregation of gliadin peptide 31-49 in enterocytes*. Gut. 2010; 59(3): 300-10. http://dx.doi.org/10.1136/gut.2008.169656

132. Luciani A, Villella VR, Vasaturo A, Giardino I, Pettoello-Mantovani M, Guido S, et al. *Lysosomal accumulation of gliadin p31-43 peptide induces oxidative stress and tissue transglutaminase-mediated PPARgamma downregulation in intestinal epithelial cells and coeliac mucosa*. 2010; Gut. 59(3): 311-9. http://dx.doi.org/10.1136/gut.2009.183608

133. Drago S, El Asmar R, Di Pierro M, Grazia Clemente M, Tripathi A, Sapone A, et al. *Gliadin, zonulin and gut permeability: Effects on celiac and non-celiac intestinal mucosa and intestinal cell lines*. Scand J Gastroenterol. 2006; 41(4): 408-19. http://dx.doi.org/10.1080/00365520500235334

134. Ali S, Mann DA. *Signal transduction via the NF-kappaB pathway: a targeted treatment modality for infection, inflammation and repair*. Cell Biochem Funct. 2004; 22(2): 67-79. http://dx.doi.org/10.1002/cbf.1082

135. Bonizzi G, Karin M. *The two NF-kappaB activation pathways and their role in innate and adaptive immunity*. Trends Immunol. 2004; 25(6): 280-8. http://dx.doi.org/10.1016/j.it.2004.03.008

136. Munz C, Steinman RM, Fujii S. *Dendritic cell maturation by innate lymphocytes: coordinated stimulation of innate and adaptive immunity*. J Exp Med. 2005; 202(2): 203-7. http://dx.doi.org/10.1084/jem.20050810

137. Calder VL, Bondeson J, Brennan FM, Foxwell BM, Feldmann M. *Antigen-specific T-cell downregulation by human dendritic cells following blockade of NF-kappaB*. Scand J Immunol. 2003; 57(3): 261-70. http://dx.doi.org/10.1046/j.1365-3083.2003.01228.x

138. Pender SL, MacDonald TT. *Matrix metalloproteinases and the gut - new roles for old enzymes*. Curr Opin Pharmacol. 2004; 4(6): 546-50.
http://dx.doi.org/10.1016/j.coph.2004.06.005

139. Ciccocioppo R, Di Sabatino A, Bauer M, Della Riccia DN, Bizzini F, Biagi F, et al. *Matrix metalloproteinase pattern in celiac duodenal mucosa*. Lab Invest. 2005; 85(3): 397-407.
http://dx.doi.org/10.1038/labinvest.3700225

140. Sanz Y, De Pama G, Laparra M. *Unraveling the ties between celiac disease and intestinal microbiota*. Int Rev Immunol. 2011; 30(4): 207-18.
http://dx.doi.org/10.3109/08830185.2011.599084

141. Nistal E, Caminero A, Vivas S, Ruiz de Morales JM, Saenz de Miera LE, Rodriguez-Aparicio LB, et al. *Differences in faecal bacteria populations and faecal bacteria metabolism in healthy adults and celiac disease patients*. Biochimie. 94(8): 1724-9.
http://dx.doi.org/10.1016/j.biochi.2012.03.025

142. De Palma G, Kamanova J, Cinova J, Olivares M, Drasarova H, Tuckova L, et al. *Modulation of phenotypic and functional maturation of dendritic cells by intestinal bacteria and gliadin: relevance for celiac disease*. J Leukoc Biol.

143. Forsberg G, Fahlgren A, Horstedt P, Hammarstrom S, Hernell O, Hammarstrom ML. *Presence of bacteria and innate immunity of intestinal epithelium in childhood celiac disease*. Am J Gastroenterol. 2004; 99(5): 894-904.
http://dx.doi.org/10.1111/j.1572-0241.2004.04157.x

144. Nadal I, Donat E, Ribes-Koninckx C, Calabuig M, Sanz Y. *Imbalance in the composition of the duodenal microbiota of children with coeliac disease*. J Med Microbiol. 2007; 56(Pt 12): 1669-74. http://dx.doi.org/10.1099/jmm.0.47410-0

145. Bernardo D, Garrote JA, Nadal I, Leon AJ, Calvo C, Fernandez-Salazar L, et al. *Is it true that coeliacs do not digest gliadin? Degradation pattern of gliadin in coeliac disease small intestinal mucosa*. Gut. 2009; 58(6): 886-7.
http://dx.doi.org/10.1136/gut.2008.167296

146. Stene LC, Honeyman MC, Hoffenberg EJ, Haas JE, Sokol RJ, Emery L, et al. *Rotavirus infection frequency and risk of celiac disease autoimmunity in early childhood: a longitudinal study*. Am J Gastroenterol. 2006; 101(10): 2333-40.
http://dx.doi.org/10.1111/j.1572-0241.2006.00741.x

147. Matysiak-Budnik T, Moura IC, Arcos-Fajardo M, Lebreton C, Menard S, Candalh C, et al. *Secretory IgA mediates retrotranscytosis of intact gliadin peptides via the transferrin receptor in celiac disease*. J Exp Med. 2008; 205(1): 143-54.
http://dx.doi.org/10.1084/jem.20071204

148. Siegel M, Strnad P, Watts RE, Choi K, Jabri B, Omary MB, et al. *Extracellular transglutaminase 2 is catalytically inactive, but is transiently activated upon tissue injury*. PLoS One. 2008; 3(3): e1861.

OmniaScience

Chapter 8

The Role of Serology in Celiac Disease Screening, Diagnosis and Follow-up

Carme Farré

Clinical Biochemistry Department, Sant Joan de Déu Pediatric University Hospital. University of Barcelona, Barcelona, Spain.

farre@hsjdbcn.org

Doi: http://www.dx.doi.org/10.3926/oms.234

How to cite this chapter

Farré C. *The Role of Serology in Celiac Disease Screening, Diagnosis and Follow-up.* In Rodrigo L and Peña AS, editors. *Celiac Disease and Non-Celiac Gluten Sensitivity.* Barcelona, Spain: Omnia-Science; 2014. p. 151-169.

Abstract

Serological markers are an essential part of the diagnostic workup for celiac disease (CD). Diverse clinical forms can be detected at any age in genetically susceptible individuals who have gluten in their diet.

Quantitative, automated IgA-class anti-tissue transglutaminase antibody testing is the recommended serological marker for CD detection, replacing the classical antiendomysial antibody test determined by indirect immunofluorescence assay. Anti-deaminated gliadin peptide antibodies improve the specificity of anti-gliadin antibodies, but lack the diagnostic efficacy of anti-transglutaminase antibodies.

Anti-transglutaminase antibodies should be determined in patients with clinical suspicion of CD, in CD-risk groups and in patients with CD-associated diseases.

Laboratories carrying out these assays must meet the following criteria: 1) Participation in quality control programs; 2) Use of appropriate reference values; 3) Quantitative monitoring of gluten-free diets; 4) Results comparable with other commercial tests, in view of the lack of a calibration standard.

The choice of a commercial test should take into account the type of antigen(s) calibrator, level of accuracy, linearity and detection limits, and any interferences.

In clinical practice, we do not recommend the use of mixed tests to screen for antibodies and isotypes, due to their contrasting significance and kinetics. Similarly, we advise against rapid immunochromatographic tests, to avoid diagnostic confusion. CD markers can also be determined using rapid point of care tests. For the time being, clinicians should be aware that these tests are expensive and they carry the risk of patients starting a GFD themselves, which then makes it harder to confirm the diagnosis.

Finally, it should be noted that anti-transglutaminase antibodies are only of limited use in adults and patients with partial villous atrophy on biopsy.

1. Introduction

A diagnosis of celiac disease (CD) is reached through an overall assessment of serology, clinical symptoms, intestinal biopsy studies, risk factors and genetic predisposition. Specific autoantibodies (serological markers) play an essential role in the diagnostic workup. These markers are requested increasingly not only by pediatricians and gastroenterologists, but also by endocrinologists, hematologists, rheumatologists, neurologists and other medical specialists.

Unlike other organ-specific autoimmune diseases, CD is unique in that it has an identified trigger (gluten), characteristic inflammatory bowel lesion staging that is a reversible, and excellent diagnostic serological markers. It can appear at any age in genetically susceptible individuals. Positive HLA-DQ2 and/or HLA-DQ8 gluten intake are necessary, but not sufficient for the clinical expression of the disease. Other key aspects are also involved that have yet to be understood, such as molecular mechanisms that control the immune response; mechanisms related to the degree of clinical severity; and the natural history of asymptomatic, untreated CD.

Serological markers are useful for detecting and monitoring CD, but intestinal histology and the response to the gluten-free diet (GFD) establishes the diagnosis. An intestinal biopsy should be requested when there is clinical suspicion and/or positive serology or even when serological tests are negative in the presence of symptoms suggestive of the disease. The diagnosis is confirmed when there is a clinical, serological and/or histological response to a gluten-free diet (GFD) and it is reinforced by the presence of genetic susceptibility markers HLA-DQ2 or HLA-DQ8.

Serological markers have played a major role in highlighting the heterogeneity of clinical presentations and they have been used to conduct prevalence studies in the general population. They have also made it possible to identify risk populations and CD-associated diseases.

2. History of Serological Markers

Celiac disease was discovered in the 1950s when the Dutch pediatrician, Dicke,[1] identified a connection between "intractable diarrhea" and the presence of wheat flour in children's diet. Years later it was found that gluten was the antigen that triggered the disease and that intestinal atrophy was reversible.

In 1970, the *European Society of Paediatric Gastroenterology and Nutrition* (ESPGAN) published the first diagnostic criteria,[2] consisting of at least three intestinal biopsies: the first at baseline, the second on a GFD and the third after a gluten challenge test.

IgA-class antigliadin antibodies (IgA-AGA) were described at the beginning of the 1980s.[3] IgA-AGA was the first serological marker available for CD, which meant that patients could be screened pre-biopsy, and other clinical forms of CD could be detected in addition to the classical presentation of diarrhea with abdominal distension. IgA-AGAs are not CD-specific. They are antibodies to gluten components in the diet, and probably reflect increased intestinal permeability, because they are also found in other gut diseases.

The sensitivity and specificity[4] of the IgA-AGA test is in the range of 70-80%. In clinical practice, lack of sensitivity (the risk of false negatives) causes more harm than the lack of specificity. The IgA-AGA test gave false negative results in 10 out of 31 CD cases among first-degree relatives of patients with CD,[5] and in 4 out of 15 CD cases in a cohort of patients with Down syndrome,[6] all of who had asymptomatic CD. This supports the strong association between IgA-AGA and digestive symptoms.

The technical advantages of using IgA-AGA markers in quantitative immunoassays has meant that they have been widely implemented in CD serological studies and in clinical practice. In fact, they are supplied commercially and form part of the serological marker panels for CD used in some laboratories.

In patients with selective IgA deficiency, IgG markers are determined instead, although IgG-class AGA markers have low specificity and are very common in the general population.

Antiendomysial antibodies (EmA) were identified[7] through their association with dermatitis herpetiformis. The high sensitivity and specificity of IgA-EmA markers (above 95%) marked a turning point in serological CD detection. Epidemiological studies that ensued showed high prevalence of CD in the general population, and diversity of its clinical forms. The 1970s triple biopsy diagnostic protocol was revised and simplified by ESPGAN in the 1990s[8] and reduced to a single initial biopsy followed by clinical improvement.

Indirect immunofluorescence (IIF) is used to determine IgA-EmA markers and other antibodies when the antigen is unknown. The immunological reaction takes place on a slide with fixed tissue slices containing the antigen. The most commonly used tissue was monkey distal esophagus. Human umbilical cord (HUC), jejunum (AJA anti-jejunal antibodies) and rat kidney (ARA, anti-reticulin antibodies) have also been used. IIF is a qualitative or semiquantitative technique using progressive serum dilutions. It can entail manual or semi-automated processing, and requires well-trained, experienced observers to interpret the patterns under a fluorescent microscope. Monkey distal esophagus slides have a high financial and ecological cost. A reasonable alternative is to use commercially available or in-house-prepared human umbilical cord, although the fluorescent pattern is harder to visualize on umbilical cord tissue.

In patients with IgA deficiency, IgG-class EmA markers are used, and their microscope image usually shows nonspecific fluorescence. This makes it harder to interpret an IgG pattern than an IgA pattern.

Anti-transglutaminase antibodies (IgA-tTG) appeared in 1997, when Dieterich[9] identified tissue transglutaminase (tTG) as the autoantigen recognized by EmA.

tTG is an enzyme protein that modifies the indigestible peptides in dietary gluten in the gut lamina propria, so that they are recognized by HLA-DQ2 molecules and are presented to CD4+ T cells, triggering an inflammatory humoral response, with the production of specific autoantibodies in patients with CD.

With the tTG antigen now available, EmA can be determined as tTG using quantitative, automatable immunoassay techniques, thus solving the technical limitations of IIF.

Quantitative determination of IgA-tTG makes it easier to monitor GFD serology and detects low autoantibody concentrations that cannot be detected using IIF. This is useful in the adult population, as explained later in this chapter. Isolated cases of falsely elevated IgA-tTG levels have been reported in patients with acute or serious diseases,[10,11] as well as small elevations of IgA-tTG, unrelated to dietary gluten, in patients with autoimmune diseases,[12] but they were considered to be nonspecific and possibly attributable to impurities in the tTG antigen.

In 2005, scientific societies[13] recommended IgA-tTG and/or IgA-EmA (with whole IgA) for serum CD detection; this was the first time that the use of IgA-AGA was discouraged.

Anti-deaminated gliadin peptide antibodies (IgA-DGP) have been developed in order to improve the efficiency of classical AGA using modified gliadin peptides as an antigen, which emulate gluten peptides in the gut lamina propria. The IgA-DGP test was found to be more effective than AGA at distinguishing patients with CD from controls in a pediatric population.[14] These observations have led to growing expectations[15] with regard to the usefulness of this new serological marker.

In 2008, the consensus document[16] issued by the *Federation of International Societies of Pediatric Gastroenterology, Hepatology, and Nutrition* did not include the IgA-DGP test in the protocol for CD serological detection, recommending that its specificity needed further study.

Children younger than two years with clinically suspected CD may have negative IgA-tTG but positive IgA-DGP. Analyzing the natural history of IgA-tTG and IgA-DGP in infants,[17] it was observed that IgA-DGP and IgA-tTG markers have different kinetics: IgA-DGPs appear before IgA-tTGs and disappear sooner when a GFD is introduced.

In infants, the sensitivity of IgA-DGP contrasts with its lack of specificity. Thus, IgA-DGP disappeared spontaneously[18] in most children under two years taking gluten who had clinical suspicion of CD and negative IgA-tTG. In these cases, intestinal biopsy was performed due to clinical suspicion rather than serology results. Another study,[19] however, surprisingly found that the diagnostic performance of IgG-DGP and IgA-tTG was comparable.

In the same context, one meta-analysis[20] of 11 studies with a total of 937 patients and 1328 controls published between 1998 and 2008, found greater discriminative power and diagnostic efficiency in IgA-tTG versus IgA-DGP.

3. Criteria for Choosing a Commercial Reagent

There is a wide range of commercial tests to determine serological markers in CD. Tests can be grouped by antibody (AGA, EmA, tTG, DGP, mixed DGP/tTG, etc.) isotype (IgA, IgG, IgA/IgG) or technique (IIF, ELISA, fluorescent immunoassay, chemiluminescence assay, etc.)

The choice of test to be used in the clinics should follow international recommendations and take into account the recent evidence-based literature. Laboratories should choose the most effective test for the context (adults, children, CD detection only, detection and follow-up). Cost should be reasonable, but should not be the only factor in the decision.

Laboratories should be involved in clinicians' decisions to modify or improve CD serology protocols. There must be a good reason for switching tests or adding a new one because this requires an adaptation period and new reference values.

Serum antibody levels are determined by quantitative and qualitative immunoassay techniques, which may be manual or automated. Analyzers are usually connected to an online system. These techniques include ELISA (enzyme-linked immunosorbent assay) with spectrophotometric reading of the final result, adapting signal amplification systems using fluorescence (e.g. fluorescent immunoassay in tTG EliA™ by Phadia) or luminescence (e.g., chemiluminescence in tTG BioflashR) to increase sensitivity.

The following technical aspects should be taken into account when choosing a test:

- The nature of the antigen(s) in the immunoassay and calibrator type (2, 3 or 6 points).
- The manufacturer's cut-off values.
- Grey or inconclusive zones, if any.
- Sensitivity and specificity in terms of histology and in the general population.
- Imprecision at different concentrations (within-run and between-run %CV), particularly at low concentrations.
- Linearity and detection limits, and any interferences or other limitations.

Pack size (e.g., 50 or 500 test pack) and reagent stability should match workload, because a laboratory must be able to offer a reasonable response time at a reasonable cost. If the test requires calibration for each analytical run, samples should be grouped to reduce calibration costs. However, if the calibration is stored in the analyzer memory, individual samples can be determined at no additional cost. Quality controls must be performed for each analytical run.

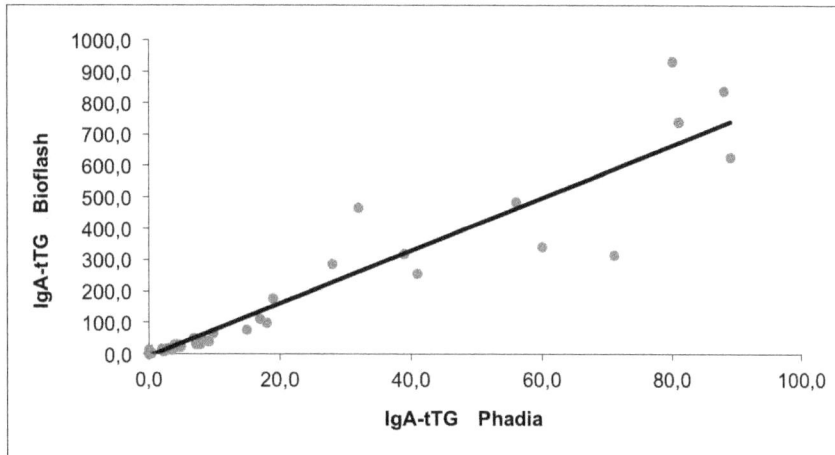

Figure 1. IgA-tTG: Fluorescent immunoassay vs. chemiluminescence, range 0-80 U/ml

Before introducing a new test, studies must be conducted on imprecision (within-run and between-run %CV) and reproducibility of results using another reference test for the same antibody. In this respect, the lack of a universal calibration standard is a major drawback, because each manufacturer defines its own arbitrary standards.

Figure 1 shows IgA-tTG results in 70 samples from patients with active CD or on a GFD, using two automated next-generation commercial tests, a fluorescent immunoassay (EliA™ by Phadia) and a chemiluminescence assay (Bioflash®). The Passing-Bablock test to analyze reproducibility of results shows that there is no constant error between tests [intercept: -0.15 (-0.45 to 0.12)] but there is a proportional error [slope: 6.190 (5.537 to 7.010)]. The results obtained using the two techniques show good correlation ($r = 0.952$), despite the proportional difference, which is explained by the differences between the manufacturers' calibrators.

Figure 2 shows the same comparison but in the grey zone (between 2 and 10 U/ml IgA-tTG in the fluorescent immunoassay taking Phadia as the reference; n=27). In this range, the regression line for the tests is [tTG Bioflash] = 5.2846 [tTG Phadia] - 0.4173. This gives a grey zone using the chemiluminescence assay of approximately 10-60 U/ml [Passing-Bablock: slope 6.000 (4.923 to 7.527); intercept -3.40 (-8.53 to 0.85)]. In clinical practice, it is important for the laboratory to identify this grey zone clearly, and to make sure that the analytical imprecision for this range is adequate.

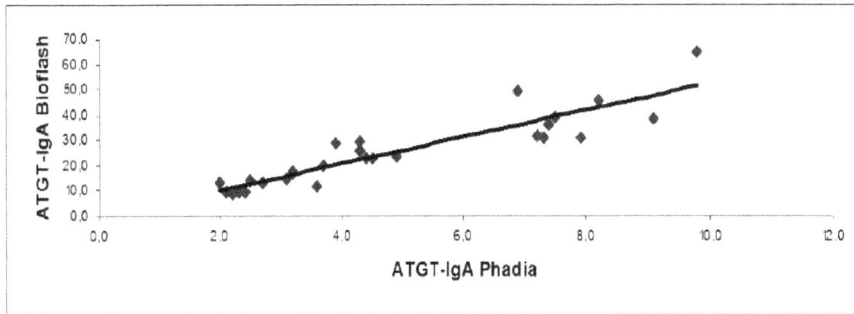

Figure 2. IgA-tTG: Fluorescent immunoassay vs. chemiluminescence, range 0-10 U/ml

In order to compare the sensitivity (SENS) and specificity (SPEC) of different representative serology strategies to detect CD, we used samples that were specifically selected from our experience of false positive (SENS) and false positive (SPEC) results. We tested 23 serum samples with high IgA-tTG in patients with asymptomatic CD diagnosed by intestinal biopsy (SENS) and 22 serum samples from children aged 1 to 2 years with diarrhea that had resolved with conventional treatment (SPEC).

The antigens used in the tests were:

1.- Recombinant human tTG (reference test);

2.- Native gliadin

3.- Synthetic Gliadin Peptide

4.- Purified erythrocyte tTG and DGP mixture (Screen)

5.- DGP-bound recombinant human tTG

6 and 7.- GAF3X peptide obtained by emulating DGP

The test results for each group (see Table 1) show that AGA and DGP are indeed less sensitive than tTG for detecting asymptomatic CD. They are also less specific than tTG in the specially selected group of children with diarrhea resolved with conventional treatment.

	Marsh III asymptomatic CD n = 23		Children aged 1-2 yeas with diarrhea n = 22	
	Positive	False Negative	False Positive	Negative
IgA-tTG	n=23	-	-	n=22
IgA-AGA	n=12	n=11	n=3	n=19
IgA-DGP	n=17	n=6	n=1	n=21
Screen IgA/IgG tTG/DGP	n=23	-	n=1	n=21
Anti-neo IgA-tTG bound DGP	n=23	-	n=2	n=20
IgA-anti-GAF3X	n=19	n=4	n=1	n=21
IgG-anti-GAF3X	n=17	n=6	n=2	n=20

Table 1. Results of different serology strategies to detect CD in selected cases

Mixed tests (used in screening) with more than one antigen (tTG and DGP) and polyvalent conjugates simultaneously detect IgA and IgG class DGP and tTG. They have good sensitivity for CD detection but they are not useful as a baseline for GFD serological monitoring, because the antibodies and isotypes have different kinetics. Likewise, caution should be exercised with some commercial tTG tests in which the tTG antigen has been "enriched" with PGD in order to increase sensitivity, as they can give false positive results due to the lack of specificity of the DGP.

CD markers can also be determined using rapid point of care (POC) tests. Pharmacies can make up these immunochromatographic tests individually to detect IgA and/or IgG tTG and/or DGP using a rapid fingerprick method. They are available as a self-testing kit and provide a quick, initial result for CD that can be carried out at the clinic or at home. The biggest disadvantage is that the test should always be followed up with a conventional analysis. A positive result needs to be confirmed using the classical diagnostic workup and a negative result also needs to be investigated if clinical suspicion persists. Furthermore, these tests are expensive and they carry the risk of patients starting a GFD themselves, which then makes it harder to confirm the diagnosis.

4. Recommendations for the Use of Serological Markers

Individuals of any age should undergo CD serological screening if they have any unexplained signs or symptoms summarized in Table 2, taken from the Working Group document on "Early Diagnosis of Celiac Disease",[21] published by the Spanish Ministry of Health and Consumer Affairs in 2008.

Age group	Symptoms	Signs
Children	Chronic Diarrhea Abdominal pain Vomiting Anorexia Apathy Moodiness	Malnutrition Abdominal bloating Failure to thrive Muscular Hypotrophy Iron deficiency Hipoproteinemia
Pre-teens and teenagers	Oligosymptomatic Abdominal pain Diarrhea-constipation Pubertal developmental delay Menstrual alterations Headaches Arthralgia	Low stature Iron deficiency Mouth ulcers Muscular weakness Osteopenia Skin and teeth alterations
Adults	Unspecific digestive symptoms: 　Dyspepsia 　Diarrhea 　Constipation 　Vomiting Weight loss Osteomuscular symptoms Infertility, repeated abortions Neurological alterations: 　Paresthesias 　Tetany 　Ataxia 　Epilepsy Psychiatric alterations: 　Depression 　Irritability 　Asthenia	Malnutrition Iron deficiency Hypoalbuminemia Coagulation alterations Vitamin deficiencies Hypertransaminasemia Peripheral neuropathy Myopathy Hyposplenism Mouth ulcers Osteoporosis and osteopenia

Based on the Working Group document on "Early diagnosis of celiac disease." Spanish Ministry of Health and Consumer Affairs. April 2008.

Table 2. Signs and symptoms of celiac disease

Individuals consider to belong to risk populations should also be screened. Risk populations consist of persons with a higher prevalence of CD than the general population, which stands at about 1%. Risk groups of note[22] are first-degree relatives (10-20%) of CD patients, patients with CD-associated diseases[22] such as type 1 diabetes mellitus (T1DM) (2-12%), Down syndrome (5-12%), autoimmune thyroid disease (up to 7%), Turner syndrome (2-5%), Williams syndrome (up to 9%), selective IgA deficiency (SigAD) (2-8%) and patients with autoimmune liver disease (12-13%).

Serological CD screening is not an urgent procedure in clinical laboratories. CD has a slow onset and it also resolves gradually. Laboratories can therefore return results in a reasonable period ranging from 1 to 7 days, depending on clinics' logistics and clinicians' expectations. Results should be assessed in a clinical-dietary-historical context and the head of the laboratory should add comments or contact the clinician, if required. Likewise, the head of the laboratory should play an active part in selecting the most appropriate markers and most appropriate patients for serological testing, in close coordination with the referring clinician. Positive tTG cases should be recorded in a database for future use. According to the latest recommendations issued by ESPGHAN,[22] IgA-tTG and/or IgA-EmA (if total serum IgA is normal) are the markers of choice for CD, while IgA-DGP markers are recommended as an additional test in children younger than two years of age with negative IgA-tTG and suspected CD. Children who are diagnosed before the age of two are candidates for a gluten challenge test, in view of the lack of knowledge of the natural course of gluten intolerance at this early disease stage.

A good clinical laboratory[22] should:

1.- Participate in internal and external quality control programs.

2.- Use tests that are validated against an EmA reference standard or histology, with >95% agreement.

3.- Use tests with a manufacturer-defined cut-off or ULN (upper limit of normal) that has been adapted according to personal experience or in view of the population studied.

4.- Express results in figures and specify immunoglobulin class. Classification as "positive" or "negative" is not sufficient because it does not provide a baseline value for GFD serological monitoring.

5.- Specify the immunoglobulin class and cut-off dilution in EmA reports, indicating whether the result is positive or negative, along with the dilution.

6.- Flag negative IgA-tTG results to avoid misinterpreting cases such as patients with IgA deficiency, children younger than two years, patients on a gluten-poor or gluten-free diet (because a few weeks of a GFD will confound a negative result), and patients receiving immunosuppressive therapy.

Depending on the test, different figures and units of measurements are used for CD serological markers. Reproducibility studies are useful for verifying whether results from such tests are comparable. Results can be expressed as multiples of the upper limit of normal (ULN) or with their respective cut-off values.

Active collaboration between clinic and laboratory undoubtedly improves the quality of care. In this respect, it is useful to set up and maintain a database with demographic, clinical, serological, genetic, histological and family data of patients with high IgA-tTG levels as an initial inclusion criterion. Mining this database may help to further our knowledge of CD and improve care protocols.

When laboratories receive a request for "CD serological markers" they should be able to offer the most appropriate screening tests available. They should not resort to a general panel of antibodies and isotypes that does not provide evidence-based additional information and is simply a burden on human and economic resources.

Serology tests precede histology in all CD diagnostic algorithms. In the latest recommendations issued by ESPGHAN,[22] the main change is the possibility of diagnosing CD without resorting to intestinal biopsy in children with compatible symptoms, genetic susceptibility and IgA-tTG serum levels >10 times the cut-off value or ULN.

However, this protocol has been subject to considerable debate,[23,24] and its opponents suggest that an initial biopsy serves as a reference for the baseline lesion, should the disease develop in an unexpected way, and that it detects discrepancies between serology and histology results. Technical disadvantages include lack of result reproducibility studies on commercial tests, lack of a universal calibration standard (as mentioned above) and the fact that the positive predictive value (PPV) of IgA-tTG tests depends on CD prevalence in the population studied.

5. The Relationship between Serology and Histology

Although the level of specific antibodies in blood is generally understood to reflect the degree of intestinal histological lesion, serology and histology results do not always match.

The sensitivity of IgA-tTG/EmA tests is lower in patients with partial villous atrophy. In fact, it has been observed that IgA-tTG/EmA markers may be negative in 60% of patients with Marsh 3a lesions.[25,26] Furthermore, negative IgA-tTG/EmA tests in patients taking a GFD do not necessarily imply histological recovery of villous architecture, especially in adults.[27,28]

Serological response to GFD varies from one patient to another. According to the ESPGHAN, a 12-month GFD is required to achieve a negative result for CD-specific antibodies, but this period can range from 3 months to 3 or 4 years, depending on the patient's gluten sensitivity. Likewise, the length of time required for a gluten challenge test (about 15 g/day in children) to achieve a positive serological result varies greatly. Blood tests should be taken every 3-6 months if there is no clear clinical response. Generally, a positive serological result is sufficient to confirm the diagnosis.

In clinical practice, dietary non-adherence can be detected by serology findings of some degree of IgA-tTG elevation in CD patients on a GFD with several previous successive negative serological controls. This is a common finding in adolescents and can be attributed to deliberate or accidental non-adherence to their GFD, which they may or may not be aware of. EmA levels determined using IIF assays are less sensitive to these minor serological variations. IgA-DGP testing is recommended[29] to detect dietary non-adherence, but its lack of specificity has a negative impact on the cost-benefit ratio.

6. Serological Markers in Adult CD

Adulthood-onset CD can occur in genetically susceptible individuals taking dietary gluten. In these cases, elevated IgA-tTG findings can confirm clinical suspicion before the histological diagnosis is reached. In some cases, late disease onset may be triggered by pregnancy, infections, trauma or stress, and it can also occur in elderly patients.

Furthermore, CD in adults may go undiagnosed due to the heterogeneity of its signs and symptoms. Serological markers have poor sensitivity because villous atrophy may be partial. An interesting study[30] of consecutive CD diagnoses across all ages showed that CD in adults has attenuated clinical symptoms, serology and intestinal histological lesions compared with CD in children. This means that it takes longer to reach a definitive diagnosis in adults than in children.

While a low-grade intestinal lesion is associated with mild clinical symptoms, a case-finding study in relatives of patients with CD[31] proved that clinical symptoms (anemia, abdominal pain or distension or bone density alterations) are as important in Marsh stage 1 as they are in Marsh stage 3. This study proposed performing an intestinal biopsy in all DQ2-positive relatives of patients with CD, regardless of serological results. The study showed that if a conventional serological screening protocol had been followed (IgA-tTG and/or IgA-EmA with the standard cut-off value), there would have been a 15.6% detection rate of cases with Marsh 1 lesions and 84.6% detection rate of cases with Marsh 3 lesions. This confirms the low sensitivity of IgA-tTG markers in adult patients with CD and low-grade intestinal lesions, in whom IgA-tTG elevations may be below the established cut-off value.

In view of these results and with the aim of increasing IgA-tTG sensitivity in the adult population, a new lower cut-off value was sought, based on the IgA-tTG level below which 98% of the general adult population belong.[32] This resulted in a cut-off value for adults four times lower than the cut-off value for children.

Applying this new cut-off value for adults in a CD case-finding study in the working population,[32] it was found that IgA-tTG had 89% sensitivity and IgA-EmA had 11% sensitivity among patients with Marsh 1 lesions, while both markers had 100% sensitivity for patients with Marsh 3 lesions.

Marsh 1 lesions are not only found in CD; they can also occur in other diseases such *Helicobacter pylori* infection, parasite infestation and other enteropathies. The suitability of the GFD in patients with Marsh 1 lesions in the absence of clinical symptoms is controversial.[33] In these cases, flow cytometry studies in gut mucosa are particularly relevant because they can detect patterns that are compatible with CD, regardless of histological changes.

7. Serological Markers in At-Risk Populations

Serological screening to detect asymptomatic CD in at-risk populations can be optimized by identifying DQ2 positive cases beforehand. The high negative predictive value of DQ2 (NPV > 99%) makes it almost impossible to diagnose CD in DQ2-negative individuals.

However, 64% of first-degree relatives of patients with CD, 57% of patients with T1DM, 29% of patients with Down syndrome and 25% of the general population are DQ2 positive.[34] In consequence, in a DQ2-positive patient with Down syndrome (6% CD prevalence), the probability of positive serology is 1:5, and in a DQ2-positive individual in the general population (1% CD prevalence), the probability is 1:25. Therefore, DQ2 is useful to select candidates for serological surveillance in at-risk populations. In these cases, there are no recommendations regarding the frequency of performing serological screening in asymptomatic individuals. In the best scenario, these individuals undergo annual serological testing.

7.1. IgA-tTG in patients with T1DM

A case-finding strategy to detect asymptomatic CD in the T1DM population consists of IgA-tTG testing when diabetes is diagnosed, and annual serological monitoring thereafter. With this strategy,[35] CD was diagnosed in 6.4% (13 out of 202) patients who had newly-diagnosed T1DM, during 6 consecutive years of systematic screening. According to the same study, CD has a strong association with early-onset T1DM and there is no preferential order of appearance between the two diseases. This is corroborated by asymptomatic CD being detected by serology at the time of the diabetes diagnosis in half the cases, whereas it was detected during serological monitoring during the next three years in the other half of cases. Inconclusive or weak positive CD serology at the onset of diabetes should be interpreted with caution, and developments should be monitored.

7.2. IgA-tTG in patients with IgA Deficiency

CD is associated with selective IgA deficiency. Serum IgA deficiency (serum IgA < 10 mg/L) is the most common of primary immunodeficiency diseases and it affects 0.2% of the general population. It is usually asymptomatic.

If selective IgA deficiency is found by chance, IgG-class tTG markers should be systematically tested. Following this strategy,[36] 6.6% (22/330) of children with absolute, partial or transient IgA deficiency (IgA < 50 mg/L) were diagnosed with CD.

Analyzing the serology findings in this population,[37] it was found that IgA deficiency was absolute in 70% of cases and that only class IgG tTG antibodies were detected. The remaining 30%, however, accounted for partial or transient IgA deficiency, and tTG antibodies of IgA and IgG classes were detected in 80% of cases.

Since IgG antibodies have a longer half-life than IgA antibodies, they take longer to disappear in GFD monitoring. Thus, IgG-tTG tests are still positive after 2 to 11 years of GFD, while IgA-tTG tests are negative after 1 to 4 years of GFD in 100% of cases.

8. Serological Markers in the General Population

CD is a common disease. It may remain undiagnosed because of the heterogeneity of clinical presentations. It has excellent diagnostic serological markers. It has effective treatment without side effects and lack of treatment is associated with negative effects.

In view of the above, CD appears to be an ideal disease to study in the general population.[38,39] However, there are drawbacks to conducting a massive study of CD in the general population such as lack of knowledge of the natural history of asymptomatic, untreated CD; lack of motivation for asymptomatic patients to adhere to a GFD; CD onset at any age, which would require repeated serological screening; and lack of cost-benefit studies.

For the same reasons, it is not recommended to add IgA-tTG screening to routine tests in healthy general population groups, such as medical check-ups at work, blood donors and pre-operative checklists for minor surgery. However, if there is an accidental finding of microcytic anemia or a slight elevation of ALT levels in blood[40] in routine tests, then systematic IgA-tTG determination would facilitate asymptomatic CD detection. Unexplained anemia or elevated transaminases are known extradigestive manifestations of asymptomatic CD.

It is accepted that CD prevalence in the general population is approximately 1:100. However, it is still widely held that CD is more prevalent in children. Epidemiological studies conducted in different age groups in the Spanish population show that prevalence ranges from 1:118 in children younger than 3 years[41] to 1:220 in primary school children[42], and 1:389 in the general population[43] with a mean age of 35 years. This apparent decreasing prevalence as age increases has recently been confirmed in an epidemiological study[44] of 4230 persons aged 1 to 90 years in the general population in Catalonia. The results from this study show that CD is 5 times more common in children than in adults, and that this increase is largely due to prevalence in the youngest children. This age-related fall in prevalence is hard to explain in view of the fact that CD is a permanent, non-resolving disease. The hypothesis of spontaneous progress to a latent state can only be investigated through longitudinal natural history studies.

References

1. Dicke WK. Coeliac disease. *Pnvestigation of the har1 ful e/ects of certain types of cereal on patients su/ering fro1 coeliac disease*. MD thesis. Utrecht: University of Utrecht, 1950.

2. Meeuwisse G. *Diagnosis criteria in coeliac disease*. Acta Paediatr Scand 1970; 59: 461-3.

3. Savilahty E, Viander M, Perkkio M, Vainio E, Kalimo K, Reunala T. *Pgl antigliadin antiUodiesHa 1 ar2er of 1 ucosal da1 age in childhood coeliac disease*. Lancet. 1983: 1(8320): 320-2. http://dx.doi.org/10.1016/S0140-6736(83)91627-6

4. Rostom A, Dube C, Cranney A, Saloojee N, Sy R, Garritty C, et al. *The diagnostic accuracy of serologic tests for celiac diseaseHa syste1 atic review*. Gastroenterology. 2005; 128: S38-46. http://www.ncbi.nlm.nih.gov/pubmed/15825125

5. Farré C, Humbert P, Vilar P, Varea V, Carballo M, Aldeguer X, Carnicer J, Gasull MA and Catalonian Coeliac Disease Study Group. *Serological k ar2ers and "M-DQ8 "aplotype I 1 ong First-Degree relatives of Celiac Patients*. Dig Dis Sci. 1999; 44(11): 2344-49. http://dx.doi.org/10.1023/A:1026685527228

6. Carnicer J, Farré C, Varea V, Vilar P, Moreno J, Artigas J. *Prevalence of coeliac disease in Down's syndro1 e*. Eur J Gastroenterol Hepatol. 2001; 13: 263-7. http://dx.doi.org/10.1097/00042737-200103000-00008

7. Chorzelsky TP, Beutner EH, Sulej J, Tchorzewska H, Jablonska S, Kumar V, et al. IgA anti-endomysium antibody. *I new i1 1 unological 1 ar2er of der1 atitis herpetifor1 is and coeliac disease*. Br J Dermatol. 1984: 111(4): 395-402. http://dx.doi.org/10.1111/j.1365-2133.1984.tb06601.x

8. Revised criteria for diagnosis of coeliac disease. Report of Working Group of European Society of Paediatric Gastroenterology and Nutrition. Arch Dis Child. 1990: 65(8): 909-11. http://dx.doi.org/10.1136/adc.65.8.909

9. Dieterich W, Ehnis T, Bauer M, Donner P, Volta U, Riecken EO, et al. *Pdentification of tissue transgluta1 inase as the autoantigen of celiac disease*. Nat Med. 1997; 3(7): 797-801. http://dx.doi.org/10.1038/nm0797-797

10. Bizzaro N, Tampoia M, Villalta, D, Platzgummer S, Liguori, M, Tozzoli, R, Tonutti, E. *Now Specificity of I nti-Tissue Transgluta1 inase I ntiUodies in Patients ff ith Pri1 ary biliary Cirrhosis*. J Clin Lab Anal. 2006; 20: 184–9. http://dx.doi.org/10.1002/jcla.20130

11. Ferrara, F, Quaglia S, Caputo I, Esposito, C, Lepretti, M, Pastore, S, Giorgi, R, Martelossi, S, Dal Molin G, Di Toro M, Ventura, A, Not, T. *I nti-transgluta1 inase antiUodies in non-coeliac children su/ering fro1 infectious diseases* Clin Exp Immunol. 2010; 159(2): 217–23. http://dx.doi.org/10.1111/j.1365-2249.2009.04054.x

12. Sárdy M, Csikós M, Geisen C, Preisz K, Kornseé Z, Tomsits E, Töx U, Hunzelmann N, Wieslander J, Kárpáti S, Paulsson M, Smyth N. *Tissue transgluta1 inase WWSI positivity in autoi1 1 une disease independent of gluten-sensitive disease*. Clinica Chimica Acta. 2007; 376: 126–35. http://dx.doi.org/10.1016/j.cca.2006.08.006

13. Hill ID, Dirks MH, Liptak GS, Colletti RB, Fasano A, Guandalini S, et al. North American Society for Pediatric Gastroenterology, Hepatology and Nutrition. *Guideline for the diagnosis and treat1 ent of celiac disease in childrenHreco1 1 endations of the North I 1 erican Society for Pediatric Gastroenterology, "epatology and Nutrition*. J Pediatr Gastroenterol Nutr. 2005 Jan; 40(1): 1-19. http://dx.doi.org/10.1097/00005176-200501000-00001

14. Schwertz E, Kahlenberg F, Sack U, Richter T, Stern M, Conrad K, Zimmer KP, Mothes T. *Serologic I ssay based on Gliadin-Related Nonapeptides as a " ighly Sensitive and Specific Diagnostic I id in Celiac Disease*. Clinical Chemistry. 2004; 50(12): 2370–5. http://dx.doi.org/10.1373/clinchem.2004.036111

15. Kaukinen K, Collin P, Laurila K, Kaartinen T, Partanen J, Mäki M. *Resurrection of gliadin antiUodies in coeliac disease. Dea1 idated gliadin peptide antiUody test provides additional diagnostic Uenefit.* Scand J Gastroenterol. 2007; 42(12): 1428-33. http://dx.doi.org/10.1080/00365520701452217

16. Fasano A, Araya M, Bhatnagar S, et al. Consensus guidelines. J. Pediatr Gastroenterol Nutr. 2008; 47(2):214-9. http://dx.doi.org/10.1097/MPG.0b013e318181afed

17. Edwin Liu et al. *Natural " istory of I ntiUodies ti Dea1 inated Gliadin Peptides and Transgluta1 inase in Wrly Childhood Celiac Disease*. J Pediatr Gastroenterol Nutr. 2007; 45: 293-300. http://dx.doi.org/10.1097/MPG.0b013e31806c7b34

18. Parizade M, Shainberg B. P*ositive Dea1 idated Gliadin Peptide I ntiUodies and Negative Tissue Transgluta1 inase PgI I ntiUodies in a Pediatric PopulationHTo biopsy or Not To biopsy.* Clin Vaccine Immunol. 2010; 17(5): 884–6. http://dx.doi.org/10.1128/CVI.00425-09

19. Vermeersch P, Geboes K, Mariën G, Hoffman I, Hiele M, Bossuyt X. *Diagnostic perfor1 ance of PgG anti-dea1 idated gliadin peptide antiUody assays is co1 paraUle to PgI anti-tTG in celiac disease.* Clinica Chimica Acta. 2010; 411: 931–5. http://dx.doi.org/10.1016/j.cca.2010.02.060

20. Levis NR, Scott BB. *k eta-analysisH Dea1 idated gliadin peptide antiUody and tissue transgluta1 inase antiUody co1 pared as screening tests for coeliac disease.* Aliment Pharmacol Ther. 2010; 31: 73–81. http://www.ncbi.nlm.nih.gov/pubmed/19664074

21. Garrote Adrados JA, Fernandez Salazar L. Protocolos de diagnóstico. Cribado de enfermedad celíaca y grupos de riesgo. *Wfer1 edad Celíaca.* (Cap 10, pp 145). Ergon 2011. ISBN: 978-8473-958-6.

22. Husby S, Koletzko S, Korponay-Szabo IR, Mearin ML, Phillips A, Shamir R, et al. *For the VßPG" I N ff or2ing Group on Coeliac Disease Diagnosis*, on behalf of the ESPGHAN Gastroenterology Committee. J Pediatr Gastroenterol Nutr. 2012; 54: 136–60. http://dx.doi.org/10.1097/mpg.0b013e31821a23d0

23. Evans KE, Sanders DS. *ff hat is the use of Uiopsy and antiUodies in coeliac disease diagnosis?* J Intern Med. 2011; 269(6): 572-81. http://dx.doi.org/10.1111/j.1365-2796.2011.02380.x

24. Fernández-Bañares F, Rosinach M, Esteve M. *Co1 1 ent to B" igh tissue-transgluta1 inase antiUody level predicts s1 all intestinal villous atrophy in adult patients at high ris2 of coeliac diseaseB.*Dig Liver Dis. 2012 Oct; 44(10): 885-6. http://dx.doi.org/10.1016/j.dld.2012.04.025

25. Rostami K, Kerckhaert JP, Tiemessen R, Meijer JW, Mulder CJ. *The relationship Uetween anti-endo1 isiu1 antiUodies and villous atrophy in celiac disease using Uoth 1 on2ey and hu1 an suUstrate.* Eur J Gastroenterol Hepatol. 1999; 11(4): 439-42. http://dx.doi.org/10.1097/00042737-199904000-00013

26. Abrams JA, Brar P, Diamond B, Rotterdam H, Green PH. *mtility in clinical practice of i1 1 unogloUulin an anti-tissue transgluta1 inase antiUody for the diagnosis of celiac disease.* Clin Gastroenterol Hepatol. 2006; 4(6): 726-30. http://dx.doi.org/10.1016/j.cgh.2006.02.010

27. Wahab PJ, Meijer J, Mulder J. *" istologic Follow-up of People ff ith Celiac Disease on a Gluten-Free Diet. Slow and Pnco1 plete Recovery.* Am J Clin Pathol. 2002; 118: 459-63. http://dx.doi.org/10.1309/EVXT-851X-WHLC-RLX9

28. Dickey W, Hughes DF, McMillan SA. *Disappearance of endo1 ysial antiUodies in treated celiac disease does not indicate indicate histological recovery*. Am J Gastroenterol. 2000; 95(3): 712-4. http://dx.doi.org/10.1111/j.1572-0241.2000.01838.x

29. Agardh D. A*ntiUodies against synthetic dea1 idated gliadin peptides and tissue transgluta1 inase for the identification of childhood celiac disease*. Clin Gastroenterol Hepatol. 2007; 5: 1276–81. http://dx.doi.org/10.1016/j.cgh.2007.05.024

30. Vivas S, Ruiz de Morales JM, Fernandez M, Hernando M, Herrero B, Casqueiro J, Gutierrez S. Age-Related Clinical, *Serological, and " istopathological Features of Celiac Disease.* Am J Gastroenterol. 2008; 103(9): 2360-5. http://dx.doi.org/10.111/j.1572-0241.2008.01977.x

31. Esteve M, Rosinach M, Fernández-Bañares F, Farré C, Salas A, Alsina M, Vilar P, Abad-Lacruz A, Forné M, Mariné M, Santaolalla R, Espinós JC, Viver JM. Barcelona Coeliac Disease Study Group. S*pectru1 of gluten-sensitive enteropathy in first degree relatives of patients with coeliac diseaseHclinical relevance of ly1 phocytic enteritis.* Gut. 2006; 55: 1739–45. http://dx.doi.org/10.1136/gut.2006.095299

32. Mariné M, Fernández-Bañares F, Alsina M, Farré C, Cortijo M, Santaolalla R, Salas A, Tomàs M, Abugattas E, Loras C, Ordás I, Viver JM, Esteve M. *I1 pact of 1 ass screening for gluten sensitive enteropathy in a wor2ing population*. World J Gastroenterol. 2009; 15 (11): 1331-8. http://dx.doi.org/10.3748/wjg.15.1331

33. Esteve M, Carrasco A, Fernandez-Bañares F. I*s a gluten-free diet necessary in k arsh P intestinal lesions in patients with " M DQ8, DQ: genotype and without gastrointestinal sy1 pto1 s?* Curr Opin Clin Nutr Metab Care. 2012; 15: 505–10. http://dx.doi.org/10.1097/MCO.0b013e3283566643

34. Farré C. *k alaltia CelíacaH1 arcadors serològics i de predisposició genètica, aspectes clínics i poUlacions de risc*. Tesi Doctoral. Universitat de Barcelona 2002.

35. Marquès T, Molero M, Tondo M, Hernández M, Vilar P, Cusi V, et al. *I sociación entre la diaUetes 1 ellitus de tipo E y la enfer1 edad celíacaH6 años de criUado serológico siste1 ático*. Rev Lab Clin. 2009; 2(2): 65–72.

36. Domínguez O, Giner MT, Alsina L, Martín MA, Lozano J, Plaza AM. *Fenotipos clínicos asociados a la deficiencia selectiva de RgI Hrevisión de 33A casos y propuesta de un protocolo de segui1 iento.* An Pediatr. 2012; 76(5): 261-7. http://dx.doi.org/10.1016/j.anpedi.2011.11.006

37. Altimira L, Marquès T, Molero M, Tondo M, Hernández M, Farré C. *¿Co1 o se co1 portan los pacientes celíacos con déficit aislado de RgI ?* V Congreso Nacional del Laboratorio Clínico. SEQC. Malaga 2011.

38. Fasano A. *Wuropean and North I 1 erican populations should Ue screened for coeliac disease*. Gut. 2003; 52(2): 168-9. http://dx.doi.org/10.1136/gut.52.2.168

39. Kumar PJ. E*uropean and North I 1 erican populations should Ue screened for coeliac disease*. Gut. 2003; 52(2): 170-1. http://dx.doi.org/10.1136/gut.52.2.170

40. Farré C, Esteve, M, Curcoy, A, Cabre E, Arranz E, Amat, Ll, et al. *" ypertransa1 inase1 ia in Pediatric Celiac Disease Patients and Rts Prevalence as a Diagnostic Clue*. Am J Gastroenterol. 2002; 97: 3176–81. http://dx.doi.org/10.1111/j.1572-0241.2002.07127.x

41. Castaño L, Blarduni E, Ortiz L, et al. *Prospective population screening for celiac diseaseH high prevalence in the first 3 years of life*. J Pediatr Gastroenterol Nutr. 2004; 39: 80–4. http://dx.doi.org/10.1097/00005176-200407000-00016

42. Cilleruelo Pascual ML, Román Riechmann E, Jiménez Jiménez J, et al. S*ilent celiac diseaseHexploring the iceⳑerg in the school-aged population*. An Esp Pediatr. 2002; 57: 321–6.
http://www.unboundmedicine.com/evidence/ub/citation/12392666/
[Silent_celiac_disease:_exploring_the_iceberg_in_the_school_aged_population]_

43. Riestra S, Fernández E, Rodrigo L, et al. *Prevalence of coeliac disease in the general population of northern Spain. Strategies of serologic screening*. Scand J Gastroenterol. 2000; 35: 398–402. http://dx.doi.org/10.1080/003655200750023967

44. Marine M, Farré C, Alsina M, Vilar P, Cortijo M, Salas A, et al. *The prevalence of coeliac disease is significantly higher in children co1 pared with adults*. Aliment Pharmacol Ther. 2011; 33: 477–486. http://dx.doi.org/10.1111/j.1365-2036.2010.04543.x

OmniaScience

Chapter 9

The Role of Endoscopy in Celiac Disease and its Complications: Advances in Imaging Techniques and Computerization

Adolfo Parra-Blanco[1], Carlos Agüero[1], Daniel Cimmino[2], Nicolás González[3], Patricio Ibáñez[1], Silvia Pedreira[4]

[1]Department of Gastroenterology, School of Medicine, Pontificia Universidad Católica de Chile (PUC), Santiago, Chile.
[2]Endoscopy Service, Hospital Alemán (HA), Buenos Aires, Argentina.
[3]Department of Gastroenterology (Prof. Henry Cohen), Faculty of Medicine, Hospital de Clínicas, Montevideo, Uruguay.
[4]Gastroenterology Service, Hospital Alemán (HA), Buenos Aires, Argentina.

parrablanco@gmail.com, carlosagueroluengo@gmail.com, danielcimmino@gmail.com, nicolasendoscopia@yahoo.es, patricio.ibanezlazo@gmail.com, spedreira@intramed.net

Doi: http://dx.doi.org/10.3926/oms.228

How to cite this chapter

Parra-Blanco A, Agüero C, Cimmino D, González N, Ibáñez P, Pedreira S. *The Role of Endoscopy in Celiac Disease and its Complications: Advances in Imaging Techniques and Computerization*. In Rodrigo L and Peña AS, editors. *Celiac Disease and Non-Celiac Gluten Sensitivity*. Barcelona, Spain: OmniaScience; 2014. p. 171-202.

A. Parra-Blanco, C. Agüero, D. Cimmino, N. González, P. Ibáñez, S. Pedreira

Abstract

Endoscopy, for many reasons, is an important technique in the diagnosis of celiac disease (CD), since it is currently the most widely used method for performing duodenal biopsies. On the other hand, certain changes in the duodenal mucosa must warn the endoscopist of a possible celiac disease. This is relevant, since it is well-known that most of the people who have this disease remain undiagnosed.

With the development of endoscopy, different markers can be used to predict the existence of villous atrophy, but a high level of suspicion is required. The correct application of guidelines performing biopsies for a celiac disease diagnosis, especially if there is a sufficient number of samples, is important to reach diagnosis. Besides, due to the fact that the spectrum of health problems related to celiac disease is quite wide, their possible association must be taken into account and the performance of duodenal biopsies must be encouraged.

This last decade's technological achievements have greatly facilitated the study of the small intestine via endoscopy. Even if these advanced techniques are generally unnecessary in most cases, there are some of them in which the video capsule and/or enteroscopy allow to achieve a diagnosis, especially in refractory celiac disease cases. Other cutting-edge techniques, such as digital chromoendoscopy, optical coherence tomography and confocal endomicroscopy could be useful to predict the existence of villous atrophy and some of them could even help the endoscopist recognize lesser degrees of celiac disease. The relevance of these techniques in daily practice remains to be dilucidated.

1. Endoscopic Findings in Celiac Disease

Endoscopy is, for several reasons, an important technique in the diagnosis of CD since it is currently the most widely used method for making duodenal biopsies. Furthermore, there are changes in the duodenal mucosa that can lead to the suspicion of CD, which may allow diagnosis in cases in which this condition has not been found. This would be relevant as it is well known that most people with CD remain undiagnosed.

The development of endoscopy allowed the description of different markers associated with CD that predict the presence of villous atrophy associated with CD. For the detection of this disease, especially when test results do not indicate the study of possible CD, a high index of suspicion by the endoscopist is required.

This last decade's technological advances have meant that the small intestine is no longer unaccesible for endoscopy. While these advanced techniques are usually not necessary in most cases, there are situations in which the video capsule and/or enteroscopy make it possible to reach a diagnosis, especially in cases of refractory CD.

Numerous authors have described endoscopic findings in the duodenum and have linked them to the presence of villous atrophy in duodenal biopsies, which could theoretically allow the prediction of CD. Those most frequently cited are reduction in the folds in the second portion of the duodenum, scalloped folds, mosaic pattern of the mucosa, nodularity of the mucosa and visualization of submucosal vessels.

The features and definition of each one of these changes in the mucosa are detailed below.

1.1. Decrease in duodenal folds (Figures 1 and 2)

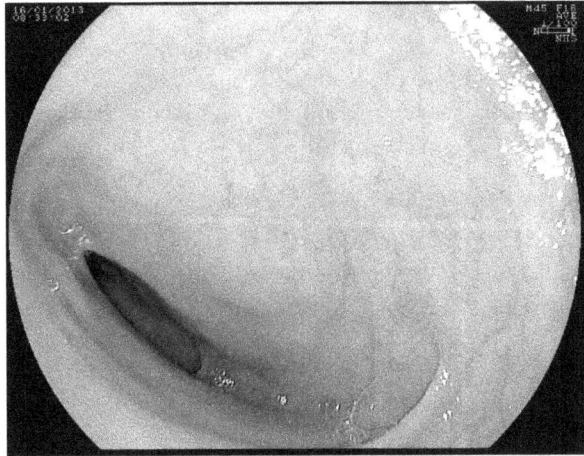

Figure 1. Duodenal mucosa with virtual disappearance of folds.

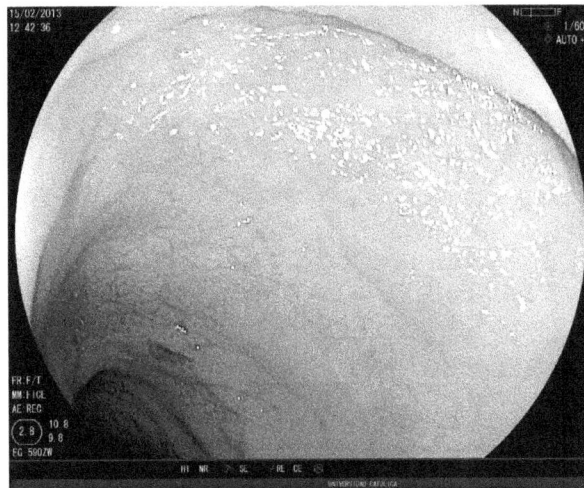

Figure 2. Duodenal mucosa with reduction of folds and granularity (a small ulcer can be observed in connection with the taking of a recent biopsy).

The loss of duodenal folds was first described in the nineteen seventies by Nicollet and Tully in radiological small intestine studies made using barium,[1] their endoscopic description being first published 1988 by Brochi et al.[2], who described loss of folds in the duodenum, defining it as the finding of only three folds in the second duodenal portion, with maximum insufflation. Evaluated in celiac disease patients, it described a sensitivity of 88% and specificity of 83%.

Subsequent studies, which defined this finding more subjectively as an obvious alteration found while performing an inspection, showed a sensitivity of 73% and a specificity of 97%.[3]

1.2. Mosaic pattern and scalloped folds (Figures 3- 6)

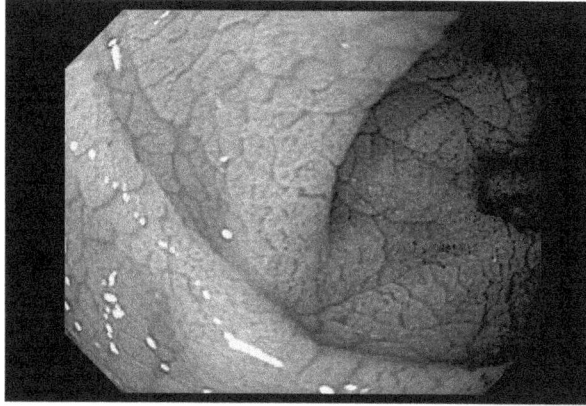

Figure 3. Duodenal mucosa with mosaic pattern (tenuous pattern).

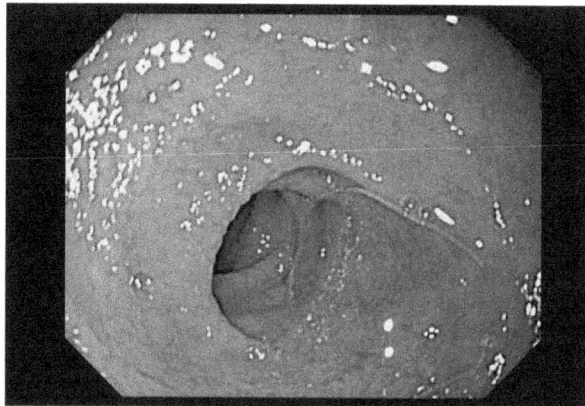

Figure 4. Duodenal mucosa with evident mosaic pattern.

The scalloped appearance of the folds was first described in 1988 in patients with celiac disease;[4] its proper inspection was described as one performed with maximum insufflation. In pediatric patients it had a sensitivity of 88% and specificity of 87% for the villous atrophy diagnosis.[5]

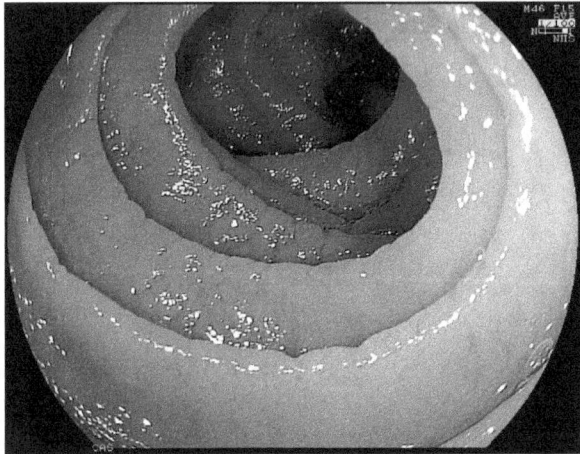

Figure 5. Scalloped appearance of the duodenal mucosa.

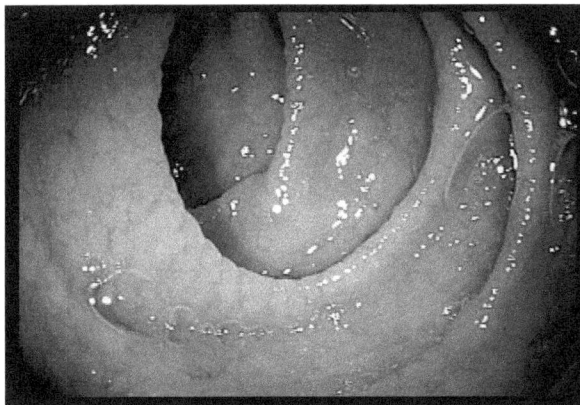

Figure 6. Scalloped appearance of the duodenal mucosa.

Duodenal mucosa grooves that seem to have a mosaic pattern between folds have also been associated with this disease and are probably manifestations of the same process that causes the scalloping of folds as the grooves advance.

Scalloped folds are not specific to celiac disease, and can be observed in patients with immunodeficiency, tropical sprue, giardiasis and eosinophilic gastroenteritis.[6]

1.3. Mucosal Nodularity (Figures 7 and 8)

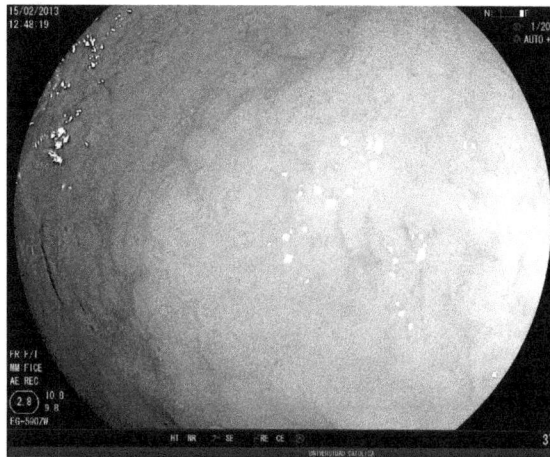

Figure 7. Nodular appearance of the bulb mucosa.

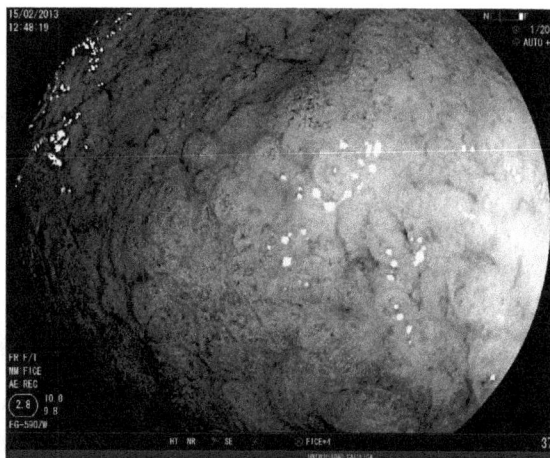

Figure 8. Same image as number 7, using computerized virtual chromoendoscopy with Fuji Intelligent Chromo Endoscopy (FICE).

In the vast majority of celiac patients studied endoscopically, the characteristic findings (mentioned above) were found in the descending duodenum. However Brocchi et al.[7] reported bulb nodularity in a 14-year-old celiac patient and no alterations in the second portion of the duodenum.

1.4. Visualization of submucosal vessels (Figures 9 and 10)

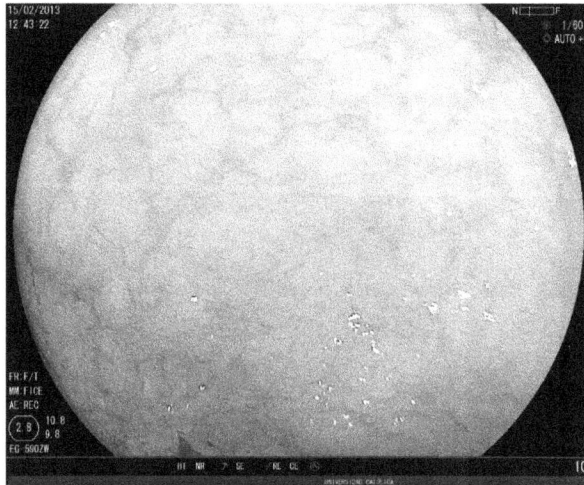

Figure 9. Prominent vessels in the bulb.

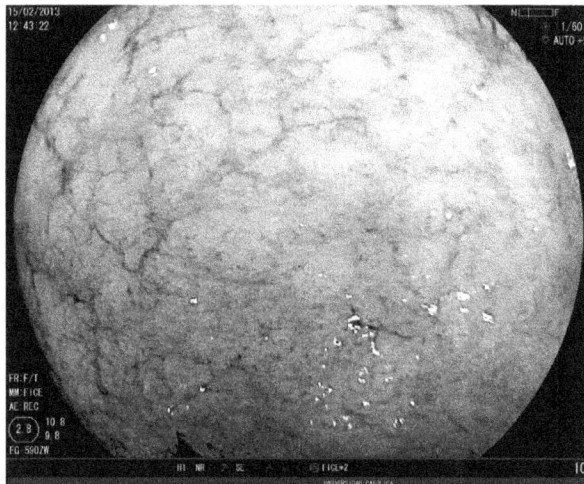

Figure 10. Same image as number 9, using computerized virtual chromoendoscopy with Fuji Intelligent Chromo Endoscopy (FICE).

The first description of this type of finding was by Stevens and McCarthy in 1976;[8] Jabbari[4] later described the prominence of duodenal submucosal vessels in celiac disease patients. Subsequent studies found for this endoscopic find a sensitivity of 2%, 5% and 14% respectively in patients who were undergoing duodenal biopsy.[9-11] Therefore, this sign seems the least relevant and reliable among those examined.

The first systematic study that globally assessed endoscopic features in celiac disease specifically encompassed 100 patients specifically referred for endoscopy in order to obtain intestinal biopsies.[9] The evaluated endoscopic findings were mosaic pattern, scalloped folds, creases and loss of blood vessel visualization. Among all the evaluated patients, 36 had a severe villous atrophy histopathological diagnosis, of which 39% had atrophic mucosal pattern, 75% loss of folds, 33% scalloped folds and 14% blood vessel visualization. The presence of at least one endoscopic finding had a sensitivity of 94% and a specificity of 92% for the celiac disease diagnosis.

Subsequently, Niveloni et al. demonstrated in a prospective study that endoscopy allowed to correctly determine which patients had celiac disease in 94% of the cases, and that chromoendoscopy with staining allowed a better outlining of the scalloped folds and mosaic pattern, with no impact on diagnosis.[10] The "interobserver" concordance was excellent for the scalloped folds (kappa 0.83) and mosaic pattern (kappa 0.76) findings and regular for loss of folds (kappa 0.41).

In patients who underwent an endoscopic duodenal biopsy, the finding of at least one endoscopic marker has a sensitivity ranging between 77% and 94%, the scalloped folds and the mosaic pattern being the most frequent in different series.[10-11]

As reviewed in other chapters of this book, many different clinical scenarios confront us with patients with suspected celiac disease (Table 1).

Clinical Scenario	Sensitivity	Specificity
Patients with celiac disease suspicion[10]	94%	99%
Patients with dyspepsia[12]	50%	99%
Patients with no celiac disease[11]	87%	100%
Patients iron deficiency anemia[15]	59 %	92%

Table 1. Endoscopic finding performance to predict villous atrophy in different celiac disease clinical scenarios.

In the differential diagnosis, iron deficiency anemia should be evaluated in the context of possible CD. About 5-12% of patients with iron deficiency anemia have celiac disease endoscopic markers and, when these are found, their sensitivity has been shown to be nearly 60% with a 92%-100% specificity. The most common findings vary according to different publications, no research has been able to show the superiority of one over the other.[12-15] When an upper endoscopy is performed in patients with iron deficiency anemia who have not been previously studied for celiac disease serological markers, the taking duodenal biopsies is recommended.[16] When said markers are negative, taking biopsies is generally not recommended except in very symptomatic patients.[16] There are, however, discrepancies regarding this subject.[17]

One controversial subject is the need for duodenal biopsy in dyspeptic patients (especially in those with the dysmotility type) without endoscopy study findings. There is a marked variability in the published series of studies on the percentage of patients in whom CD symptoms can be confirmed, with a range of 1-19%.[18,19]

The unexpected find of an endoscopic marker in a patient without an *a priori* indication from a duodenal biopsy has also been evaluated and results in this setting have shown mixed concordances between identification of endoscopic markers and pathologic correlation with a sensitivity of 50% and a specificity of 99.6%.[12,20]

Summing up, several studies have shown a high degree of correlation between the above findings and the presence of villous atrophy due to celiac disease. The high specificity of these signs warrants endoscopic biopsies in its presence, therefore, the endoscopist should be actively seek them out in the course of exploring, even in patients not referred for suspected CD.

2. Advanced Diagnostic Techniques: Chromoendoscopy, Magnification, Computerized Virtual Chromoendoscopy with *Fuji Intelligent Chromo Endoscopy (FICE)*, Narrow Band Image (NBI) Optical Coherence Tomography, Confocal Endomicroscopy and Endocytoscopy

In order to improve the endoscopic detection of villous atrophy, various diagnostic methods have been implemented, among them, magnification endoscopy with or without chromoendoscopy, computerized virtual chromoendoscopy obtained with *Fuji* color enhancement technology, Narrow Band Imaging (NBI), optical coherence tomography and ultra-magnification techniques such as endocytoscopy and confocal endomicroscopy.

These technological innovations would be potentially useful to identify atrophy sites with patchy distribution, thus allowing the taking of targeted biopsies in suspicious areas, improving diagnostic efficiency compared with random biopsies. Another potentially relevant use of endoscopic-microscopic techniques is their possible ability to discern milder degrees of histological damage (Marsh 1 and 2).

2.1. Magnification Endoscopy and Chromoendoscopy (Table 2 and Figures 11- 14)

Badreldin et al. included CD patients in treatment, and sought to evaluate this technique not regarding its ability to predict villous atrophy existence, to determine its degree.[22] Concordance between endoscopic and histological according to atrophy degree was fair-good (kappa 0.631), positive and negative predictive value to predict villous atrophy was 83% and 77% respectively.

Magnification endoscopy has been considered in the diagnosis and evaluation of the degree of CD villous atrophy; some classification schemes attempt to characterize the various endoscopic villi patterns (Table 2). As it is known, this technique can increase image size by pressing a button on the endoscope controls, which is helpful in predicting histological diagnosis. However, regarding CD, the number of studies is small and the results obtained are contradictory.

In a descriptive prospective study, Cammarota et al. studied patients referred for duodenal biopsies, in which magnification endoscopy was used.[21] The evaluation was performed without and with the water immersion technique. Results were excellent, with sensitivity, specificity, positive and negative predictive values for villous atrophy at 95%, 99%, 95% and 99%, respectively, values which did not improve using water technique.

	Technique	Patients (n)	Sensitivity	Specificity
Maurino 1993[9]	CE	100	94%	92%
Dickey 2001[11]	CE	129	77%	-
Cammarota 2004[21]	ME	191	95%	99%
Badreldin 2005[22]	ME	53	77%	63%
Iovino 2010[24]	ME + IC	50	98%	100%
Singh 2010[25]	ME + NBI	21	93%	98%

CE: Conventional endoscopy; ME: Magnification endoscopy; IC: Indigo carmine; NBI Narrow Band Imaging

Table 2. Sensitivity and specificity of conventional and magnification endoscopy in duodenal atrophy diagnosis.

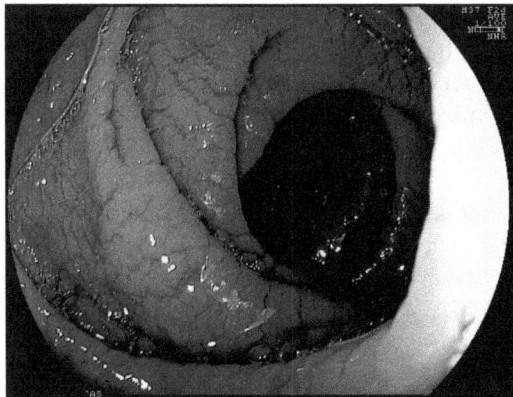

Figure 11. Mosaic pattern, with indigo carmine.

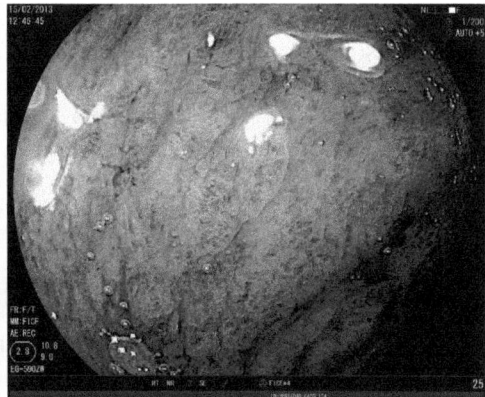

Figure 12. Bulb mosaic pattern, shown with computerized virtual chromoendoscopy using Fuji color enhancement technology (FICE).

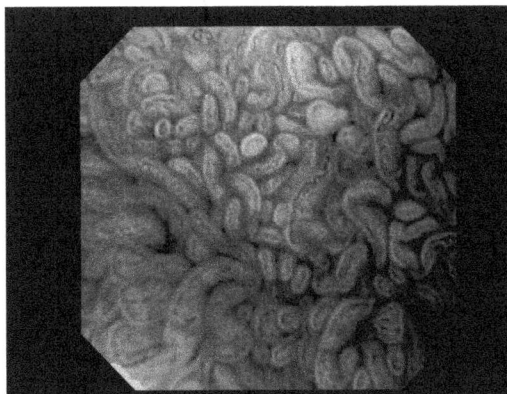

Figure 13. Normal duodenal mucosa view obtained using narrow band imaging and magnification.

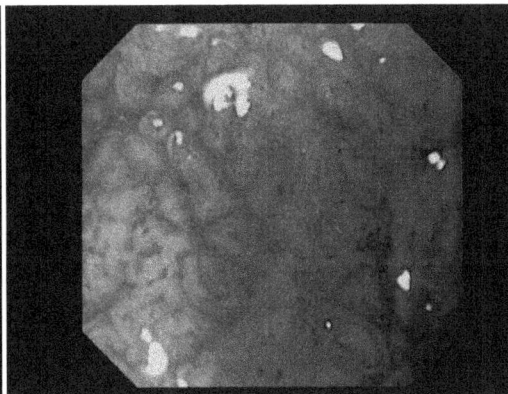

Figure 14. Duodenal mucosa with partial to total villous atrophy view obtained with narrow band imaging and magnification.

In a study of 12 CD patients, which compared the use of magnification associated with 3% acetic acid versus conventional endoscopy, sensitivity was higher for the combined technique compared to the standard (100% versus 58%).[23] Furthermore, magnification endoscopy identified patchy areas of villous atrophy in 5 patients, while conventional endoscopy did not identify them in any case.

Another recent study evaluated the usefulness of magnification endoscopy (*Fujinon*, Omiya, Japan EG 490 ZW) associated with indigo carmine staining to recognize duodenal villi pattern changes in patients with difficult CD diagnosis.[24] This was defined as a lack of concordance between diagnostic tests or as a result of beginning the study at a stage in which gluten had already been removed from the diet. In the control group, 100% of cases were diagnosed accurately; in the group of CD patients the accuracy was of 97%. However, in the group of difficult diagnosis, sensitivity was only 67%.

A system has been proposed for classifying villous atrophy using magnification endoscopic associated to narrow band imaging.[25] Twenty one patients (3 with CD and 18 controls) were studied and a simple classification was used:

1) Normal pattern (normal villi with finger-like projections),

2) Atrophy pattern (cerebroid/shortened villi or their absence).

The sensitivity and specificity required to correctly distinguish the presence or absence of villi were of 93.3% and 97.8%, respectively; furthermore, the sensitivity and specificity required to differentiate partial or total atrophy were of 83.3% and 100%, respectively.

Magnification endoscopy provides high-quality images, and the results of available studies are promising; however, large, well-designed studies aiming at confirming that it is more effective than conventional endoscopic examination are necessary.

2.2. Optical coherence tomography (Table 3)

Author, year	OTC	CEM	Endocystoscopy	Patients (n)	Sensitivity	Specificity
Leong, 2008[34]	-	Yes	-	31	94%	92%
Masci, 2009[28]	Yes	-	-	134	82%	100%
Venkatesh, 2010[32]	-	Yes	-	19	100%	80%
Günther, 2010[33]	-	Yes	-	60	74%	100%
Matysiak-Budnik, 2010[37]	-	-	Yes	23	83%	100%

TOC: Optical coherence tomography, EMC: Confocal endomicroscopy.

Table 3. Sensitivity and specificity of optical coherence tomography, confocal endomicroscopy and endocytoscopy in duodenal atrophy diagnosis.

Optical coherence tomography is an imaging technique that allows the histological study of tissue inserting a probe through the working channel of the endoscope *in vivo* and *in situ*, which has led to the term *optical biopsy*.[26] This technique was first demonstrated in 1991 with an axial resolution of ~30 μm. With every generation the technique has progressed to a higher resolution; in 2001 optical coherence tomography achieved submicron resolution due to the introduction of wide-band light sources (emitting wavelengths over a range of ~100 nm); currently there exists ultra-high resolution equipment. At present, the optical coherence tomography is widely accepted, providing a penetration of a 2-3mm depth with axial and lateral resolution of a micrometric range (1 to 3 microns).

In 2006, Masci et al., presented a preliminary report on the usefulness of optical coherence tomography (*Pentax; Lightlab Imaging*, Westford, Massachusetts, USA) in CD.[27] They included 18 CD patients and 22 controls, optical coherence tomography was performed in all cases and biopsies were simultaneously taken. Subsequently, the images and histological findings were evaluated in the blind by an independent gastroenterologist with experience in optical coherence tomography, who was not informed of the clinical data and the endoscopic appearance of the duodenal mucosa, and also by an anatomopathologist. There was 100% concordance between optical coherence tomography and histology in determining the villous morphology in both groups.

In a more recent study by the same group, 134 pediatric patients were prospectively included, 67 with serological CD suspicion (group 1) and 67 with negative histology for atrophy (group 2).[28] In all cases, an optical coherence tomography was also performed in the second duodenal portion;

biopsies were taken in the area where the optical coherence tomography had been performed. Three patterns were considered: Pattern 1 with no atrophy, pattern 2 with mild atrophy and pattern 3 with marked atrophy. OCT Concordance with histology was of 100%, 94% and 92% respectively for patterns 1, 2 and 3. Sensitivity and specificity were of 82% and 100% respectively. In the control group, there was a 100% concordance between optical coherence tomography and histology.

According to these results, optical coherence tomography appears to be a promising method to correctly identify villous atrophy and can be of help in the selection of intestinal biopsy patients.

2.3. Confocal Endomicroscopy (Table 3)

Confocal endomicroscopy is a new imaging technique which allows the observation of cell morphology at the time of endoscopic examination (*in vivo* histology). Confocal microscopy uses a fine laser beam to scan the specimen. Currently, a miniaturized confocal microscope was developed to be integrated into the distal tip of a conventional endoscope (a joint venture between *Pentax*, Japan and *Optiscan*, Australia).[29] This technology allows simultaneous conventional white light endoscopy and confocal microscopy. More importantly, the working channel allows biopsies guided by endomicroscopy and/or immediate and specific endoscopic therapy.

Conventional endoscopes provide an optical magnification of 50x, while confocal endomicroscopy a magnification of 1000x.[30] Therefore, the use of this technology requires that the endoscopist have basic anatomopathologic knowledge of the mucosal to recognize and interpret the findings. With this technique, it is possible to obtain deep images down to the lamina propria, approximately 250µm.[31] Confocal endomicroscopy requires the use of an excitable fluorescent contrast agent which has emission spectra in the blue light range (excitation wavelength of 488nm). The most widely used contrast agent is sodium fluorescein, which is administered intravenously, is not toxic and is distributed throughout the tissues in a few seconds.[30]

The results of confocal endomicroscopy in CD were described in a pediatric trial of 9 patients with suspected CD comparing the findings with paired controls.[32] Endoscopists and anatomopathologists were blinded to the diagnosis. 1384 pictures of the patients were obtained and 5 images per patient were selected and compared with a biopsy sample from the same site. According to the data provided by this study, confocal endomicroscopy sensitivity was 100%, specificity 80% and positive predictive value of 81%, the relatively low specificity was related to the score employed to define the suspected CD diagnosis according to findings according to confocal endomicroscopy. With more stringent criteria, the specificity would have been of 100%.

In a clinical trial in 30 adult patients with CD, including 6 with disease refractory to the gluten-free diet, the sensitivity of confocal endomicroscopy was useful for the detection of increased intraepithelial lymphocytes (81%), but decreased for villous atrophy diagnosis of (74%) and for crypt hyperplasia (52%).[33] In the same study, 30 patients without CD who underwent confocal endomicroscopy and duodenal biopsies showed, in all cases, normal architecture under endomicroscopy confocal and in histology, resulting in a specificity of 100%. It must be pointed out that for the intraepithelial lymphocyte (semiquantitative) determination is necessary, by means of applying a second contrast staining agent (topical acriflavine).

In the widest study, 31 patients (17 with CD, 14 controls) were evaluated and over 7,000 confocal endomicroscopy images were compared with 326 pairs of biopsy samples.[34] Diagnosis sensitivity for CD was of 94% with a specificity of 92% and good correlation with Marsh scoring system. This study also concludes that by aiming biopsies at microscopically abnormal regions, confocal endomicroscopy may be a promising approach to investigate patients with clinical CD suspicion and with negative biopsies.

According to the results provided by the few published studies, confocal endomicroscopy seems to be a technique with high sensitivity and specificity for the diagnosis of villous atrophy and can also evaluate intraepithelial lymphocytes and crypt features, although the diagnostic yield for this last purpose is not so elevated.

2.4. Endocytoscopy (Table 3)

Endocytoscopy is a form of ultra-high magnification, which allows visualization of the epithelial surface architecture at cellular and subcellular levels, being able to establish cell abnormalities, and other features such as cell density, cell size and organization, shape of the nuclei, staining pattern as well as the nucleus/cytoplasm ratio. This is a microscopy technique where physical contact with the mucosal surface is required for imaging (Figures 15-18).[35]

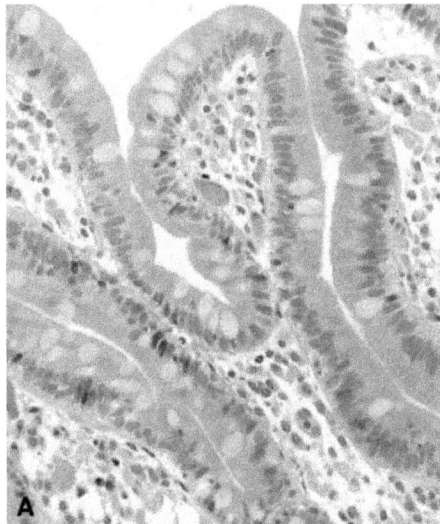

Figure 15. Microscopy image of normal duodenum with hematoxylin eosin staining (reprinted with permission from Elsevier, reference 38).

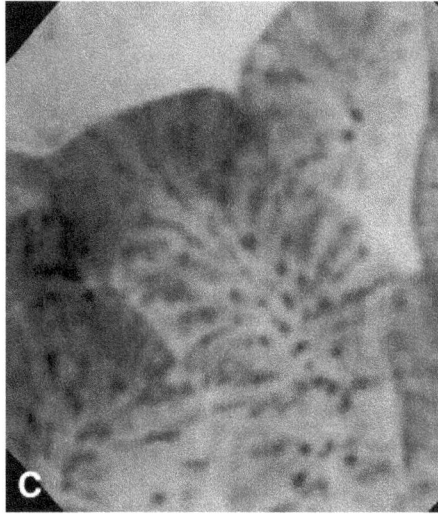

Figure 16. Normal duodenum endocytoscopy image (same case as W) (x450).
The mucous layer shows long, thin villi, and epithelium with low
stromal/epithelial ratio and normal vellositary capillaries (reproduced with
permission from Elsevier, reference 38).

The use of a contrast agent for visualizing subcellular entities is necessary. For the proper performance of this technique, the mucosa must be pre-treated with a mucolytic agent, such as N-acetylcysteine after which staining can be performed directly with 0.5%-1% methylene blue or 0.25% toluidine blue.[36]

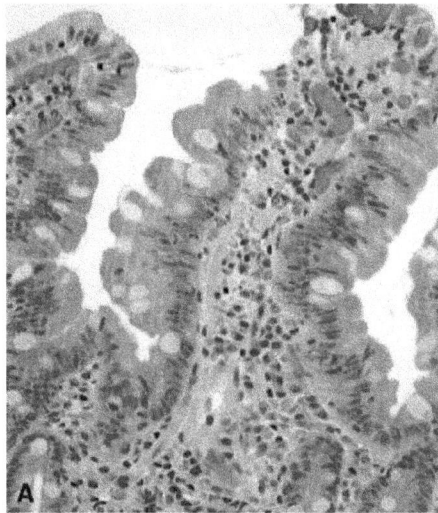

Figure 17. Duodenal mucosa with Marsh III compatible villous atrophy (staining:
hematoxylin-eosin) (reproduced with permission from Elsevier, reference 38).

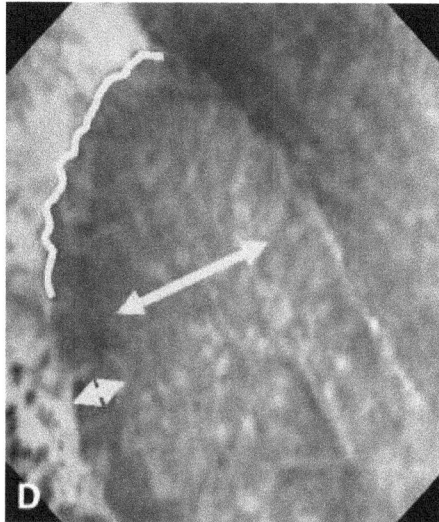

Figure 18. Image endocytoscopy (x450). The mucosa shows irregular atrophic villi, absence of large villi, irregular epithelium (short arrow), with a high stroma/epithelium ratio (long arrow), and absence of vellositary capillaries (reproduced with permission from Elsevier, reference 38).

Endocytoscopy is limited by its ability to image only the superficial layer of the mucosa and is therefore not a suitable technique for lesion depth analysis.

There are two types of endocytoscopy tools, although they are currently not commercially available: one based on probes (*Olympus*, Tokyo, Japan; *Xec-120* and *Xec-300* models) and another based on the endoscope (*Olympus* models *XGIF-Q260EC1* and *XCF-Q260EC1*). The two probe-based models provide a 450x magnification, which means a 300 μm x 300 μm field of view. The endoscopic models use an endocytoscope integrated to the endoscope and provide a 580x magnification.

Applied to CD, endocystoscopy has demonstrated the presence of three different *in vivo* histopathological patterns: normal pattern, subtotal villous atrophy pattern and total duodenal atrophy pattern.[37]

In a clinical trial of 40 patients (32 with known CD and 8 with CD suspicion) 166 endocytoscopy recordings were prospectively obtained and compared with histopathology (Marsh classification).[38] One endocytoscope with a 450x magnification was used; prediction was accurate for moderate to severe atrophy (Marsh III), however it was not reliable in detecting atrophy in its early stages (Marsh I). The use of the endocytoscope with a 1100x magnification provided no additional diagnostic value.

Another recent study, in which an endocytoscope with a 450x magnification was used, encompassed 16 patients with CD diagnosis and 7 controls.[39] In this study, the three abovementioned patterns were also identified. Sensitivity and specificity for the villous atrophy diagnosis, calculated by patients, was of 88% and 100% respectively. However, it was not possible to determine the presence of intraepithelial lymphocytes.

Therefore, according to the results of the existing studies, endocytoscopy permits real time visualization of the duodenal mucosa and villous architecture characterization; thus, it can be considered a promising method for in vivo duodenal mucosa evaluation for villous atrophy diagnosis. Nevertheless, it has limitations when it comes to displaying intraepithelial lymphocytes and crypt hyperplasia; therefore, the endocytoscopic early-stage diagnosis of celiac disease is not possible currently.

Technique	Intraepithelial lymphocytes	Crypt Hyperplasia	Vellositary atrophy
Magnification	-	-	+++
CEM	++	+	+++
OCT	No data	No data	+++
Endocytoscopy	-	-	++

CEM: Confocal endomicroscopy; OCT: Optical coherence tomography; (-) Bad; (+) Regular; (++) Good; (+++) Very good.
Table 4. Diagnostic utility of the various techniques for the visualization of intraepithelial lymphocytes, crypt hyperplasia and villous atrophy.

To sum up: new endoscopy techniques allow high-accuracy prediction of villous atrophy, but are less accurate for determining histologic of injury grade (Table 4). Although, in difficult cases or in those without histological confirmation they would be potentially useful for directing biopsies, studies are needed to evaluate their utility and cost-effectiveness in the overall diagnosis and management of CD.

3. Biopsies: How, Where and Whom to Biopsy?

To confirm the CD diagnosis biopsies should be taken from duodenum while the patient consumed a diet containing gluten. It has been established that 4-6 biopsies must be taken to make the diagnosis, including samples from the duodenal bulb.[40]

Formerly, biopsies were obtained by peroral suction techniques (Watson´s and Crosby's capsules, and multipurpose tube). Several studies demonstrated that duodenal endoscopic biopsy was comparable to that of the capsule to detect vellositary atrophy.[41-45] The recommended biopsy site was the second portion of the duodenum distal to the bulb, due to the presence of Brunner's glands or duodenitis, which may interfere with recognition of vellositary atrophy.[46] Later research showed that changes attributed to celiac disease may occur in the duodenal bulb[7] and that this may even be the only site with atrophy.[47,48]

The multiple biopsy strategy is suggested to reduce the risk of false negatives, since mucosal damage may be irregularly distributed, a condition known as "patchy villous atrophy." That is why, as stated before, for best results, the recommendation is to take 4-6 biopsies, one or two from the bulb and the rest of the second duodenal portion (Table 5).[49-53]

Subsequent studies showed that by using immersion techniques and magnification endoscopy it is feasible to take directed biopsies;[54,55] in this sense, the technological advances mentioned above (narrow band imaging, computed virtual chromoendoscopy obtained with *Fuji* color enhancement technology *(FICE)*, confocal endomicroscopy) guide us in the taking of endoscopic samples, improving the diagnostic yield. Future studies should confirm the practical utility of such techniques in relation to random sampling.[56,57]

The orientation of the duodenal biopsy is fundamental for an appropriate histopathological study. The uppermost placement of the luminal surface of the biopsy and the blood side surface on filter paper facilitates the correct orientation of the specimen avoiding tangential cutting and allowing accurate diagnosis of vellositary atrophy.[58]

Regarding the issue of whom to biopsy, the concept changed over time. More than two decades ago, biopsy was done only in patients with clear symptoms (diarrhea, weight loss or abdominal distension) or significant laboratory abnormalities (mineral, protein or lipid deficits) or with positive antibodies. In recent years, with the emergence of new, more sensitive antibodies and the spread of the disease towards other specialties, the duodenal biopsy prescription increased continuously. Intestinal biopsy must be performed whenever celiac disease is suspected and before eliminating dietary gluten.[59,60] Although this is mentioned in other chapters, it is necessary to remember those situations in which biopsy should be considered in order to rule out CD: chronic diarrhea (the most common symptom), weight loss, anemia, abdominal bloating. Non-gastrointestinal symptoms/alterations: dermatitis herpetiformis, peripheral neuropathy, reduced bone density, unexplained infertility. Also, folic acid, iron and vitamin B12 deficiencies, reduced serum albumin, hypertransaminasemia with no hepatic origin. In patients at increased risk: first- and second-degree relatives (5-15%), HLA-DQ2 or HLA-DQ8 bearers (10-30%), Down's syndrome (12%), autoimmune thyroid disease (5%), chronic active hepatitis, diabetes mellitus type 1 (5-6%), lymphocytic colitis (15-27%), chronic fatigue syndrome (2%) and irritable bowel syndrome. Biopsy is also indispensable when an incidental finding by an endoscopist detects the suspicious signs described above.

In conclusion, there are many situations that lead to duodenal biopsy in search of celiac disease, and, despite the fact that it is the diagnostic "gold standard", we must not forget the existence of patchy celiac disease; therefore, multiple distal duodenal sampling and duodenal bulb sampling must be performed since this will help avoid underdiagnosis (Table 5).

Author	Patients (n)	Antibodies	HLA	Biopsies	Patchy vellositary atrophy	Bulb only atrophy	Sensitivity
Bonámico, 2004[48]	95	EMA + tTGA +	DQ 2+ DQ 8 +	Bulb (1) Distal duodenum (4)	13/95 (13.7%)	4/95 (4.2%)	–
Ravelli, 2005[49]	112	EMA + tTGA +	110 DQ 2+ DQ8 +	Bulb (1) Duodenum (3) proximal - intermediate - distal)	8/110 (7.2%)	–	–
Hopper, 2007[51]	56	EMA + tTGA +	–	Bulb (1) Proximal duodenum (4) Distal duodenum (4)	10/53 (18.8%)	1/53 (1.8%)	100% (3 biopsies)
Gonzalez, 2010[53]	40	–	–	Bulb (2) Proximal duodenum (4)	5/40 (12.5%)	5/40 (12.5%)	72%

EMA (antiendomisium antibodies), tTGA (Antitransglutaminase antibodies), DQ 2 (HLA-DQ 2 gene), DQ 8 (HLA-8 gene).

Table 5. Performance of biopsies using different protocols.

4. The Role of Capsule Endoscopy in Celiac Disease

The endoscopic capsule has allowed the exploration of the small intestine, which, by its anatomical location and characteristics, has previously been limited and less accessible to traditional endoscopic studies; capsule endoscopy has become a useful diagnostic tool for diseases that affect this segment of the digestive tube.[61-63] Numerous publications show that the capsule's endoscopic ability is superior to imaging techniques traditionally used to detect small intestinal lesions.[64-66] Capsule endoscopy was first used in humans in 1999; in 2001 it was approved for clinical use by the Federal Drug Administration.[67] Capsule endoscopy takes 2 frames per second, has a 8x magnification lens and has an optical dome in close contact with the mucosa allowing a very good evaluation of the villous pattern. The main indication for this study is gastrointestinal bleeding of obscure origin, though there are numerous studies that seek to understand the capsule's value in other small intestinal pathologies.[68]

Serological CD markers, such as endomysial antibodies and anti-transglutaminase, have shown a very good performance, with positive and negative predictive values of near 96%. However, the objectification of villous atrophy identified by means of a histopathological study in duodenal samples are the diagnostic standard.[50,69]

Capsule endoscopy in the context of CD has been the subject of a growing interest to investigate its use; there are several possible scenarios for its use, each of them will be discussed below.

4.1. CD Diagnosis (Table 6)

Publication	n	Sensitivity %	Specificity %	NPV %	PPV %
Petroniene, 2005[74]	10	70	100	77	100
Hopper, 2007[75]	21	85	100	89	100
Rondonotti, 2007[76]	32	87	90	71	96
Biagi, 2006[77]	26	90	63	77	100
Maiden, 2009[78]	19	67	100	60	100
Lidums, 2011[79]	22	93	100	89	100
Total	130	82	92.1	77.1	99

Table 6. Summary of sensitivity and specificity studies and NPV and PPV for capsule endoscopy in celiac disease.

As mentioned earlier, the determination of villous atrophy is a central event in CD diagnosis. Endoscopic methods have made progress regarding image quality, since they are able to distinguish alterations that suggest CD and allow the endoscopist to decide on whether to take biopsies according to certain findings. Capsule endoscopy, by having an 8x magnification and an optical dome which allows a direct view of the mucosa, helps to distinguish alterations which have a high correlation with a CD diagnosis , previously referred to in this chapter.[70]

The findings of capsule endoscopy show good correlation with serological and histological diagnosis, but there are inter-observer variations that may limit this method in terms of reliability and reproducibility. A study made on a cohort of CD patients evaluated the utility of capsule endoscopy in patients with equivocal CD diagnosis (defined as the presence of villous atrophy with negative or inconclusive antibodies with Marsh 1 or 2 histological changes), compared with the diagnostic yield of capsule endoscopy in a cohort of patients with a confirmed CD diagnosis and persistent symptoms. Authors found in the first group of patients a diagnostic utility of 28% (9/32) in the atrophy and negative marker subgroup and of 7% (2/30) in the patients with mild subgroup histological findings.[71,72]

In a retrospective series of 8 patients evaluated using capsule endoscopy for suspected CD, but with non-diagnostic biopsy or with the impossibility of performing an endoscopy, the characteristic capsule endoscopy findings were followed by the initiation of a gluten-free diet; improvement of symptoms and/or serological markers was demonstrated in 7 of the 8 patients.[73]

Overall published studies in this area deal with a limited number of patients and have a high degree of diagnostic suspicion and show an average sensitivity of 82%, a specificity of 92% and positive and negative predictive values of 99% and 77% respectively (Table 6).[74-79]

4.2. Evaluation of the Extent of CD Damage

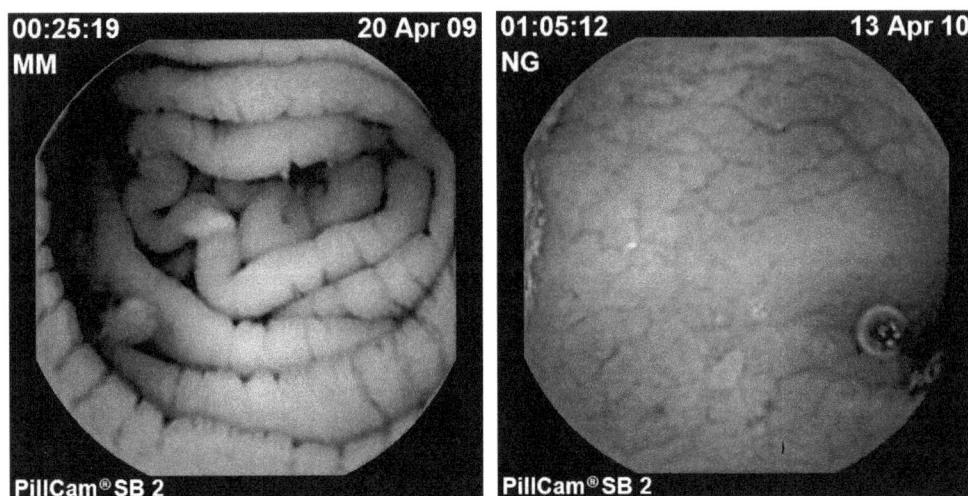

Capsule endoscopy, by allowing a complete evaluation of the small intestine, can help determine whether the extent of mucosal involvement is limited to the duodenum, if it reaches the jejunum or if it involves the entire small intestine and can also identify areas or patches of involvement with atrophy which can explain or support the diagnosis. The clinical implications of the extension are not yet well defined, there is controversy between different studies, and some suggest that there is a correlation between the severity or intensity of symptoms of CD and the extension in the mucosa, while Murray's publication does not support this view.[80] In a publication by Barret et al., a positive correlation between CD extent and albumin levels was found (Figures 19-20).[73,80-82]

4.3. Evaluation in Patients with Refractory CD or a Poor Response to Gluten-Free Diet (Table 7)

Author	Country	n	Tumors found
Maiden 2009[85]	UK	19	No
Kurien 2013[86]	UK	69	2
Daum 2007[84]	Germany	14 (7 type I,7 type II)	1 T-cell Lymphoma
Barret 2012[73]	France	37 (11 type I y 26 type II)	2 T-cell Lymphoma

Table 7. Utility of capsule endoscopy in patients with refractory CD or with no response to gluten-free diet.

In this clinical scenario, the main cause for suspicion is the appearance of CD complications such as small intestinal adenocarcinoma, T-cell lymphomas and ulcerative jejunitis. In a retrospective study of 14 patients with refractory CD (including 7 CD type 2 refractory) capsule endoscopy identified 2 patients with T-cell lymphomas (Figure 21).

In a study where 47 patients with a high suspicion of CD complications were evaluated, based on symptoms such as weight loss or abdominal pain, lesions were found in up to 50% of patients by means of capsule endoscopy.[83] In a recent publication on 37 patients with refractory CD, capsule endoscopy had a higher correlation with histology in comparison with conventional endoscopic studies (Table 7).[84-86]

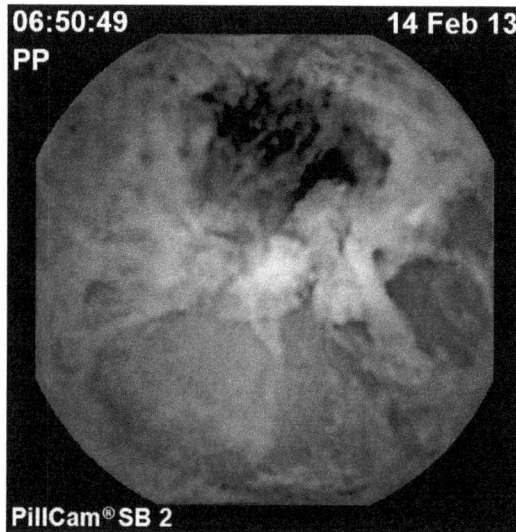

Figure 21. Capsule Image (GIVEN): Ulcerative jejunitis (T lymphoma) in a patient with refractory celiac disease.

4.4. Monitoring Malignancy Development in Patients with Established CD

It is unclear which CD patients ought to be tested and when they ought to have tests made to monitor the development of neoplasias. It is conceivable that patients with long-standing CD or irregular monitoring could benefit from the detection of tumors in early stages.

4.5. Limitations of the Studies by Capsule Endoscopy in Patients with CD

The limitations of capsule endoscopy in the context of CD patients are dictated primarily by variations or inter-observer discrepancies that make this exam operator-dependent if those clinicians conducting the capsule endoscopy evaluation are not familiar with the changes that can be found in CD. Another limitation is the inability to evaluate the entire small intestine.[84]

Published studies show that there is a good correlation with celiac disease diagnosis. However, these have mostly been conducted in patients with high pretest probability, such as patients with suggestive symptoms and/or positive serological markers or contrasted with CD patients with advanced histological stages (Marsh III). In mild villous alteration stages (Marsh I or II) diagnostic difficulty may be higher. With this in mind, a valuation is being made of the potential usefulness of computerized assessment systems, looking for differences in surface brightness patterns of the mucosa in CD patients compared to healthy ones, or of the spectral analysis of images obtained by capsule endoscopy.[73,87]

Finally, it must be pointed out that capsule endoscopy is, for the time being, a complementary test that can be used in the evaluation of CD patients in the previously discussed scenarios.

5. Push Enteroscopy in Celiac Disease Diagnosis

Just over a decade ago, most widely used endoscopic method for the study of the small intestine was push enteroscopy (length 2000 mm, diameter 9.8 mm). However, the procedure was often frustrating, even though it was possible to use overtubes, by the inability to advance far enough into the small intestine. With the new millennium, capsule endoscopy and double-balloon push enteroscopy were developed (2001).[88]

Double-balloon enteroscopy uses enteroscopes that measure 2000 mm and 8.5 mm (diagnostic) or 9.3 mm (therapeutic) and an overtube 12.2-13.2 mm in diameter, which allows to advance deeper than push enteroscopy.[89] Single balloon enteroscopy single obtains similar results, but spiral enteroscopy, which employs an overtube shaped as the name implies, is not able to penetrate so deeply.[90]

Few studies have evaluated the effectiveness of enteroscopy in the study of celiac disease, and these are not extensive series. A recent systematic review showed that of the existing publications on double-balloon enteroscopy up to 2010 only in 51 (0.4%) of 12,000 explorations the indication was of celiac disease.[91]

The usefulness of enteroscopy in CD would rest, on one hand, on the possibility of taking multiple intestinal biopsies from distal portions to the second portion of the duodenum in patients with clinical suspicion but negative biopsies. In a study (published in abstract form) push enteroscopy was performed on 20 pediatric patients with serological celiac disease suspicion, with biopsies from the bulb, second and fourth portion of the duodenum and proximal jejunum (30 cm from the Angle of Treitz) and distal (60 cm from the Ligament of Treitz).[92] The aim was to map the histological lesion thus evaluate the patchy distribution. Histological celiac injury was found in 90%, 90%, 95%, 90% and 90% respectively at different locations. Bulb involvement was never the exclusive location. In one patient (5%) the diagnosis could only be confirmed by proximal jejunum biopsy.

Another study evaluated the usefulness of push enteroscopy for a confirmatory CD diagnosis in patients with positive serology, but negative biopsies.[93] Out of 31 patients, 23 were positive for anti-gliadin antibodies and enteroscopy with new duodenal and jejunum biopsies did not offer a histological CD diagnosis. However, in 5/8 with antiendomisium, CD was diagnosed from the new biopsies and 3/5 were positive only in the jejunal samples.

A further potential use for enteroscopy, probably the most important, would be the study of refractory celiac disease. Push enteroscopy was useful in patients with refractory CD in one study; out of 8 patients, enteroscopy showed ulcerative jejunitis in five; in 7/8 there was severe duodenal villous atrophy, in all them in the jejune.[94]

In another study, double-balloon enteroscopy and biopsies were performed in 21 patients with a refractory celiac disease indication.[95] In 5 patients (24%) jejunal ulcerations were found whose examination revealed T-cell lymphoma, one of them associated with stenosis. In 3/5 cases the proximal mucosa exhibited Marsh grade III injury. Two patients (9%) had ulcers without lymphoma, which were diagnosed as ulcerative jejunitis. In the 14 (66%) remaining patients, mucosal changes compatible with celiac disease were observed, and were diagnosed as refractory disease. In all of them, duodenal biopsies revealed a Marsh III lesion, but only 8/14 had histological lesions in more distal sections. In two patients with lymphoma, a follow-up double balloon enteroscopy was performed. Based on these studies, enteroscopy should be considered to be a front-line technique in the study of refractory celiac disease by combining imaging and biopsy.

Double-balloon enteroscopy has also been used in patients with malabsorption of unknown origin, and the biopsy procedure allowed a new diagnosis in 33% of cases (Crohn's disease, amyloidosis, and primary intestinal lymphangiectasia).[96]

Acknowledgements

The authors wish to thank Associate Professor Rajvinder Singh (University of Adelaide, Australia) for allowing the use of his excellent images; Professor Kenshi Yao (University of Fukuoka, Japan), Dr. Krish Ragunath (University of Nottingham, UK) (Figures 13 and 14), Professor Daniel Baumgardt (Department of Gastroenterology, Charité Medical Center-Virchow Hospital, Berlin, Germany) (Figures 15-18, from ref. 38, reproduced with permission from Elsevier) and Assistant Professor Carolina Olano Gossweiler, Department of Gastroenterology ("Prof. Henry Cohen"), Hospital de Clinicas, Montevideo, Uruguay (Figures 19-21).

References

1. Nicolette CC, Tully TE. *The duodenum in celiac sprue.* Am J Roentgenol Radium Ther Nucl Med. 1971; 113: 248-54. http://dx.doi.org/10.2214/ajr.113.2.248
2. Brocchi E, Corazza G, Caletti G, Treggiari EA, Barbara L, Gasbarrini U. *Endoscopic demonstration of loss of duodenal folds in the diagnosis of celiac disease.* N Engl J Med. 1988; 319: 741-4. http://dx.doi.org/10.1056/NEJM198809223191202
3. McIntyre AS, Ng DP, Smith JA, Amoah J, Long RG. *The endoscopic appearance of duodenal folds is predictive of untreated adult celiac disease.* Gastrointest Endosc. 1992; 38: 148-51. http://dx.doi.org/10.1016/S0016-5107(92)70380-0
4. Jabbari M, Wild G, Goresky CA et al. *Scalloped valvulae conniventes: an endoscopic marker of celiac sprue.* Gastroenterology. 1988; 95: 1518-22.
5. Corazza GR, Caletti GC, Lazzari R, Collina A, Brocchi E, Di Sario A, et al. *Scalloped duodenal folds in childhood celiac disease.* Gastrointest Endosc. 1993; 29: 543-5. http://dx.doi.org/10.1016/S0016-5107(93)70167-4
6. Hazar M, Brandt LJ, Tanaka KE, Berkowitz D, Cardillo M, Weidenheim K. *Congo-red negative amyloid with scalloping of the valvulae conniventes.* Gastrointestinal Endosc. 2001; 53: 653-5. http://dx.doi.org/10.1067/mge.2001.113581
7. Brocchi E, Corazza GR, Brusco G, Mangia L, Gasbarrini G. *Unsuspected celiac disease diagnosed by endoscopic visualization of duodenal bulb micronodules.* Gastrointest Endosc. 1996; 44: 610-1. http://dx.doi.org/10.1016/S0016-5107(96)70020-2
8. Stevens FM, McCarthy CF. *The endoscopic demonstration of coeliac disease.* Endoscopy. 1976; 8: 177-80. http://dx.doi.org/10.1055/s-0028-1098406
9. Maurino E, Capizzano H, Niveloni S, Kogan Z, Valero J, Boerr L et al. *Value of endoscopic markers in celiac disease.* Dig Dis Sci. 1993; 38: 2028-33. http://dx.doi.org/10.1007/BF01297080
10. Niveloni S, Fiorini A, Dezi R, Pedreira S, Smecuoi E, Vazquez H et al. *Usefulness of videoduodenoscopy and vital dye staining as indicators of mucosal atrophy of celiac disease: assess- ment of interobserver agreement.* Gastrointest Endosc. 1998; 47: 223-9. http://dx.doi.org/10.1016/S0016-5107(98)70317-7
11. Dickey W, Hughes D. *Disappointing sensitivity of endoscopic markers for villous atrophy in a high-risk population: implications for celiac disease diagnosis during routine endoscopy.* Am J Gastroenterol. 2001; 96: 2126-8. http://dx.doi.org/10.1111/j.1572-0241.2001.03947.x
12. Dickey W, Hughes D. *Prevalence of celiac disease and its endoscopic markers among patients having routine upper gastrointestinal endoscopy.* Am J Gastroenterol. 1999; 94: 2182-6. http://dx.doi.org/10.1111/j.1572-0241.1999.01348.x
13. Dickey W. *Diagnosis of coeliac disease at open-access endoscopy.* Scand J Gastroenterol. 1998; 33: 612-5. http://dx.doi.org/10.1080/00365529850171882
14. Bardella MT, Minoli G, Radaelli F, Quatrini M, Bianchi PA, Conte D. *Reevaluation of duodenal endoscopic markers in the diagnosis of celiac disease.* Gastrointest Endosc. 2000; 51: 714-6. http://dx.doi.org/10.1067/mge.2000.104653
15. Oxentenko AS, Grisolano SW, Murray JA, Burgart LJ, Dierkhising RA, Alexander JA. *The Insensitivity of Endoscopic Markers in Celiac Disease.* Am J Gastroenterol. 2002; 97: 933-8. http://dx.doi.org/10.1111/j.1572-0241.2002.05612.x

16. Goddard AF, James MW, McIntyre AS, Scott BB. *Guidelines for the management of iron deficiency anemia.* Gut. 2011; 60: 1309-16. http://dx.doi.org/10.1136/gut.2010.228874

17. Ishaq S, Mahmood R, Vilannacci V, Bassotti G, Rostami K. *Avoiding biopsy in iron deficiency anemia is not a cost-effective approach.* Rev Esp Enferm Dig. 2012; 104: 334-5. http://dx.doi.org/10.4321/S1130-01082012000600013

18. Santolaria S, Alcedo J, Cuartero B et al. *Spectrum of gluten-sensitive enteropathy in patients with dysmotility-like dyspepsia.* Gastroenterol Hepatol. 2013; 36: 11-20. http://dx.doi.org/10.1016/j.gastrohep.2012.07.011

19. Santolaria-Piedrafita S, Fernández-Bañares F. *Enteropatía sensible al gluten y dispepsia funcional.* Gastroenterol Hepatol. 2012; 35: 78-88. http://dx.doi.org/10.1016/j.gastrohep.2011.10.006

20. Radaelli F, Minoli G, Bardella MT, Conte D. *Celiac Disease Among Patients Referred for Routine Upper Gastrointestinal Endoscopy: Prevalence and Diagnostic Accuracy of Duodenal Endoscopic Markers.* Am J Gastroenterol. 2000; 95: 1089-90. http://dx.doi.org/10.1111/j.1572-0241.2000.01948.x

21. Cammarota G, Martino A, Pirozzi G, Cianci R, et al. *Direct visualisation of intestinal villi by high resolution magnifying upper endoscopy: a validation study.* Gastrointest Endosc. 2004; 60: 732-8. http://dx.doi.org/10.1016/S0016-5107(04)02170-4

22. Badreldin R, Barrett P, Woolf DA, Mansfield J, Yiannakou Y. *How good is zoom endoscopy for assessment of villous atrophy in coeliac disease?* Endoscopy. 2005; 37: 994-8. http://dx.doi.org/10.1055/s-2005-870245

23. Lo A, Guelrud M, Essenfeld H, Bonis P. *Classification of villous atrophy with enhanced magnification endoscopy in patients with celiac disease and tropical sprue.* Gastrointest Endosc. 2007; 66: 377-82. http://dx.doi.org/10.1016/j.gie.2007.02.041

24. Iovino P, Pascariello P, Russo I, Galloro G, Pellegrini L, Ciacci C. *Difficult diagnosis of celiac disease: diagnostic accuracy and utility of chromo-zoom endoscopy.* Gastrointestinal Endoscopy. 2013; 77: 233-40. http://dx.doi.org/10.1016/j.gie.2012.09.036

25. Singh R, Nind G, Tucker G, Nguyen N, Holloway R, Bate J, et al. *Narrow-band imaging in the evaluation of villous morphology: a feasibility study assessing a simplified classification and observer agreement.* Endoscopy. 2010; 42: 889-94. http://dx.doi.org/10.1055/s-0030-1255708

26. Zysk AM, Nguyen FT, Oldenburg AL, Marks DL, Boppart SA. *Optical coherence tomography: a review of clinical development from bench to bedside.* J Biomedical Optics. 2007; 12: 051403. http://dx.doi.org/10.1117/1.2793736

27. Masci E, Mangiavillano B, Albarello L, Mariani A, Doglioni C, Testoni PA. *Optical coherence tomography in the diagnosis of coeliac disease: a preliminary report.* Gut. 2006; 55: 579-92. http://dx.doi.org/10.1136/gut.2005.081364

28. Masci E, Mangiavillano B, Barera G, Parma B, Albarello L, Mariani A et al. *Optical coherence tomography in pediatric patients: a feasible technique fordiagnosing celiac disease in children with villous atrophy.* Dig Liver Dis. 2009; 4: 639-43. http://dx.doi.org/10.1016/j.dld.2009.02.002

29. Kiesslich R, Burg J, Vieth M et al. *Confocal laser endoscopy for diagnosing intraepithelial neoplasias and colorectal cancer in vivo.* Gastroenterology. 2004; 127: 706-13. http://dx.doi.org/10.1053/j.gastro.2004.06.050

30. Wallace MB, Kiesslich R. *Advances in endoscopic imaging of colorrectal neoplasia.* Gastroenterology. 2010; 138: 2140-50. http://dx.doi.org/10.1053/j.gastro.2009.12.067

31. Leong RW, Chang D, Merrett ND, Biankin AV. *Taking optical biopsies with confocal endomicroscopy.* J Gastroenterol Hepatol. 2009; 24: 1701-3. http://dx.doi.org/10.1111/j.1440-1746.2009.06011.x

32. Venkatesh K, Abou-Taleb A, Cohen M et al. *Role of confocal endomicroscopy in the diagnosis of celiac disease.* J Pediatr Gastroenterol Nutr. 2010; 51: 274-9.

33. Günther U, Daum S, Heller F et al. *Diagnostic value of confocal endomicroscopy in celiac disease.* Endoscopy. 2010; 42: 197-202. http://dx.doi.org/10.1055/s-0029-1243937

34. Leong RW, Nguyen NQ, Meredith CG et al. *In vivo confocal endomicroscopy in the diagnosis and evaluation of celiac disease.* Gastroenterology. 2008; 135: 1870-6. http://dx.doi.org/10.1053/j.gastro.2008.08.054

35. Dekker E, Fockens P. *Advances in colonic imaging: new endoscopic imaging methods.* Eur J Gastroenterol Hepatol. 2005; 17: 803-8. http://dx.doi.org/10.1097/00042737-200508000-00004

36. Kwon RS, Wong Kee Song LM, Adler DG, Conway JD, Diehl DL, Farraye FA et al. *Endocytoscopy.* Gastrointest Endosc. 2009; 70: 610-3. http://dx.doi.org/10.1016/j.gie.2009.06.030

37. Matysiak-Budnik T, Coron E, Mosnier JF, Le Rhun M, Inoue H, Galmiche JP. *In vivo real-time imaging of human duodenal mucosal structures in celiac disease using endocytoscopy.* Endoscopy. 2010; 42: 191-6. http://dx.doi.org/10.1055/s-0029-1243838

38. Pohl H, Rösch T, Tanczos BT, Rudolph B, Schlüns K, Baumgart DC. *Endocytoscopy for the detection of microstructural features in adult patients with celiac sprue: a prospective, blinded endocytoscopy-conventional histology correlation study.* Gastrointest Endosc. 2009; 70: 933-41. http://dx.doi.org/10.1016/j.gie.2009.04.043

39. Matysiak-Budnik T, Coron E, MosnierJF, Le Rhun M, Inoue H, Galmiche JP. *In vivo real-time imaging of human duodenal mucosal structures in celiac disease using endocytoscopy.* Endoscopy. 2010; 42: 191-6. http://dx.doi.org/10.1055/s-0029-1243838

40. Ludvigsson JF, Leffler DA, Bai JC et al. *The Oslo definitions for coeliac disease and related terms.* Gut. 2013; 62: 43-52. http://dx.doi.org/10.1136/gutjnl-2011-301346

41. Achkar E, Carey WD, Petras R et al. *Comparison of suction capsule and endoscopic biopsy of small bowel mucosa.* Gastrointest Endosc. 1986; 32: 278-81. http://dx.doi.org/10.1016/S0016-5107(86)71846-4

42. Gillberg R, Ahren C. *Coeliac disease diagnosed by means of duodenoscopy and endoscopic duodenal biopsy.* Scand J Gastroenterol. 1977; 12: 911-6. http://dx.doi.org/10.3109/00365527709181349

43. Mee AS, Burke M, Vallon AG et al. *Small bowel biopsy for malabsorption: comparison of the diagnostic adequacy of endoscopic forceps and capsule biopsy specimens.* BMJ. 1985; 291: 769-72. http://dx.doi.org/10.1136/bmj.291.6498.769

44. Meijer JW, Wahab PJ, Mulder CJ. *Small intestinal biopsies in celiac disease: duodenal or jejunal?* Virchows Arch. 2003; 442: 124-8. http://dx.doi.org/10.1007/s00428-002-0709-7

45. Thijs WJ, van Baarlen J, Kleibeuker JH, Kolkman JJ. *Duodenal versus jejunal biopsies in suspected celiac disease.* Endoscopy. 2004; 36: 993-6. http://dx.doi.org/10.1055/s-2004-825954

46. Shidrawi RG, Przemioslo R, Davies DR et al. *Pitfalls in diagnosing coeliac disease.* J Clin Pathol. 1994; 47: 693-4. http://dx.doi.org/10.1136/jcp.47.8.693

47. Vogelsang H, Hanel S, Steiner B, Oberhuber G. *Diagnostic duodenal bulb biopsy in celiac disease.* Endoscopy. 2001; 33: 336-40. http://dx.doi.org/10.1055/s-2001-13702

48. Bonamico M, Mariani P, Thanasi E et al. *Patchy villous atrophy of the duodenum in childhood celiac disease.* J Pediatr Gastroenterol Nutr. 2004; 38: 204-7. http://dx.doi.org/10.1097/00005176-200402000-00019

49. Ravelli A, Bolognini S, Gambarotti M, Villanacci V. *Variability of histologic lesions in relation to biopsy site in glutensensitive enteropathy.* Am J Gastroenterol. 2005; 100: 177-85. http://dx.doi.org/10.1111/j.1572-0241.2005.40669.x

50. Rostom A, Murray JA, Kagnoff MF. *American Gastroenterological Association (AGA) Institute technical review on the diagnosis and management of celiac disease.* Gastroenterology. 2006; 131: 1981-2002. http://dx.doi.org/10.1053/j.gastro.2006.10.004

51. Hopper AD, Cross SS, Sanders DS. *Patchy villous atrophy in adult patients with suspected glutensensitive enteropathy: is a multiple duodenal biopsy strategy appropriate?* Endoscopy. 2008; 40: 219-24. http://dx.doi.org/10.1055/s-2007-995361

52. Pais WP, Duerksen DR, Pettigrew NM et al. *How many duodenal biopsy specimens are required to make a diagnosis of celiac disease?* Gastrointest Endosc. 2008; 67: 1082-7. http://dx.doi.org/10.1016/j.gie.2007.10.015

53. Gonzalez S, Gupta A, Cheng J et al. *Prospective study of the role of duodenal bulb biopsies in the diagnosis of celiac disease.* Gastrointest Endosc. 2010; 72: 758-65. http://dx.doi.org/10.1016/j.gie.2010.06.026

54. Cammarota G, Martino A, Pirozzi GA et al. *Direct visualization of intestinal villi by high-resolution magnifying upper endoscopy: a validation study.* Gastrointest Endosc. 2004; 60: 732-8. http://dx.doi.org/10.1016/S0016-5107(04)02170-4

55. Gasbarrini A, Ojetti V, Cuoco L et al. *Lack of endoscopic visualization of intestinal villi with the "immersion technique" in overt atrophic celiac disease.* Gastrointest Endosc. 2003; 57: 348-51. http://dx.doi.org/10.1067/mge.2003.116

56. Singh R, Nind G, Tucker G et al. *Narrow-band imaging in the evaluation of villous morphology: a feasibility study assessing a simplified classification and observer agreement.* Endoscopy. 2010; 42: 889-94. http://dx.doi.org/10.1055/s-0030-1255708

57. Cammarota G, Cesaro P, Cazzato A et al. *Optimal band imaging system: a new tool for enhancing the duodenal villous pattern in celiac disease.* Gastrointest Endosc. 2008; 68: 352-7. http://dx.doi.org/10.1016/j.gie.2008.02.054

58. Serra S, Jani PA. *An approach to duodenal biopsies.* J Clin Pathol. 2006; 59: 1133-50. http://dx.doi.org/10.1136/jcp.2005.031260

59. Bai JC, Fried M, Corazza GR et al. *World gastroenterology organisation global guidelines on celiac disease.* J Clin Gastroenterol. 2013; 47(2). http://dx.doi.org/10.1097/MCG.0b013e31827a6f83

60. Husby S, Koletzko S, Korponay-Szabo IR. *European Society for Pediatric Gastroenterology, Hepatology, and Nutrition Guidelines for the Diagnosis of Coeliac Disease.* J Pediatr Gastroenterol Nutr. 2012; 54: 136-60. http://dx.doi.org/10.1097/MPG.0b013e31821a23d0

61. Krevsky B. *Enteroscopy: exploring the final frontier.* Gastroenterology. 1991; 100: 838-9.

62. Appleyard M, Fireman Z, Glukhovsky A et al. *A randomized trial comparing wireless capsule endoscopy with push enteroscopy for the detection of small-bowel lesions.* Gastroenterology. 2000; 119: 1431-8. http://dx.doi.org/10.1053/gast.2000.20844

63. Marmo R., Rotondano G, Rondonotti E, de Franchis R, D Inca R, Vettorato M et al. *Capsule enteroscopy vs. other diagnostic procedures in diagnosing obscure gastrointestinal bleeding: a cost-effectiveness study.* Eur J Gastroenterol Hepatol. 2007; 19: 535-42. http://dx.doi.org/10.1097/MEG.0b013e32812144dd

64. Voderholzer WA, Ortner M, Rogalla P, Beinholzl J, Lochs H. *Diagnostic yield of wireless capsule enteroscopy in comparison with computed tomography enteroclysis.* Endoscopy. 2003; 35: 1009-14. http://dx.doi.org/10.1055/s-2003-44583

65. Costamagna G, Shah SK, Riccioni ME et al. *A prospective trial comparing small bowel radiographs and video capsule endoscopy for suspected small bowel disease.* Gastroenterology. 2002; 123: 999-1005. http://dx.doi.org/10.1053/gast.2002.35988

66. Eliakim R, Fischer D, Suissa A et al. *Wireless capsule video endoscopy is a superior diagnostic tool in comparison to barium follow-through and computerized tomography in patients with suspected Crohn's disease.* Eur J Gastroenterol Hepatol. 2003; 15: 363-7. http://dx.doi.org/10.1097/00042737-200304000-00005

67. Iddan G, Meron G, Glukhovsky A, Swain P et al. *Wireless capsule endoscopy.* Nature. 2000; 405: 417. http://dx.doi.org/10.1038/35013140

68. Sanhueza Bravo E, Ibáñez P, Araya R et al. *Experience with capsule endoscopy diagnostic tool for the small intestine.* Rev Med Chil. 2010; 138: 303-8.

69. Green PH, Cellier C. *Celiac disease.* N Engl J Med. 2007; 357: 1731-43. http://dx.doi.org/10.1056/NEJMra071600

70. Ersoy O, Akin E, Ugras S, Buyukasik S, Selvi E, Guney G. *Capsule Endoscopy Findings in Celiac Disease.* Dig Dis Sci. 2009; 54: 825-9. http://dx.doi.org/10.1007/s10620-008-0402-z

71. Kurien M, Evans KE, Aziz I et al. *Capsule endoscopy in adult celiac disease: a potential role in equivocal cases of celiac disease?* Gastrointest Endosc. 2013; 77: 221-32. http://dx.doi.org/10.1016/j.gie.2012.09.031

72. Chang M, Rubin M, Lewis SK et al. *Diagnosing celiac disease by video capsule endoscopy (VCE) when esophogastroduodenoscopy (EGD) and biopsy is unable to provide a diagnosis: a case series.* BMC Gastroenterology. 2012, 12: 90. http://dx.doi.org/10.1186/1471-230X-12-90

73. Barret M, Malamut G, Rahmi G et al. *Diagnostic Yield of Capsule Endoscopy in Refractory Celiac Disease.* Am J Gastroenterol. 2012; 107: 1546-55. http://dx.doi.org/10.1038/ajg.2012.199

74. Petroniene R, Dubcenco E, Baker JP et al. *Given capsule endoscopy in celiac disease: evaluation of diagnostic accuracy and interobserver agreement.* Am J Gastroenterol. 2005; 100: 685-94. http://dx.doi.org/10.1111/j.1572-0241.2005.41069.x

75. Hopper AD, Sidhu R, Hurlstone DP, McAlindon ME, Sanders DS. *Capsule endoscopy: an alternative to duodenal biopsy for the recognition of villous atrophy in coeliac disease?* Dig Liver Dis. 2007; 39: 140-5. http://dx.doi.org/10.1016/j.dld.2006.07.017

76. Rondonotti E, Spada C, Cave D et al. *Video capsule enteroscopy in the diagnosis of celiac disease: a multicenter study.* Am J Gastroenterol. 2007; 102: 1624-31. http://dx.doi.org/10.1111/j.1572-0241.2007.01238.x

77. Biagi F, Rondonotti E, Campanella J et al. *Video capsule endoscopy and histology for small-bowel mucosa evaluation: a comparison performed by blinded observers.* Clin Gastroenterol Hepatol. 2006; 4: 998-1003. http://dx.doi.org/10.1016/j.cgh.2006.04.004

78. Maiden L, Elliott T, McLaughlin SD, Ciclitira P. *A blinded pilot comparison of capsule endoscopy and small bowel histology in unresponsive celiac disease.* Dig Dis Sci. 2009; 54: 1280-3. http://dx.doi.org/10.1007/s10620-008-0486-5

79. Lidums I, Cummins AG, Teo E. *The role of capsule endoscopy in suspected celiac disease patients with positive celiac serology.* Dig Dis Sci. 2011; 56: 499-505.
http://dx.doi.org/10.1007/s10620-010-1290-6

80. Murray JA, Rubio-Tapia A, van Dyke CT et al. *Mucosal atrophy in celiac disease: extent of involvement, correlation with clinical presentation, and response to treatment.* Clin Gastroenterol Hepatol. 2008; 6: 186-93. http://dx.doi.org/10.1016/j.cgh.2007.10.012

81. Petroniene P, Dubcenco E, Baker JP et al. *Given capsule endoscopy in celiac disease.* Gastrointest Endosc Clin N Am. 2004; 14: 115-27.
http://dx.doi.org/10.1016/j.giec.2003.10.005

82. Lidums I, Teo E, Field J, Cummins AG. *Capsule Endoscopy: A Valuable Tool in the Follow-Up of People With Celiac Disease on a Gluten-Free Diet.* Clin and Transl Gastroenterol. 2011; 2: e4. http://dx.doi.org/10.1038/ctg.2011.3

83. Culliford A, Daly J, Diamond B, Rubin M, Green PH. *The value of wireless capsule endoscopy in patients with complicated celiac disease.* Gastrointest Endosc. 2005; 62: 55-61. http://dx.doi.org/10.1016/S0016-5107(05)01566-X

84. Daum S, Wahnschaffe U, Glasenapp R, Borchert M, Ullrich R, Zeitz M, et al. *Capsule endoscopy in refractory celiac disease.* Endoscopy. 2007; 39: 455-8.
http://dx.doi.org/10.1055/s-2007-966239

85. Maiden L, Elliott T, McLaughlin SD et al. *A blinded pilot comparison of capsule endoscopy and small bowel histology in unresponsive celiac disease.* Dig Dis Sci. 2009; 54: 1280-3. http://dx.doi.org/10.1007/s10620-008-0486-5

86. Kurien M, Evans K, Aziz I, Sidhu R et al. *Capsule endoscopy in adult celiac disease: a potential role in equivocal cases of celiac disease?* Gastrointest Endosc. 2013; 77: 227-32. http://dx.doi.org/10.1016/j.gie.2012.09.031

87. Ciaccio XX et al. *Classification of videocapsule endoscopy image patterns: comparative analysis between patients with celiac disease and normal individuals.* BioMedical Engineering On Line. 2010; 9: 44. http://dx.doi.org/10.1186/1475-925X-9-44

88. Tennyson CA, Lewis BS. *Enteroscopy: an overview.* Gastrointest Endosc Clin N Am. 2009; 19: 315-24. http://dx.doi.org/10.1016/j.giec.2009.04.005

89. Matsumoto T, Moriyama T, Esaki M, Nakamura S, Iida M. *Performance of antegrade double-balloon enteroscopy: comparison with push enteroscopy.* Gastrointest Endosc. 2005; 62: 392-8. http://dx.doi.org/10.1016/j.gie.2005.04.052

90. Messer I, May A, Manner H, Ell C. *Prospective, randomized, single-center trial comparing double-balloon enteroscopy and spiral enteroscopy in patients with suspected small-bowel disorders.* Gastrointest Endosc. 2013; 77: 241-9.
http://dx.doi.org/10.1016/j.gie.2012.08.020

91. Xin L, Liao Z, Jiang YP, Li ZS. *Indications, detectability, positive findings, total enteroscopy, and complications of diagnostic double-balloon endoscopy: a systematic review of data over the first decade of use.* Gastrointest Endosc. 2011; 74: 563-70.
http://dx.doi.org/10.1016/j.gie.2011.03.1239

92. Di Nardo G, Oliva S, Ferrari F et al. *Usefulness of single balloon enteroscopy in pediatric Crohn's disease.* Gastroenterology. 2011; 140: S-197.

93. Höroldt BS, McAlindon ME, Stephenson TJ, Hadjivassiliou M, Sanders DS. *Making the diagnosis of coeliac disease: is there a role for push enteroscopy?* Eur J Gastroenterol Hepatol. 2004; 16: 1143-6. http://dx.doi.org/10.1097/00042737-200411000-00010

94. Cellier C, Cuillerier E, Patey-Mariaud de Serre N. *Push enteroscopy in celiac sprue and refractory sprue.* Gastrointest Endosc. 1999; 50: 613-7.
http://dx.doi.org/10.1016/S0016-5107(99)80007-8

95. Hadithi M, Al-toma A, Oudejans J, van Bodegraven AA, Mulder C, Jacobs M. *The value of double-balloon enteroscopy in patients with refractory celiac disease.* Am J Gastroenterol. 2007; 102: 987-96.
http://dx.doi.org/10.1111/j.1572-0241.2007.01122.x

96. Fry LC, Bellutti M, Neumann H, Malfertheiner P, Mönkemüller K. *Utility of double-balloon enteroscopy for the evaluation of malabsorption.* Dig Dis. 2008; 26: 134-9.
http://dx.doi.org/10.1159/000116771

Chapter 10

Small Intestine Biopsy and its Interpretation: Preliminary Results in Costa Rica

Fernando Brenes-Pino[1], Adelita Herrera[2]

[1] Laboratory of Pathology, Hospital CIMA San José, San José, Costa Rica.

[2] Molecular Diagnosis Unit, Sáenz Renauld Laboratories, San José, Costa Rica.

ferbrenes@gmail.com, adelitaherrerae@gmail.com

Doi: http://dx.doi.org/10.3926/oms.229

How to cite this chapter

Brenes-Pino F, Herrera A. *Small Intestine Biopsy and its Interpretation: Preliminary Results in Costa Rica*. In Rodrigo L and Peña AS, editors. *Celiac Disease and Non-Celiac Gluten Sensitivity*. Barcelona, Spain: OmniaScience; 2014. p. 203-218.

Abstract

Celiac disease is an autoimmune disease with diverse histopathological changes of the small intestine which are fundamental for the diagnosis of the disease. The main changes are intraepithelial lymphocytic infiltration of the intestinal mucosa, with or without villous atrophy. The number of biopsies has to be adequate, at least six, because the histopathological abnormalities often have a patchy distribution. The disease may exhibit only minimal alterations along with the intraepithelial lymphocytic infiltrate, which can be shared with other non-celiac entities. We recommend the use of the Corazza-Villanacci classification because it has demonstrated a better correlation among pathologists.

We present the results of 258 patients (108 male and 150 female) with celiac disease in Costa Rica with lymphocytic duodenitis and villous atrophy. Mean age was 48.3 years, ranging between 16 and 90 years. Furthermore, in 35 patients, HLA-DQ2 and HLA-DQ8 genotyping was performed; 11 cases were positive for HLA-DQ2, 7 for HLA-DQ8, and 3 for both HLA-DQ2 and HLA-DQ8. 15 cases were negative, but had only lymphocytic duodenitis, which should be studied further and are currently being followed-up.

1. Introduction

The interpretation of celiac disease biopsies for CD diagnosis has evolved due to the knowledge of reliable genetic and serological markers. Correct and timely diagnosis of celiac disease is necessary to start a gluten-free diet and reduce the risk of chronic complications.

Serological tests are useful for detecting gluten intolerance, and include IgA anti tissue transglutaminase antibodies, IgA anti endomysial antibodies and IgA and IgG anti-gliadin, plus IgA anti reticulin. Of these, the first two have optimal sensitivity and specificity, with a high positive predictive value.[1] However, it has been observed that up to 5-15% of all patients with celiac disease may have normal values and up to 30% in cases with minor mucosal changes.[2-4] This is associated with the fact that between 20 to 50% of the patients have no obvious malabsorption symptoms.[5] Duodenal and jejunal biopsies remain for the time being the "gold standard" necessary to confirm the celiac disease diagnosis.

The classic histopathological small intestine mucosal alterations, such as flattening of the villi, were described originally by Paulley in 1954 in surgically obtained samples.[6] This villous atrophy was considered for many years as the main criterion needed for the celiac disease diagnosis. Subsequently, the recognition of subtler changes, specially the intraepithelial inflammatory infiltrate and in the lamina propria, acquired importance to help understand the histological features of the disease.[7] For these reasons, Marsh classified histological patterns of mucosal damage in the small intestine.[8] These changes, which represent progressive stages, include increased intraepithelial lymphocyte infiltration, even in an intestinal mucosa with no atrophy, followed by the varying degrees of atrophy in four categories (1 to 4), together with the increase in the lamina propria inflammation and a progressive alteration of the mucosa. These criteria were modified by Oberhüber in 1999,[8] who, in turn, divided the type 3 lesion into three subgroups based on the severity of atrophy and eliminated type 4. Villous atrophy belonging to type 3A is of a mild degree, type 3B is defined by moderate or subtotal atrophy and type 3C by a totally flat mucosa. This classification is now being used routinely by many pathologists.

2. Location and Amount of Biopsies

Small bowel biopsies have increased significantly in recent years, mainly because clinicians are aware of the existence of less severe forms of celiac disease; likewise, the number of endoscopic procedures of the upper gastrointestinal tract has increased. The new endoscopes allow a more detailed view of the villi, but in most patients, if there is no marked atrophy, changes are not visible. The features of "patchy" villous atrophy have been discussed in the literature in relation to the number of samples to be taken and the optimal place for taking biopsies.[9-12] The American Gastroenterological Association (AGA) recommends taking at least 6 biopsies in the second duodenal, or more distal, portion in order to search for celiac disease.[12] In daily practice, it is suggested that a total of 6 biopsies be taken: 4 biopsies from the distal duodenum, 2 from the duodenal bulb, to reduce the possibility of error attributable to the existence of an irregular or non-homogeneous distribution of the disease.[10,13]

3. Normal Small Bowel Mucosa

The small intestinal mucosa should be assessed based on normal morphology, which must be known by the pathologist who will diagnose this organ biopsies. The villi biopsies under analysis must be properly oriented, the entire villi should be observable with an adequate view of the muscularis mucosae. The presence of the muscularis mucosae in the biopsy itself is critical, because it allows a comprehensive assessment and without it, the biopsy cannot be regarded as adequate for evaluation. In daily practice, the villi are not always arranged vertically and upwards but tend to bend in different directions. Furthermore, when there is lymphoid hyperplasia, villi tend to flatten, due to the effect to the lamina propria injury. To avoid interpretation problems, it has been proposed that biopsies of the small intestine should be considered representative when at least four tall villi are observed and aligned in any serial biopsy cut.[14]

The upper region of normal ends in an arrow shape, which occurs gradually in the villi's upper third. Groups of 3 to 5 well-oriented villi ought to be evaluated in order to define their ratio in relation to the crypts. The villi height should be of at least 3 to 1, even 5 to 1, in relation to the crypts, depending on the biopsy site (Figure 1). Shorter villi are proximally found in the duodenum, while their height increases distally from the jejunum towards the ileum, where they shorten again.

The orientation of biopsy specimens is essential to proper interpretation and analysis. Some authors have suggested that biopsies be placed on a support surface, such as filter paper, in order to achieve an appropriate vertical orientation.[15] Pathologists must help histotechnicians become aware of these facts and educate them about the importance of biopsy orientation in order to obtain a proper evaluation. Magnifying glasses must be routinely used for gastrointestinal biopsy inclusions since this helps identify the sample's base due to the presence of dark spots, which correspond to the blood vessels cut transversally during sampling. This helps the technician guide biopsy vertically into the paraffin inclusion.[16]

The crypts' volume also defines the existence of a lesion since they normally will not exceed two gland's thickness, so that any increase should be considered as abnormal and therefore should be carefully evaluated in all aspects. Its increase implies a lengthening of the crypts of Lieberkühn within a progressive process that usually precedes the onset of villous atrophy.

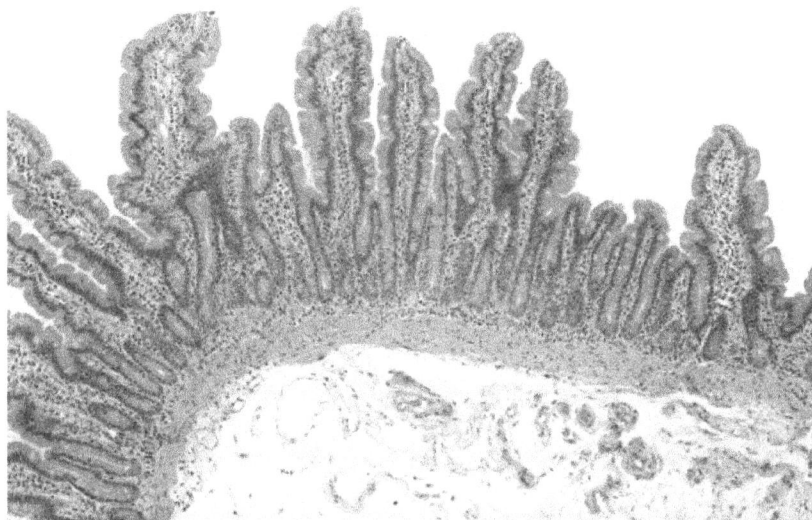

Figure 1. Well-oriented normal duodenal mucosa with proper 3:1-4:1 villi/crypts ratio, with intraepithelial lymphocytes showing the pattern of progressive decrease towards the apical part.

The enterocytes lining the villi show a slightly eosinophilic cytoplasm, homogeneous in appearance. Special attention must be paid to the enterocytes found in the upper third since, should there be immune injury, the cytoplasm tends to have vacuoles.

At the lamina propria level, the normal inflammatory infiltrate is mild, including lymphocytes, plasma cells and some eosinophils against a background where light areas are still observed, without inflammation; this covers about a third of the bottom of the lamina propria.[17] If there is an increased inflammatory infiltrate, these clear zones tend to disappear and the lamina propria fills with inflammatory mononuclear cells. Occasionally, neutrophils can be observed; this has been described in relation to the existence of activity in the disease's inflammatory process.[18]

4. Histological Changes of Celiac Disease

Celiac disease symptoms are thought to be more related to the extent of affected bowel than to the intensity of the lesion.[19] The severity of the injury is also greater in the proximal small intestine than in the distal; however, in many cases, patients who are being studied due to diarrhea first undergo a colonoscopy, so terminal ileum biopsies are frequently taken to rule out the possibility of celiac disease. The pathologist must be aware for mucosal alterations in the terminal ileum, since in the literature they are described as mild, but changes such as increased intraepithelial lymphocytes may be an important sign that leads to suspect the presence of an associated celiac disease.[20-21]

The morphological alterations to be evaluated are architecture abnormalities (such as shortening of the villi), crypt hyperplasia, increased presence of intraepithelial lymphocytes and expansion of the lamina propria's inflammatory mononuclear infiltrate. However, these characteristics, both individually as well as combined, may be nonspecific.

5. Intraepithelial Lymphocytic Infiltrate

Celiac disease is an immune process, therefore intraepithelial lymphocytes are responsible for the epithelial injury. This is the first change and the most sensitive indicator of the effects of gluten on the small intestine mucosa: type T lymphocytes, mainly cytotoxic.[22] Furthermore, the lamina propria also will respond immunologically and a significant increase of lymphocytes, plasma cells and macrophages is observed.

Counts greater than 40 intraepithelial lymphocytes per 100 enterocytes were formerly considered abnormal. Over the years, this value been tweaked with the lowering of this threshold down to the point where today 20 intraepithelial lymphocytes per 100 enterocytes is considered to be normal, that is to say, a ratio of one lymphocyte per 5 enterocytes.[23] One of the reasons for this lies in the fact that the place where biopsies are taken has gradually changed, which has led to the observation that normal jejunal mucosa has a greater count of intraepithelial lymphocytes than the duodenal mucosa. When a specific anti-CD3 lymphocyte immunohistochemistry is performed, due to a higher sensitivity than that observed with hematoxylin-eosin, a limit of 25 intraepithelial lymphocytes per 100 enterocytes ought to be considered.[23] Immunohistochemistry should not be used routinely in the evaluation of biopsies to screen for celiac disease, but it must be insisted that the pathologist must analyze the largest possible number of duodenal biopsies to become familiar with the normal number of intraepithelial lymphocytes. The cost of this biopsy evaluation should not be increased, nor should the pathologist's time be wasted or else delay diagnosis with this technique; it would be wiser rather to seek a second opinion or recommend a serological test.

In daily practice, the intraepithelial lymphocyte count can be a little impractical since it involves counting from 300 to 500 enterocytes. It should be performed in a well-oriented villi, excluding the base crypts. According to experience, a duodenal villus of mean height contains 90 to 110 enterocytes, so, while analyzing 3-5 villi, the total enterocyte count may be disregarded and only count the intraepithelial lymphocytes. The distribution pattern of normal lymphocyte density in the villi is higher towards the base and decreases as it reaches the luminal end (Figure 1).[19]

In recent literature, a more practical way to perform celiac disease screening in small bowel biopsies has been proposed, in which the intraepithelial lymphocytes in tips of five well-oriented villi are counted; each tips has about 20 enterocytes each (Figure 2). The normal intraepithelial lymphocyte average count using the tip counting method is equal to or less than 5 per each 20 enterocytes, while a larger number is considered suggestive of or compatible with the existence of gluten intolerance.[24,25] It must always be borne in mind that there are a variety of entities which can also lead to an increased intraepithelial lymphocyte count, so that this change cannot be considered as an exclusive diagnostic criteria for celiac disease, but should be included within a range of differential diagnoses.

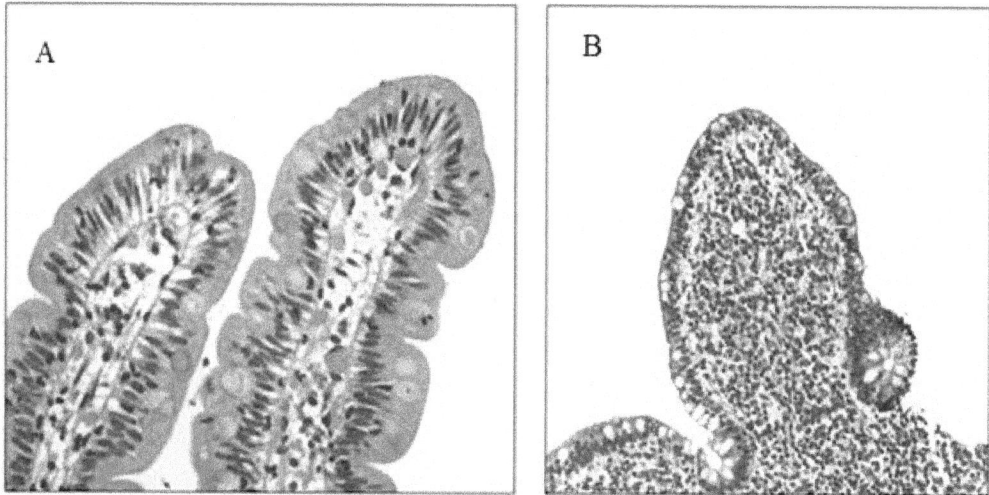

Figure 2. A. The villi exhibit sharp or pointed ends, with the presence of less than 5 intraepithelial lymphocytes (hematoxylin-eosin, x400). B. The villus has a significant increase in intraepithelial lymphocytes, greater than 5 (hematoxylin-eosin, x400).

Besides celiac disease, there is a group of disorders that have a morphology similar to early celiac disease, including normal villous architecture with increased intraepithelial lymphocytes (greater than 5 per 20 enterocytes) morphology. These conditions are described below (Table 1).[26]

* Gluten sensitivity
* Hipersensitivity to gluten-free foods: Cow milk protein, rice, chicken, fish, other cereals, etc.
* Infections: Helicobacter pylori, giardiasis and criptosporidiosis
* Bacterial overgrowth
* Non-steroidal anti-inflammatory drugs (NSAIDs)
* Immunological deficiencies: common variable immunodeficiency, IgA deficiency
* Immunological alterations: Hashimoto's Thyroiditis, rheumatoid arthritis and systemic lupus erythematous
* Intestinal inflammatory disease

Table 1. Causes of intraepithelial lymphocytosis in a small intestine with normal villous architecture (Brown, 2006).[26]

Among these, hypersensitivity to various foods may be included, among which milk proteins, rice, chicken, fish and other cereals stand out, besides the presence of infections such as *Helicobacter pylori, giardiasis* and *cryptosporidiosis*. *Giardiasis* also produces a significant increase in mononuclear inflammation of the lamina propria, including the presence of lymphoid follicles, which are relatively rare in celiac disease. Also, bowel bacterial overgrowth syndrome is secondary to various viral and bacterial enteritis.

An important issue is enteric damage related to the toxicity of various drugs, such as non-steroidal anti-inflammatory drugs (NSAIDs), which has been confirmed, since upon withdrawal of the drug, symptoms and histological features become normalized. Immune deficiencies such as common variable immunodeficiency (CVID), which is marked by minimal presence or complete absence of plasma cells level of the lamina propria cells, which can be corroborated through immunohistochemistry. Other immune disorders may include such as Hashimoto's thyroiditis, rheumatoid arthritis (RA) and systemic lupus erythematous (SLE). Chronic inflammatory bowel disease (IBD), can also cause lymphocytic duodenitis, particularly in cases with Crohn's disease.

6. Villous Atrophy

The assessment of villous atrophy should be done only in well-oriented histological sections. These changes may be focalized, so if enough fragments were not analyzed, the result may be a false negative. If the received fragments are few (less than 4), new cuts can be made, which could show areas with alterations. It must be pointed out that diagnostic reliability is crucial because low reliability can mean a significant number of misclassified cases.

Villous atrophy has been considered as one of the most characteristic alterations in the diagnosis of celiac disease.[8] However, pathologists should be aware that there are other diseases to include in the differential diagnosis, which may include various degrees of atrophy, which are listed below (Table 2).

• Autoimmune enteropathy
• Microvillus inclusions disease
• Tropical sprue
• Collagenous sprue
• Radiochemotherapy
• Graft vs host disease
• Nutritional deficiencies
• Chronic pancreatitis
• T-cell lymphoma induced enteropathy

Table 2. Causes of atrophy and flattening of the villi (Ensari, 2010).[33]

7. Crypt Hyperplasia

Crypt hyperplasia produces elongation, a process that initially precedes villous atrophy. This is a change secondary to enterocyte loss on the villi surface, as an expression of immunological injury caused by celiac disease. The crypts contain cells capable of renewing enterocytes and it is common to observe the presence of significant mitotic activity at this level, which under normal conditions is rare, but not a reliable indicator of crypt hyperplasia.[7]

8. Histological Classification of Celiac Disease

In 1992 Marsh designed a system to classify morphological changes secondary to gluten sensitivity enteropathy, which was later amended by Oberhüber in 1999.[8] This system integrated celiac disease pathophysiology with its histological alterations morphological changes, grading the presence of immunological disorders in conjunction with architectural changes of the mucosa (Table 3).

Marsh-Oberhuber Classification		Corazza-Villanacci Classification	
Type 1	Villi and normal crypt architecture with ≥30 IELs/100 enterocytes	Grade A	No atrophy, normal villous architecture with or without crypt hyperplasia and ≥25 IELs/100 enterocytes
Type 2	Normal villous architecture, crypt hyperplasia and ≥30 IELs/100 enterocytes		
Type 3a	Partial villous atrophy with crypt/villi ratio of <3:1 or 2:1, crypt hyperplasia and ≥30 IELs/100 enterocytes	Grade B1	Atrophic, with villi/crypt ratio of <3:1, 2:1 or 1:1, villi still detectable and ≥25 IELs/100 enterocytes
Type 3b	Subtotal villous atrophy with villi/crypt of <1:1, crypt hyperplasia and ≥30 IELs/100 enterocytes		
Type 3c	Total villous atrophy (flat mucosa) with marked crypt hyperplasia and ≥30 IELs/100 enterocytes	Grade B2	Completely flat atrophic mucosa, no observable villi and ≥25 IELs/100 enterocytes
Type 4	Hypoplastic atrophic lesion (flat mucosa) with only a few crypts and near-normal IEL count	Eliminated	

Table 3. Comparison of histopathological classifications of mucosal changes associated with celiac disease (Bao, 2012).[34]

However, this classification have had the problem that type 1 and 2 mucosal alterations are often not recognized and, in subtype 3, there is a great variability between observers, even among expert gastrointestinal pathologists.[27] Therefore, in 2005, Corazza and Villanacci proposed a simplified classification scheme in order to reduce the possibility of disagreement in assessing celiac disease biopsies.[28] Their proposal was to reduce the original five Marsh-Oberhüber classification categories to three (Table 3). This includes two simple categories: First, Grade A, comprising lesion without atrophy and, second, Grade B comprising atrophic lesion (Figure 3). B grade lesions are subsequently subdivided into types B1 and B2, which depend on atrophy with the presence or absence of villi. This classification is based on the recognition of type 2 Marsh-Oberhüber injury; types 3a and 3b are not essential for the diagnosis and monitoring of celiac disease.[27]

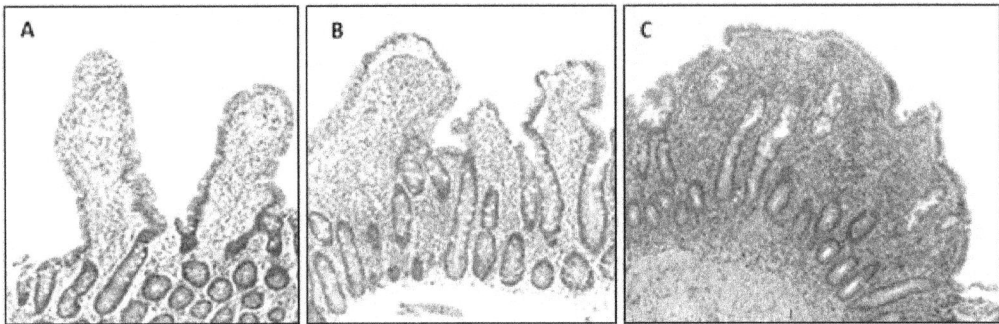

Figure 3. Different degrees of duodenal injury. A: Normal villous height and ratio, with increased intraepithelial lymphocytic infiltrate corresponding to Corazza Villanacci Grade-A (Marsh type 2) (hematoxylin-eosin, x100). B: Moderate villous atrophy and diffuse intraepithelial lymphocyte infiltration, corresponding to Corazza-Villanacci Grade B1 (Marsh type 3b) (hematoxylin-eosin, x100). C: Marked villus atrophy with diffuse intraepithelial lymphocyte infiltration, Corazza-Villanacci Grade B2 (Marsh 3c) (hematoxylin-eosin, x100).

The simplification of histopathological classifications has been shown to increase concordance among pathologists, as it has happened with low grade and high grade dysplasia classification.[29]

When the degree of diagnostic agreement or concordance on celiac disease between pathologists was compared, it rose from 0.35 according to the Marsh-Oberhüber classification to 0.55 with the new Corazza-Villanacci classification.[27] Therefore, its use is recommended since it facilitates the correct interpretation of the histological lesions and it reduces the possibility of disagreement on gluten enteropathy, thus benefiting the diagnosis and management of patients.

9. Celiac Disease in Costa Rica

The preliminary results of celiac disease studies in Costa Rica are presented, from 2006 to 2012, from an open endoscopy service at CIMA Hospital and from private Endoscopy Clinics sent to the Pathology Laboratory. Biopsies were submitted with an application with the patients' data, including age and gender as well as clinical data including studies on chronic diarrhea, abdominal pain or celiac disease. Cases with a lymphocytic duodenitis diagnosis were searched for in the laboratories' databases, up to a total of 643 patients with their respective biopsies. These biopsies were taken from the duodenum and were analyzed by one of the authors (F.B.), classifying them using the Corazza-Villanacci system of atrophy degree definition.[27] However, serological results in Costa Rica using anti-transglutaminase have, in daily practice, often have been negative, which was demonstrated in a previous work that used an IgA and IgG anti-transglutaminase detection system. Since the expected results were not reliable and, since we only found 15% positivity in biopsies with some degree of atrophy,[30] these were excluded from analysis in this preliminary work.

Only those patients with some degree of villous atrophy were included, including Corazza-Villanacci B1 and B2 and which responded to the gluten-free diet; a total of 258 patients (Table 4).

Characteristics	Number (%)
Average age ± SD (range)	48.3 ± 16.5 (16-90)
Gender	
• Male	108 (41.9)
• Female	150 (58.4)
Corazza classification	
• B1	246 (95.3)
• B2	12 (4.7)
Number of Biopsies ± SD (range)	4.6 ± 1.7 (2-14)

Table 4. Characteristics of 258 patients with celiac disease in Costa Rica.

The average age was 48.3 years, with slight female predominance (58.4%) over males (41.9%). Most patients corresponded to grade B1 Corazza-Villanacci classification (mild to moderate atrophy) (95.3%). Severe atrophy (B2 level), was only observed in a small group of 12 patients (4.7%).

Since duodenal endoscopic studies were initiated in Costa Rica, special emphasis was placed on the importance of the number of biopsies taken, which is reflected in the average number of fragments, which was of 4.6 per case.

Regarding the number of cases diagnosed during the observed period, it is noteworthy that, during the first two years, the number was relatively lower than in later years probably because of the generalized idea that celiac disease was rare in our environment (Figure 4). Approximately

50% of the cases classified as grade B1 were under 50 years of age, while B2 cases, 67%, were over 50 years of age; this is compatible with a longer disease evolution. However, these data will be complete when they are analyzed and all studies are finished (Figure 5).

Regarding another issue related to these patients, peripheral blood samples were taken from a group of 36, from which DNA was extracted, and the HLA-DQ2 and DQ8 genotypes were detected with HLA-DQA1, HLA-DQB1 and HLA-DRB1 exon 2 amplification using the CeliacStrip® system from Operon (Zaragoza, Spain) as per the manufacturer's instructions. The results were displayed in a hybridization nylon membrane.[31] The cases described responded to the GFD. This group took into account all biopsies of the total original group independently the presence or absence of an atrophy. They accounted for 29 female patients (78.4%) and 8 males (21.6%) with a mean age of 46.2 (range 18-79 years, SD 14.7 years). Most of the cases, 23 were under 50 years of age 50, 64%. The Corazza-Villanacci classification found 27 grade A cases and 9 B1 cases, with no cases of severe atrophy.

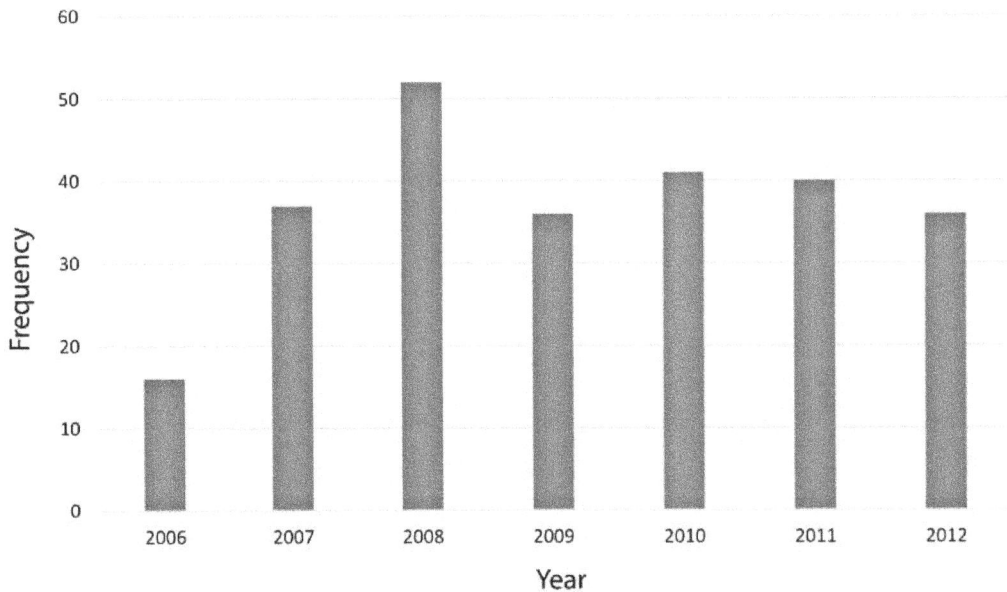

Figure 4. Annual distribution of celiac disease cases in Costa Rica.

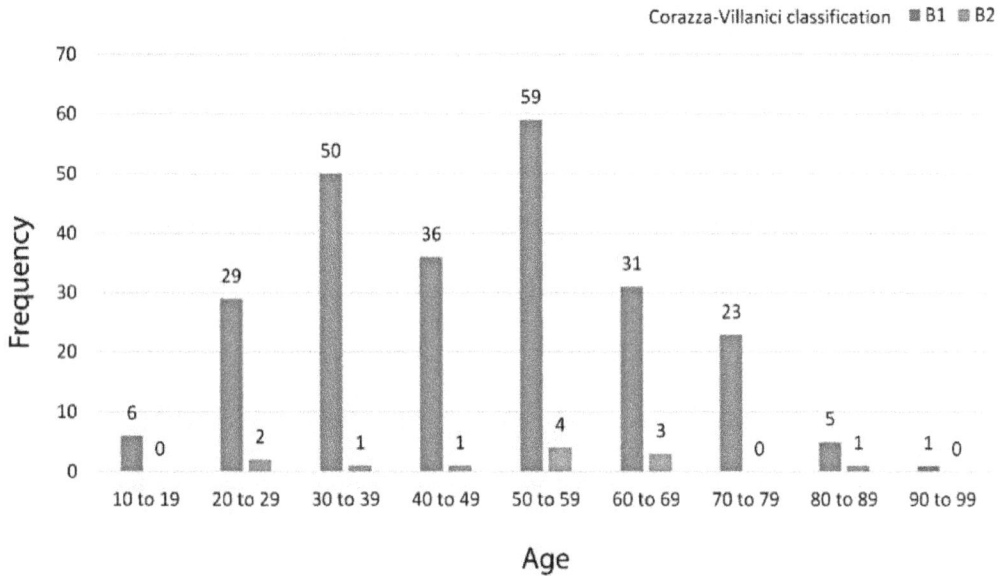

Figure 5. Age distribution of celiac disease cases in Costa Rica classified as Corazza-Villanacci B1 and B2.

Out of 36 cases, 20 were carriers of risk haplotypes, distributed in 11 cases HLA-DQ2 (+), 7 HLA-DQ8 (*) cases and 3 cases with simultaneous HLA-DQ2 and HLA-DQ8 (+). In addition, 15 cases were negative for these haplotypes, however, further studies are required to complete these data.

Most of the cases were of biopsies without villous atrophy. These included the 11 cases which were negative for risk haplotypes, which subsequently make it imperative to corroborate whether they were celiac patients or not (Table 5).[32]

HLA	Grade A	Grade B1
DQ2 +	8	3
DQ8 +	6	1
DQ2 + y DQ8 +	2	1
DQ2 – y DQ8 –	11	4

Table 5. HLA-DQ2 and HLADQ8 duodenal biopsies from 36 Costa Rican patients classified according to Corazza-Villanacci.

10. Conclusions

Celiac disease is an immune process, which causes highly variable morphological alterations in the small intestine in genetically susceptible individuals. The small intestinal biopsy still remains the gold standard for the diagnosis of celiac disease. Small intestinal biopsies can confirm the diagnosis when clinical and serological assays suggest this disease, or else suggest it when patients have subclinical or atypical presentations or else when serology fails to support the diagnosis. Once the diagnosis is established, histological evaluation is an important appraisal of adherence to the gluten-free diet when response to it is unsatisfactory, as well as to detect possible gastrointestinal involvement. The pathologist who examines the biopsy should be aware of possible differential diagnoses of morphological changes, especially in the early stages of celiac disease.

The experience of celiac disease diagnosis in Costa Rica demonstrates that patients ought to be comprehensively analyzed by a team of professionals including gastroenterologists with adequate training for duodenal biopsies, in conjunction with pathologists able to interpret tissue-level changes, since biopsies could be the first wake-up call for further studies of the patient's case. Serology for anti-endomysium and anti-transglutaminase antibodies are essential in addressing the patient and must have adequate quality control so that results are reliable. Finally, HLA-DQ2 studies should be a basic part of the celiac disease tests, however, the characteristics of the Latin American population have not been fully studied yet and it is necessary to seek other haplotypes that may also be related to the appearance of disease.

References

1. Hopper AD, Hadjivassiliou M, Hurlstone DP, Lobo AJ, McAlindon ME, Egner W et al. *What is the role of serologic testing in celiac disease? A prospective, biopsy-confirmed study with economic analysis.* Clini Gastroenterol Hepatol. 2008; 6: 314-20. http://dx.doi.org/10.1016/j.cgh.2007.12.008

2. Tursi A, Brandimarte G, Giorgetti GM. *Prevalence of antitissue transglutaminase antibodies in different degrees of intestinal damage in celiac disease.* J Clin Gastroenterol. 2003;36:219–21. http://dx.doi.org/10.1097/00004836-200303000-00007

3. Murray JA, Herlein J, Mitros F, Goeken JA. *Serologic Testing for Celiac Disease in the United States: Results of a Multilaboratory Comparison Study.* Clin and Vac Immunol. 2000; 7: 584-7. http://dx.doi.org/10.1128/CDLI.7.4.584-587.2000

4. Abrams JA, Diamond B, Rotterdam H, Green PHR. *Seronegative Celiac Disease: Increased Prevalence with Lesser Degrees of Villous Atrophy.* Dig Dis Sci. 2004; 49: 546-50. http://dx.doi.org/10.1023/B:DDAS.0000026296.02308.00

5. Verdu EF, Armstrong D, Murray JA. *Between celiac disease and irritable bowel syndrome: the "no man's land" of gluten sensitivity.* The American journal of gastroenterology. 2009; 104: 1587-94. http://dx.doi.org/10.1038/ajg.2009.188

6. Paulley JW. *Observation on the aetiology of idiopathic steatorrhoea; jejunal and lymph-node biopsies.* BMJ. 1954; 2(4900): 1318-21. http://dx.doi.org/10.1136/bmj.2.4900.1318

7. Goldstein NS, Underhill J. *Morphologic features suggestive of gluten sensitivity in architecturally normal duodenal biopsy specimens.* Am J Clin Pathol. 2001; 116: 63-71. http://dx.doi.org/10.1309/5PRJ-CM0U-6KLD-6KCM

8. Oberhuber G, Granditsch G, Vogelsang H. *The histopathology of coeliac disease: time for a standardized report scheme for pathologists.* Eur J Gastroenterol Hepatol. 1999; 11: 1185-94. http://dx.doi.org/10.1097/00042737-199910000-00019

9. Ravelli A, Bolognini S, Gambarotti M, Villanacci V. *Variability of histologic lesions in relation to biopsy site in gluten-sensitive enteropathy.* Am J Gastroenterol. 2005; 100: 177-85. http://dx.doi.org/10.1111/j.1572-0241.2005.40669.x

10. Mangiavillano B, Parma B, Brambillasca MF, Albarello L, Barera G, Mariani A et al. *Diagnostic bulb biopsies in celiac disease.* Gastrointest Endosc. 2009; 69: 388-9. http://dx.doi.org/10.1016/j.gie.2008.06.014

11. Pais WP, Duerksen DR, Pettigrew NM, Bernstein CN. *How many duodenal biopsy specimens are required to make a diagnosis of celiac disease?* Gastrointest Endosc. 2008: 67: 1082-7. http://dx.doi.org/10.1016/j.gie.2007.10.015

12. AGA Institute. *AGA Institute Medical Position Statement on the Diagnosis and Management of Celiac Disease.* Gastroenterol. 2006; 131: 1977-80. http://dx.doi.org/10.1053/j.gastro.2006.10.003

13. Bonamico M, Thanasi E, Mariani P, Nenna R, Luparia RPL, Barbera C et al. *Duodenal Bulb Biopsies in Celiac Disease: A Multicenter Study.* J Ped Gastroenterol and Nutr. 2008; 47: 618-22. http://dx.doi.org/10.1097/MPG.0b013e3181677d6e

14. Perera DR, Weinstein WM, Rubin CE. *Small intestinal biopsy.* Hum Pathol. 1975; 6: 157-217. http://dx.doi.org/10.1016/S0046-8177(75)80176-6

15. Babbin BA, Crawford K, Sitaraman SV. *Malabsorption work-up: utility of small bowel biopsy.* Clin Gastroenterol Hepatol. 2006; 4: 1193-8.
http://dx.doi.org/10.1016/j.cgh.2006.07.022

16. Brenes F. Observación personal.

17. Serra S, Jani PA. *An approach to duodenal biopsies.* J Clin Pathol. 2006; 59: 1133-50.
http://dx.doi.org/10.1136/jcp.2005.031260

18. Hällgren R, Colombel JF, Dahl R, Fredens K, Kruse A, Jacobsen NO et al. *Neutrophil and eosinophil involvement of the small bowel in patients with celiac disease and Crohn's disease: Studies on the secretion rate and immunohistochemical localization of granulocyte granule constituents.* Am J Med. 1989; 86: 56-64.
http://dx.doi.org/10.1016/0002-9343(89)90230-1

19. Goldstein NS. *Proximal small-bowel mucosal villous intraepithelial lymphocytes.* Histopathol. 2004; 44: 199-205. http://dx.doi.org/10.1111/j.1365-2559.2004.01775.x

20. Hopper AD, Hurlstone DP, Leeds JS, McAlindon ME, Dube AK, Stephenson TJ et al. *The occurrence of terminal ileal histological abnormalities in patients with coeliac disease.* Dig Liver Dis. 2006; 38: 815-9. http://dx.doi.org/10.1016/j.dld.2006.04.003

21. Trecca A, Gaj F, Gagliardi G, Calcaterra R, Battista S, Silano M. *Role of magnified ileoscopy in the diagnosis of cases of coeliac disease with predominant abdominal symptoms.* Scand J Gastroenterol. 2009; 44: 320-4.
http://dx.doi.org/10.1080/00365520802538237

22. Antonioli DA. *Celiac disease: a progress report.* Mod Pathol. 2003; 16: 342-6.
http://dx.doi.org/10.1097/01.MP.0000062997.16339.47

23. Veress B, Franzén L, Bodin L, Borch K. *Duodenal intraepithelial lymphocyte-count revisited.* Scand J Gastroenterol. 2004; 39: 138-44.
http://dx.doi.org/10.1080/00365520310007675

24. Järvinen TT, Collin P, Rasmussen M, Kyrönpalo S, Mäki M, Partanen J et al. *Villous tip intraepithelial lymphocytes as markers of early-stage coeliac disease.* Scand J Gastroenterol. 2004; 39: 428-33. http://dx.doi.org/10.1080/00365520310008773

25. Biagi F, Luinetti O, Campanella J, Klersy C, Zambelli C, Villanacci V et al. *Intraepithelial lymphocytes in the villous tip: do they indicate potential coeliac disease?* J Clin Pathol. 2004; 57: 835-9.http://dx.doi.org/10.1136/jcp.2003.013607

26. Brown I, Mino-Kenudson M, Deshpande V, Lauwers GY. *Intraepithelial lymphocytosis in architecturally preserved proximal small intestinal mucosa: an increasing diagnostic problem with a wide differential diagnosis.* Arch Pathol Lab Med. 2006; 130: 1020-5.

27. Corazza GR, Villanacci V, Zambelli C, Milione M, Luinetti O, Vindigni C et al. *Comparison of the interobserver reproducibility with different histologic criteria used in celiac disease.* Clin Gastroenterol Hepatol. 2007; 5: 838-43.
http://dx.doi.org/10.1016/j.cgh.2007.03.019

28. Corazza GR, Villanacci V. *Coeliac disease. Some considerations on the histological diagnosis.* J Clin Pathol. 2005; 58: 573-4. http://dx.doi.org/10.1136/jcp.2004.023978

29. Rugge M, Correa P, Dixon MF, Hattori T, Leandro G, Lewin K et al. *Gastric dysplasia: the Padova international classification.* Am J Surg Pathol. 24: 167-76.
http://dx.doi.org/10.1097/00000478-200002000-00001

30. Barahona R. *Utilidad de los anticuerpos Antitransglutaminasa y su relación con la Enfermedad Celiaca en pacientes del Hospital San Juan de Dios de enero del 2008 al 2010.* Sistema de Estudios de Posgrado, Escuela de Medicina, Universidad de Costa Rica, San José. Tesis, 2010.

31. *Operon.* Manual de usuario del CeliacStrip. Zaragoza, España; 2012.

32. Karell K, Louka AS, Moodie SJ, Ascher H, Clot F, Greco L et al. *HLA types in celiac disease patients not carrying the DQA1*05-DQB1*02 (DQ2) heterodimer: results from the European Genetics Cluster on Celiac Disease.* Hum Immunol. 2003; 64: 469-77. http://dx.doi.org/10.1016/S0198-8859(03)00027-2

33. Ensari A. *Gluten-sensitive enteropathy (celiac disease): controversies in diagnosis and classification.* Arch Pathol Lab Med. 2010; 134: 826-36.

34. Bao F, Bhagat G. *Histopathology of celiac disease.* Gastrointest Endosc Clin North Am. 2012; 22: 679-94. http://dx.doi.org/10.1016/j.giec.2012.07.001

Chapter 11

Celiac Disease in Children

Isabel Polanco Allué

Full Professor of Pediatrics, School of Medicine, Autonomous University of Madrid

Head of Gastroenterology and Pediatric Nutrition Service, La Paz University Children's Hospital, Madrid, España.

ipolanco.hulp@salud.madrid.org

Doi: http://dx.doi.org/10.3926/oms.227

How to cite this chapter

Polanco I. *Celiac Disease in Children.* In Rodrigo L and Peña AS, editors. *Celiac Disease and Non-Celiac Gluten Sensitivity.* Barcelona, Spain: OmniaScience; 2014. p. 221-233.

Abstract

Celiac Disease (CD) is an immune-mediated systemic disorder caused by gluten and related prolamins in genetically susceptible individuals, characterized by the presence of a variable combination of gluten-dependent clinical manifestations, CD-specific antibodies, HLA-DQ2 or HLA-DQ8 haplotypes and enteropathy. CD-specific antibodies comprise autoantibodies against TGt2, including endomysial antibodies (EMA) and antibodies against deamidated forms of gliadin peptides (DGP).

To diagnose children and adolescents without intestinal biopsy, the following conditions are imperative: signs or symptoms suggestive of CD, high anti-TG2 levels (>10 times UNL), verified by EMA and positive HLA-DQ2 and/or DQ8. Only then the intestinal biopsy can be avoided, the CD diagnosis made and the child started on a gluten-free diet (GFD).

In childhood and adolescence, intestinal biopsy can be omitted in symptomatic subjects with high anti-TG2-IgA levels (>10 times normal values), verified by EMA and positive HLA-DQ2 and/or HLA-DQ8. In these cases, a GFD can be started. In all other cases, intestinal biopsies should be perform first before starting a GFD to avoid misdiagnosis.

1. Introduction

Celiac disease (CD) is a systemic disorder with an immunological basis, caused by the ingestion of gluten and similar proteins (gliadins, secalins, hordeins and possibly avenines), which affects people with genetic predisposition. It is characterized by a variety of clinical manifestations dependent on gluten ingestion: CD-specific antibodies, HLA-DQ2 and/or HLA-DQ8 haplotypes and enteropathy. Specific antibodies are tissue transglutaminase (AAtTG) autoantibodies, endomysial antibodies (EMA) and deamidated gliadin peptide antibodies (DGP).[1]

It appears that the absence of breastfeeding, ingestion of excessive amounts of gluten and the early introduction of these cereals in the diet of susceptible people are risk factors for its development. A strict gluten-free diet, leads to the disappearance of clinical symptoms, as well as to the normalization of the intestinal mucosa and prevents complications.

The contact of the intestinal mucosa with gluten leads to the appearance of mucosal damage, whose spectrum ranges from cases where there is only a slight increase in the population of intraepithelial lymphocytes (lymphocytic enteritis) to advanced forms of villous atrophy.[1-3] Any of the histological forms of the disease, even milder forms, may run their course with various states of deficiency, including anemia, osteopenia or osteoporosis and a wide range of digestive and extradigestive symptoms.[4] All these manifestations and serological and histological alterations disappear when gluten is removed from the diet and reappear when it is reintroduced in the diet. The only effective treatment for celiac disease is a strict, indefinite gluten-free diet.

CD affects both children and adults and the female/male ratio is 2:1. It is present in both in Europe and in countries populated by people of European descent, as well as in the Middle East, Asia, South America and North Africa. It may affect up to 1% of the population in Western countries and up to 5% of the native population of sub-Saharan Africa.[5] However, it is considered that CD epidemiology can be likened to an iceberg, and that its prevalence may be much higher, since a significant percentage of the cases remains undetected.[6] Today it is thought that subclinical forms are more frequent than symptomatic forms; their diagnosis constitutes a challenge for the general health system.

2. Symptoms

Clinical history and physical examination are the diagnostic cornerstones in the primary care field[7,8] and should be based on knowledge of different patterns of disease presentation, including atypical, paucisymptomatic or monosymptomatic forms, certainly the most prevalent today (Table 1).

2.1. Classic Forms

Classic symptoms include chronic diarrhea, vomiting, mood swings, poor appetite, failure to thrive and growth retardation. Prominent abdomen and flattened buttocks complete the distinctive appearance of these patients and can easily lead to suspect the diagnosis.

Children	Adolescents	Adults
Symptoms		
Diarrhea	Frequently asymptomatic	Dyspepsia
Anorexia	Abdominal pain	Chronic diarrhea
Vomiting	Headache	Abdominal pain
Abdominal pain	Arthralgia	Irritable intestine syndrome
Irritability	Delayed menarche	Bone and articular pain
Apathy	Menstrual irregularities	Infertility, recurrent abortions
Introversion	Constipation	Paresthesia, tetany
Sadness	Irregular bowel habit	Anxiety, depression, epilepsy, ataxia
Signs		
Malnutrition	Canker sores	Malnutrition with/without weight loss
Abdominal bloating	Enamel hypoplasia	Peripheral edemas
Muscular hypotrophy	Abdominal bloating	Short stature
Failure to thrive	Muscular weakness	Peripheral neuropathy
Iron deficiency anemia	Low stature	Proximal Myopathy
	Arthritis, osteopenia	Iron deficiency anemia
	Follicular keratosis	Hypertransaminasemia
	Iron deficiency anemia	Hyposplenism

Table 1. Clinical manifestations according to age of presentation

When the disease is left untreated, serious manifestations may appear (celiac crisis), comprising dermic or gastrointestinal hemorrhages (due to a defect in default vitamin K synthesis and other intestinal-dependent factors), hypocalcaemic tetany and edema due to hypoalbuminemia. There may be severe hypotonic dehydration along with great abdominal distention marked hypokalemia; extreme malnutrition may also occur. A state of celiac crisis arises if no proper diagnosis or treatment have been made.

2.2. Nonclassical Forms

Digestive symptoms may be absent or in the background (Table 1). Sometimes, in older children, it takes the form of constipation, associated or not with abdominal cramping, bloating or sudden onset of edema, usually coinciding with a precipitating factor (infection, surgery, etc.). Delayed puberty or height increase can also be evocative data. Another isolated manifestation occurs through iron deficiency anemia caused by iron and folate malabsorption in the jejunum. In untreated celiac disease, enamel hypoplasia has been described.

The epileptic triad has also been described as well as bilateral occipital intracranial calcifications and celiac disease, which responds to treatment with gluten-free diet.

2.3. Subclinical Forms

The disease may be asymptomatic for several years, even with high levels of specific antibodies, compatible HLA and enteropathy, as it has been proved in first-degree relatives of celiac patients. Therefore, careful clinical follow-up of these relatives is necessary, including serological markers (transglutaminase IgA antibodies) and even intestinal biopsy, if necessary.

2.4. Potential Forms

The term "potential celiac disease" should be reserved for those individuals who, while consuming gluten, with or without symptoms, have a normal jejunal biopsy, or else just increased intraepithelial lymphocytes, but positive celiac serology. As it progresses, it could include intestinal villi atrophy with anatomic normalization after withdrawing dietary gluten from the diet and reappearance of injuries after its reintroduction. These patients are usually first-degree relatives of celiac patients and, given their high risk of developing the disease, should be monitored regularly.

3. Risks Groups

3.1. First-Degree Relatives

They are a high-risk group in which celiac disease prevalence of wavers between 10 and 20%. They may remain clinically asymptomatic or exhibit mild clinical forms.

3.2. Associated Diseases

They usually precede celiac disease, but may also occur simultaneously with it and even its after diagnosis (Table 2). Patients who suffer from them are considered risk groups since their association occurs with a frequency higher than expected. The following are the most representative:

Dermatitis herpetiformis. It occurs in older children, adolescents and young adults in the form of pruritic vesicular lesions in normal skin, or macular plaques located symmetrically head, elbows, knees and thighs. Diagnosis is made by means of direct immunofluorescence demonstration of the granular IgA deposits in the dermal-epidermal junction in healthy skin; it means, in most cases, severe damage to the intestinal mucosa.

Diabetes mellitus type 1. Approximately 8% of patients with type 1 diabetes are associated with celiac disease.

Selective IgA deficiency. Approximately 4% of celiac patients also have selective IgA deficiency.

Down's syndrome. The association with celiac disease is higher than 15%.

Thyroid diseases. The association of celiac disease with autoimmune thyroiditis is frequent, about 4%, both in children and in adults.

Liver disease. Elevated transaminase is a common finding in up to 10% of active celiac patients. Its gradual normalization should be monitored after starting a gluten-free diet.

First-Degree relatives	
Patients with associated diseases	
Autoimmune diseases	Neurological and psychiatric disorders
Dermatitis herpetiformis	Progressive encephalopathy
Type I diabetes	Cerebellar syndromes
Selective IgA deficit	Dementia with cerebral atrophy
Thyroiditis	Leucoencephalopathy
Inflammatory bowel disease	Epilepsy and calcifications
Sjögren's syndrome	Other associations:
Systemic lupus erythematous	Down's syndrome
Addison's disease	Cystic fibrosis
IgA nephropathy	Turner's syndrome
Chronic hepatitis	Williams' syndrome
Primary biliary cirrhosis	Hartnup's disease
Rheumatoid arthritis	Cystinuria
Psoriasis, vitiligo and alopecia areata	

Table 2. Risk groups.

4. Diagnosis

4.1. Serum Markers

Serum markers are quite useful as indicators of CD, provided that their interpretation is correct (age, gluten intake, immunosuppressive drug treatment, etc.). They aid in selecting the individuals most likely to develop it, being particularly useful in patients without gastrointestinal symptoms, in patients with diseases associated with CD and in searching for first-degree relatives of diagnosed CD patients.[9-11] It ought to be considered, however, that the negativity of these markers does not definitively exclude diagnosis, being sometimes necessary to resort to more complex tests[12] (genetic study) when clinical suspicion is high.

Human tissue transglutaminase IgA antibodies (AAtTG) have proven to be most useful, cheap and cost-effective in screening for the disease; they must be systematically indicated, along with total serum IgA plasma levels of when faced with clinical suspicion of CD. It is not unusual to find IgA deficit in the celiac population, which could lead to a "false negative" while testing for antibodies. In such a situation, AAtTG IgG can be analyzed and only if they yield negative results can serology be considered to be negative.

Recently, an interesting study of 5,000 Italian schoolchildren has been published, suggesting that that celiac disease could be detected by the determination of tissue transglutaminase IgA antibodies in saliva.[13] Although this is a simple and safe screening test that could allow early diagnosis of the disease, with the undoubted benefits that its application could entail, further studies are needed to confirm the sensitivity and specificity of salivary antibodies.[14] In any case, they also have the limitation of not being detectable in patients with isolated IgA deficiency.

Gliadin antibodies (AGA) were the first to be used. Those belonging to IgA class are preferred and their effectiveness in CD screening is higher in children than in adults. They are sensitive but very nonspecific, so at present they are not indicated for use in CD screening. Determination of deamidated gliadin peptide antibodies (DGP) could be of more interest, although their specificity is no higher than that of AAtTG or EMA.[15]

The detection of IgA endomysial antibodies (EMA) is also used. Its sensitivity and specificity vary according to age. They have the disadvantages of being difficult to determine, of their subjective interpretation and their high cost. However, levels greater than 10 times the normal limit value can be regarded as highly specific for CD even when AAtTG are negative.[1]

In practice, serology results determine what course to take, making it necessary to consider the following situations:[1, 9-11]

- Serology sensitivity is very high (close to 100%), especially in people with advanced histological lesions (villous atrophy). Therefore, only in very specific cases and under specialized care, when faced with the presence of very suggestive symptoms, clearly positive serology (levels higher than 100 U, 10 times the normal limit, validated by EMA) and demonstrated genetic susceptibility (HLA DQ2 or DQ8 positive individuals), could gluten be removed from the diet without performing bowel biopsy. Favorable clinical response would definitely confirm the diagnosis.[1]

- In the remaining cases, that is to say, whenever there is any degree of diagnostic uncertainty, intestinal biopsy performed in a specialized environment is still the definitive diagnostic criterion. If morphological alterations are compatible, gluten must be removed from the diet.

- Recent evidence suggests that negative serology does not definitely exclude celiac disease. This is particularly true for patients with mild histological lesions (Marsh 1 and 2). On the other hand, low-relevance morphological alterations (lymphocytic enteritis without villous atrophy) do not preclude the patient from having clinically evident symptoms and signs of disease (asthenia, flatulence, anemia, osteopenia, etc.). For this reason, when faced with suspicious symptoms and negative serology, especially in risk groups, the possibility of evaluating the case in a specialized environment must be considered.

4.2. Genetic Studies

Genetic studies (HLA-DQ2/DQ8) are useful in the management of celiac disease[12], since almost all celiac patients are HLA-DQ2 or DQ8 positive. 90% of CD patients are HLA-DQ2 positive while only 20-30% of individuals in the general population express it. The rest of celiac patients have allelic variants encoding HLA-DQ8 without HLA-DQ2 (6%) or a single HLA-DQ2 allele. Therefore, the absence of HLA-DQ2 and HLA-DQ8 makes the diagnosis of CD is highly unlikely. Genetic testing has therefore, a high negative predictive value, allowing the exclusion of CD with 99% certainty.

Genetic testing has clinical utility in some of the following situations:

- Excluding genetic susceptibility in first-degree relatives of celiac patients.

- Excluding CD in symptomatic patients with negative serology and a normal biopsy.

- Selecting high-risk individuals among relatives of celiac patients, patients with CD-associated diseases (type I diabetes, Down's syndrome, autoimmune thyroid disease, etc.), with positive autoantibodies and normal biopsies.

- In patients with intestinal biopsy consistent with CD and doubtful or negative serology.

- Latent celiac disease.

- Asymptomatic patients for whom gluten has been withdrawn and with no intestinal biopsy.

- People with positive antibodies who reject having a biopsy made.

4.3. Intestinal Biopsy

The gold standard for definitive diagnosis is making a biopsy of the proximal duodenum or jejunum (a more habitual procedure in children), although the need to perform it in every case is being reviewed.[1,15,16] It ought to be conducted prior to the removal of gluten from the diet. It is necessary to have a prior coagulation study, since some patients may have a prothrombin deficiency secondary to vitamin K malabsorption.

In the Marsh[17] classification of small bowel lesions (Figure 1) the pathologic criteria are: Marsh 0 (preinfiltrative mucosa); Marsh 1 (an increase in the number of intraepithelial lymphocytes); Marsh 2 (crypt hyperplasia); Marsh 3 (partial villous atrophy 3a, subtotal 3b, total 3c) and Marsh 4 (hypoplasia).

Since histological lesions may be patchy, it is advised that, at least, four samples be taken for histological analysis.[2] Anatomopathologic study allows confirmation of compatible lesions and establishing the lesion type (Marsh classification).[17] The spectrum of histological lesions in these patients is broad and ranges from varieties with lymphocytic enteritis, in which there is only an increase of the population of intraepithelial lymphocytes (>25%, Marsh 1) to severe forms of mucosal atrophy (Marsh 3). Since hematoxylin-eosin staining could not be conclusive, it is important to have anti-CD3 monoclonal antibody immunostaining in order to count intraepithelial lymphocytes. Only in this way can lymphocytic enteritis be diagnosed with any reasonable certainty (>25 lymphocytes/100 epithelial cells).

Any of the abovementioned histological forms is compatible with the disease, but none of them is specific. Hence the importance of serology and genetic studies (should there be negative serology and high clinical suspicion), in order to enhance the diagnosis and to verify clinical improvement following the removal of gluten from the diet. Regarding the gluten challenge, it ought to be done when there is doubt about the accuracy of the diagnosis.

In the Marsh[17] classification of small bowel lesions (Figure 1) the pathologic criteria are: Marsh 0 (preinfiltrative mucosa); Marsh 1 (an increase in the number of intraepithelial lymphocytes); Marsh 2 (crypt hyperplasia); Marsh 3 (partial villous atrophy 3a, subtotal 3b, total 3c) and Marsh 4 (hypoplasia).

The diversity and different sensitivity and specificity of the methods used in the diagnosis of CD has led to their being comprehensively appraised, especially while looking for new, noninvasive diagnostic strategies.

It is necessary to clinically monitor patients in order to observe the progression of symptoms and monitor growth in children and diet compliance. Determining AAtTG is useful for assessing proper adherence to the diet when serology is positive. In those patients who continue having symptoms or relapses despite the gluten-free regime, a deliberate search for hidden sources of dietary gluten or minimal transgressions must to be conducted. Both situations account for most cases which remain symptomatic or have maintained high serum marker levels.

5. Treatment

There are no pharmacological treatments for CD. The only effective treatment for this disease is a strict, lifelong gluten-free diet.[18-19] Improvement of symptoms is achieved after approximately two weeks, serological standardization between takes between 6 and 12 months and recovery of the intestinal villi around 2 years after starting treatment.

In recent years, other possible therapeutic strategies have been studied, other than the gluten-free diet.[20] However, before their clinical application, their efficacy and safety compared to the gluten-free diet should be demonstrated.

Dietary suppression of all gluten-bearing products includes flour made from barley, rye, wheat and possibly oats, as well as their derivatives. Although the toxicity of oats has been questioned, there are no conclusive studies on the subject.

After excluding gluten from the diet, complete histological recovery does not occur immediately; in adults it may even take more than 2 years and it does not occur in children before one year after the beginning of dietary treatment. Therefore, it may be necessary to temporarily exclude dietary lactose, until the intestinal wall enzymes have recovered, especially lactase. Also, depending on the malabsorption and/or malnutrition degree in the patient's initial dietary treatment, it may be necessary to recommend a high-calorie or low-fiber diet. Iron supplements and/or other minerals are usually not necessary, except in situations of significant nutritional deterioration.

Table 3 shows food that is either unsuitable or suitable for celiac patients. Keep in mind that flours are widely used in the food industry.

Gluten-free food	Gluten-bearing food	Food which may contain gluten
Milk and dairy products: cheese, curd, cream, natural yoghurt and whey	Bread and wheat, rye, barley, oats and triticale flour	All kinds of sausages, black pudding, etc.
All sorts of meat and fresh entrails, frozen, naturally preserved, or dried; ham, high-quality cooked ham	Industrial products which include any of the abovementioned flours in any form; starches, modified starches, and their proteins	Delicatessen food
Fresh and frozen fish, fresh seafood, preserved or in oil	Pastries, cakes, cookies, pies and all sweet and salty baked products	Flavored yoghurt with pieces of fruit
Eggs	Pasta (macaroni, noodles, etc.) and wheat meal	Melted and flavored cheeses
Vegetables, tubers	Milk shakes	Pâté
Fruit	Distilled or fermented drinks made from cereals: beer, barley water, some liquors, etc.	Canned meat
Rice, corn (maize) and tapioca as well as their derivates		Canned fish with sauce
Sugar and honey		Candy (all types)
Oil and butter		Coffee substitutes and other machine-dispensed drinks
Coffee (grains or ground), tea and fruit juice		Dried, fried and toasted fruit with salt
All kinds of wine and bubbly drinks		Ice cream
Raw dried fruit		Chocolate substitutes
Salt, wine vinegar, all natural, fresh spices (fresh leaves or grains)		Food coloring

Table 3. Food that is either unsuitable or suitable for celiac patients.

The Official Journal of the European Union has recently the Regulations for the composition and labeling of foodstuffs suitable for people intolerant to gluten[21], whose contents are summarized below:

5.1 Composition and Labeling of Foodstuffs for People Intolerant To Gluten

1- Foodstuffs for people intolerant to gluten, consisting of one or more ingredients from wheat, rye, barley, oats or their crossbred varieties, which have been especially processed to reduce gluten, shall not contain a gluten level exceeding 100 mg/kg in foods as sold to the final consumer.

2- The labeling, advertising and presentation of the products referred to in paragraph 1 shall bear the words very low gluten content. They may bear the term "gluten-free" if the gluten content does not exceed 20 mg/kg, based on the food as sold to the final consumer.

3- Oats contained in food for people intolerant to gluten must be produced, prepared or treated specially in order to avoid contamination by wheat, rye, barley, or their crossbred varieties and the gluten content shall not exceed 20 mg/kg.

4- Foodstuffs for people intolerant to gluten, consisting of one or more ingredients that substitute wheat, rye, barley, oats or their crossbred varieties shall not contain a gluten level exceeding 20 mg/kg in the food as sold to the final consumer. The labeling, presentation and advertising of these products must include the phrase "gluten-free".

5- In the case of foodstuffs for people intolerant to gluten that contain ingredients which substitute wheat, rye, barley, oats or their crossbred varieties as well as ingredients from wheat, rye varieties, barley, oats or their crossbred varieties which have been especially processed to reduce gluten, paragraphs 1, 2 and 3 shall apply and paragraph 4 shall not apply.

6- The terms "very low gluten content" or "gluten-free" referred to in paragraphs 2 and 4 shall appear in proximity to the product's commercial name.

References

1. Husby S, Koletzko S, Korponay-Szabo IR, et al. E*uropean Society for Paediatric Gastroenterology, Hepatology, and Nutrition Guidelines for the Diagnosis of Coeliac Disease*. J Ped Gastroenterol Nutr. 2012; 54: 136-60.
   http://dx.doi.org/10.1097/MPG.0b013e31821a23d0

2. Polanco I, Grupo de Trabajo sobre "Diagnóstico precoz de la enfermedad celíaca". *Diagnóstico precoz de la enfermedad celíaca*. Madrid: Ministerio de Sanidad y Consumo; 2008.

3. Polanco I, Ribes C. *Enfermedad celíaca*. En: SEGHNP-AEP, ed. Protocolos diagnóstico-terapéuticos de gastroenterología, hepatología y nutrición pediátrica. Madrid: Ergon; 2010: 37-46.

4. Polanco I, Mearin ML. *Enfermedad celíaca*. En: Argüelles F, et al, eds. Tratado de gastroenterología, hepatología y nutrición pediátrica aplicada de la SEGHNP. Madrid: Ergon; 2011: 284-91.

5. Lohi S, Mustalahti K, Kaukinen K, Laurila K, Collin P, Rissanen H, et al. *Increasing prevalence of coeliac disease over time*. Aliment Pharmacol Ther. 2007; 26: 1217-25.
   http://dx.doi.org/10.1111/j.1365-2036.2007.03502.x

6. West J, Logan RFA, Hill PG, Lloyd A, Lewis S, Hubbard R et al. *Seroprevalence, correlates, and characteristics of undetected coeliac disease in England*. Gut. 2003; 52: 960-5.
   http://dx.doi.org/10.1136/gut.52.7.960

7. Polanco I, Roldán B, Arranz M. *Documento técnico protocolo de prevención secundaria de la enfermedad celíaca*. Madrid: Dirección General Salud Pública y Alimentación; 2006.

8. Catassi C,, Kryszak D, Louis-Jacques O, Duerksen DR, et al. *Detection of Celiac Disease in Primary Care: A Multicenter Case-Finding Study in North America*. Am J Gastroenterol. 2007; 102: 1454-60. http://dx.doi.org/10.1111/j.1572-0241.2007.01173.x

9. Rostom A, Murray JA, Kagnoff MF. *American Gastroenterological Association (AGA) Institute technical review on the diagnosis and management of celiac disease*. Gastroenterology. 2006; 131: 1981-2002.
   http://dx.doi.org/10.1053/j.gastro.2006.10.004

10. Rostom A, Dube C, Cranney A, Saloojee N, Sy R, Garritty C, et al. T*he diagnostic accuracy of serologic tests for celiac disease: a systematic review*. Gastroenterology. 2005; 128 (4 Suppl 1): S38-46. http://dx.doi.org/10.1053/j.gastro.2005.02.028

11. Polanco I, Román E. *Marcadores serológicos en la Enfermedad Celíaca*. An Pediatr Contin. 2006; 4:176-9. http://dx.doi.org/10.1016/S1696-2818(06)73607-1

12. Wolters VM, Wijmenga C. *Genetic background of celiac disease and its clinical implications*. Am J Gastroenterol. 2008; 103: 190-5.
    http://dx.doi.org/10.1111/j.1572-0241.2007.01471.x

13. Bonamico M, Nenna R, Montuori M, Luparia RP, Turchetti A, Mennini M, et al. *First salivary screening of celiac disease by detection of ant-transglutaminase autoantobody radioimmunoassay in 5000 Italian primary schoolchildren*. J Pediat Gastroenterol Nutr. 2011; 52: 17-20. http://dx.doi.org/10.1097/MPG.0b013e3181e6f2d0

14. Green PHR, Cellier C. *Celiac Disease*. N Eng J Med. 2007; 357: 1731-43.
    http://dx.doi.org/10.1056/NEJMra071600

15. Lindfors K, Koskinen O, Kaukinen K. *An update on the diagnostics of celiac disease*. Int Rev Immunol. 2011; 30: 185-96. http://dx.doi.org/10.3109/08830185.2011.595854

16. *Guideline for the Diagnosis and Treatment of Celiac Disease in Children: Recommendations of the North American Society for Pediatric Gastroenterology, Hepatology and Nutrition*. J Pediat Gastroenterology Nutr. 2005; 40: 1-19.
http://dx.doi.org/10.1097/00005176-200501000-00001

17. Marsh MN. *Gluten, major histocompatibility complex, and the small intestine. A molecular and immunobiologic approach to the spectrum of gluten sensitivity ('celiac sprue')*. Gastroenterology. 1992; 102: 330-54.

18. Case S. *The gluten-free diet: How to provide effective education and resources*. Gastroenterology. 2005; 128: S128-S134.
http://dx.doi.org/10.1053/j.gastro.2005.02.020

19. Polanco I. *Libro Blanco de la Enfermedad Celíaca*. Ed: ICM. Madrid: Consejería de Sanidad de la Comunidad de Madrid; 2008.

20. Polanco I, Arranz E. *Nuevos avances en el tratamiento de la Enfermedad Celíaca*. An Pediatr Contin. 2006; 4: 46-9. http://dx.doi.org/10.1016/S1696-2818(06)73587-9

21. *Reglamento (CE) No 41/2009 de la Comisión de 20 de enero de 2009 sobre la composición y etiquetado de productos alimenticios apropiados para personas con intolerancia al gluten. Diario Oficial de la Unión Europea 21.1.2009*.
http://eur-lex.europa.eu/LexUriServ/LexUriServ.do?uri=OJ:L:2009:016:0003:0005:ES:PDF

Chapter 12

Celiac Disease in Adults

Miguel Montoro Huguet[1,2], Manuel Domínguez Cajal[1]

[1]Gastroenterology and Hepatology Unit, San Jorge Hospital, Huesca, Spain.

[2]Department of Medicine. University of Zaragoza, Spain.

maimontoro@gmail.com

Doi: http://dx.doi.org/10.3926/oms.233

How to cite this chapter

Montoro M, Domínguez Cajal M. *Celiac Disease in Adults*. In Rodrigo L and Peña AS, editors. *Celiac Disease and Non-Celiac Gluten Sensitivity.* Barcelona, Spain: OmniaScience; 2014. p. 235-287.

Abstract

Celiac disease (CD) is a common condition affecting up to 1% of the adult population of Caucasoid origin. It arises from an inflammatory response to dietary gluten in the small intestine in genetically predisposed individuals.

Its clinical presentations are grouped into four categories: 1) Classic celiac disease, defined on the basis of diarrhea with failure to thrive or weight loss (a rare occurrence in contemporary adult presentation in); 2) "Atypical" gastrointestinal presentation, defined on the basis of a set of nonspecific and persistent gastrointestinal symptoms, often misdiagnosed as a digestive functional disorder; 3) Extraintestinal presentation, defined on the basis of signs or symptoms outside the gastrointestinal tract, such as iron deficiency anemia or short stature and 4) Silent presentation. The latter is identified through testing due to a family history of CD or a celiac disease-associated condition (i.e. type 1 diabetes mellitus).

The CD diagnosis is confirmed if at least 4 of the following 5 criteria are satisfied: typical CD symptoms, serum-positive celiac disease class-A immunoglobulin autoantibodies at high titers, presence of HLA-DQ2 and/or-DQ8, celiac enteropathy in small bowel biopsy and response to the gluten-free diet. Seronegative CD is likely to be underestimated due to the tendency to perform small intestinal biopsies only in patients with positive celiac disease serum markers. Whilst the majority of patients will respond to a gluten-free diet, a significant minority will continue to be symptomatic. In such cases, it is essential that a systematic follow-up approach be adopted.

> *"If the stomach be irretentive of the food and if it pass through undigested and crude and nothing ascends into the body, we call such persons coeliacs..."*

Adams F. (trans.), *The Extant Works of Aretaeus the Capadocian*
London, London Sydenham Society, 1856:350

1. Introduction

The introduction of gluten-bearing cereals with the advent of agriculture, about 10,000 years ago, generated the necessary conditions for the development of a set of immune disorders due to gluten exposure, among which basically are wheat allergy and celiac disease (CD).[1] Although the first descriptions of this condition date back to the time of Aretaeus of Cappadocia, in ancient Ionian Greece (today's Turkey), it was not until the 1940-1950 decade when Dicke, a Dutch pediatrician, established a relationship between the gluten content in wheat and the symptoms of this disease.[2] Since the first consensus definitions were established in 1970[3], in which the diagnosis of the disease required the demonstration of severe villous atrophy, which retreats following the removal of gluten from the diet and reappears after allowing again the ingestion of these cereals, more than 40 years have elapsed. During the last decade, further evidence has accumulated to suggest that dietary gluten intake can cause a wide spectrum of symptoms, in some cases with no evidence of duodenal histological lesion (DHL). All this has stirred great controversy in the scientific community regarding the nomenclature to be used in each situation.[4] Three consensus conferences have been published recently, whose reading is highly recommended in order to understand the true dimensions of this problem.[1-5,6] In recent years, consumption of gluten-free foods has increased exponentially, not only among celiac patients, but in many other patients previously diagnosed with a functional gastrointestinal disorder (FGD) who finally found relief when gluten was permanently removed from their diet, either because they actually suffered from a hitherto unsuspected CD[7] or else because they suffered from non-celiac gluten sensitivity (NCGS)[8] or even due to the placebo effect involved in any diet. This chapter is primarily restricted to CD and, to that end, it will use the concepts defined by the recent guidelines established by ESPGHAN[5], as well as those established by the Oslo[6] and London[1] consensus meetings, all of them published in 2012.

2. Definitions and Nomenclature

CD forms part of a gluten-related disorder spectrum including those of a clearly immune etiology (CD, dermatitis herpetiformis and gluten-related ataxia), others of an IgE-mediated allergic etiology (wheat allergy) and others which do not depend on allergy or acquired immunity, such as NCGS (Figure 1).[1] The definitions of the different gluten-related clinical conditions[1,4,5,6] are described below.

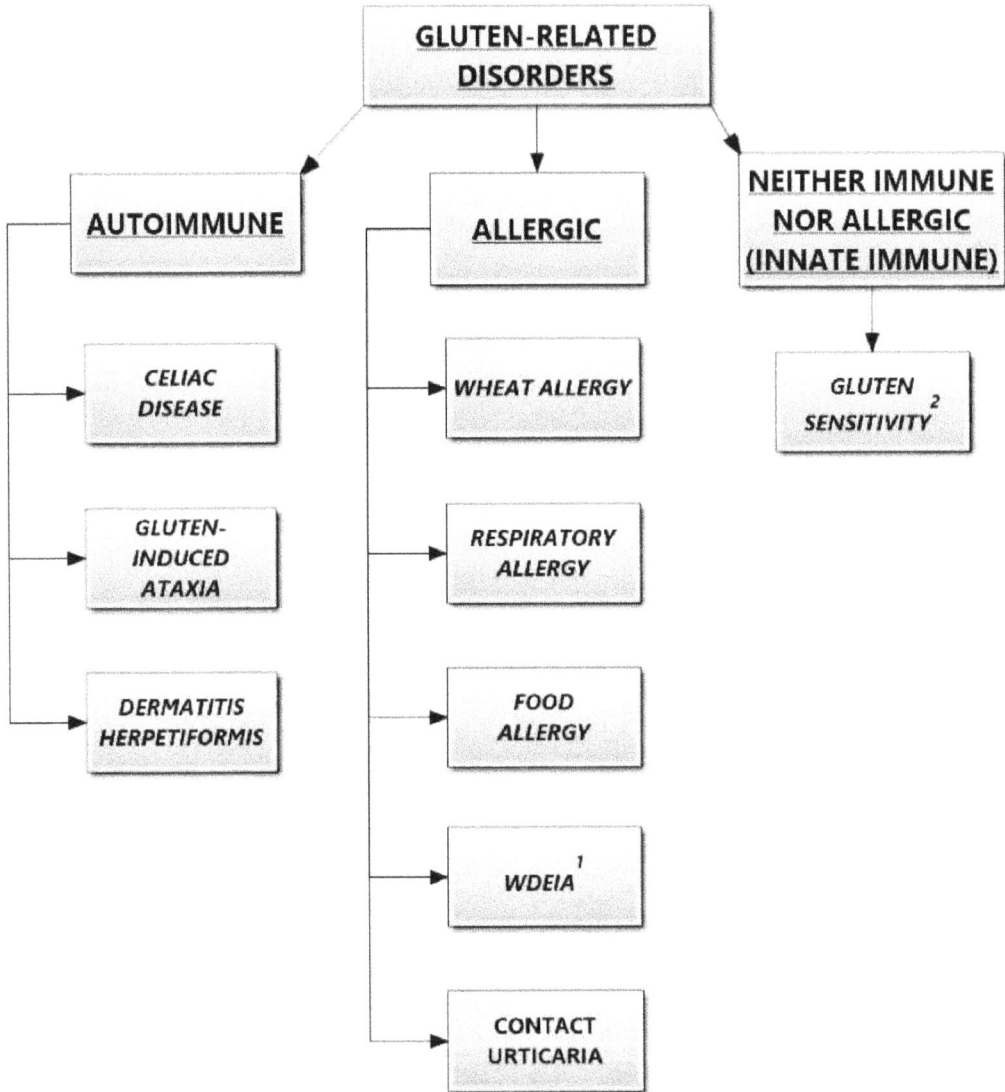

Figure 1. Classification of gluten-related disorders.

1) WDEIA: wheat-dependent exercise-induced anaphylaxis.

2) Term admitted by the London Consensus, but not by the Oslo Consensus, the latter encourages the use of the term "non-celiac gluten sensitivity".

Celiac disease. According to the ESPGHAN guide published in 2012[5], CD is defined as a systemic disease mediated by the immune system and precipitated by contact between the intestinal mucosa and gluten and other related prolamins in genetically susceptible individuals. The disorder is characterized by a variable combination of symptoms and signs depending on gluten intake, CD-specific antibodies (anti-transglutaminase-2, antiendomysial and deamidated gliadin anti-peptides), the presence of HLA DQ2 or DQ8 haplotypes and varying degrees of enteropathy.

Formerly, other equivalent terms have been used to refer to the same disease, including terms such as *sprue, celiac sprue, gluten-sensitive enteropathy, gluten intolerance, nontropical sprue* and *idiopathic steatorrhea*. None of these terms is, at this time, universally accepted, so their use cannot be recommended.[6]

Classic celiac disease. This term refers to those patients whose disease presents a clear-cut pattern of malabsorption with chronic diarrhea, steatorrhea, weight loss or delayed growth.[9] This pattern is often seen in children, in whom loss of muscular mass, loss of appetite, anemia, abdominal bloating and irritability are frequently observed; these symptoms, however, are exceptional in adults, hence the term "typical" celiac disease is not recommended at present, since both conditions (classical and typical) are not coincident. The common (typical) presentation of the disease in adults is the manifestation of nonspecific symptoms and signs that do not resemble those of a state of malabsorption with emaciation.[10,11]

Non-classic celiac disease. This definition applies to those who have symptoms and signs not associated with a state of florid malabsorption. This includes cases of patients with symptoms that mimic those of "functional" dyspepsia[8], irritable bowel syndrome (IBS) or chronic constipation and those with extraintestinal manifestations, whose presentation under monosymptomatic forms is not uncommon. This section will, therefore, include cases of thyroid dysfunction (hyper or hypo)[12], neurological symptoms[13], depression[14], fertility disorders[15,16], aphthous stomatitis[17-20], skeletal[21] or dermal[22] alterations or transaminitis.[23] Again, the term "atypical" celiac disease should be discouraged, because, at the present time, these symptoms and signs appear to be most common presentation.[6]

Asymptomatic celiac disease. This patient subgroup does not have symptoms that may suggest a diagnosis, even after being interviewed using structured questionnaire. These are often patients in whom the diagnosis has been established while conducting a screening population study or while studying bearers of comorbidities associated with a high risk of CD. It is not uncommon that, after removing gluten, the patient reveals a clear improvement of a hitherto unrecognized asthenia case. According to the Oslo Consensus, the term "silent celiac" is consistent with and equivalent to "asymptomatic" and should be abandoned.

Subclinical celiac disease. Today, this term is reserved for those patients with a set of symptoms or signs that are not considered sufficient to lead to clinical suspicion and which are below the threshold required to encourage clinical research to confirm or rule out the disease.[6,24]

Symptomatic celiac disease. This term refers to a CD patient who has any of the symptoms included in the wide manifestation spectrum attributable to the disease, whether it means gastrointestinal symptoms (dyspepsia, diarrhea, bloating) as well as extraintestinal symptoms (fatigue, depression or canker sores).

Latent celiac disease and potential celiac disease. At least 5 different senses or meanings have been in the literature for the term "latent"[6], the most accepted being probably that of a patient who consumes gluten, has "normal" intestinal mucosa at the time of its evaluation, but who, in an earlier or later time suffered (or will develop) a typical intestinal lesion. Regarding the term "potential", the Oslo group's recommendation is that it should be used referring to a patient with "normal" intestinal mucosa and an increased risk of developing CD after detecting positive CD serology, especially if the patient has the HLA DQ2 or DQ8 haplotypes.[25,26]

Refractory celiac disease. This term applies to those patients diagnosed with CD who maintain persistent malabsorption symptoms or signs (i.e., diarrhea with involuntary weight loss, low hemoglobin levels or hypoalbuminemia), with persistent villous atrophy despite a strict diet without gluten (GFD) for more than 12 months, after excluding other causes of villous atrophy or the presence of malignancy. This category includes those patients with severe and persistent symptoms, regardless of the GFD duration. It is obvious that not all patients who do not respond to the GFD can be labeled as refractory, since in many cases the persistence of symptoms can be explained by an unorthodox compliance of the diet or by the presence of conditions associated with CD that explain the persistence of symptoms (lactose or fructose intolerance, intestinal bacterial overgrowth, exocrine pancreatic insufficiency or microscopic colitis).

Genetic risk for celiac disease. The concept of "individual with genetic risk of CD" should be limited to relatives of CD patients who share the DQ2 and/or DQ8 HLA haplotypes, elevating the risk to 20-25% when it comes to first-degree relatives.

Dermatitis herpetiformis (DH). DH is a cutaneous expression of the enteropathy precipitated by dietary gluten (CD). It appears in 1 out of 10,000 people of Caucasoid and European descent and its incidence is of 0.98 cases per 100,000 inhabitants per year.[6,32,33] DH is rare in other continents such as Africa and Asia. The disease shares the same HLA haplotypes DQ2 (90%) and DQ8 (5%)[34] and it predominates in males (1.5 to 1.9:1). There is a clear family aggregability and the average age of onset is of about 40 years.[1] It manifests typically by the appearance of small erythematous macules which soon become intensely pruritic papules, finally bursting to form scabs. The distribution of lesions is symmetrical, affecting the elbows in 90% of cases. Other affected areas include the face, scalp, neck, shoulders, trunk, sacral region, buttocks and knees.[1] Its progression is chronic and recurrent. Although only 10% of its patients report gastrointestinal symptoms, nearly two thirds have some degree of villous atrophy in the intestinal mucosa.[6,20] The remaining cases may have normal mucosa or increased type γ/δ intraepithelial lymphocytes as an unequivocal expression of gluten sensitization. In these patients' serum the same CD autoimmunity biomarkers (anti-TG, anti-endomysium and PGD) can be identified and, in fact, they are not infrequently associated with other autoimmune diseases. Its diagnosis is based on serological evidence of these markers by immunofluorescent demonstration of granular IgA deposits in the dermal papillae. Since DH is the equivalent of CD in the skin, intestinal biopsy is not an obligatory requirement. Once diagnosed, it is essential to start a GFD; some patients require treatment with *dapsone*. In the long term, almost half of the patients who adhere well to the diet may interrupt the treatment with this neutrophil inhibitor.[35-38]

Gluten-related ataxia (GA). GA is defined as an autoimmune disease associated with the presence of antigliadin antibodies (AGA) in the serum, which can cause damage to the cerebellum resulting in a case of ataxia, all this regardless of the presence or absence of enteropathy.[1,39-43] Clinically, it is expressed as a case of pure cerebellar ataxia, or more rarely in combination with myoclonus and palatal tremor. Its onset is insidious, with a mean onset age of 53 years.[44,45] As is the case with DH, less than 10% of patients report gastrointestinal symptoms, but up to 1/3 show different degrees of enteropathy with IgA deposits in the duodenal mucosa.[45] The pathogenesis of this disorder is not clear, but in these patients anti-TG deposits have been identified around the brain vessels, these being more pronounced in the cerebellum and the spinal cord. Also, antibodies against transglutaminase-6, a transglutaminase which is mainly expressed in the brain, have been detected.[46] The current recommendation is that patients presenting progressive cerebellar ataxia should be tested for AGA, for IgG and IgA-type antibodies, anti-TG2 and anti-TG 6 (IgG and IgA) antibodies. If any of these serological tests is positive, a duodenal biopsy is recommended. If the diagnosis is made late, when there has already been a marked loss of Purkinje cells, the response to gluten withdrawal may be poor.[1]

Wheat allergy. Wheat allergy (WA) is an adverse immune reaction to wheat proteins and includes classic food allergy, the origin of gastrointestinal, skin and respiratory symptoms; it also includes wheat-dependent exercise-induced anaphylaxis (WDEIA), occupational asthma (baker's asthma) and contact urticaria (Figure 1). The pathogenesis of these disorders is mediated by IgE antibodies against various protein components from wheat grains (α-gliadin, β-gliadin, γ-gliadin, ϖ-gliadin and other high-molecular weight subunits) and its overall prevalence ranges between 1-3%.[47] Its diagnosis is based on skin prick tests and on *in vitro* IgE determination for various allergens. Often, challenge tests become necessary.[1]

Non-celiac gluten sensitivity (NCGS). A growing proportion of people have a set of gastrointestinal symptoms (some attributed to an IBS)[7] which improve or disappear entirely after removing gluten from the diet, reappearing upon ingesting again cereals that contain this ingredient. When these patients are investigated, they do not have specific antibodies to gluten and no histological lesions in the duodenal mucosa, which is why they cannot be classified as celiac patients.[5] This clinical condition was first recognized more than 30 years ago[27] and it is named by some as "gluten sensitivity"[1] or, even better, as non-celiac gluten sensitivity (NCGS)[4], a term accepted by most authorities on this subject.[7,27,28] Both diseases (CD and NCGS) share the presence of nonspecific symptoms that improve after establishing a GFD, but differ by the fact that in the latter (NCGS) no allergic or autoimmune mechanisms, alterations in intestinal permeability or morphological changes in the duodenal mucosa can be identified.[29,30] There is some evidence that this disorder may affect up to 6% of the population, being commonly associated with abdominal pain (68%), skin symptoms like rush and/or eczema (40%), headache (35%), confusion (34%), fatigue (33%), diarrhea (33%), depression (22%), anemia (20%), numb legs, hands and fingers (20%) and joint pain (11%).[1] DQ2 gene prevalence (50%) is lower than that observed in CD patients and somewhat higher than that observed in the general population.[31] It is an exclusion diagnosis, in which one of the criteria (symptomatic improvement after introducing the GFD) should be validated in a blinded fashion to avoid the placebo effect inherent to any diet.

Gluten intolerance. This term lacks specificity, which can lead to confusion and contradictions. In the light of current knowledge it may not be synonymous with CD and moreover, the symptoms often attributed to gluten may be a consequence of other components of the grain, so today this expression is inappropriate and is not subject to consensus.

Having clarified these terms (Figure 1), essential to avoid labeling a patient as CD patient when he or she may have another disorder, hereinafter we will exclusively discuss issues related to CD.

3. Epidemiology

The prevalence of CD depends on many factors including the historical moment in which studies have been conducted[48-52], the geographical area where they have been carried out[50-55], the procedures used for screening (serology, intestinal biopsy or both) and the type of population studied (asymptomatic persons, individuals with genetic risk or healthy volunteers).[48] Studies of population-based cohorts performed on healthy volunteers in the U.S., UK and other European countries allow a prevalence estimate of 0.5-1%, which leads to consider CD as the most frequent chronic intestinal disease.[51,53] When screening studies stratify different populations, CD prevalence is estimated at 1 in 22 in first-degree relatives, 1 in 56 in symptomatic patients and 1 out of every 133 people without high risk of developing the disease.[51] Despite these high prevalence rates, the identified cases are just the tip of an iceberg, beneath which is a large contingent of undiagnosed patients (>75%).[8,55,57] The prevalence of CD in the general population is increasing.[58-64] The reasons for this phenomenon cannot be attributed solely to improved screening methods and diagnosis but also to environmental and geographical factors. In Asian countries, for example, where the prevalence has traditionally been low, the number of new cases is increasing due to changes in eating patterns introduced in urban areas, where wheat flour, used in the preparation of fast food, has begun to replace other traditional cereals like rice.[1,60] In India, there is a region where a typical syndrome known as "summer diarrhea" coincides with the season where maize crops are temporarily replaced by wheat.[65] It must be borne in mind that, in most prevalence studies, the diagnosis has been carried out based on a positive result in the determination of specific antibodies. Serology, however, has low sensitivity in patients with mild histological lesions (slight enteropathy). Not indicating a duodenal biopsy in patients with nonspecific gastrointestinal symptoms and negative serology may lead to underestimate the true prevalence of CD, especially when these patients bear the HLA system DQ2 and DQ8 haplotypes.[8,66,67] Finally, 15% of new diagnoses of CD are made in people over 65 years, most of which suffer its symptoms for a period of 11±19 years.[68] A Finnish study demonstrated a prevalence of biopsy-proven CD in 2% of the population between 52 and 74 years.[69] The pattern of presentation has also changed over time, so that in adults, a debut with severe diarrhea and malabsorption today is unusual.[64,67-71]

4. Pathogeny

CD responds to a multifactorial model of interaction between genetic and environmental factors[72,73] involving adaptive (acquired) and innate immunity.[74-81]

- **Adaptive Immunity:** Gluten contains immunogenic peptides which, after crossing the epithelium and undergoing transglutaminase-2 deamidation, are presented by dendritic cells to CD4 lymphocytes in the lamina propria, in the presence of HLA DQ2-DQ8 molecules. Activation of these lymphocytes promotes the release of proinflammatory cytokines that lead to tissue damage, which provide, as well, a signal to the TG2-specific B cells for the synthesis of anti-transglutaminase-2 antibodies.[74]

- **Innate immunity:** The innate immunity mechanisms that lead to the activation of intraepithelial lymphocytes (LIEs) are less well understood. In short, certain gluten peptides such as p31-43/49 (α-gliadin) can directly damage the epithelium by activating innate immunity-dependent mechanisms and the production of (IL)-15 interleukin, responsible, ultimately, for alterations in the permeability of intercellular junctions (intestinal barrier) and of enterocyte apoptosis. IL-15 induces proliferation and activation of CD8+ IELs, while promoting the production of interferon (IFN-γ) by IELs and cytolytic-protein-dependent epithelial cytotoxicity.[74]

Summing up: the tissular damage that occurs in the intestinal mucosa of CD patients is the sum of the activation mechanisms of the lamina propria T CD4+ lymphocytes (adaptive immunity-dependent) and intraepithelial CD8+ lymphocytes (innate immunity-dependent). Both mechanisms are necessary and contribute to trigger a response dominated by Th1 IFN-γ, the T bet transcription factor and other pro-inflammatory cytokines (tumor necrosis factor [TNF]-α, IL-18, IL-21), accompanied by a decrease of immunosuppressive cytokines (IL-10 and TGF-β35-37), which normally help to maintain tolerance to dietary antigens and the production of IL-15 by enterocytes. This pro-inflammatory profile eventually activates the effector mechanisms of tissue damage, such as keratinocyte growth factor (KGF) and matrix metalloproteinases (MMPs) involved in the extracellular matrix degradation and the mucosal transformation.[74-76] All these mechanisms are disabled when the patient is in remission. Note that, although the presence of DQ2 or DQ8 haplotypes is necessary for the development of the disease, there are other multiple genes involved, without which the disease may not appear in an individual.[77-87] A good proof of this is that genes linked to the HLA are present in 25-35% of the general population, while CD appears only 1% (Figure 2).

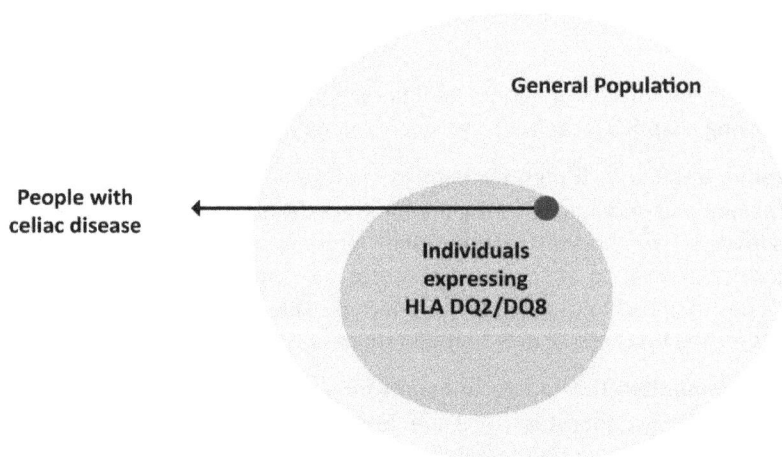

Figure 2. Prevalence of celiac disease and its relationship to the HLA DQ2 heterodimers. *Celiac disease affects approximately 0.5-1% of the general population. Except in special cases, it mostly affects patients expressing the HLA DQ2 (95%) or DQ8 (5%) heterodimers. However, not all HLA DQ2/DQ8 people develop the disease. Therefore, this seems a necessary, but not sufficient, condition. The involvement of other genes is required.*

5. Pathology

The changes in the small intestine of CD patients are usually confined to the mucosa while the submucosa, muscularis and serosa are preserved.[88,89] In a healthy intestine, villi constitute 65-80% of the total thickness of the mucosa, while crypts occupy the rest. The epithelium is composed of tall columnar cells with a crisp edge "brush" and a basal core. The crypts are lined by undifferentiated cells which, through a process of division, migration and maturation, replace the mature absorptive cells which are continually lost at the tips of the villi.[88] In CD, the toxic effect of gliadin peptides on enterocyte maturation results in premature loss of the same in the intestinal lumen, leading to a compensating increase of their replication in the crypts ("enteropoiesis").[90,91] This central mechanism explains most morphological changes observed in CD.

- **Changes in mucosal architecture:** In CD, there is a shortening of the villi, which seem to be wider; at the same time, there is an elongation of and hyperplasia of the crypts, which seem to be branched, with increased mitosis. In most cases, mucosal thickness is normal or only discretely reduced, because the shortening of the villi is compensated by crypt hyperplasia.[88,92] These architectural changes lead to a reduction in the anatomical absorption surface.

- **Changes in the epithelium lining:** the remaining absorptive cells lose their columnar arrangement and appear cuboidal or scaly, while the nuclei lose their basal polarity. The cytoplasm becomes more basophilic and the brush border appears markedly attenuated. Changes observable by electron microscopy include increased ribosomes and degenerative changes including cytoplasmic and mitochondrial vacuolization, plus an increase in the number and size of lysosomes. The increase in intercellular junctions explains the increased permeability of the intestinal mucosa and the barrier's impaired function.[91] The minor activity in the endoplasmic reticulum reflects the low level of digestive enzyme synthesis (discaridases and peptidases), which supports the idea that there is not only a decrease in the number of absorptive cells, but also in their function.[88,90] An increase in the number of cells containing secretin and CCK has also been observed, which is due to an abnormality in these hormones' release mechanisms, which favors the appearance of pancreatic exocrine insufficiency. In contrast to absorptive epithelial cells, the cytological and immunohistochemical characteristics of crypt cells do not differ from their normal status. In fact, some studies suggest that, in patients with untreated CD, crypt-dependent enteropoiesis is 6 times higher than that observed in normal conditions.[91]

- **Cellularity changes:** The lamina propria cellularity is significantly increased in CD, mainly at the expense of the plasma cells that produce IgA, IgG and IgM (particularly IgA) and activated CD4 (helper/inducer) lymphocytes.[92] Other cellular components that contribute to the dense lamina propria infiltration are polymorphonuclear leukocytes (PMN), eosinophils and mastocytes.[89] Meanwhile, in the epithelium, an increased number of intraepithelial lymphocytes (IELs), which besides being real, is also the result of the proportional reduction in the anatomical absorption surface. Therefore it is fitting to express this phenomenon as a numeric value based on an absorptive area unit (100 epithelial cells).[93] In this case, these are CD8+ cells (cytotoxic/suppressors). Marsh hypothesized that morphological changes appeared described in a sequential and progressive manner.[94] Thus, starting from a normal mucosa (preinfiltrative, stage 0), the first observable morphological change would be LIE increase, followed by a lymphocytic infiltration of the lamina propria (stage I). Crypt hyperplasia (stage II) precedes villous atrophy (stage 3), a phenomenon that is observed only in the presence of a marked lymphocytosis in the lamina propria, thereby suggesting that IELs are not sufficient to induce the architectural changes described in CD. Oberhüber amended this classification by stratifying different degrees of atrophy (mild, moderate and severe). Some drawbacks of these classifications, derived from a bias introduced by interobserver variations, have been avoided largely with Corazza's simplified version (Table 1).[93]

Marsh	Morphology		IELs%
Type 0	No change in inflammatory cells or in the crypt/villi relation (preinfiltrative).		< 40
Type 1	Increase in the number of intraepithelial lymphocytes.		> 40
Type 2	Intraepitelial lymphocytosis, increase of crypt/villi relation (hyperplastic).		> 40
Type 3	Intense inflammation, villous atrophy, crypt hyperplasia (destructive).		> 40
Oberhuber			
Type 0	Normal mucosa.		< 40
Type 1	IEL increase, normal villous architecture, normal crypt height.		> 40
Type 2	Normal villous architecture, IEL increase, crypt hyperplasia.		> 40
Type 3	Destructive, with variable atrophy degrees, elongated crypts and inflammatory cells.		> 40
3a	Mild partial atrophy; widened and shortened villi with a V/C: 1.1 relation.		> 40
3b	Subtotal atrophy, atrophic villi, but separated and still recognizable.		> 40
3c	Total atrophy; rudimentary or absent villi; mucosa similar to that of the colon.		> 40
Type 4	Atrophic hypoplastic lesion, flat mucosa with normal crypt height. Barely perceptible inflammatory cellularity. Normal IEL count.		< 40
Corazza	**Morphology**	**Marsh-Oberhuber equivalence**	
Grade A	Normal architecture without atrophy.	Type 1 and type 2; type 0 discarded.	> 25
Grade B1	Atrophic with villus/crypt relation of <3:1.	Type 3a and type 3b.	> 25
Grade B2	Atrophic with no detectable villi.	Type 3c; Type 4 is not included.	> 25

IELs: Intraepithelial Lymphocytes

Table 1. Comparison between Marsh-Oberhuber/Corazza classifications.[93]

None of the described alterations is pathognomonic for CD, hence the different findings described need necessarily be harmonized by an expert clinician able to make a correct differential diagnosis. This is particularly important when the histological lesions are circumscribed to Marsh-Oberhuber types 1 and 2 (Corazza grade A) and Marsh-Oberhuber types 3a and 3b (Corazza grade B), lesions that can be shared by entities other than CD (Table 2). The distribution of lesions typical of CD has some relation to the severity of symptoms. In fact, a global intestinal alteration, from the proximal duodenum to the terminal ileum can only be seen in clinically severe forms of the disease. In the remaining cases, there is usually a lesion severity gradient; the more intense lesions are generally observed in the proximal duodenum.[88,89] The ileum and, in some cases, the jejunum, may be lesion-free, these being confined to the duodenum. In some cases, villous atrophy can only be seen in the duodenal bulb.[96]

Primary	Secondary	

• Gluten-induced enteropathy
• Hypersensitivity to proteins unrelated to gluten:
  - Cow milk
  - Cereals
  - Eggs
  - Peanuts
  - Soy
• Others:
  - Acute gastroenteritis
  - Autolimited enteritis
  - Collagenous duodenitis
  - Tropical sprue
  - Autoimmune enteropathy
  - Graft vs host disease
	Autoimmune diseases
	
	• Autoimmune thyroiditis
	• Hashimoto's thyroiditis
	• Type 1 diabetes
	• Graves' disease
	• Rheumatoid Arthritis
	• Psoriasis
	• Multiple sclerosis
	• Systemic lupus erythematous
	• Hemolytic anemia
		Other immune disorders
		
		• Glomerulonefritis
		• IgA hypogammaglobulinemia or variable common immunodeficiency (they may coexist with celiac disease).

	Chronic inflammatory disorders • Inflammatory bowel disease • Ulcerative colitis • Crohn's disease • Microscopic colitis • Collagenous colitis • Glycogenic deposit disease	***Neoplastic diseases*** • T Cell lymphoma associated enteropathy • CD4+ lymphoproliferative disease • Immunoproliferative small intestinal disease (IPSID) • Thymoma • Refractory sprue
	Drugs • Non-steroidal anti-inflammatory drugs (NSAIDs) • Proton pump inhibitors • Chemotherapy • Idiosyncrasy due to other drugs	***Infections*** • *Giardia Lamblia* • *Criptosporidium* • Viral • Tropical sprue • *Helicobacter Pylori* • Bacterial overgrowth

Table 2. Lymphocytic enteropathy causes.

The introduction of a gluten-free diet (GFD) leads to a marked and significant improvement of CD lesions (Figure 3). Absorptive epithelial cells regain their columnar morphology and the polarity of their nuclei basal and their characteristic brush border. The intraepithelial lymphocyte density tends to decrease and recover villous architecture tends to recover, as does the lymphoplasmacytic infiltrate density in the lamina propria. Usually, the mucosa of the distal small intestine recovers before the more proximal segments, which are more severely affected. In some patients it can take years to observe a complete or nearly complete histologic recovery. Not infrequently, some degree of intraepithelial lymphocytosis may persist, especially when the patient is committing voluntary or unintentional transgressions.[95,97-100]

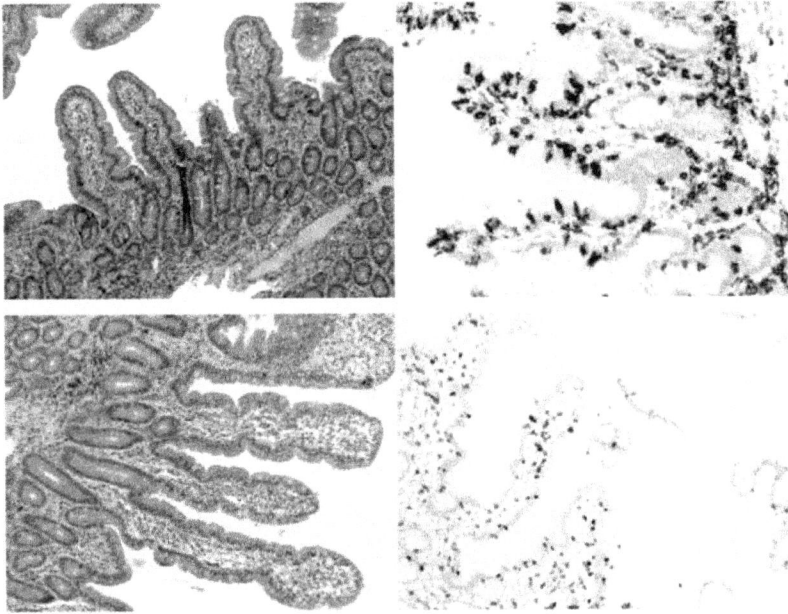

Figure 3. Histological images of a biopsy from the duodenal 2nd portion of a 21-year-old male with symptoms of postprandial distress syndrome dyspepsia (postprandial fullness and bloating) long-term, no response to empiric treatment with prokinetics and antisecretories (PPI). Anti-TG: 2.1 U/mL/[positive DQA1*05, DQB1*02 positive].

In the upper image (left) mild focal villous atrophy can be seen; to the right immunostaining for CD3 shows an IEL count of 31%, with a predominant localization at the tip of the villi (Marsh-Oberhuber 3a; Corazza B1). At the bottom of the images obtained 18 months later, after a GFD. To the left, the villi have recovered their height with an adequate villus/crypt relation. The right image shows immunohistochemical results, with normal IEL count (8%) (Marsh-Oberhuber 0). Courtesy of Dr. Vera, Pathological Anatomy Service, San Jorge Hospital, Huesca.

6. Clinical Presentation

The mean age of CD presentation in adults is 42-45 years (range 18-74 years), with a clear female predominance (1:3).[89] In some cases, a history of growth retardation is discovered or else other symptoms suggestive of unrecognized childhood CD. Some patients regained their growth rhythm in adolescence until it equaled that of the general population. Other patients always had a normal stature, while others show a higher body-mass index, even obesity. Factors associated with the disease onset, after a long silent period, are surgery involving accelerated gastric emptying (gastrectomy, pyloroplasty), the postpartum period, gastrointestinal infection or period of emotional stress. In the authors' unit, up to 56% of the patients diagnosed with CD as adults had been previously diagnosed with a FGD, including refractory pyrosis, "functional" dyspepsia, irritable bowel or chronic constipation. Approximately 15-25% of the cases are diagnosed at an age equal to or greater than 65 years.

6.1. Gastrointestinal Symptoms

In adults, the classic florid presentation of the disease with malabsorption, diarrhea, steatorrhea, weight loss and flatulence is rare (<25%); "atypical" unspecific gastrointestinal symptoms are more common.[56,101-103] This is particularly applicable to patients in whom intestinal involvement is limited to the proximal small intestine.[89] Table 3 shows the set of pathophysiological changes which explain these patients' diarrhea and their multifactorial origin. Although these are generally diurnal stools (often postprandial), it is also not uncommon for them to wake the patient at night. The stool volume may be increased due to loss of nutrients (fats, carbohydrates, proteins and electrolytes) or else rather watery stools and mixed with abundant gas, the result of bacterial fermentation of unabsorbed sugars. This fact is compounded because 2/3 of CD patients have intestinal bacterial overgrowth (SIBO) and/or lactose intolerance, which contribute to H_2, CO_2 and CH_4 production. Some patients have bouts of diarrhea alternating with periods of normalcy, or else constipation, simulating the typical IBS behavior.[101] A history of inveterate chronic constipation does not, in any way, exclude the disease. The presence of refractory pyrosis to antisecretory drugs should encourage considering CD in the differential diagnosis. A subset of these patients suffer from gaseous reflux and PPI administration may contribute to increased intra-abdominal pressure by favoring SIBO and gas production. In this context, it is not unusual for the "refractory" pyrosis in these patients to disappear completely after removing gluten from the diet. The authors have seen some cases with this peculiarity. Some patients with dyspepsia and apparent functionality criteria (absence of alarming symptoms and negative endoscopy) have, in fact, CD or NCGS, erroneously labeled as "functional" dyspepsia, as some recent studies have shown.[8,103-110] The same applies to a subset of patients with symptoms of "functional" chronic diarrhea, or IBS-D subtype.[111-116] Some of these patients cannot be categorized as celiac and correspond more closely to NCGS criteria.[1,6,115] A not uncommon clinical profile is that of patients, usually female, who complain of repeated episodes of severe epigastric pain which can simulate a "biliary colic", without any organicity being evident in additional tests. Some experience a significant improvement in the frequency and intensity of seizures after starting a GFD. No link has been established, beyond any doubt, about the possible relationship between CD and the absence of relaxation in the sphincter of Oddi, although there is a documented relationship between idiopathic acute pancreatitis and CD.[117] Gliadinic shock prevalence, a condition characterized by uncontrollable vomiting, abdominal pain and peripheral collapse signs, 2-4 hours after gluten ingestion, is exceptional in adults.[88]

Osmotic mechanism
• Lactose malabsorption due to secondary disacaridase deficit.

Secretory mechanism
• Protein, fat and carbohydrate absorption inhibition (steatorrhea, creatorrhea). • Water and electrolyte secretion stimulus. • Exocrine pancreatic insufficiency due to duodenal mucosa secretion of secretin and CCK.[1] • Cathartic effect of unabsorbed fatty acids hydroxilated by bacteria. • Cathartic effect of bile salts hydroxilated by bacteria (only in cases with ileal involvement).

Motility alterations
• Failure in the clearing up of bacteria which leads to intestinal bacterial overgrowth.[2]

Inflammatory mechanism
• The probability of inflammatory bowel disease is 10 times higher among CD patients. • In refractory CD cases complicated with ulcerative jejunoileitis there is an exudation of blood, mucus and proteins. • Some CD patients have microscopic colitis (lymphocytic or collagenous).

[1] *May even appear in cases without villous atrophy.*[252,261-263]
[2] *May explain persistent diarrhea and flatulence in CD patients who adhere to the GFD.*

Table 3. Factors which contribute to diarrhea in CD.

6.2. Extraintestinal symptoms

The prevalence of extraintestinal manifestations in CD is very high among adult patients, especially if a specific search is performed.[13-22] In the authors' experience, more than 90% of the patients have systemic signs or symptoms, the most frequent being fatigue and lassitude, iron deficiency anemia, canker sores, dysthymia, osteoporosis and skin lesions. Not infrequently, this is one of the reasons for initial consultation, as some minor digestive symptoms may have gone unnoticed and were never serious enough to consult a physician. Sometimes, these symptoms and signs are conditioned by nutrient malabsorption and in others, the relationship with malabsorption may not be as clear (Table 4).

Implicated organ or system	Mechanism
Hematological	
Anemia	Iron, Folate or Vitamin B12 malabsorption or pyridoxine deficiency.
Hemorrhagic diathesis	Vitamin K deficit. Thrombocytopenia due to folate deficit. There is an epidemiological association between CD and idiopathic thrombocytopenia purpura .[211-217]
Thrombocytosis	Hyposplenism.
Skeletal	
Osteopenia/osteoporosis	Calcium and vitamin D malabsorption.
Pathological fractures	Osteopenia / osteoporosis.
Muscular	
Atrophy	Malabsorption-induced malnutrition/osteoporosis.
Tetany	Calcium, vitamin D and magnesium malabsorption.
Weakness	Muscular atrophy, hypokalemia.
Dermal	
Dermatitis herpetiformis	Dermal equivalent to CD.
Edema	Hipoproteinemia.
Ecchymosis and petechia	Vitamin K malabsorption.
Follicular Hyperkeratosis	Vitamin A and B-complex malabsorption.
Psoriasiform lesions	Associated disease of immune origin.
Neurological	
Peripheral neuropathy	Vitamin B12 and thiamine deficiencies.
Ataxia	Cerebellar and posterior columnar damage.
Demyelinating lesions of the central nervous system.	Unknown mechanism.
Vertigo	Unknown mechanism.
Endocrinological	
Amenorrhea, infertility, impotence	Malnutrition, hypothalamus-hypophysis dysfunction.
Secondary hyperparatiroidism	Calcium and vitamin D absorption deficit.
Hepatological	
Aminotransferase increase	Unknown mechanism.

[1] *May appear even in cases without villous atrophy.[252,261-263]*
[2] *May explain persistent diarrhea and flatulence in CD patients who adhere to the GFD.*

Table 4. Extraintestinal CD symptoms and signs, grouped according to organs and systems.

6.3. Anemia

Anemia is a common finding among celiac patients; its origin is often associated with iron or folate malabsorption when the proximal intestine is affected.[88,118] In some cases, there is also vitamin B-12 malabsorption when there is a concomitant involvement of the ileum or when there is SIBO. There is a special difficulty involving the assessment of iron deficiency anemia, when the histological lesion is limited to lymphocytic enteropathy (>25% IELs) (Marsh 1; Corazza) associated with *H. pylori* (*Hp*) infection. The difficulty lies in that *Hp* infection is a recognized cause of iron deficiency which may disappear when the infection is eradicated.[119-121] Distinguishing both situations can be difficult in patients with negative serology and positive DQ2-DQ8, which makes a specialized assessment imperative. Figure 4 shows the case of a patient with iron deficiency anemia, lymphocytic enteropathy and Hp infection, whose histological lesion did not abate definitively until gluten was removed the diet. In severe cases, anemia can result from a hemorrhagic diathesis due to vitamin K malabsorption or gastrointestinal bleeding secondary to ulcerative jejunoileitis or lymphoma.

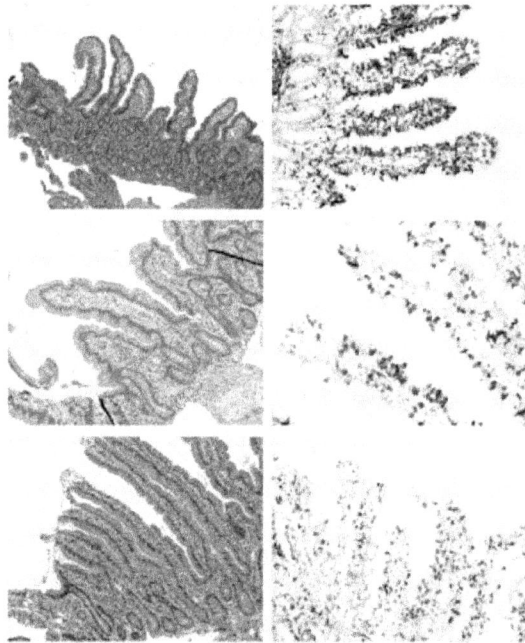

Figure 4. Images from a 45-year-old male with dyspepsia and flatulence
Anti TG: 1.8 U/mL.[DQA1*05 positive; DQB1*02 positive] Above (left) mild focal villous atrophy can be appreciated. Immunohistochemistry (right) shows an IEL count of 35%. Below, the results of the eradication of the Helicobacter Pylori *infection, can be seen, 4 months later. To the left, mild focal villous atrophy persists. The image on the right shows a decrease in the IEL count (19%). Further down (left) complete mucosal architecture and villous recovery can be seen, one year after withdrawing dietary gluten. To the right, the effect of the GFD on the IEL count can be appreciated, which is of 15%. Courtesy of Dr. Vera, Pathological Anatomy Service, San Jorge Hospital, Huesca.*

6.4. Osteopenia and Osteoporosis

The prevalence of osteopenia and osteoporosis among CD patients is high, both in children and in adults[88,122,123] and it is the result of a combination of factors, such as deficiencies in calcium ion transport across the intestinal mucosa, vitamin D malabsorption, secondary hyperparathyroidism which promotes bone calcium mobilization aggravating osteopenia and the effect of the inflammatory mediators. Note that osteopenia and risk of fractures also occur in patients with mild forms of enteropathy, even without villous atrophy.[124-130] There is evidence that suggests that children with a CD diagnosis who dropped the gluten-free diet and remained asymptomatic, later developed osteoporosis as adults, proof that the diet should be lifelong.[126] Figure 5 shows the case of a boy with childhood growth delay and mild gastrointestinal symptoms, who presented a vertebral fracture at age 34 ignoring that he suffered from CD. Several studies agree that the GFD allows significant bone mass recovery in children. This benefit is lesser in the adult population, but still evident.[131-135] One study showed that magnesium supplements improved bone mass in adults with CD.[136]

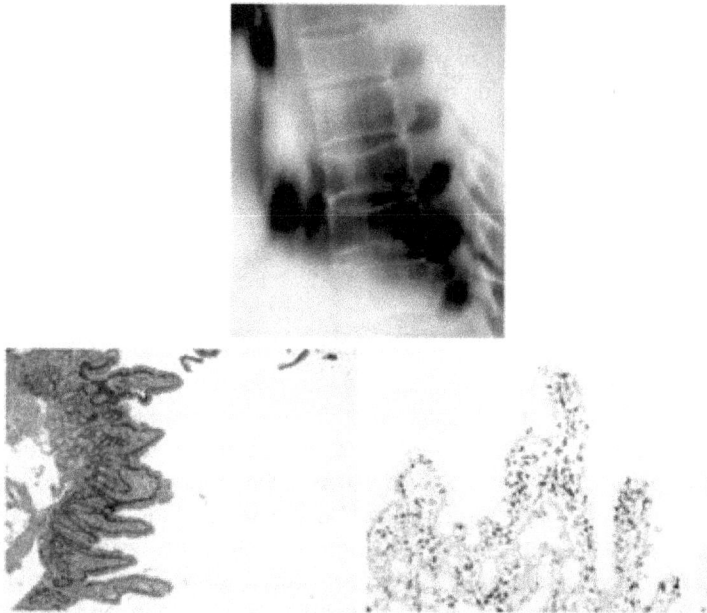

Figure 5. Histological images corresponding to a 51-year-old male with a history of unstudied childhood delay.

At 34 years of age a flattening of the 10th dorsal vertebra (backbone x-ray) occurred due to a slight fall, which led to a "young adult's idiopathic osteoporosis" diagnosis. Nine years later, a jejunal biopsy using a Crosby capsule was performed, which yielded a report of normalcy. Said biopsy was evaluated 9 years later by an expert pathologist who reported a focal mild villous atrophy and an IEL count of 24% (below right). One first-degree relative and two second-degree relatives were later diagnosed with CD; all of them were HLA-DQ2 positive. Courtesy of Dr. Vera, Pathological Anatomy Service, San Jorge Hospital, Huesca.

6.5. Neurological Symptoms

The association between CD and neurological disorders has been widely documented.[137-144] Some CD patients may develop neurological symptoms due to malabsorption of vitamin B1 (thiamine), B2 (riboflavin), B3 (niacin), B6 (pyridoxine), B12 (cobalamin) and vitamin E.[88] These deficiencies are unusual except in cases with severe and extensive intestinal involvement. Other neurological symptoms frequently observed in CD patients include headache, dizziness and peripheral neuropathy, consisting of burning, numbness and tingling in the hands and legs, symptoms that may occur in up to 50% of them before diagnosis.[13] The association of cerebellar ataxia and various forms of epilepsy is well known[145-149], but it is not always related to the presence of cerebral calcifications.[149] Their prognosis is variable, ranging from mild cases to intractable forms which evolve to severe encephalopathy, including progressive myoclonic epilepsy.[149]

6.6. Psychiatric Symptoms

It has been usually described that CD patients, especially children, exhibit irritability and mood swings. The association of CD with depression in adults is unclear, as an independent variable of other clinical conditions.[14,150-152] A Swedish study involving 13,776 CD patients and 66,815 controls found a higher depression prevalence in the first group.[151] These data, however, have not been reproduced in other studies.[152] Another study has shown, in patients diagnosed with CD one year after removing dietary gluten, improvement in anxiety levels, but not in depression.[153]

6.7. Infertility and Menstrual Disorders

Women with untreated CD have a higher incidence of menstrual abnormalities, including delayed menarche, early menopause, secondary amenorrhea, unwanted abortions, infertility and intrauteral growth retardation of children.[152-159] A case-control study of women of childbearing age showed a CD prevalence of 6.7% among those who reported unwanted abortions, 5.7% among those with a history of stillbirths, 5.6% in those with infertility and 9.3% in those with intrauterine fetal growth retardation. In the same study, CD prevalence in the control group was 1.3%. These figures could be underestimated because the CD diagnosis was made on the basis of serological studies without duodenal biopsy.[159] In males, sperm abnormalities have been documented regarding morphology and motility and resistance to the effects of androgens, manifested by elevated testosterone levels and LDH which become normalized sometime after starting the GFD.[160-161]

7. Associated Clinical Conditions

A set of diseases are more prevalent among CD patients. Besides dermatitis herpetiformis, already mentioned, the following can be highlighted.

7.1. Type I Diabetes Mellitus

Diabetes mellitus type 1 shares some HLA system haplotypes (HLA-DR3, HLA DQ2, and HLA-DQ8) and other genetic CD variants.[162-165] This explains the fact that 2-8% of type 1 DM patients have anti-TG2 antibodies.[166-167] One study showed that one third of type 1 DM patients who bore HLA-DQ2 had anti-TG2, while the prevalence of these antibodies in the population of type 1 diabetic without this haplotype was of 2%.[168] Although there are conflicting views[169], CD does not seem to be a contributing factor to the development of type-1 diabetes, since anti-TG2 usually appears after onset of diabetes.[170] It is not clear if instituting a GFD improves the development of type 1 DM and of its insulin requirements.

7.2. Liver Disease

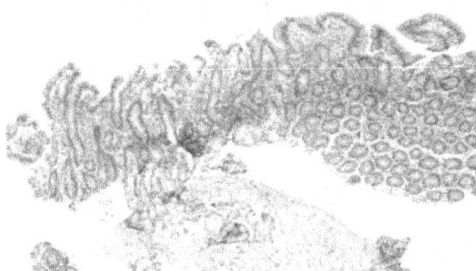

Figure 6. Histological image from a 53-year-old woman formerly diagnosed with primary biliary cirrhosis, autoimmune hypothyroidism, Sjögren's syndrome and follicular porokeratosis.

She had suffered, for several years, from dyspepsia and flatulence with no other associated gastrointestinal symptoms. The biopsy shows a marked disorganization of the mucosal villous architecture, with severe villous atrophy, crypt hyperplasia and an IEL count of 63%. A first-degree relative was later diagnosed with EC. Courtesy of Dr. Vera, Pathological Anatomy Service, San Jorge Hospital, Huesca.

Up to 25% of patients have a nonspecific transaminase elevation (<3 UNL) at the time of CD diagnosis, which returns to normal in 65-90% of the cases, after instituting a GFD.[171-175] In fact, the probability of CD among patients with chronic liver disease is 10 times higher than that observed in the population.[173-176] There is also a well-documented association with primary biliary cirrhosis (PBC), primary sclerosing cholangitis (PSC), congenital hepatic fibrosis (CHF) and massive steatosis. Figure 6 illustrates the case of a patient with primary biliary cirrhosis who referred dyspepsia as the only gastrointestinal manifestation of the illness. The recognition both diseases in the same patient is important since both can lead to osteoporosis. One study identified the presence of CD in 4% of patients who received a liver transplant; these were patients with autoimmune hepatitis, PBC, PSC and CHF.[177-179] In some patients, the beginning of a GFD has led to a decrease of advanced liver disease.[180,182] Other authors have shown there is a decrease of steatosis associated with a metabolic syndrome.[182]

7.3. Thyroid Disease

The probability of autoimmune thyroid disease (particularly hypothyroidism) is higher among CD patients.[183,184]

7.4. Selective IgA Deficiency

The prevalence of CD among patients with this immune deficit is as high as 8%. In turn, the prevalence of selective IgA deficiency in CD patients reaches 1-2%.[185-187]

7.5. Down's Syndrome

There is a well-established association between CD and Down's syndrome, reaching, in some studies, a prevalence of up to 16%, a value 20 times higher than in the general population.[188-189] In Spain, the prevalence of intestinal biopsy-confirmed CD 286 patients was of 6.5%; most of them related both gastrointestinal symptoms as well as extraintestinal manifestations.[190]

7.6. Inflammatory Bowel Disease

The probability that a CD patient will develop or suffer from a concomitant IBD is 10 times higher than in the general population, especially for ulcerative colitis (UC).[191-193] In turn, UC is 5 times more common among the relatives of a CD patient.[194] This could be related to the fact that both share a receptor gene polymorphism for IL-23 which determines a proinflammatory state.[195-196] An association between CD, UC and PSC has been described.[199] In contrast, the prevalence of CD between IBD patients does not seem to be higher than that of the general population.

7.7. Eosinophilic Esophagitis

Several studies agree that the prevalence of eosinophilic esophagitis is higher in children or adults with CD. This should be firmly considered in celiac patients with persistent pyrosis or dysphagia.[198-200]

7.8. Pancreatitis

A study of 14,000 CD patients has shown that the prevalence of every type of pancreatitis is higher among adult CD patients (OR 3.2, 95% CI 2.5-4.3, P <.001). The risk of developing chronic pancreatitis is also higher (OR 7.3, 95% CI 4.0-13.5, P <.001). This risk was not dependent on socioeconomic status, drinking habits or the presence of gallstones.[201]

7.9. Atrophic Glossitis

Various reports agree on a higher prevalence of atrophic glossitis[17,202] and other oral symptoms among CD patients, which usually improve after starting a GFD.

7.10. Heart Disease

Other associations described for CD include autoimmune myocarditis and dilated cardiomyopathy, which also improve after starting a GFD, whether or not immunosuppressive medications are taken (most of the cases have iron deficiency).[203-205] Some studies suggest a higher incidence of ischemic cardiopathic disease.[206-208]

7.11. Idiopathic Thrombocytopenic Purpura

As with other autoimmune diseases, there are isolated reports of an association between idiopathic thrombocytopenic purpura and CD.[209-215] It is not uncommon to find a triple association with other immunoregulation disorders, including thyroiditis,[211] multiple sclerosis,[212] selective IgA deficiency,[213] ranulomatous hepatititis[216] and myositis.[215] Figure 7 shows the duodenal biopsy of one of our patients with ITP, Sjögren's syndrome and CD. There are reports that establish a relationship between Sicca's syndrome and CD.[216-218]

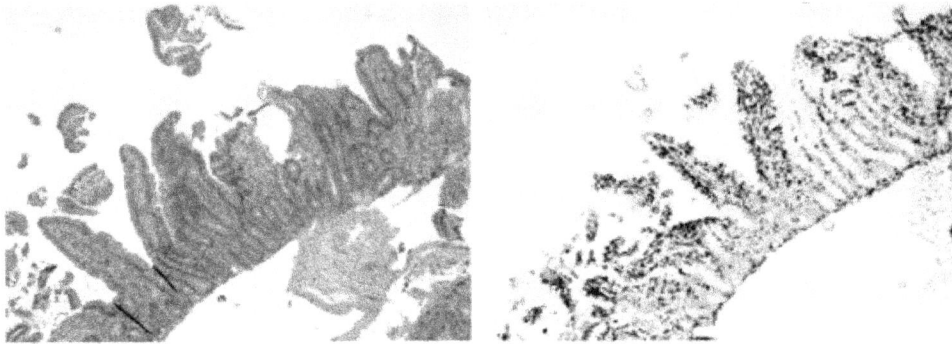

Figure 7. Images from a 45-year-old woman of low height, suffering from autoimmune thrombocytopenia, dryness of the mouth and eyes with a marked anti-Ro and anti-SSLab increase compatible with Sjögren's Syndrome.

She only reported nonspecific gastrointestinal symptoms. Anti-TG: 2 U/mL. HLA-DQ2 positive (DQAI*05/DQB1*02). The image shows a mild focal villous atrophy (left) and an IEL count of 35% (right). Courtesy of Dr. Vera, Pathological Anatomy Service, San Jorge Hospital, Huesca.

8. Diagnosis

8.1. Suspicion Index

The suspicion index for CD is extremely low and, in fact, at least 75% of the cases remain undiagnosed.[8-9] Data obtained from the ARETAEA registry allow establishing that the time between the onset of symptoms and diagnosis is, on average, of 10 years (unpublished observations); up to 60% of these patients have been diagnosed with one or more FGD over time and more than half have been subjected to various radiological or endoscopic studies, which are of no benefit to the clinical development of their disease.

These data are explained by several considerations:

1) The classic pattern of CD presentation, based on a florid case of malabsorption, is exceptional in adults (<20%), lesser or nonspecific gastrointestinal symptoms being the more frequent presentation;[56,101-103] a significant proportion of these patients fail to consult with a physician and those who do it are often anxiety-laden, due to the persistence and recurrence of their symptoms, leading the physician to issue a preconceived judgment of neurosis, hypochondria or somatization.[219]

2) According to the Rome Criteria, the diagnosis of a FGD is based on the presence of a set of symptoms, needing no further testing, save when there exist the so called "warning signs". The presence of pyrosis, postprandial fullness, bloating, abdominal discomfort or frequent changes in bowel habit (common symptoms in adult CD), are not sufficient to indicate a specific evaluation, unless there is anemia, vomiting, fever, rectal bleeding or weight loss.

3) Some antecedents, such as growth retardation in childhood, a history of iron deficiency, delayed menarche, early menopause, unwanted abortions, infertility, fractures due to minimal trauma, recurrent oral ulcers, psoriasiform skin lesions, are often overlooked, because the gastroenterologist's questions have focused exclusively on gastrointestinal symptoms, forgetting that CD is a disorder with a multisystemic expression.[5]

4) Experts participating in regular meetings of the Roman Committees are particularly incisive in the deliberate search for warning signs ("red flags"), aimed at the exclusion of malignancies, but are not as aware of the need to define a context favorable to the suspicion of CD (including the coexistence of other autoimmune diseases).[220,221]

5) Most IBS experts agree that an endomysial or anti-TG2 determination is useful for screening CD in IBS of the diarrheal subtype[222,223] but few consider that negative serology is quite common in patients with mild forms enteropathy (Marsh 1, 2 and 3a),[8,224-227] which excludes the patient from a fuller investigation.

6) Finally, current clinical practice guidelines do not include the need to biopsy the duodenum in patients with dyspepsia and negative endoscopy.

Besides, the application of specific immunostaining for CD3 is not standard practice, thus losing many cases of lymphocytic enteropathy that may be clinically relevant.[8,228] The Ministry of Health of Spain, promoted in 2008 development of an early diagnosis protocol as well as a decalogue of recommendations in order to increase the CD index of suspicion.[229] The Spanish Gastroenterology Association's AEGastrum recommendations project o draft recommendations of the Spanish Gastroenterological Association for clinical practice in primary care provides a number of key points for suspecting celiac disease in the field of primary health care (www.aegastro.es).

8.2. Approach to the Patient with Clinical Suspicion of CD

The diagnostic approach to a patient with suspected CD is complex, especially in adults, given the diversity of possible clinical settings.[230-231] It should be considered that, in any case, serology, genetic testing or duodenal biopsy results are pathognomonic. This means that in, certain cases, it is extremely difficult to confirm or rule out the disease. ESPGHAN published in 2012 a guide to clinical practice[5] and its readers can consult as well the Oslo[6] and London[1] Consensuses' recommendations as well as the recent criteria proposed by Catassi and Fasano[232], which emphasize the application of rigid algorithms, but do not cover the entire spectrum of situations, which makes preferable application of simple rules, which, in the hands of an experienced gastroenterologist, may be equally efficient (Table 5). Briefly we shall mention the most recommendable attitude for the two scenarios most often seen in adults. It always takes it as given that, in the face of clinical suspicion, a specific antibodies test (Anti-TG-2, antiendomysial or anti-DGP) should be the first test to be performed.

	At least 4 out of 5, or 3 out of 4 if there are no HLA genotypes
1	Typical CD symptoms.[1]
2	IgA-class specific antibodies for celiac disease at adult-level titers.[2]
3	HLA DQ2 or DQ8 genotypes.[3]
4	Celiac disease compatible enteropathy in intestinal biosy.[4]
5	Response to gluten-free diet.[5]

Note: A family history of celiac disease adds evidence to the diagnosis; in asymptomatic patients, particularly in children, it is advisable to confirm positive serology in 2 or more blood samples with a difference of at least 3 months; in selected cases a challenge test may be necessary, at least 2 years after the gluten-free diet.

[1] Examples of typical symptoms are chronic diarrhea, growth delay (children) or weight loss (adults) or iron deficiency anemia.

[2] IgA anti-TG or IgA antiendomisium in patients with no IgA or IgG anti-TG or anti-endomysium deficit, in patients with IgA deficit. The finding of IgG deaminated gliadin antipeptides adds evidence to the diagnosis.

[3] Positive HLA-DQ2 includes subjects with half the heterodimer (positive HLA-DQB1*02).

[4] Includes type 3 Marsh-Oberhuber lesions, Marsh Oberhuber types 1-2 associated to the presence of CD-specific antibodies or Marsh-Oberhuber types 1-3 associated with subepithelial IgA deposits.

[5] Histologic response is required of patients with negative serology or associated with IgA deficit.

Table 5. Criteria proposed by Catassi for the diagnosis of CD.

8.2.1. Symptomatic Patients with Positive Anti-TG-2

In a situation like this, if anti-TG titers are more than 10 times higher than the UNL, the intestinal biopsy could be excluded (fully accepted criterion in children), since the probability of detecting villous atrophy is quite high.[5] Before taking this decision it is prudent to investigate and confirm the presence of anti-endomysial antibodies (performing the extraction at a different time of the first time) and checking for HLA DQ2 or DQ8 heterodimers, since a positive result reinforces the diagnosis.[233] In contrast, antiTG2 antibodies titers are of <10 UNL, duodenal biopsies must be performed (2 bulb biopsies and 4 duodenal 2nd portion biopsies) to detect enteropathy. If the result is positive, a GFD should be started. If the duodenal biopsy reveals no abnormalities and the genetic test is positive, we face "potential" CD. Some authors recommend a GFD in this circumstance, to treat the symptoms and to prevent future complications.[232,234]

8.2.2. Seronegative Patients with Specific Antibodies and High Suspicion

This is a matter of crucial importance, especially in the adult population. In fact, the true prevalence of CD in this population has been underestimated, because both in population screening programs, as in symptomatic or high genetic risk people, intestinal biopsy is indicated only for positive serology.[237,238] However, there is evidence that the sensitivity of different antibodies is considerably lower in the absence of histological gravity.[225-227,237-240] Thus, once some of the causes of false negative serology have been taken into account (selective IgA deficiency, immunosuppressive treatments, low-gluten diet)[187] and having a well-founded clinical suspicion of CD, the clinician should not hesitate to request a duodenal biopsy[230,240] since there is evidence that the GFD provides symptomatic relief and reversion of lesions even in mild enteropathy cases.[8,241,243]

8.2.3. Important Considerations for Patients with Negative Serology and Mild Enteropathy

The presence of a minor histologic injury (slight enteropathy) (Marsh-Oberhuber 1 and 2) represents a difficult to interpret "gray area". It should be noted that this type of injury is nonspecific and that the symptomatic improvement seen in some patients, after removing gluten, may reflect changes in bowel function, the placebo effect or a combination of both. These patients should be managed with caution.

Some considerations strengthen the hypothesis of a gluten-induced enteropathy:

A) According to Catassi's criteria (Table 5) the presence of mild enteropathy (Marsh 1 and 2), negative serology and IgA subendothelial deposits clearly reinforce the CD diagnosis.[234,245]

B) Other suggestive characteristics are the predominance of γ/δ lymphocyte populations in the epithelial lining and the preferential localization of IELs at the tips of the villi.[245]

C) Lymphocytic enteropathy (LE) can be caused by peptic duodenitis, Helicobacter pylori (*Hp*) infection, frequent NSAID intake, SIBO, viral infections, Crohn's disease or some other autoimmune disease (Table 2). All these causes should be seriously considered for the differential diagnosis. For example, an LE (also known as lymphocytic duodenosis) can reverse after eradicating an Hp infection or curing an iron deficiency anemia, which otherwise could have been wrongly attributed to CD.[119-121]

D) In all these cases, information on the major determinants of CD genetic susceptibility can be a valuable aid, given its high negative predictive value. Over 95% of CD patients share HLA DQ2 heterodimers either in the *cis* position (encoded by HLA-DR3-DQA1*0501-DQB1*0201) or in *trans* (encoded by HLA-DR11-DQA1*0505 DQB1*0201 DQB1 0301/DR7-DQA1 0202). Most of the remaining ones are HLA-DQ8 (encoded by DQA1*0301-DQB1*0302). Either HLA-DQ2 or HLA-DQ8 expression is necessary, but not sufficient, for development of this disease. In fact, these haplotypes are present in 30-40% of the Caucasoid population, while CD is only present in 1% of it.

On the other hand, a negative genetic test virtually excludes the possibility of CD, but cases have been reported without these haplotypes (0.4%).[244] We follow the criteria proposed by Catassi (the "4 out of 5" rule) stressing the importance of a deliberate search of compatible symptoms and signs and the need for a correct differential diagnosis in mild enteropathies.[245]

9. CD Patient Follow-up

Treatment of CD is based on a strict GFD to be maintained for life. In most situations, this will be sufficient to induce an improvement in symptoms, while normalizing serology and reverting lesions. Several studies agree that, in adults, a complete regression of mucosal lesions is the exception rather than the rule, even if the symptoms have abated.[224,246,247] Patients with more severe villous atrophy often suffer from an associated secondary lactase deficiency, making it necessary to recommend the temporary withdrawal of dairy products. Some patients with significant malnutrition states may require temporary nutritional supplements and multivitamins. Patients with osteopenia or osteoporosis require additional calcium and vitamin D supplements (it must be noted that some commercial calcium preparations contain gluten); patients with anemia, oral ferrous salts and, in some cases, folic acid and vitamin B12 depending on the type of identified deficit. Cases of refractory or oral iron-intolerant anemia can benefit from i.v. carboxymaltose iron administration. Once clinical stabilization is achieved, patients can be evaluated by their primary care physician, with the recommendation to undergo a voluntary annual check-up, monitor weight and diet compliance as well as some basic analytical parameters, including iron metabolism.

10. Procedure to be Followed for Patients with Persistent Symptoms

The persistence of symptoms in a patient diagnosed with CD forces a revaluation in which two distinct situations must be discerned:

1) Lack of initial response to GFD and

2) Refractory CD (RCD).[248]

The reader can obtain further information on the diagnosis and management of RCD, as well as on the serious complications of CD (nongranulomatous jejunoileitis and CD associated T cell lymphoma) in another section of this work (Figures 8 and 9). This last condition is defined by the persistence of malabsorption symptoms and villous atrophy despite a strict GFD, with anti-TG2 and negative AEM, which persists for >12 months.[249] This is a rare condition (8-18% of patients referred to a tertiary hospital to investigate the lack of response to diet).[250-252] The situation is different for patients who initially respond to the GFD once the hypothesis of CD has been established. The three most common causes for this situation are:

1) Incorrect initial diagnosis,

2) The patient, voluntary or inadvertently, violates the diet and

3) There is a clinical condition associated with CD which explains the persistence of symptoms.[248]

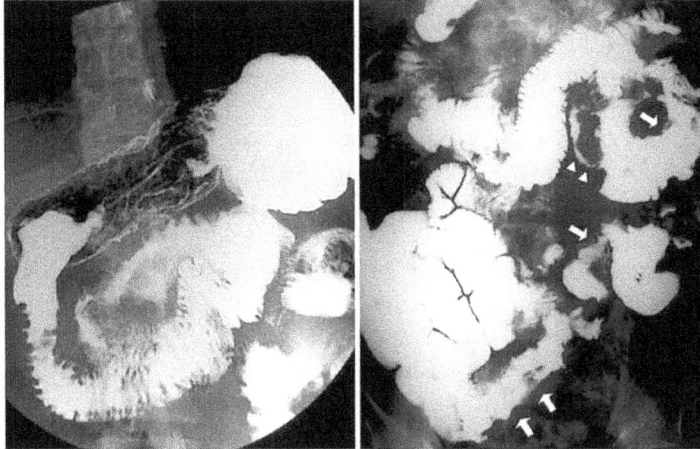

Figure 8. Lymphomas can complicate the CD patient's progress.
Barium radiography of a CD patient affected by a lymphoma. Courtesy of Dr. Domínguez, San Jorge Hospital. Reproduced by permission of Jarpyo Publishing, *from the 2nd edition of the book* Problemas Comunes en la Práctica Clínica *("Common Problems in Daily Clinical Practice") (Montoro, M. and García Pagan, JC (eds) (Copyright 2012).*

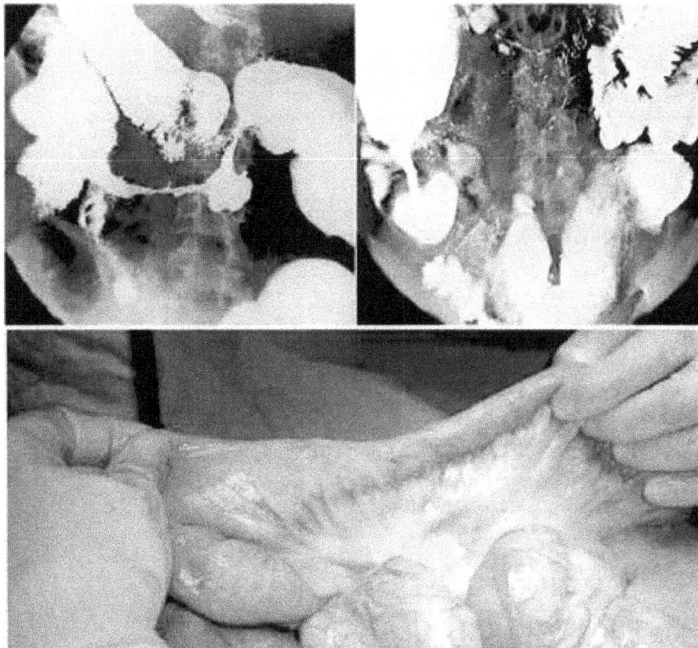

Figure 9. Ulcerative jejunoileitis in a patient with celiac disease and schizophrenia.
The radiological images show areas with stenosis and dilation in the small intestine. There is observable stenosis in the small intestine during laparotomy. Courtesy of Drs. Domínguez and Ligorred, San Jorge de la Huesca Hospital. Reproduced by permission of Jarpyo Publishing, *from the 2nd edition of the book* Problemas Comunes en la Práctica Clínica *("Common Problems in Daily Clinical Practice") (Montoro, M. and García Pagan, JC (eds) (Copyright 2012).*

10.1. Incorrect Initial Diagnosis

This can affect patients with mild enteropathy and negative serology as well as patients with villous atrophy (with or without positive serology). Some of these patients have experienced a transient improvement in their symptoms after starting the GFD, which reappear later. In both situations, an experienced pathologist should review the biopsies, including an assessment of villi orientation, atrophy degree, crypt elongation, villus/crypt ratio and degree of intraepithelial lymphocytosis. In some cases, it is advisable to repeat the biopsy to assess the presence of subendothelial IgA deposits and obtain a flow cytometry intraepithelial lymphangiogram to search for presence of an immunophenotype characteristic to CD (clear γ/δ lymphocyte predominance). In 55 patients referred to a tertiary center, the biopsy reviewed by an expert pathologist helped to finally dismiss a CD diagnosis in 6 cases.[250] The involvement of other etiologic agents in mild enteropathy forms (Table 2) has already been mentioned. Ultimately, it must be remembered that Catassi's criteria require the demonstration of a regression (or marked improvement) of histological lesions regarding seronegative enteropathies, a key issue in the validation of the diagnosis. Under special circumstances, a challenge test may be required.[5] Finally, the clinician and the pathologist ought not to forget there is a list of clinical conditions that may present villous atrophy, including allergies to different gluten proteins (chicken, cow's milk, egg, fish and soy), SIBO, hypogammaglobulinemia, giardiasis and autoimmune enteropathy, among others (Table 6).[70,248]

- Tropical sprue
- Parasitosis (*Giardia Lamblia*)
- Common variable immunodeficiency
- Lymphoma
- Whipple's disease
- Mastocytosis
- Abetalipoproteinemia.
- Vasculitis
- Amyloidosis
- Crohn's disease
- Eosinophilic gastroenteritis
- Autoimmune enteropathy
- Dietary protein intolerance (cow milk, egg, etc.)
- Infectious gastroenteritis
- Graft vs patient disease
- Small intestine chronic ischemia
- IgA deficit

Table 6. Diseases which manifest villous atrophy.

10.2. Noncompliant Patients

The first step in evaluating a patient who initially responded the GFD is to assess the degree of compliance with the diet, even if the patient assures that he or she does comply properly with it.[250] Certainly, complete lack of compliance with the GFD is unusual (<5% in most studies with a range of 0-32%),[253] but estimates of a really effective adherence to the GFD have a range of 42-91%.[253-255] The usual dietary gluten content oscillates around 13 g per day for a healthy person. Many people with CD can tolerate small amounts of gluten, but there is evidence that as little as 10 mg per day are capable of inducing mucosal abnormalities (international regulatory legislation provides that a gluten-free food must contain an amount of <20-100 parts per million (ppm)) and some patients are extremely sensitive.[248,256] Therefore, some patients, especially those with a strong drive to comply with the diet can benefit from advice provided by a nutritionist or a patients' association, making their symptoms disappear completely, particularly if they are very sensitive.[248] It is important to note that the persistence of some histological injury degree after starting the GFD in asymptomatic individuals is not an unusual occurrence and should not necessarily be considered as an indicator of dietary transgression. At this point it should be remembered that lesion reversion begins in the more distal portions of the intestine while the duodenum anatomical region is the last to experience a definitive cure.[257]

10.3. Associated Clinical Conditions which Explain the Persistence of Symptoms

Some CD patients who comply well with the diet show persistent symptoms, even in the presence of a significant improvement in their histological injuries.[258,259] Such cases may present a set of associated conditions that explain the persistence of diarrhea, either by an alteration in the small intestine's pathophysiology related to CD itself, or the existence of a concomitant disease, whose prevalence is higher among the CD patient population.[250,260] Lactose intolerance should be considered among the first,[255] fructose deficiency (an often underdiagnosed entity),[248] SIBO is probably related to microinflamatory changes which compromise the intestinal of bacterial clearing mechanisms[261-266] and pancreatic exocrine insufficiency due to a defect in the perception of the signal which activates pancreatic enzymes secretion after the release of endogenous secretin by the duodenal mucosa.[250,259-261] One or more of these pathophysiological abnormalities may contribute to persistent diarrhea after a successfully launched GFD. An H2 breath test, a culture of duodenal aspirate or, failing that, a Glucose-H2 as well as fecal elastase determination can be of valuable help in this context and allow taking specific measures aimed at controlling these mechanisms (lactose or fructose suppression, rifaximin or pancreatic enzymes). Note: pancreatic exocrine insufficiency may be present even in patients without severe villous atrophy, as has been shown in some studies where patients agreed to conduct a duodenal biopsy before prescribing pancreatic ferments.[250,259-261] The other category of patients comprises those suffering from a clinical condition whose prevalence is higher than that of the general population. Such is the case of microscopic colitis,[267] anal sphincter dysfunction,[259] intestinal inflammatory disease[191-193] or IBS itself[230,248] an entity whose prevalence in the general population[267-268] reaches 8-12%. Some patients labeled as IBS may improve after introducing the gluten-free regimen[7] others, however, may relate having constipation and swelling fostered by eating less fiber.[248] The frequent association between CD and microscopic colitis (50 times higher than expected in the general population)[267] requires a colonoscopy with biopsies performed in cases of watery refractory diarrhea.[269]

11. Emerging Therapies

Voluntary or inadvertent dietary transgressions pose a significant handicap for CD patients. Hence, in recent years different lines of research have been developed whose primary objective is to promote effective alternatives for prevention and symptom control. Briefly, these emerging therapies include dietary modifications, aimed at developing wheat grains without harmful gluten epitopes by transgenic technology[270-271] or the addition of proteolytic enzymes (prolylendopeptidase) designed to degrade proline-rich peptides which may be finally hydrolyzed by intestinal endopeptidases.[272-276] Gluten-capturing polymers have also been tested as well as permeability modulating agents, including inhibitors for zonulin (a human protein that acts on intercellular junctions causing disruption epithelial barrier and whose expression is increased by exposure to gliadin in celiac patients).[277-278] AT-1001 (Lazarotide acetate) is an octapeptide derived from a protein secreted by *Vibrio Cholerae* that binds to zonulin, acting as a competitive antagonist and inducing inhibition of epithelial cell reordering. Its use in a double blind case-control study showed a decrease in the permeability of gamma interferon levels and gastrointestinal symptoms without significant adverse effects.[278] Other advanced therapies include targeting agents which block antigen presentation by means of tissular transglutaminase inhibitors[279-283] or agents which block the intervention of the DQ2 or DQ8 HLA system haplotypes in antigen presentation.[284-285] Advanced therapies for disease control would include different monoclonal antibodies for inflammation modulation.[286-291] It is well known that T cell activation induces IFN-γ and TNF-α secretion, these are the inflammatory response and proteolytic cascade mediators responsible for tissular damage. Good results have been reported with *infliximab* in grave refractory CD cases.[288] Other IFN-γ antibodies (*fontolizumab*) could be tested in the future.[287] This advanced therapy spectrum is completed by agents that block the overexpression of IL-15, which is responsible for epithelial cell apoptosis induced by cytotoxic lymphocytes[289-290] and by substances that selectively inhibit lymphocyte adhesion including *natalizumab*[291] as well as other molecules directed against α4-integrin and α4β7-integrin and agents that block the chemokine ligand interaction,[25] secreted by intestinal epithelium cells and CCR9, located on the lymphocyte surface. Table 7 summarizes the aforementioned emerging therapies.

Treatment	Overview
Dietary modifications	
Enzyme therapies	Prolil-endopeptidases which collaborate to degrade gluten through proteolysis, diminishing its immunogenicity.
Wheat alteration	Development of wheat grains with low or null immunogenic peptide content and high nutritional quality.
Permeability modulation	
Zonulin inhibitors	Competitive zonulin agonist which inhibits the intestinal permeability increase it produces.
Antigen Presentation Blockage	
TG2 Inhibition	Deamination process blockage, avoiding effective gluten antigen presentation.
HLA Inhibition	Blockage of the HLA DQ2 and/or DQ8 gluten peptide linkage places.
Inflammation Modulation	
Anti-Interferon-γ and anti TNF-α antibodies	Blockage of aberrant inflammatory response provoked by these cytokines.
Anti IL-15 antibodies	Stops cytotoxic T-lymphocyte proliferation.
Lymphocyte adhesion inhibition	Selective inhibition of lymphocyte adhesion in order to impede their migration to inflamed tissues.
Others	
Vaccine	Desensitation by means of repeated gluten solution injections.
Parasites	Use of intestinal parasites as immune system modulators.

Table 7. Emerging therapies for celiac disease.

References

1. Sapone A, Bai JC, Ciacci C, Dolinsek J, Verde PH, Hadjivassiliou M et al. *Spectrum of gluten-related disorders: consensus on new nomenclature and classification.* BMC Med. 2012; 10: 13. http://dx.doi.org/10.1186/1741-7015-10-13

2. van Berge-Henegouwen GP, Mulder CJ. *Pioneer in the gluten free diet: Willem-Karel Dicke 1905 e 1962, over 50 years of gluten free diet.* Gut. 1993; 34: 1473-5. http://dx.doi.org/10.1136/gut.34.11.1473

3. Meeuwisse GW. *Round table discussion. Diagnostic criteria in coeliac disease.* Acta Paediatr. 1970; 59: 461-3.

4. Maki M. *Lack of consensus regarding definitions of coeliac disease.* Nature Reviews Gastroenterology & Hepatology. 2012; 9: 305-6. http://dx.doi.org/10.1038/nrgastro.2012.91

5. Husby S, Koletzko S, Korponay-Szabo IR, Mearin ML, Phillips A, Shamir R et al. *European Society for Pediatric Gastroenterology, Hepatology, and Nutrition guidelines for the diagnosis of coeliac disease.* J Pediatr Gastroenterol Nutr. 2012; 54: 136-60. http://dx.doi.org/10.1097/MPG.0b013e31821a23d0

6. Ludvigsson JF, Leffler DA, Bai JC, Biagi F, Fasano A, Green PH et al. *The Oslo definitions for coeliac disease and related terms.* Gut. 2013; 62: 43-52. http://dx.doi.org/10.1136/gutjnl-2011-301346

7. Biesiekiersky JR, Newnham ED, Irving PM, Barrett JS, Haines M, Doecke JD. *Gluten causes gastrointestinal symptoms in subjects without celiac disease: a double-blind randomized placebo-controlled trial.* Am. J. Gastroenterol. 2011; 106: 508-14. http://dx.doi.org/10.1038/ajg.2010.487

8. Santolaria S, Alcedo J, Cuartero B, Díez I, Abascal M, García-Prats D et al. *Spectrum of gluten-sensitive enteropathy in patients with dysmotility-like dyspepsia.* Gastroenterol Hepatol, 2013; 36(1): 11-20. http://dx.doi.org/10.1016/j.gastrohep.2012.07.011

9. Farrell RJ, Kelly CP. *Diagnosis of celiac sprue.* Am J Gastroenterol. 2001; 96: 3237-46. http://dx.doi.org/10.1111/j.1572-0241.2001.05320.x

10. Wahab PJ, Meijer JW, Goerres MS, Mulder CJ. *Coeliac disease: changing views on gluten-sensitive enteropathy.* Scand J Gastroenterol Suppl. 2002; 236: 60-5. http://dx.doi.org/10.1080/003655202320621472

11. Mulder CJ, Cellier C. *Coeliac disease: changing views.* Best Pract Res Clin Gastroenterol. 2005; 19: 313-21. http://dx.doi.org/10.1016/j.bpg.2005.01.006

12. Elfstrom P, Montgomery SM, Kampe O, Ekbom A, Ludvigsson JF. *Risk of thyroid disease in individuals with celiac disease.* J Clin Endocrinol Metab. 2008; 93: 3915-21. http://dx.doi.org/10.1210/jc.2008-0798

13. Ludvigsson JF, Olsson T, Ekbom A, Montgomery SM. *A population-based study of coeliac disease, neurodegenerative and neuroinflammatory diseases.* Aliment Pharmacol Ther. 2007; 25: 1317-27. http://dx.doi.org/10.1111/j.1365-2036.2007.03329.x

14. Ciacci C, Iavarone A, Mazzacca G, De Rosa A. *Depressive symptoms in adult coeliac disease.* Scand J Gastroenterol. 1998; 33: 247-50. http://dx.doi.org/10.1080/00365529850170801

15. Zugna D, Richiardi L, Akre O, Stephansson O, Ludvigsson JF. *A nationwide population-based study to determine whether coeliac disease is associated with infertility.* Gut. 2010; 59: 1471-5. http://dx.doi.org/10.1136/gut.2010.219030

16. Santonicola A, Iovino P, Cappello C, Capone P, Andreozzi P, Ciacci C. *From menarche to menopause: thefertile life span of celiac women.* Menopause. 2011; 18: 1125-30. http://dx.doi.org/10.1097/gme.0b013e3182188421

17. Cheng J, Malahias T, Brar P, Minaya MT, PH Verde. *The association between celiac disease, dental enamel defects, and aphthous ulcers in a United States cohort.* J Clin Gastroenterol. 2010; 44: 191-4. http://dx.doi.org/10.1097/MCG.0b013e3181ac9942

18. Ludvigsson JF, Lindelof B, Zingone F, Ciacci C. *Psoriasis in a nationwide cohort study of patients with celiac disease.* J Invest Dermatol. 2011; 131: 2010-16. http://dx.doi.org/10.1038/jid.2011.162

19. Pastore L, Lo Muzio L, Serpico R. *Atrophic glossitis leading to the diagnosis of celiac disease.* N Engl J Med. 2007; 356: 2547. http://dx.doi.org/10.1056/NEJMc070200

20. Zone JJ. *Skin manifestations of celiac disease.* Gastroenterology. 2005; 128(4 Suppl 1): S87-91. http://dx.doi.org/10.1053/j.gastro.2005.02.026

21. Collin P, Korpela M, Hallstrom O, Viander M, Keyriläinen O, Mäki M. *Rheumatic complaints as a presenting symptom in patients with coeliac disease.* Scand J Rheumatol. 1992; 21: 20-3. http://dx.doi.org/10.3109/03009749209095057

22. Caproni M, Bonciolini V, D'Errico A, Antiga E, Fabbri P. *Gastroenterol Res Pract. Celiac disease and dermatologic manifestations: many skin clue to unfold gluten-sensitive enteropathy.* 2012. http://dx.doi.org/10.1155/2012/952753

23. Volta U, Granito A, De Franceschi L, Petrolini N, Bianchi FB. *Anti tissue transglutaminase antibodies as predictors of silent coeliac disease in patients with hypertransaminasaemia of unknown origin.* Dig Liver Dis. 2001; 33: 420-5. http://dx.doi.org/10.1016/S1590-8658(01)80014-1

24. Bottaro G, Cataldo F, Rotolo N, Spina M, Corazza GR. *The clinical pattern of subclinical/silent celiac disease: an analysis on 1026 consecutive cases.* Am J Gastroenterol. 1999; 94: 691-6. http://dx.doi.org/10.1111/j.1572-0241.1999.00938.x

25. Gonzalez S, Gupta A, Cheng J, C Tennyson, Lewis SK, Bhagat G et al. *Prospective study of the role of duodenal bulb biopsies in the diagnosis of celiac disease.* Gastrointest Endosc. 2010; 72: 758-65. http://dx.doi.org/10.1016/j.gie.2010.06.026

26. Kurien M, Evans KE, Hopper AD, Hale MF, Cross SS, Sanders DS. *Duodenal bulb biopsies for diagnosing adult celiac disease: is there an optimal biopsy site?* Gastrointest Endosc. 2012; 75: 1190-6. http://dx.doi.org/10.1016/j.gie.2012.02.025

27. Cooper BT, Holmes GK, Ferguson R, Thompson RA, Allan RN, Cooke WT. *Gluten-sensitive diarrhea without evidence of celiac disease.* Gastroenterology. 1980; 79: 801-6.

28. Verdu EF. *Editorial: Can gluten contribute to irritable bowel syndrome?* Am J Gastroenterol. 2011; 106: 516-8. http://dx.doi.org/10.1038/ajg.2010.490

29. Sapone A, Lammers KM, Mazzarella G, Mikhailenko I, Cartenì M, Casolaro V et al. *Differential mucosal IL-17 expression in two gliadin-induced disorders: gluten sensitivity and the autoimmune enteropathy celiac disease.* Int Arch Allergy Immunol. 2010, 152: 75-80. http://dx.doi.org/10.1159/000260087

30. Sapone A, Lammers KM, Casolaro V, Cammarota M, Giuliano MT, De Rosa M et al. *Divergence of gut permeability and mucosal immune gene expression in two gluten-associated conditions: celiac disease and gluten sensitivity.* BMC Med. 2011; 9: 23. http://dx.doi.org/10.1186/1741-7015-9-23

31. Monsuur AJ, Wijmenga C. *Understanding the molecular basis of celiac disease: what genetic studies reveal.* Ann Med. 2006; 38: 578-91. http://dx.doi.org/10.1080/07853890600989054

32. Smith JB, Tulloch JE, Meyer LJ, Zone JJ. *The incidence and prevalence of dermatitis herpetiformis in Utah.* Arch Dermatol. 1992; 128: 1608-10.
http://dx.doi.org/10.1001/archderm.1992.04530010046006

33. Bolotin D, Petronic-Rosic V. *Dermatitis herpetiformis. Part I. Epidemiology, pathogenesis, and clinical presentation.* J Am Acad Dermatol. 2011; 64: 1017-24.
http://dx.doi.org/10.1016/j.jaad.2010.09.777

34. Collin P, Reunala T. *Recognition and management of the cutaneous manifestations of celiac disease: a guide for dermatologists.* Am J Clin Dermatol. 2003; 4: 13-20.
http://dx.doi.org/10.2165/00128071-200304010-00002

35. Caproni M, Antiga E, Melani L, Fabbri P. *Italian Group for Cutaneous Immunopathology. Guidelines for the diagnosis and treatment of dermatitis herpetiformis.* J Eur Acad Dermatol Venereol. 2009; 23: 633-8.
http://dx.doi.org/10.1111/j.1468-3083.2009.03188.x

36. Reunala T, Blomqvist K, Tarpila S, Halme H, Kangas K. *Gluten-free diet in dermatitis herpetiformis.Clinical response of skin lesions in 81 patients.* Br J Dermatol. 1977; 97: 473-80. http://dx.doi.org/10.1111/j.1365-2133.1977.tb14122.x

37. Garioch JJ, Lewis HM, Sargent SA, Leonard JN, Fry L. *25 years' experience of a gluten-free diet in the treatment of dermatitis herpetiformis.* Br J Dermatol. 1994; 131: 541-5.
http://dx.doi.org/10.1111/j.1365-2133.1994.tb08557.x

38. Herrero-González JE. *Clinical guidelines for the diagnosis and treatment of dermatitis herpetiformis.* Actas Dermosifiliogr. 2010; 101: 820-6.
http://dx.doi.org/10.1016/j.ad.2010.06.018

39. Hadjivassiliou M, Grunewald RA, Chattopadhyay AK, Davies-Jones GA, Gibson A, Jarratt JA et al. *Clinical, radiological, neurophysiological and neuropathological characteristics of gluten ataxia.* Lancet. 1998; 352: 1582-5.
http://dx.doi.org/10.1016/S0140-6736(98)05342-2

40. Hadjivassiliou M, Gibson A, Davies-Jones GAB, Lobo AJ, Stephenson TJ, Milford-Ward A. *Does cryptic gluten sensitivity play a part in neurological illness?* Lancet. 1996; 347: 369-371. http://dx.doi.org/10.1016/S0140-6736(96)90540-1

41. Pellecchia MT, Scala R, Filla A, De Michele G, Ciacci C, Barone P. *Idiopathic cerebellar ataxia associated with celiac disease: lack of distinctive neurological features.* J Neurol Neurosurg Psychiatry. 1999; 66: 32-35. http://dx.doi.org/10.1136/jnnp.66.1.32

42. Luostarinen LK, Collin PO, Peräaho MJ, Mäki MJ, Pirttilä TA. *Coeliac disease in patients with cerebellar ataxia of unknown origin.* Ann Med. 2001, 33: 445-9.
http://dx.doi.org/10.3109/07853890108995958

43. Bürk K, Bösch S, Müller CA, Melms A, Zühlke C, Stern M. *Sporadic cerebellar ataxia associated with gluten sensitivity.* Brain. 2001; 124: 1013-9.
http://dx.doi.org/10.1093/brain/124.5.1013

44. Cooke WT, Smith WT. *Neurological disorders associated with adult coeliac disease.* Brain. 1966; 89: 683-722. http://dx.doi.org/10.1093/brain/89.4.683

45. Hadjivassiliou M, Maki M, Sanders DS, Williamson CA, Grünewald RA, Woodroofe NM et al. *Autoantibody targeting of brain and intestinal transglutaminase in gluten ataxia.* Neurology. 2006; 66: 373-7. http://dx.doi.org/10.1212/01.wnl.0000196480.55601.3a

46. Hadjivassiliou M, Aeschlimann P, Strigun A, Sanders DS, Woodroofe N, Aeschlimann D. *Autoantibodies in gluten ataxia recognize a novel neuronal transglutaminase.* Ann Neurol. 2008; 64: 332-43. http://dx.doi.org/10.1002/ana.21450

47. Zuidmeer L, Goldhahn K, Rona RJ, Gislason D, Madsen C, Summers C et al. *The prevalence of plant food allergies: a systematic review.* J Aller Clin Immunol. 2008; 121: 1210-8. http://dx.doi.org/10.1016/j.jaci.2008.02.019

48. Schuppan D, Dieterich W. *Pathogenesis, epidemiology, and clinical manifestations of celiac disease in adults.* Uptodate. 2012.

49. Fasano A. *Where have all the American celiacs gone?* Acta Paediatr Suppl. 1996; 412: 20-4. http://dx.doi.org/10.1111/j.1651-2227.1996.tb14242.x

50. Not T, Horvath K, Hill ID, Hammed A, Magazzu G, Fasano A. *Celiac disease risk in the USA: high prevalence of antiendomysium antibodies in healthy blood donors.* Scand J Gastroenterol. 1998; 33: 494-8.http://dx.doi.org/10.1080/00365529850172052

51. Fasano A, Berti I, Gerrarduzzi T, T No, Colletti RB, Drago S et al. *Prevalence of celiac disease in at-risk and not-at-risk groups in the United States: a large multicenter study.* Arch Intern Med. 2003; 163: 286-92. http://dx.doi.org/10.1001/archinte.163.3.286

52. West J, Logan RF, Hill PG, Lloyd A, Lewis S, Hubbard R et al. *Seroprevalence, correlates, and characteristics of undetected coeliac disease in England.* Gut. 2003; 52: 960-5. http://dx.doi.org/10.1136/gut.52.7.960

53. Green PH, Jabri B. *Coeliac disease.* Lancet. 2003; 362(9381): 383-91. http://dx.doi.org/10.1016/S0140-6736(03)14027-5

54. Catassi C, Kryszak D, Bhatti B, Sturgeon C, Helzlsouer K, Clippet SL et al. *Natural history of celiac disease autoimmunity in a USA cohort followed since 1974.* Ann Med. 2010; 42: 530-8. http://dx.doi.org/10.3109/07853890.2010.514285

55. Catassi C, Fabiani E, Rätsch IM, GV Coppa, PL Giorgi, Pierdomenico R et al. *The coeliac iceberg in Italy. A multicentre antigliadin antibodies screening for coeliac disease in school-age subjects.* Acta Paediatr Suppl. 1996; 412: 29-35. http://dx.doi.org/10.1111/j.1651-2227.1996.tb14244.x

56. Green PH. *The many faces of celiac disease: clinical presentation of celiac disease in the adult population.* Gastroenterology. 2005; 128(4 Suppl 1): S74-8. http://dx.doi.org/10.1053/j.gastro.2005.02.016

57. Fasano A, Catassi C. *Current approaches to diagnosis and treatment of celiac disease: an evolving spectrum.* Gastroenterology. 2001; 120: 636-51. http://dx.doi.org/10.1053/gast.2001.22123

58. Lohi S, Mustalahti K, Kaukinen K, Laurila K, Collin P, Rissanen H et al. *Increasing prevalence of coeliac disease over time.* Aliment Pharmacol Ther. 2007; 26: 1217-25. http://dx.doi.org/10.1111/j.1365-2036.2007.03502.x

59. Rubio-Tapia A, Kyle RA, Kaplan EL, Johnson DR, W Page, Erdtmann F et al. *Increased prevalence and mortality in undiagnosed celiac disease.* Gastroenterology. 2009; 137: 88-93. http://dx.doi.org/10.1053/j.gastro.2009.03.059

60. Catassi C, Gobellis G. *Coeliac disease epidemiology is alive and kicking, especially in the developing world.* Dig Liver Dis. 2007; 39: 908-10. http://dx.doi.org/10.1016/j.dld.2007.07.159

61. Catassi C, Kryszak D, Louis-Jacques O, Duerksen DR, Hill I, Crowe SE et al. *Detection of Celiac disease in primary care: a multicenter case-finding study in North America.* Am J Gastroenterol. 2007; 102: 1454-1460. http://dx.doi.org/10.1111/j.1572-0241.2007.01173.x

62. Mäki M, Mustalahti K, Kokkonen J, Kulmala P, Haapalahti M, Karttunen T et al. *Prevalence of Celiac disease among children in Finland.* N Engl J Med. 2003; 348: 2517-4. http://dx.doi.org/10.1056/NEJMoa021687

63. Reilly NR, Green PH. *Epidemiology and clinical presentations of celiac disease. Semin Immunopathol.* 2012; 34: 473-8. http://dx.doi.org/10.1007/s00281-012-0311-2

64. Lee SK, Green PH. *Celiac sprue (the great modern-day imposter).* Curr Opin Rheumatol. 2006; 18: 101-7. http://dx.doi.org/10.1097/01.bor.0000198008.11439.c9

65. Sher KS, Fraser RC, Wicks AC, Mayberry JF. *High risk of coeliac disease in Punjabis. Epidemiological study in the south Asian and European populations of Leicestershire.* Digestion 1993; 54: 178-82. http://dx.doi.org/10.1159/000201035

66. Esteve M, Rosinach M, Fernandez-Bañares F, Farre C, Salas A, Alsina M et al. *Spectrum of gluten-sensitive enteropathy in first-degree relatives of patients with coeliac disease: clinical relevance of lymphocytic enteritis.* Gut. 2006; 55: 1739-45.
http://dx.doi.org/10.1136/gut.2006.095299

67. Esteve M, Carrasco A, Fernandez-Bañares F. *Is a gluten-free diet necessary in Marsh I intestinal lesions in patients with HLADQ2, DQ8 genotype and without gastrointestinal symptoms?* Current Opinion in Clinical Nutrition & Metabolic Care. 2012; 15: 505-10.
http://dx.doi.org/10.1097/MCO.0b013e3283566643

68. Patel D, Kalkat P, Baisch D, Zipser R. *Celiac disease in the elderly.* Gerontology. 2005; 51: 213-4. http://dx.doi.org/10.1159/000083996

69. Vilppula A, Collin P, Mäki M et al. *Undetected coeliac disease in the elderly: a biopsy-proven population-based study.* Dig Liver Dis. 2008; 40: 809-13.
http://dx.doi.org/10.1016/j.dld.2008.03.013

70. Vivas S, Santolaria S. *Enfermedad Celiaca.* En Ponce J, Castells A, Gomollon F (eds.). Tratamiento de las Enfermedades Gastroenterológicas. 3ª ed. Barcelona: Asociación Española de Gastroenterologia. 2010; 265-78.

71. Santolaria S, Fernandez-Banares F. *Gluten-sensitive enteropathy and functional dyspepsia.* Gastroenterol Hepatol. 2012; 35: 78-88.
http://dx.doi.org/10.1016/j.gastrohep.2011.10.006

72. Kagnoff MF. *Celiac disease. A gastrointestinal disease with environmental, genetic, and immunologic components.* Gastroenterol Clin North Am. 1992; 21: 405-25.

73. Schuppan D. *Current concepts of celiac disease pathogenesis.* Gastroenterology. 2000; 119: 234-42. http://dx.doi.org/10.1053/gast.2000.8521

74. Arranz E. *Inmunología de la enfermedad celíaca. ¿Qué debe saber el clínico?* GH continuada. 2010; 9: 124-6.

75. Jabri B, Sollid LM. *Mechanisms of disease: immunopathogenesis of celiac disease.* Nat Clin Pract Gastroenterol Hepatol. 2006; 3: 516-25.
http://dx.doi.org/10.1038/ncpgasthep0582

76. Kagnoff MF. *Celiac disease: pathogenesis of a model immunogenetic disease.* J Clin Invest. 2007; 117: 41-9. http://dx.doi.org/10.1172/JCI30253

77. Sollid LM, Lie BA. *Celiac disease genetics: current concepts and practical applications.* Clin Gastroenterol Hepatol. 2005; 3: 843-51.
http://dx.doi.org/10.1016/S1542-3565(05)00532-X

78. Wolters VM, Wijmenga C. *Genetic Background of Celiac Disease and Its Clinical Implications.* Am J Gastroenterol. 2008; 103: 190-5.
http://dx.doi.org/10.1111/j.1572-0241.2007.01471.x

79. Lundin KE, Scott H, Hansen T, Paulsen G, Halstensen TS, Fausa O et al. *Gliadin-specific, HLA-DQ (alpha 1*0501, beta 1*0201) restricted T cells isolated from the small intestinal mucosa of celiac disease patients.* J Exp Med. 1993; 178: 187-96.
http://dx.doi.org/10.1084/jem.178.1.187

80. Molberg O, McAdam SN, Korner R, Quarsten H, Kristiansen C, Madsen L et al. *Tissue transglutaminase selectively modifies gliadin peptides that are recognized by gut-derived T cells in celiac disease.* Nat Med. 1998; 4: 713-7.
http://dx.doi.org/10.1038/nm0698-713

81. Meresse B, Chen Z, Ciszewski C, Tretiakova M, Bhagat G, Krausz TN et al. *Coordinated induction by IL15 of a TCR-independent NKG2D signaling pathway converts CTL into lymphokine-activated killer cells in celiac disease.* Immunity. 2004; 21: 357-66.
http://dx.doi.org/10.1016/j.immuni.2004.06.020

82. Petronzelli F, Bonamico M, Ferrante P et al. *Genetic contribution of the HLA region to the familial clustering of coeliac disease.* Ann Hum Genet. 1997; 61: 307.
http://dx.doi.org/10.1017/S0003480097006258

83. Houlston RS, Ford D. *Genetics of coeliac disease.* QJM. 1996; 89: 737-43.
http://dx.doi.org/10.1093/qjmed/89.10.737

84. Houlston RS, Tomlinson IP, Ford D, Seal S, Marossy AM, Ferguson A et al. *Linkage analysis of candidate regions for coeliac disease genes.* Hum Mol Genet. 1997; 6: 1335-9. http://dx.doi.org/10.1093/hmg/6.8.1335

85. Greco L, Corazza G, Babron MC, Clot F, Fulchignoni-Lataud MC, Percopo S et al. *Genome search in celiac disease.* Am J Hum Genet. 1998; 62: 669-75.
http://dx.doi.org/10.1086/301754

86. Romanos J, van Diemen CC, Nolte IM, Trynka G, Zhernakova A, Fu J et al. *Analysis of HLA and non-HLA alleles can identify individuals at high risk for celiac disease.* Gastroenterology. 2009; 137: 834-40. http://dx.doi.org/10.1053/j.gastro.2009.05.040

87. Kaukinen K, Partanen J, Mäki M, Collin P. *HLA-DQ typing in the diagnosis of celiac disease.* Am J Gastroenterol. 2002; 97: 695-9.
http://dx.doi.org/10.1111/j.1572-0241.2002.05471.x

88. Cooke WT, Holmes GKT. *Enteropatía inducida por el gluten (celiaquía).* En Berk JE, Haubrich WS, Kalser M, Roth JL, Schafnner F (eds.). Gastroenterología 4ª edición. Barcelona: Salvat Editores. 1987; 1897-38.

89. Farrell RJ, Kelly CP. *Celiac Disease, and refractory Celiac Disease.* En Feldman M, Friedmann L, Brandt LJ (eds.). Sleisenger-Fordtran 9th Gastrointestinal and Liver Disease. Philadelphia: Saunders. 2010: 1797-820.

90. Rubin CE, Brandborg LL, Phelps PC, Taylor HC Jr. *Studies of celiac disease: I. The apparent identical and specific nature of the duodenal and proximal jejunal lesion in celiac disease and idiopathic sprue.* Gastroenterology. 1960; 38: 28.

91. Madara JL, Trier JS. *Structural abnormalities of jejunal epithelial cell membranes in celiac sprue.* Lab Invest. 1980; 43: 254-61.

92. Baklien K, Brandtzaeg P, Fausa O. *Immunoglobulins in jejunal mucosa and serum from patients with adult coeliac disease.* Scand J Gastroenterol. 1977; 12: 149.

93. Walker MM, Murray JA. *An update in the diagnosis of coeliac disease.* Histopathology. 2011; 59: 166-79. http://dx.doi.org/10.1111/j.1365-2559.2010.03680.x

94. Marsh MN. *Gluten, major histocompatibility complex, and the small intestine: A molecular and immunobiologic approach to the spectrum of gluten sensitivity ("celiac sprue").* Gastroenterology. 1992; 102: 330-54.

95. Grefte JM, Bouman JG, Grond J, Jansen W, Kleibeuker JH. *Slow and incomplete histological and functional recovery in adult gluten-sensitive enteropathy.* J Clin Pathol. 1988; 41: 886-91.

96. MacDonald RM. *A importance of duodenal bulb biopsies in children for diagnosis of celiac disease in clinical practice.* Gastroenterol. BMC. 2009; 9: 78.
http://dx.doi.org/10.1186/1471-230X-9-78

97. Mahadeva S, Wyatt JI, Howdle PD. *Is a raised intraepithelial lymphocyte count with normal duodenal villous architecture clinically relevant?* J Clin Pathol. 2002; 55: 424-8.
http://dx.doi.org/10.1136/jcp.55.6.424

98. Vande Voort JL, Murray JA, Lahr BD, Van Dyke CT, Kroning CM, Moore SB et al. *Lymphocytic duodenosis and the spectrum of celiac disease.* Am J Gastroenterol. 2009; 104: 142-8. http://dx.doi.org/10.1038/ajg.2008.7

99. Pellegrino S, Villanacci V, Sansotta N, Scarfì R, Bassotti G, Vieni G et al. *Redefining the intraepithelial lymphocytes threshold to diagnose gluten sensitivity in patients with architecturally normal duodenal histology.* Aliment Pharmacol Ther. 2011; 33: 697-706.
http://dx.doi.org/10.1111/j.1365-2036.2011.04578.x

100. Owens SR, Greenson JK. *The pathology of malabsorption: current concepts.* Histopathology. 2007; 50: 64-82. http://dx.doi.org/10.1111/j.1365-2559.2006.02547.x

101. Sanders DS, Carter MJ, Hurlstone DP, Pearce A, Ward AM, McAlindon ME. *Association of adult coeliac diseasewith irritable bowel syndrome: a case-control study in patients fulfilling ROME IIcriteria referred to secondary care.* Lancet. 2001; 358(9292): 1504–8.
http://dx.doi.org/10.1016/S0140-6736(01)06581-3

102. Sanders DS, Hurlstone DP, Stokes RO, Rashid F, Milford-Ward A, Hadjivassiliou M et al. *Changing face of adult coeliac disease: experience of a single university hospital in South Yorkshire.* Postgrad Med J. 2002;78(915): 31-3.
http://dx.doi.org/10.1136/pmj.78.915.31

103. Green PHR, Stavropoulos SN, Panagi SG, Goldstein SL, Mcmahon DJ, Absan H et al. *Characteristics of adult celiac disease in the USA: results of a national survey.* Am J Gastroenterol. 2001; 96: 126-31. http://dx.doi.org/10.1111/j.1572-0241.2001.03462.x

104. Santolaria-Piedrafita S, Fernandez-Banares F. *Gluten-sensitive enteropathy and functional dyspepsia.* Gastroenterol Hepatol. 2012; 35: 78-88.
http://dx.doi.org/10.1016/j.gastrohep.2011.10.006

105. Ford AC, Ching E, Moayyedi P. *Meta-analysis: yield of diagnostic tests for coeliac disease in dyspepsia.* Aliment Pharmacol Ther. 2009; 30: 28-36.
http://dx.doi.org/10.1111/j.1365-2036.2009.04008.x

106. Dickey W. *Diagnosis of coeliac disease at open-access endoscopy.* Scand J Gastroenterol. 1998; 33: 612-5. http://dx.doi.org/10.1080/00365529850171882

107. Bardella MT, Minoli G, Ravizza D, Radaelli F, Velio P, Quatrini M et al. *Increased prevalence of celiac disease in patients with dyspepsia.* Arch Intern Med. 2000; 160: 1489-91. http://dx.doi.org/10.1001/archinte.160.10.1489

108. Cammarota G, Pirozzi GA, Martino A, Zuccala G, Cianci R, Cuoco L et al. *Reliability of the "immersion technique" during routine upper endoscopy for detection of abnormalities of duodenal villi in patients with dyspepsia.* Gastrointest Endosc. 2004; 60: 223-8.
http://dx.doi.org/10.1016/S0016-5107(04)01553-6

109. Lima VM, Gandolfi L, Pires JA, Pratesi R. *Prevalence of celiac disease in dyspeptic patients.* Arq Gastroenterol. 2005; 42: 153-6.
http://dx.doi.org/10.1590/S0004-28032005000300005

110. Giangreco E, D'Agate C, Barbera C, Puzzo L, Aprile G, Naso P et al. *Prevalence of celiac disease in adult patients with refractory functional dyspepsia: value of routine duodenal biopsy.* World J Gastroenterol. 2008; 14: 6948-53. http://dx.doi.org/10.3748/wjg.14.6948

111. Sanders DS, Carter MJ, Hurlstone DP, Pearce A, Ward AM, McAlindon ME et al. *Association of adult coeliac disease with irritable bowel syndrome: a case-control study in patients fulfilling ROME II criteria referred to secondary care.* Lancet. 2001; 358: 1504-8. http://dx.doi.org/10.1016/S0140-6736(01)06581-3

112. Shahbazkhani B, Forootan M, Merat S, Akbari MR, Nasserimoghadam S, Vahedi H et al. *Coeliac disease presenting with symptoms of irritable bowel syndrome.* Aliment Pharmacol Ther. 2003; 18: 231-5. http://dx.doi.org/10.1046/j.1365-2036.2003.01666.x

113. Ford AC, Chey WD, Talley NJ, Malhotra A, Spiegel BMR, Moayyedi P. *Yield of Diagnostic Tests for Celiac Disease in Individuals With Symptoms Suggestive of Irritable Bowel Syndrome Systematic Review and Meta-analysis.* Archives of Internal Medicine. 2009; 169: 651-58. http://dx.doi.org/10.1001/archinternmed.2009.22

114. Fernandez-Bañares F, Esteve M, Salas A, Alsina M, Farre C, Gonzalez C et al. *Systematic evaluation of the causes of chronic watery diarrhea with functional characteristics.* Am J Gastroenterol. 2007; 102: 2520-8. http://dx.doi.org/10.1111/j.1572-0241.2007.01438.x

115. Verdu EF, Armstrong D, Murray JA. *Between Celiac Disease and Irritable Bowel Syndrome: The "No Man's Land" of Gluten Sensitivity.* Am J Gastroenterol. 2009; 104: 1587-94. http://dx.doi.org/10.1038/ajg.2009.188

116. Mearin F, Montoro M. *Síndrome de intestino irritable.* En Montoro M, García Pagan J, (eds.). Gastroenterologia y Hepatología: Problemas comunes en la práctica clínica. Barcelona: Jarpyo. 2011; 523-68.

117. Patel RS, Johlin FC Jr, Murray JA. *Celiac disease and recurrent pancreatitis.* Gastrointest Endosc. 1999; 50: 823-7. http://dx.doi.org/10.1016/S0016-5107(99)70166-5

118. Rodrigo L, Fuentes D, Pérez I, Álvarez N, Niño P, de Francisco R. *Anemia ferropénica refractaria e intolerancia al gluten: respuesta a la dieta sin gluten.* Rev Enf Digest. 2011; 103: 349-54.

119. Nahon S, Patey-Mariaud De Serre N, Lejeune O, Huchet FX, Lahmek P, Lesgourgues B et al. *Duodenal intraepithelial lymphocytosis during Helicobacter pylori infection is reduced by antibiotic treatment.* Histopathology. 2006; 48: 417-23. http://dx.doi.org/10.1111/j.1365-2559.2006.02358.x

120. Qu XH, Huang XL, Xiong P, Zhu CY, Huang YL, Lu LG et al. *Does Helicobacter pylori infection play a role in iron deficiency anemia? A meta-analysis.* World J Gastroenterol. 2010; 16: 886-96. http://dx.doi.org/10.3748/wjg.v16.i7.886

121. Kurekci AE, Atay AA, Sarici SU, Yesilkaya E, Senses Z, Okutan V et al. *Is there a relationship between childhood Helicobacter pylori infection and iron deficiency anemia?* Trop Pediatr. 2005; 51: 166-9. http://dx.doi.org/10.1093/tropej/fmi015

122. Szymczak J, Bohdanowicz-Pawlak A, Waszczuk E, Jakubowska J. *Low bone mineral density in adult patients with coeliac disease.* Endokrynol Pol. 2012; 63: 270-6.

123. Meyer D, Stavropolous S, Diamond B, Shane E, Green PH. *Osteoporosis in a north american adult population with celiac disease.* Am J Gastroenterol. 2001; 96: 112-9. http://dx.doi.org/10.1111/j.1572-0241.2001.03507.x

124. Zanini B, Caselani F, Magni A, Turini D, Ferraresi A, Lanzarotto F et al. *Celiac disease with mild enteropathy is not mild disease.* Clin Gastroenterol Hepatol. 2012 Sep 27. Pii: S1542-3565(12)01142-1. http://dx.doi.org/10.1016/j.cgh.2012.09.027

125. Kurppa K, Collin P, Sievänen H, Huhtala H., Mäki M, Kaukinen K. *Gastrointestinal symptoms, quality of life and bone mineral density in mild enteropathic coeliac disease: A prospective clinical trial.* Scand J Gastroenterol. 2010; 45: 305-14. http://dx.doi.org/10.3109/00365520903555879

126. Cellier C, Flobert C, Cormier C, Roux C, Schmitz J. *Severe osteopenia in symptom-free adults with a childhood diagnosis of coeliac disease.* Lancet. 2000; 355: 806. http://dx.doi.org/10.1016/S0140-6736(99)04855-2

127. Moreno ML, Vazquez H, Mazure R, Smecuol E, Niveloni S, Pedreira S et al. *Stratification of bone fracture risk in patients with celiac disease.* Clin Gastroenterol Hepatol. 2004; 2: 127-34. http://dx.doi.org/10.1016/S1542-3565(03)00320-3

128. Vasquez H, Mazure R, Gonzalez D, Flores D, Pedreira S, Niveloni S et al. *Risk of fractures in celiac disease patients: a cross-sectional, case-control study.* Am J Gastroenterol. 2000; 95: 183-9. http://dx.doi.org/10.1111/j.1572-0241.2000.01682.x

129. Ludvigsson JF, Michaelsson K, Ekbom A, Montgomery SM. *Coeliac disease and the risk of fractures — a general population-based cohort study.* Aliment Pharmacol Ther. 2007; 25: 273-85. http://dx.doi.org/10.1111/j.1365-2036.2006.03203.x

130. West J, Logan RF, Card TR, Smith C, Hubbard R. *Fracture risk in people with celiac disease: a population-based cohort study.* Gastroenterology. 2003; 125: 429-36. http://dx.doi.org/10.1016/S0016-5085(03)00891-6

131. Vilppula A, Kaukinen K, Luostarinen L, Krekelä I, Patrikainen H, Valve R et al. *Clinical benefit of gluten-free diet in screen-detected older celiac disease patients.* BMC Gastroenterol. 2011: 11: 136. http://dx.doi.org/10.1186/1471-230X-11-136

132. Kemppainen T, Kroger H, Janatuinen E, Arnala I, Lamberg-Allardt C, Kärkkäinen M et al. *Bone recovery after a gluten-free diet: a 5-year follow-up study.* Bone. 1999; 25: 355-60. http://dx.doi.org/10.1016/S8756-3282(99)00171-4

133. Capriles VD, Martini LA, Arêas JA. *Metabolic osteopathy in celiac disease: importance of a gluten-free diet.* Nutr Rev. 2009; 67: 599-606. http://dx.doi.org/10.1111/j.1753-4887.2009.00232.x

134. Blazina S, Bratanic N, Campa AS, Blagus R, Orel R. *Bone mineral density and importance of strict gluten-free diet in children and adolescents with celiac disease.* Bone. 2010; 47: 598-603. http://dx.doi.org/10.1016/j.bone.2010.06.008

135. Kemppainen T, Kröger H, Janatuinen E, Arnala I, Lamberg-Allardt C, Kärkkäinen M et al. *Bone recovery after a gluten-free diet: a 5-year follow-up study.* Bone. 1999; 25: 355-60. http://dx.doi.org/10.1016/S8756-3282(99)00171-4

136. Rude RK, Olerich M. *Magnesium Deficiency: Possible Role in Osteoporosis Associated with Gluten-Sensitive Enteropathy.* Osteoporos Int. 1996; 6: 453-61. http://dx.doi.org/10.1007/BF01629578

137. Chin RL, Sander HW, Brannagan TH, Verde PH, Hays AP, Alaedini A et al. *Celiac neuropathy.* Neurology. 2003; 60: 1581-5. http://dx.doi.org/10.1212/01.WNL.0000063307.84039.C7

138. Freeman HJ. *Neurological disorders in adult celiac disease.* Can J Gastroenterol. 2008; 22: 909-11.

139. Grossman G. *Neurological complications of coeliac disease: what is the evidence?* Pract Neurol. 2008; 8: 77-89. http://dx.doi.org/10.1136/jnnp.2007.139717

140. Hadjivassiliou M, Sanders DS, Grünewald RA, Woodroofe N, Boscolo S, Aeschlimann D. *Gluten sensitivity: from gut to brain.* Lancet Neurol. 2010; 9: 318-30.
http://dx.doi.org/10.1016/S1474-4422(09)70290-X

141. Hernández-Lahoz C, Mauri-Capdevila G, Vega-Villar J, Rodrigo L. *Neurogluten: patología neurológica por intolerancia al gluten.* Rev Neurol. 2011; 53: 287-300.

142. Hernández-Lahoz C, Rodrigo L. *Gluten sensitivity and the CNS: diagnosis and treatment.* Lancet Neurol. 2010; 9: 653-4. http://dx.doi.org/10.1016/S1474-4422(10)70149-6

143. Hernández-Lahoz C, Rodríguez S, Tuñón A, Saiz A, Santamarta E, Rodrigo L. *Remisión clínica sostenida en paciente con esclerosis múltiple tipo remitente-recurrente y enfermedad celíaca con dieta sin gluten durante 6 años.* Neurologia. 2009; 24: 213-5.

144. Wills AJ, Unsworth DJ. *The neurology of gluten sensitivity: separating the wheat from the chaff.* Curr Opin Neurol. 2002; 15: 519-23.
http://dx.doi.org/10.1097/00019052-200210000-00001

145. Gobbi G, Bouquet F, Greco L, Lambertini A, Tassinari CA, Ventura A et al. *Coeliac disease, epilepsy, and cerebral calcifications. The Italian Working Group on Coeliac Disease and Epilepsy.* Lancet. 1992; 340: 439.
http://dx.doi.org/10.1016/0140-6736(92)91766-2

146. Ferroir JP, Fénelon G, Billy C, Huon R, Herry JP. *Epilepsy, cerebral calcifications, and celiac disease.* Rev Neurol. 1997; 153: 354.

147. Gobbi G. *Coeliac disease, epilepsy and cerebral calcifications.* Brain Dev. 2005; 27: 189-200. http://dx.doi.org/10.1016/j.braindev.2004.05.003

148. Johnson AM, Dale RC, Wienholt L, Hadjivassiliou M, Aeschlimann D, Lawson JA. *Coeliac disease, epilepsy, and cerebral calcifications: association with TG6 autoantibodies.* Rev Med Child Neurol. 2013; 55: 90-3.
http://dx.doi.org/10.1111/j.1469-8749.2012.04369.x

149. Licchetta L, Bisulli F, Di Vito L, La Morgia C, Naldi I, Volta U et al. *Epilepsy in coeliac disease: not just a matter of calcifications.* Neurol Sci. 2011; 32: 1069-74.
http://dx.doi.org/10.1007/s10072-011-0629-x

150. Ludvigsson JF, Reutfors J, Osby U, Ekbom A, Montgomery SM. *Coeliac disease and risk of mood disorders--a general population-based cohort study.* J Affect Disord. 2007; 99: 117-26. http://dx.doi.org/10.1016/j.jad.2006.08.032

151. Garud S, Leffler D, Dennis M, Edwards-George J, Saryan D, Sheth S et al. *Interaction between psychiatric and autoimmune disorders in coeliac disease patients in the Northeastern United States.* Aliment Pharmacol Ther. 2009; 29: 898-905.
http://dx.doi.org/10.1111/j.1365-2036.2009.03942.x

152. Addolorato G, Capristo E, Ghittoni G, Valeri C, Mascianà R, Ancona C et al. *Anxiety but not depression decreases in coeliac patients after one-year gluten-free diet: a longitudinal study.* Scand J Gastroenterol. 2001; 36: 502-6.

153. Soni S, Badawy SZ. *Celiac disease and its effect on human reproduction: a review.* J Reprod Med. 2010; 55(1-2): 3-8.

154. Meloni GF, Dessole S, Vargiu N, Tomasi PA, Musumeci S. *The prevalence of coeliac disease in infertility.* Hum Reprod. 1999; 14: 2759-61.
http://dx.doi.org/10.1093/humrep/14.11.2759

155. Sher KS, Mayberry JF. *Female fertility, obstetric and gynaecological history in coeliac disease: a case control study.* Acta Paediatr Suppl. 1996; 412: 76.
http://dx.doi.org/10.1111/j.1651-2227.1996.tb14258.x

156. Choi JM, Lebwohl B, Wang J, Lee SK, Murray JA, Sauer MV et al. *Increased prevalence of celiac disease in patients with unexplained infertility in the United States.* J Reprod Med. 2011: 199-203.

157. Tata LJ, Card TR, Logan RF, Hubbard RB, Smith CJ, West J. *Fertility and pregnancy-related events in women with celiac disease: a population-based cohort study.* Gastroenterology. 2005; 128: 849-55. http://dx.doi.org/10.1053/j.gastro.2005.02.017

158. Sher KS, Jayanthi V, Probert CS, Stewart CR, Mayberry JF. *Infertility, obstetric and gynaecological problems in coeliac sprue.* Dig Dis. 1994; 12: 186-90.
http://dx.doi.org/10.1159/000171452

159. Kumar A, Meena M, Begum N, Kumar N, Gupta RK, Aggarwal S et al. *Latent celiac disease in reproductive performance of women.* Fertil Steril. 2011; 95: 922-7.
http://dx.doi.org/10.1016/j.fertnstert.2010.11.005

160. Farthing MJ, Edwards CR, Rees LH, Dawson AM. *Male gonadal function in coeliac disease: 1. Sexual dysfunction, infertility, and semen quality.* Gut. 1982; 23: 608-14.
http://dx.doi.org/10.1136/gut.23.7.608

161. Farthing MJ, Rees LH, Edwards CR, Dawson AM. *Male gonadal function in coeliac disease: 2. Sex hormones.* Gut. 1983; 24: 127-35.
http://dx.doi.org/10.1136/gut.24.2.127

162. Kota SK, Meher LK, Jammula S, Kota SK, Modi KD. *Clinical profile of coexisting conditions in type 1 diabetes mellitus patients.* Diabetes Metab Syndr. 2012;6:70-6.
http://dx.doi.org/10.1016/j.dsx.2012.08.006

163. Kumar N, Sharma G, Kaur G, Tandon N, Bhatnagar S, Mehra N. *Major histocompatibility complex class I chain related gene-A microsatellite polymorphism shows secondary association with type 1 diabetes and celiac disease in North Indians.* Tissue Antigens. 2012;80:356-62. http://dx.doi.org/10.1111/j.1399-0039.2012.01931.x

164. Marchese A, Lovati E, Biagi F, Corazza GR. *Coeliac disease and type 1 diabetes mellitus: epidemiology, clinical implications and effects of gluten-free diet.* Endocrine. 2013;43:1-2. http://dx.doi.org/10.1007/s12020-012-9758-0

165. Smyth DJ, Plagnol V, Walker NM, Cooper JD, Downes K, Yang JH et al. *Shared and distinct genetic variants in type 1 diabetes and celiac disease.* N Engl J Med. 2008; 359: 2767-77. http://dx.doi.org/10.1056/NEJMoa0807917

166. Seissler J, Schott M, Boms S, Ostendorf B, Morgenthaler NG, Scherbaum WA. *Autoantibodies to human tissue transgutaminase identify silent coeliac disease in Type I diabetes.* Diabetologia. 1999; 42: 144-1.

167. Kordonouri O, Dieterich W, Schuppan D, Webert G, Müller C, Sarioglu N et al. *Autoantibodies to tissue transglutaminase are sensitive serological parameters for detecting silent coeliac disease in patients with Type 1 diabetes mellitus.* Diabet Med. 2000; 17: 441-4. http://dx.doi.org/10.1046/j.1464-5491.2000.00291.x

168. Bao F, Yu L, Babu S, Wang T, Hoffenberg EJ, Rewers M et al. *One third of HLA DQ2 homozygous patients with type 1 diabetes express celiac disease-associated transglutaminase autoantibodies.* J Autoimmun. 1999; 13: 143-8.
http://dx.doi.org/10.1006/jaut.1999.0303

169. Galli-Tsinopoulou A, Nousia-Arvanitakis S, Dracoulacos D, Dracoulacos D, Xefteri M, Karamouzis M. *Autoantibodies predicting diabetes mellitus type I in celiac disease.* Horm Res. 1999; 52: 119-24. http://dx.doi.org/10.1159/000023447

170. Saukkonen T, Savilahti E, Reijonen H, Ilonen J, Tuomilehto-Wolf E, Akerblom HK. *Coeliac disease: frequent occurrence after clinical onset of insulin-dependent diabetes mellitus. Childhood Diabetes in Finland Study Group.* Diabet Med. 1996; 13: 464-70. http://dx.doi.org/10.1002/(SICI)1096-9136(199605)13:5<464::AID-DIA101>3.0.CO;2-R

171. Sainsbury A, Sanders DS, Ford AC. *Meta-analysis: Coeliac disease and hypertransaminasaemia.* Aliment Pharmacol Ther. 2011; 34: 33-40. http://dx.doi.org/10.1111/j.1365-2036.2011.04685.x

172. Prasad KK, Debi U, Sinha SK, Nain CK, Singh K. *Hepatobiliary disorders in celiac disease: an update.* Int J Hepatol. 2011; 2011: 438184. http://dx.doi.org/10.4061/2011/438184

173. Abdo A, Meddings J, Swain M. *Liver abnormalities in celiac disease.* Clin Gastroenterol Hepatol. 2004; 2: 107-12. http://dx.doi.org/10.1016/S1542-3565(03)00313-6

174. Rubio-Tapia A, Murray JA. *Liver involvement in celiac disease.* Minerva Med. 2008; 99: 595-604.

175. Duggan JM, Duggan AE. *Systematic review: the liver in coeliac disease.* Aliment Pharmacol Ther. 2005; 21: 515-18. http://dx.doi.org/10.1111/j.1365-2036.2005.02361.x

176. Ludvigsson JF, Elfström P, Broomé U, Ekbom A, Montgomery SM. *Celiac disease and risk of liver disease: a general population-based study.* Clin Gastroenterol Hepatol. 2007; 5: 63-9. http://dx.doi.org/10.1016/j.cgh.2006.09.034

177. Kingham JG, Parker DR. *The association between primary biliary cirrhosis and coeliac disease: a study of relative prevalences.* Gut. 1998; 42: 120-2. http://dx.doi.org/10.1136/gut.42.1.120

178. Dickey W, McMillan SA, Callender ME. *High prevalence of celiac sprue among patients with primary biliary cirrhosis.* J Clin Gastroenterol. 1997; 25: 328-9. http://dx.doi.org/10.1097/00004836-199707000-00006

179. Bardella MT, Quatrini M, Zuin M, Podda M, Cesarini L, Velio P et al. *Screening patients with celiac disease for primary biliary cirrhosis and vice versa.* Am J Gastroenterol. 1997; 92: 1524-6.

180. Stevens FM, McLoughlin RM. *Is coeliac disease a potentially treatable cause of liver failure?* Eur J Gastroenterol Hepatol. 2005; 17: 1015-7. http://dx.doi.org/10.1097/00042737-200510000-00002

181. Kaukinen K, Halme L, Collin P, Färkkilä M, Mäki M, Vehmanen P et al. *Celiac disease in patients with severe liver disease: gluten-free diet may reverse hepatic failure.* Gastroenterology. 2002; 122: 881-8. http://dx.doi.org/10.1053/gast.2002.32416

182. García-Manzanares A, Lucendo AJ, González-Castillo S, Moreno-Fernández J. *Resolution of metabolic syndrome after following a gluten free diet in an adult woman diagnosed with celiac disease.* World J Gastrointest Pathophysiol. 2011; 2: 49-52. http://dx.doi.org/10.4291/wjgp.v2.i3.49

183. Counsell CE, Taha A, Ruddell WS. *Coeliac disease and autoimmune thyroid disease.* Gut. 1994; 35: 844-6. http://dx.doi.org/10.1136/gut.35.6.844

184. Badenhoop K, Dieterich W, Segni M, Hofmann S, Hüfner M, Usadel KH et al. *HLA DQ2 and/or DQ8 is associated with celiac disease-specific autoantibodies to tissue transglutaminase in families with thyroid autoimmunity.* Am J Gastroenterol. 2001; 96: 1648-9. http://dx.doi.org/10.1111/j.1572-0241.2001.03821.x

185. Meini A, Pillan NM, Villanacci V, Monafo V, Ugazio AG, Plebani A. *Prevalence and diagnosis of celiac disease in IgA-deficient children.* Ann Allergy Asthma Immunol. 1996; 77: 333-6. http://dx.doi.org/10.1016/S1081-1206(10)63329-7

186. Cataldo F, Marino V, Bottaro G, Greco P, Ventura A. *Celiac disease and selective immunoglobulin A deficiency.* J Pediatr. 1997; 131: 306-8.
http://dx.doi.org/10.1016/S0022-3476(97)70172-0

187. Cataldo F, Marino V, Ventura A, Bottaro G, Corazza GR. *Prevalence and clinical features of selective immunoglobulin A deficiency in coeliac disease: an Italian multicentre study. Italian Society of Paediatric Gastroenterology and Hepatology (SIGEP) and "Club del Tenue" Working Groups on Coeliac Disease.* Gut. 1998; 42: 362-5.
http://dx.doi.org/10.1136/gut.42.3.362

188. Gale L, Wimalaratna H, Brotodiharjo A, Duggan JM. *Down's syndrome is strongly associated with coeliac disease.* Gut. 1997; 40: 492-6.
http://dx.doi.org/10.1136/gut.40.4.492

189. Carlsson A, Axelsson I, Borulf S, Bredberg A, Forslund M, Lindberg B et al. *Prevalence of IgA-antigliadin antibodies and IgA-antiendomysium antibodies related to celiac disease in children with Down syndrome.* Pediatrics. 1998; 101: 272-5.
http://dx.doi.org/10.1542/peds.101.2.272

190. Carnicer J, Farré C, Varea V, Vilar P, Moreno J, Artigas J. *La prevalencia de la enfermedad celíaca en el síndrome de Down.* Eur J Gastroenterol Hepatol. 2001; 13: 263-7.
http://dx.doi.org/10.1097/00042737-200103000-00008

191. Breen EG, Coghlan G, Connolly EC, Stevens FM, McCarthy CF. *Increased association of ulcerative colitis and coeliac disease.* Ir J Med Sci. 1987; 156: 120-1.
http://dx.doi.org/10.1007/BF02954635

192. Falchuk KR, Falchuk ZM. *Selective immunoglobulin a deficiency, ulcerative colitis, and gluten-sensitive enteropathy--a unique association.* Gastroenterology. 1975; 69: 503-6.

193. Leeds JS, Höroldt BS, Sidhu R, Hopper AD, Robinson K, Toulson B et al. *Is there an association between coeliac disease and inflammatory bowel diseases? A study of relative prevalence in comparison with population controls.* Scand J Gastroenterol. 2007; 42: 1214-20. http://dx.doi.org/10.1080/00365520701365112

194. Shah A, Mayberry JF, Williams G, Holt P, Loft DE, Rhodes J. *Epidemiological survey of coeliac disease and inflammatory bowel disease in first-degree relatives of coeliac patients.* Q J Med. 1990; 74: 283-8.

195. Einarsdottir E, Koskinen LL, Dukes E, Kainu K, Suomela S, Lappalainen M et al. *IL23R in the Swedish, Finnish, Hungarian and Italian populations: association with IBD and psoriasis, and linkage to celiac disease.* BMC Med Genet. 2009; 10: 8.
http://dx.doi.org/10.1186/1471-2350-10-8

196. Glas J, Stallhofer J, Ripke S, Wetzke M, Pfennig S, Klein W et al. *Novel genetic risk markers for ulcerative colitis in the IL2/IL21 region are in epistasis with IL23R and suggest a common genetic background for ulcerative colitis and celiac disease.* Am J Gastroenterol. 2009; 104: 1737-44. http://dx.doi.org/10.1038/ajg.2009.163

197. Wurm P, Dixon AD, Rathbone BJ. *Ulcerative colitis, primary sclerosing cholangitis and coeliac disease: two cases and review of the literature.* Eur J Gastroenterol Hepatol. 2003; 15: 815-7. http://dx.doi.org/10.1097/01.meg.0000059152.68845.53

198. Thompson JS, Lebwohl B, Reilly NR, Talley NJ, Bhagat G, Green PH. *Increased incidence of eosinophilic esophagitis in children and adults with celiac disease.* J Clin Gastroenterol. 2012; 46: e6-e11. http://dx.doi.org/10.1097/MCG.0b013e318221aefd

199. Ooi CY, Day AS, Jackson R, Bohane TD, Tobias V, Lemberg DA. *Eosinophilic esophagitis in children with celiac disease.* J Gastroenterol Hepatol. 2008; 23: 1144-8.
http://dx.doi.org/10.1111/j.1440-1746.2007.05239.x

200. Leslie C, Mews C, Charles A, Ravikumara M. *Celiac disease and eosinophilic esophagitis: a true association.* J Pediatr Gastroenterol Nutr. 2010; 50: 397-9.
http://dx.doi.org/10.1097/MPG.0b013e3181a70af4

201. Ludvigsson JF, Montgomery SM, Ekbom A. *Risk of pancreatitis in 14,000 individuals with celiac disease.* Clin Gastroenterol Hepatol. 2007; 5: 1347-53.
http://dx.doi.org/10.1016/j.cgh.2007.06.002

202. Lähteenoja H, Toivanen A, Viander M, Mäki M, Irjala K, Räihä I et al. *Oral mucosal changes in coeliac patients on a gluten-free diet.* Eur J Oral Sci. 1998; 106: 899-906.
http://dx.doi.org/10.1046/j.0909-8836.1998.eos106501.x

203. Frustaci A, Cuoco L, Chimenti C, Pieroni M, Fioravanti G, Gentiloni N. *Celiac disease associated with autoimmune myocarditis.* Circulation. 2002; 105: 2611-8.
http://dx.doi.org/10.1161/01.CIR.0000017880.86166.87

204. Curione M, Barbato M, De Biase L, Viola F, Lo Russo L, Cardi E. *Prevalence of coeliac disease in idiopathic dilated cardiomyopathy.* Lancet. 1999; 354: 222-3.
http://dx.doi.org/10.1016/S0140-6736(99)01501-9

205. Curione M, Barbato M, Viola F, Francia P, De Biase L, Cucchiara S. *Idiopathic dilated cardiomyopathy associated with coeliac disease: the effect of a gluten-free diet on cardiac performance.* Dig Liver Dis. 2002; 34: 866-9.
http://dx.doi.org/10.1016/S1590-8658(02)80258-4

206. Ludvigsson JF, Montgomery SM, Ekbom A, Brandt L, Granath F. *Small-intestinal histopathology and mortality risk in celiac disease.* JAMA. 2009; 302: 1171-8.
http://dx.doi.org/10.1001/jama.2009.1320

207. Ludvigsson JF, James S, Askling J, Stenestrand U, Ingelsson E. *Nationwide cohort study of risk of ischemic heart disease in patients with celiac disease.* Circulation. 2011; 123: 483-90. http://dx.doi.org/10.1161/CIRCULATIONAHA.110.965624

208. Ludvigsson JF, de Faire U, Ekbom A, Montgomery SM. *Vascular disease in a population-based cohort of individuals hospitalised with coeliac disease.* Heart. 2007; 93: 1111-5.
http://dx.doi.org/10.1136/hrt.2006.097097

209. Olén O, Montgomery SM, Elinder G, Ekbom A, Ludvigsson JF. *Increased risk of immune thrombocytopenic purpura among inpatients with coeliac disease.* Scand J Gastroenterol. 2008; 43: 416-22. http://dx.doi.org/10.1080/00365520701814028

210. Stenhammar L, Ljunggren CG. *Thrombocytopenic purpura and coeliac disease.* Acta Paediatr Scand. 1988; 77: 764-6.
http://dx.doi.org/10.1111/j.1651-2227.1988.tb10749.x

211. Dogan M, Sal E, Akbayram S, Peker E, Cesur Y, Oner AF. *Concurrent celiac disease, idiopathic thrombocytopenic purpura and autoimmune thyroiditis: a case report.* Clin Appl Thromb Hemost. 2011; 17: E13-6. http://dx.doi.org/10.1177/1076029610378502

212 Yamout B, Usta J, Itani S, Yaghi S. *Celiac disease, Behçet, and idiopathic thrombocytopenic purpura in siblings of a patient with multiple sclerosis.* Mult Scler. 2009; 15: 1368-71. http://dx.doi.org/10.1177/1352458509345908

213. Mulder CJ, Gratama JW, Trimbos-Kemper GC, Willemze R, Pena AS. *Thrombocytopenic purpura, coeliac disease and IgA deficiency.* Neth J Med. 1986; 29: 165-6.

214. Kahn O, Fiel MI, Janowitz HD. *Celiac sprue, idiopathic thrombocytopenic purpura, and hepatic granulomatous disease. An autoimmune linkage?* J Clin Gastroenterol. 1996; 23: 214-6. http://dx.doi.org/10.1097/00004836-199610000-00012

215. Williams SF, Mincey BA, Calamia KT. *Inclusion body myositis associated with celiac sprue and idiopathic thrombocytopenic purpura.* South Med J. 2003; 96: 721-3. http://dx.doi.org/10.1097/01.SMJ.0000051148.97720.69

216. Roblin X, Helluwaert F, Bonaz B. *Celiac disease must be evaluated in patients with Sjögren syndrome.* Arch Intern Med. 2004;164: 2387. http://dx.doi.org/10.1001/archinte.164.21.2387-b

217. D'Onofrio F, Miele L, Diaco M, Santoro L, De Socio G, Montalto M et al. *Sjogren's syndrome in a celiac patient: searching for environmental triggers.* Int J Immunopathol Pharmacol. 2006; 19: 445-8.

218. Fracchia M, Galatola G, Corradi F, Dall'Omo AM, Rovera L, Pera A et al. *Coeliac disease associated with Sjögren's syndrome, renal tubular acidosis, primary biliary cirrhosis and autoimmune hyperthyroidism.* Dig Liver Dis. 2004; 36: 489-91. http://dx.doi.org/10.1016/j.dld.2003.10.022

219. Locke III GR, Weaver AL, Melton III LJ, Talley NJ. *Psycochocial factors in functional gastrointestinaldisorders.* Am J Gastroenterol. 2004; 99: 350-7.

220. American College of Gastroenterology Task Force on Irritable Bowel Syndrome, Brandt LJ, Chey WD, Foxx-Orenstein AE, Schiller LR, Schoenfeld PS et al. *An evidence-based position statement on the management of irritable bowel syndrome.* Am J Gastroenterol. 2009; 104(Suppl 1): S1-35.

221. Irritable bowel syndrome in adults: diagnosis and management of irritable bowel syndrome in primary care. 2008. Disponible en: http://guidance.nice.org.uk/CG61/NICEGuidance/pdf/English. Fecha último acceso: 21 Enero 2011.

222. Fasano A, Berti I, Gerarduzzi T, Not T, Colletti RB, Drago S. *Prevalence of celiac disease in atrisk and not at-risk groups in the United States. A large multicenter study.* Arch Intern Med. 2003; 163: 286-92. http://dx.doi.org/10.1001/archinte.163.3.286

223. Ford AC, Chey WD, Talley NJ, Malhotra A, Spiegel BM, Moayyedi P. *Yield of diagnostic tests for celiac disease in individuals with symptoms suggestive of irritable bowel syndrome.* Arch Intern Med. 2009; 169: 651-8. http://dx.doi.org/10.1001/archinternmed.2009.22

224. Hopper AD, Cross SS, Hurlstone DP, McAlindon ME, Lobo AJ, Hadjivassiliou M et al. *Pre-endoscopy serological testing for coeliac disease: evaluation of a clinical decision tool.* BMJ. 2007; 334(7596): 729. http://dx.doi.org/10.1136/bmj.39133.668681.BE

225. Tursi Λ, Brandimarte G, Giorgetti G, Gigliobianco A, Lombardi D, Gasbarrini G. *Low prevalence of antigliadin and antiendomysium antibodies in subclinical/silent celiac disease.* Am J Gastroenterol. 2001; 96: 1507-10. http://dx.doi.org/10.1111/j.1572-0241.2001.03744.x

226. Dickey W, Hughes DF, McMillan SA. *Reliance on serum endomysial antibody testing underestimates the true prevalence of coeliac disease by one fifth.* Scand J Gastroenterol 2000; 35: 181-3. http://dx.doi.org/10.1080/003655200750024362

227. Salmi TT, Collin P, Korponay-Szabó IR, Laurila K, Partanen J, Huhtala H et al. *Endomysial antibody-negative coeliac disease: clinical characteristics and intestinal autoantibody deposits.* Gut. 2006; 55: 1746-53. http://dx.doi.org/10.1136/gut.2005.071514

228. Alcedo J, Montoro M. *El enfermo con dispepsia.* En Montoro M, García Pagan J (eds.). Gastroenterologia y Hepatología: Problemas comunes en la práctica clínica. 2 ed. Barcelona: Jarpyo, 2011: 37-60.

229. Protocolo de diagnóstico precoz del Ministerio de Sanidad y Consumo de España. Disponible en: http://bit.ly/13lVaO6

230. Evans KE, Sanders DS. *Celiac Disease.* Gastroenterolol Clin North Am. 2012; 41: 639-50. http://dx.doi.org/10.1016/j.gtc.2012.06.004

231. Evans KE, Hadjivassiliou M, Saunders D. *Recognising Coeliac Disease in Eastern Europe-the Hidden Epidemic in our Midst?* J Gastrointest Liver Dis. 2011; 20: 117-8.

232. Catassi C, Fasano A. *Celiac disease diagnosis: simple rules are better than complicated algorithms.* Am J Med. 2010; 123: 691-3. http://dx.doi.org/10.1016/j.amjmed.2010.02.019

233. Hill PG, Holmes GK. *Coeliac disease: a biopsy is not always necessary for diagnosis.* Alimen Pharmacol Ther. 2008; 27: 572-7. http://dx.doi.org/10.1111/j.1365-2036.2008.03609.x

234. Salmi TT, Collin P, Järvinen O, Haimila K, Partanen J, Laurila K et al. *Immunoglobulin A autoantibodies against transglutaminase 2 in the small intestinal mucosa predict forthcoming celiac disease.* Aliment Pharmacol Ther. 2006; 2: 541-52. http://dx.doi.org/10.1111/j.1365-2036.2006.02997.x

235. Abrams JA, Diamond B, Rotterdam H, Green PH. *Seronegative celiac: increased prevalence with lesser degrees of villous atrophy.* Dig Dis Sci. 2004; 49: 456-0. http://dx.doi.org/10.1023/B:DDAS.0000026296.02308.00

236. Lewis NR, Scott BB. *Systematic review: the use of serology to exclude or diagnose coeliac disease (a comparison of the endomysial and tissue transglutaminase antibody tests).* Aliment Pharmacol Ther. 2006; 24: 47-54. http://dx.doi.org/10.1111/j.1365-2036.2006.02967.x

237. Tursi A, Giorgetti G, Brandimarte G, Rubino E, Lombardi D, Gasbarrini G. *Prevalence and clinical presentation of subclinical/silent celiac disease in adults: an analysis on a 12-year observation.* Hepatogastroenterology. 2001; 48: 462-4.

238. Tursi A, Brandimarte G, Giorgetti GM. *Prevalence of antitissue transglutaminase antibodies in different degrees of intestinal damage in celiac disease.* J Clin Gastroenterol. 2003; 36: 219-21. http://dx.doi.org/10.1097/00004836-200303000-00007

239. Rostami K, Kerckhaert J, Tiemessen R, von Blomberg BM, Meijer JW, Mulder CJ. *Sensitivity of antiendomysium and antigliadin antibodies in untreated celiac disease: disappointing in clinical practice.* Am J Gastroenterol. 1999; 94: 888-94. http://dx.doi.org/10.1111/j.1572-0241.1999.983_f.x

240. Evans KE, Sanders DS. *What is the use of biopsy and antibodies in coeliac disease diagnosis?* J Intern Med. 2011; 269: 572-81. http://dx.doi.org/10.1111/j.1365-2796.2011.02380.x

241. Kurppa K, Collin P, Viljamaa M, Haimila K, Saavalainen P, Partanen J. *Diagnosing mild enteropathy celiac disease: a randomized, controlled clinical study.* Gastroenterology. 2009; 136: 816-23. http://dx.doi.org/10.1053/j.gastro.2008.11.040

242. Tursi A, Brandimarte G. *The symptomatic and histologic response to a gluten-free diet in patients with borderline enteropathy.* J Clin Gastroenterol. 2003; 36: 13-7. http://dx.doi.org/10.1097/00004836-200301000-00006

243. Salmi TT, Collin P, Reunala T Mäki M, Kaukinen K. *Diagnosis methods beyond conventional histology.* Dig Liver Dis. 2010; 42: 28-32.
http://dx.doi.org/10.1016/j.dld.2009.04.004

244. Karell K, Louka AS, Moodie SJ, Ascher H, Clot F, Greco L et al. *HLA type in celiac disease patients not carrying the DQA1*05-DQB1*02 (DQ2) heterodimer: results from the European Genetics Cluster on Celiac Disease.* Hum Immunol. 2003; 64: 469-477.
http://dx.doi.org/10.1016/S0198-8859(03)00027-2

245. Biagi F, Bianchi PI, Campanella J, Badulli C, Martinetti M, Klersy C et al. *The prevalence and the causes of minimal intestinal lesions in patients complaining of symptoms suggestive of enteropathy: a follow-up study.* J Clin Pathol. 2008; 61: 1116-8.
http://dx.doi.org/10.1136/jcp.2008.060145

246. Rubio-Tapia A, Rahim MW, See JA, Lahr BD, Wu TT, Murray JA. *Mucosal recovery and mortality in adults with celiac disease after treatment with a gluten-free diet.* Am J Gastroenterol. 2010; 105: 1412-20. http://dx.doi.org/10.1038/ajg.2010.10

247. Lanzini A, Lanzarotto F, Villanacci V, *Complete recovery of intestinal mucosa occurs very rarelyet al. Complete recovery of intestinal mucosanoccurs very rarely in adult coeliac patients despite adherence to gluten-free diet.* Aliment Pharmacol Ther. 2009; 29: 1299-308. http://dx.doi.org/10.1111/j.1365-2036.2009.03992.x

248. Mooney PD, Evans KE, Singh S, Sanders DS. *Treatment failure in coeliac disease: a practical guide to investigation and treatment of non-responsive and refractory coeliac disease.* J Gastrointestin Liver Dis. 2012; 21: 197-203.

249. Rubio-Tapia A, Murray JA. *Classification and management of refractory coeliac disease.* Gut. 2010; 59: 547-57. http://dx.doi.org/10.1136/gut.2009.195131

250. Abdulkarim AS, Burgart LJ, See J, Murray JA. *Etiology of nonresponsive celiac disease: results of a systematic approach.* Am J Gastroenterol. 2002; 97: 2016-21.
http://dx.doi.org/10.1111/j.1572-0241.2002.05917.x

251. Leffler DA, Dennis M, Hyett B, Kelly E, Schuppan D, Kelly CP. *Etiologies and predictors of diagnosis in nonresponsive celiac disease.* Clin Gastroenterol Hepatol. 2007; 5: 445-50.
http://dx.doi.org/10.1016/j.cgh.2006.12.006

252. Roshan B, Leffler DA, Jamma S, Dennis M, Sheth S, Falchuk K et al. *The incidence and clinical spectrum of refractory celiac disease in a North American referral center.* Am J Gastroenterol. 2011; 106: 923-8. http://dx.doi.org/10.1038/ajg.2011.104

253. Hall NJ, Rubin G, Charnock A. *Systematic review: adherence to a gluten-free diet in adult patients with coeliac disease.* Aliment Pharmacol Ther. 2009; 30: 315-30.
http://dx.doi.org/10.1111/j.1365-2036.2009.04053.x

254. O'Leary C, Wieneke P, Healy M, Cronin C, O'Regan P, Shanahan F. *Celiac disease and the transition from childhood to adulthood: a 28-year follow-up.* Am J Gastroenterol. 2004; 99: 2437-41. http://dx.doi.org/10.1111/j.1572-0241.2004.40182.x

255. Leffler DA, Edwards-George J, Dennis M, Schuppan D, Cocinero F, Franko DL et al. *Factors that influence adherence to a gluten-free diet in adults with celiac disease.* Dig Dis Sci. 2008; 53: 1573-81. http://dx.doi.org/10.1007/s10620-007-0055-3

256. Akobeng AK, Thomas AG. *Systematic review: tolerable amount of gluten for people with coeliac disease.* Aliment Pharmacol Ther. 2008; 27: 1044-52.
http://dx.doi.org/10.1111/j.1365-2036.2008.03669.x

257. Bardella MT, Velio P, Cesana BM, Prampolini L, Casella G, Di Bella C et al. *Coeliac disease: a histological follow-up study.* Histopathology. 2007; 50: 465-71.
http://dx.doi.org/10.1111/j.1365-2559.2007.02621.x

258. Evans KE, Sanders DS. *Joint BAPEN and British Society of Gastroenterology Symposium on 'Coeliac disease: basics and controversies'. Coeliac disease: optimising the management of patients with persisting symptoms?* Proc Nutr Soc. 2009; 68: 242-8.
http://dx.doi.org/10.1017/S0029665109001360

259. Fine KD, Meyer RL, Lee EL. *The prevalence and causes of chronic diarrhea in patients with celiac sprue treated with a gluten-free diet.* Gastroenterology. 1997; 112: 1830-38.
http://dx.doi.org/10.1053/gast.1997.v112.pm9178673

260. Leeds JS, Hopper AD, Hurlstone DP, Edwards SJ, McAlindon ME, Lobo AJ et al. *Is exocrine pancreatic insufficiency in adult coeliac disease a cause of persisting symptoms?* Aliment Pharmacol Ther. 2007; 25: 265-71.
http://dx.doi.org/10.1111/j.1365-2036.2006.03206.x

261. Carroccio A, Iacono G, Lerro P, Cavataio F, Malorgio E, Soresi M et al. *Role of pancreatic impairment in growth recovery during gluten-free diet in childhood celiac disease.* Gastroenterology. 1997; 112: 1839-44.
http://dx.doi.org/10.1053/gast.1997.v112.pm9178674

262. Tursi A, Brandimarte G, Giorgetti G. *High prevalence of small intestinal bacterial overgrowth in celiac patients with persistence of gastrointestinal symptoms after gluten withdrawal.* Am J Gastroenterol. 2003; 98: 839-43.
http://dx.doi.org/10.1111/j.1572-0241.2003.07379.x

263. Riordan SM, McIver CJ, Walker BM, Duncombe VM, Bolin TD, Thomas MC. *The lactulose breath hydrogen test and small intestinal bacterial overgrowth.* Am J Gastroenterol. 1996; 91: 1795-803.

264. Corazza GR, Strocchi A, Gasbarrini G. *Fasting breath hydrogen in celiac disease.* Gastroenterology. 1987; 93: 53-8.

265. Rubio-Tapia A, Barton SH, Rosenblatt JE, Murray JA. *Prevalence of small intestine bacterial overgrowth diagnosed by quantitative culture of intestinal aspirate in celiac disease.* J Clin Gastroenterol. 2009; 43: 157-161.
http://dx.doi.org/10.1097/MCG.0b013e3181557e67

266. Chang MS, Minaya MT, Cheng J, Connor BA, Lewis SK, Green PH et al. *Double-blind randomized controlled trial of rifaximin for persistent symptoms in patients with celiac disease.* Dig Dis Sci. 2011; 56: 2939-46. http://dx.doi.org/10.1007/s10620-011-1719-6

267. Stewart M, Andrews CN, Urbanski S, Beck PL, Storr M. *The association of coeliac disease and microscopic colitis: a large population-based study.* Aliment Pharmacol Ther. 2011; 33: 1340-9. http://dx.doi.org/10.1111/j.1365-2036.2011.04666.x

268. O'Mahony S, Howdle PD, Losowsky MS. *Review article: management of patients with non-responsive coeliac disease.* Aliment Pharmacol Ther. 1996; 10: 671-80.
http://dx.doi.org/10.1046/j.1365-2036.1996.66237000.x

269. Gomollón F. *Enfermedad celíaca.* En Montoro M, García Pagán JC et al (eds). Gastroenterología y Hepatología. Problemas Comunes en la Práctica Clínica (2ª ed.). Barcelona: Jarpyo editores. 2012: 331-46.

270. Molberg O, Uhlen AK, Jensen T, Flaete NS, Fleckenstein B, Arentz-Hansen H et al. *Mapping of gluten T-cell epitopes in the bread wheat ancestors: implications for celiac disease.* Gastroenterology. 2005; 128: 393-401.
http://dx.doi.org/10.1053/j.gastro.2004.11.003

271. van den Broeck HC, van Herpen TW, Schuit C et al. *Removing celiac disease-related gluten proteins from bread wheat while retaining technological properties: a study with Chinese Spring deletion lines.* BMC Plant Biol. 2009; 9: 41. http://dx.doi.org/10.1186/1471-2229-9-41

272. Piper JL, Gray GM, Khosla C. *Effect of prolyl endopeptidase on digestive-resistant gliadin peptides in vivo.* J Pharmacol Exp Ther. 2004; 311: 213-9. http://dx.doi.org/10.1124/jpet.104.068429

273. Shan L, Marti T, Sollid LM, Gray GM, Khosla C. *Comparative biochemical analysis of three bacterial prolyl endopeptidases: implications for coeliac sprue.* Biochem. 2004; 383: 311-8. http://dx.doi.org/10.1042/BJ20040907

274. Marti T, Molberg O, Li Q, Gray GM, Khosla C, Sollid LM. *Prolyl endopeptidase-mediated destruction of T cell epitopes in whole gluten: chemical and immunological characterization.* J Pharmacol Exp Ther. 2004; 312: 19-26. http://dx.doi.org/10.1124/jpet.104.073312

275. Pyle GG, Paaso B, Anderson BE, Allen DD, Marti T, Li Q. *Effect of pretreatment of food gluten with prolyl endopeptidase on gluten induced malabsorption in celiac sprue.* Clin Gastroenterol Hepatol. 2005; 3: 687-94. http://dx.doi.org/10.1016/S1542-3565(05)00366-6

276. Tye-Din JA, AndersonRP, FfrenchRA, Brown GJ, Hodsman P, Siegel M. *The effects of ALV003 pre-digestion of gluten on immune response and symptoms in coeliacdisease in vivo.* Clin Immunol. 2010; 134: 289-95. http://dx.doi.org/10.1016/j.clim.2009.11.001

277. Fasano A, Not T, Wang W, Uzzau S, Berti I, Tommasini A et al. *Zonulin, a newly discovered modulator of intestinal permeability, and its expression in coeliac disease.* Lancet. 2000; 355: 1518-9. http://dx.doi.org/10.1016/S0140-6736(00)02169-3

278. Paterson BM, Lammers KM, Arrieta MC, Fasano A, Meddings JB. *The safety, tolerance, pharmacokinetic and pharmacodynamic effects of single doses of AT-1001 in celiac disease subjects: a proof of concept study.* Aliment Pharmacol Ther. 2007; 26: 757-66. http://dx.doi.org/10.1111/j.1365-2036.2007.03413.x

279. Szondy Z Nemeth T, Piacentini M, Mastroberardino PG. *Transglutaminase 2–/– mice reveal a phagocytosis-associated crosstalk between macrophages and apoptotic cells.* Proc Natl Acad Sci. 2003; 100: 7812-7. http://dx.doi.org/10.1073/pnas.0832466100

280. Choi K, Siegel M, Piper J, Nemeth T, Piacentini M, Mastroberardino PG et al. *Chemistry and biology of dihydroisoxazole derivatives: selective inhibitors of human transglutaminase 2.* Chem Biol. 2005; 12: 469-75. http://dx.doi.org/10.1016/j.chembiol.2005.02.007

281. Shweke N, Boulos N, Jouanneau C, Vandermeersch S, Melino G, Dussaule JC. *Tissue transglutaminase contributes to interstitial renal fibrosis by favoring accumulation of fibrillar collagen through TGF-beta activation and cell infiltration.* Am J Pathol. 2008; 173: 631-42. http://dx.doi.org/10.2353/ajpath.2008.080025

282. Shao M, Cao L, Shen C, Vandermeersch S, Melino G, Dussaule JC et al. *Epithelial-to-mesenchymal transition and ovarian tumor progression induced by tissue transglutaminase.* Cancer Res. 2009; 69: 9192-201. http://dx.doi.org/10.1158/0008-5472.CAN-09-1257

283. Ruan Q, Johnson GV. *Transglutaminase 2 in neurodegenerative disorders.* Front Biosci. 2007; 12: 891-904. http://dx.doi.org/10.2741/2111

284. Xia J, Siegel M, Bergseng E, Sollid LM, Khosla C. *Inhibition of HLA-DQ2-mediated antigen presentation by analogues of a high affinity 33-residue peptide from alpha2-gliadin.* J Am Chem Soc. 2006; 128: 1859-67. http://dx.doi.org/10.1021/ja056423o

285. Jüse U, van de Wal Y, Koning F, Sollid LM, Fleckenstein B. *Design of new high-affinity peptide ligands for human leukocyte antigen-DQ2 using a positional scanning peptide library.* Hum Immunol. 2010; 71: 475-81.
http://dx.doi.org/10.1016/j.humimm.2010.01.021

286. Schuppan D, Junker Y, Barisani D. *Celiac disease: from pathogenesis to novel therapies.* Gastroenterology. 2009; 137: 1912-33. http://dx.doi.org/10.1053/j.gastro.2009.09.008

287. Reinisch W, de Villiers W, Bene L, Simon L, Rácz I, Katz S et al. *Fontolizumab inmoderate to severe Crohn's disease: a phase 2, randomized, double-blind, placebo-controlled, multiple-dose study.* Inflamm Bowel Dis. 2010; 16(2): 233-42.
http://dx.doi.org/10.1002/ibd.21038

288. Costantino G, della Torre A, Lo Presti MA, Caruso R, Mazzon E, Frites W et al. *Treatment of life threatening type I refractory celiac disease with long-term infliximab.* Dig Liver Dis. 2008; 40: 74-7. http://dx.doi.org/10.1016/j.dld.2006.10.017

289. Di Sabatino A, Ciccocioppo R, Cupelli F, Cinque B, Millimaggi D, Clarkson MM et al. *Epithelium derived interleukin 15 regulates intraepithelial lymphocyte Th1 cytokine production, cytotoxicity, and survival in coeliac disease.* Gut. 2006; 55: 469-77. http://dx.doi.org/10.1136/gut.2005.068684

290. Malamut G, El Machhour R, Montcuquet N, Martin-Lannerée S, Dusanter-Fourt I, Verkarre V et al. *IL-15 triggers an antiapoptotic pathway in human intraepithelial lymphocytes that is a potential new target in celiac disease associated inflammation and lymphomagenesis.* J Clin Invest. 2010; 120: 2131-43.
http://dx.doi.org/10.1172/JCI41344

291. Ghosh S, Goldin E, Gordon FH, Malchow HA, Rask-Madsen J, Rutgeerts P et al. *Natalizumab for active Crohn's disease.* N Engl J Med. 2003; 348: 24-32.
http://dx.doi.org/10.1056/NEJMoa020732

Chapter 13

Type 1 Marsh Celiac Disease: Diagnosis and Response

Fernando Fernández Bañares, Meritxell Mariné, Mercè Rosinach, Anna Carrasco, Maria Esteve

Gastroenterology Service, Hospital Universitari Mutua Terrassa, University of Barcelona, CIBERehd, Terrassa, Barcelona, Spain.

ffbanares@mutuaterrassa.es, mmarine@mutuaterrassa.es, mrosinach@mutuaterrassa.es, acarrasco@mutuaterrassa.es, mariaesteve@mutuaterrassa.es

Doi: http://dx.doi.org/10.3926/oms.214

How to cite this chapter

Fernández Bañares F, Mariné M, Rosinach M, Carrasco A, Esteve M. *Type 1 Marsh Celiac Disease: Diagnosis and Response.* In Rodrigo L and Peña AS, editors. *Celiac Disease and Non-Celiac Gluten Sensitivity.* Barcelona, Spain: OmniaScience; 2014. p. 289-302.

F. Fernández Bañares, M. Mariné, M. Rosinach, A. Carrasco, M. Esteve

Abstract

The histological Marsh classification distinguishes three types of lesion, among which gluten-sensitive enteropathy with a Type 1 Marsh lesion is the most difficult to diagnose. Unlike Marsh 3 lesion, which almost always corresponds to celiac disease, Marsh 1 lesion has a wider differential diagnosis. This is further compounded by the absence of celiac disease-specific antibodies in up to 80% of the patients with a Marsh 1 lesion. For all these reasons, gluten-sensitive enteropathy diagnosis in Marsh type 1 lesions has become a challenge for clinicians. In recent years, new diagnostic techniques have emerged in order to distinguish gluten-dependent from non-gluten dependent Marsh 1 lesions. In this sense, the presence of transglutaminase IgA subepithelial deposits or increased intraepithelial lymphocytes expressing TCR gamma/delta in the duodenal mucosa strongly suggest the diagnosis of celiac disease. Another important issue is to determine which patients with a Marsh type 1 lesion should be treated. It should be noted that up to 50% of patients with minimal lesions present the same symptoms as those with Marsh 3 lesion, which suggests that they will benefit from a Gluten-Free Diet (GFD). Ultimately, the diagnosis of celiac disease cannot rely on the results of a single test and requires a good understanding of clinical, serological, genetic and histological criteria and of the GFD response.

1. Introduction

Celiac disease (CD) is an enteropathy caused by an immune reaction triggered by dietary gluten, a protein found in wheat, rye and barley, that manifests in genetically predisposed individuals. Since the first morphological lesion description by John Paulley in 1954, CD diagnosis was based precisely on the demonstration of the characteristic, gluten-dependent small intestinal lesion. This basic general concept is still valid. However, in recent decades, the discovery of accurate diagnostic methods (serological and genetic), through mass screening techniques or evaluating risk groups, has allowed the identification of large numbers of patients with silent or paucisymptomatic forms. This has afforded the knowledge that CD is not a rare disease, that its spectrum of clinical manifestations, both in type and severity, is very wide, and that there is not always a correlation between the severity of the histological lesion and intensity of the clinical manifestations. In this regard, an important change in CD diagnostic criteria has been the gradual acceptance that histologically mild enteropathy forms (type 1 Marsh lesions, also called lymphocytic enteritis, lymphocytic enteropathy or lymphocytic duodenosis) are also part of the CD spectrum and are to be treated as such when they produce clinically relevant symptoms or signs.

2. Histological Spectrum of Celiac Disease

In 1992 Michael N. Marsh published a classification scheme of histological lesion degrees based on the results of dynamic studies on gluten challenge which allowed to describe the whole histological injury spectrum.[1] This classification, subsequently modified by Oberhuber, Granditsch and Vogelsang, is the most widely accepted one among clinicians and patologists.[2] However, simpler schemes have been proposed, with fewer categories, allowing a greater degree of consistency and reproducibility between pathologists (Table 1).[3,4] In these more recent classifications type 2 or crypt hyperplasia has been eliminated, as this histological lesion phase is very unstable (fleetingly detected during lesion's progression towards atrophy)[1] and type 4 (related to CD refractory forms) which is usually diagnosed with cytometric and immunohistochemical techniques, showing an aberrant clonal expansion,[4] has also been eliminated.

In the most recent classification scheme, Ensari proposes maintaining Corazza's classification of lesion severity levels, but exchanges the term "degree" for "type", in order to avoid using a term which pathologists use for grading tumors.[4]

Thus, the most recent classification scheme foresees 3 levels of lesion severity:

Type 1: Preserved villous structure with increased intraepithelial lymphocytes (lymphocytic enteropathy, lymphocytic duodenosis or lymphocytic enteritis) and the few detected cases of crypt hyperplasia.
Type 2: Villi shortening (<3:1 or <2:1 in duodenal bulb) plus type 1 findings.
Type 3: Complete flattening of the villi plus type 1 findings.

An essential aspect of anatomopathological diagnosis is to establish the normal limits of the intestinal mucosa, this is particularly important in lesions with preserved villous architecture. The generally accepted limit of normality for the amount intraepithelial lymphocytes is of 25 for each 100 epithelial cells[5-7] and it is advisable to systematically perform CD3 immunostaining which allows for a better differentiation between lymphocytes and epithelial cell nuclei.[4] To facilitate cell count it has been proposed to examine 20 enterocytes on 5 well-oriented villi considering the normal limit to be of less than 5 lymphocytes per each 20 enterocytes.[4]

Marsh 1992[1]	Oberhuber et al. 1999[2]	Corazza & Villanaci 2005[3]	Ensari 2010[4]
Type 1 Infiltrative lesion	Type 1 Infiltrative lesion	Grade A Infiltrative lesion	Type 1 Infiltrative lesion
Type 2 Crypt hyperplasia	Type 2 Crypt hyperplasia	Discarded Incorporated into Grade A	Discarded Incorporated into Type 1
Type 3 Atrophy	Type 3: Atrophy Type 3A: Partial Type 3B: Subtotal Type 3C: Total	Atrophy Grade B1 Grade B1 Grade B2	Atrophy Type 2 Type 2 Type 3
Type 4 Destructive lesion	Type 4 Destructive lesion	Obsolete	Obsolete

Table 1. Classification schemes for the histopathological evaluation of gluten-sensitive enteropathy.

3. Definition of Marsh Type 1 Lesions and Differential Diagnosis of Lymphocytic Enteropathy

The gluten-sensitive enteropathy spectrum of histopathological lesion is not pathognomonic to this entity, since other entities may produce indistinguishable microscopic lesions (Table 2).[4,8,9] The differential diagnosis is even broader for minimal lesions with conserved architecture than for villous atrophy. Lymphocytic enteropathy-type lesions can result from an unspecific and transient response of the intestine to multiple lesions (allergic, infectious, and toxic). In many cases the frequency of these alterations and their clinical relevance are not well established. However, in cases where there have been systematic studies to determine the frequency and severity of a lesion associated with specific agents, such as the parasite *Giardia lamblia*, it has been observed that atrophy and intraepithelial lymphocytosis are rarely produced by this parasite.[10]

Villous atrophy-causing diseases, besides CD, are generally too infrequent, such as microvillus inclusion disease, neonatal enteropathy or autoimmune enteropathy, which primarily affect children. In developed countries, gastrointestinal atrophy-causing infections are also much less frequent than in developing countries. On the other hand, the differential diagnosis with lymphocytic enteropathy is more difficult.[11-16] Lymphocytic enteropathy caused by *Helicobacter pylori* is a challenging diagnosis and, in much the same way as that produced by gluten sensitivity, it may be clinically relevant. Therefore, reaching an etiologic diagnosis is essential. Other common lymphocytic enteropathy causes to be ruled out are NSAIDs lesion, food hypersensitivity in children, *Blastocystis hominis* parasitosis and Crohn's disease. Currently, an etiologic diagnosis can take a long time, since the response to sequential treatments must be determined and this requires a great deal of motivation, discipline and acceptance by both the patient and the physician.[15-17] Research in this field is nowadays focusing on finding cell markers (immunohistochemical and cytometric) and/or molecular which may allow the establishment of a baseline etiologic diagnosis without having to wait for the response to a specific treatment.

Intraepithelial lymphocytosis (Type 1)	Atrophy (Types 2 and 3)
• Gastroduodenitis caused by *H. pylori* • Hipersensitivity to food • Infections (viral, parasitic, bacterial) • Bacterial overgrowth • Pharmacological drugs (mainly NSAIDs) • IgA deficit • Common variable immunodeficiency • Crohn's disease	• Microvillus inclusion disease • Autoimmune enteropathy • Tropical sprue • Collagenous sprue • Refractory celiac disease (including enteropathy associated T cell lymphoma). • Lesions due to irradiation and/or chemotherapy. • Graft vs host disease • Nutritional deficits

Table 2. Histopathological differential diagnosis of gluten-sensitive enteropathy.[4,8,9,11-17]

4. Diagnostic Criteria for Celiac Disease Patients with Lymphocytic Enteropathy-Type Lesion

Recently, it has been considered that, to reach a CD diagnosis, 4 out of 5 of the diagnostic criteria described in Table 3 are needed. This is what has been called the "4 out of 5" rule.[18] According to these criteria, patients with type 1 Marsh lesions can be diagnosed with CD upon finding of typical CD serum antibodies (IgA anti-endomysium, IgA anti-transglutaminase or deamidated anti-gliadin) or, if there is negative serology, when subepithelial IgA transglutaminase deposits can be found. Recent ESPGHAN diagnostic criteria for CD in children and adolescents are plentiful in this sense.[19]

However, it is well known that celiac serology is often negative in the milder forms of CD: in 30% of the patients with partial villus atrophy and up to 80% of those with Marsh 1 lesions.[20,21] Gluten challenges have been performed in these patients in order to determine if this tends to worsen the histologic lesion or if antibodies become positive[15,22], which would lead to a CD diagnosis. Furthermore, the presence of subepithelial IgA transglutaminase deposits or increased intraepithelial lymphocytes expressing gamma/delta TCR has been considered suggestive of celiac disease.[19,23,24] To benefit from these new diagnostic techniques it is necessary to obtain duodenal mucosa samples which must be immediately frozen in liquid nitrogen and processed by immunofluorescence under confocal microscopy to determine subepithelial deposits or by means of immunohistochemistry for TCR gamma/delta.

• Typical celiac disease symptoms[*1]
• High titers of IgA-class celiac disease serum antibodies[*2]
• HLA-DQ2 o DQ8 haplotypes[*3]
• Celiac type enteropathy in small intestinal biopsy[*4]
• Response to the GFD[*5]

[*1]Examples: chronic diarrhea, growth delay in children or weight loss in adults, iron deficit anemia.
[*2]10 x times the normal value (IgG-class in subjects with IgA deficit).
[*3]Also with only half the heterodimer (positive HLA-DQB1*02).
[*4]Including Marsh 1 to 3 lesions associated with positive celiac serology with high/low titers and Marsh 1 to 3 lesions associated to IgA subepithelial deposits.
[*5]Clinical and histologic response in patients with negative serology.

Table 3. Celiac disease diagnostic criteria: "4 out of 5" rule.[18]

Response to the GFD is an important diagnostic criterion in patients with type Marsh 1 lesions and it is still essential to document the histological response in patients with negative serology for proper diagnosis of CD. In research studies our group has used the following criteria in order to define whether a complete or partial histological response to the GFD is occurring:[25] a) Complete response: Evolution of Marsh-Oberhuber types 3, 2 and 1 to type 0, or, in type 1, at least a reduction of over 50% in the number of intraepithelial lymphocytes in relation to a baseline biopsy; b) Partial response: Improvement of the atrophy degree (Marsh-Oberhuber type 3C to 3B-3A or Ensari type 3 to type 2) and in the case of patients with a type 1 baseline biopsy, at least an intraepithelial lymphocyte reduction of 25% to 50% in relation to the baseline biopsy. Given the possible existence of a patchy lesion and to properly assess the response it is necessary to clearly identify the location (bulb, distal duodenum or jejunum) for the taking of samples in both the basal biopsy and in posterior control biopsies. These criteria may be useful and applicable in routine clinical practice.

The adequate time to carry out the follow-up biopsy after starting the gluten-free diet has not yet been well established, even in patients with villous atrophy. In a recent systematic review of the literature it has been recommended not to perform it before 1-2 years have elapsed after beginning of the diet.[26] If there is mucosal healing, there is no justification for further biopsies, except for the appearance of changes in clinical status. If histological improvement is incomplete, it would probably be necessary to perform a new control 1-2 years later.

4.1. Usefulness of Intraepithelial γδ+ Determination

The γδ+ intraepithelial lymphocyte determination is considered useful in doubtful or difficult cases.[27] In CD patients these γδ+ T cells are increased in all stages of the disease, both in untreated CD and under the gluten-free diet.[27] It has also seen that they are increased both in potential and latent CD.[28,29] This increase in γδ+ T cells has not been observed in other common intestinal diseases, thus it is possible to affirm that CD is the only disease in which they are systematically, permanently and intensely increased.[27]

An increase in this type of cells has been detected in most patients with mild enteropathy.[30] Therefore, their determination may be useful in the differential diagnosis of lymphocytic enteropathy.

4.2. Diagnostic Utility of Tissue IgA Transglutaminase Subepithelial Deposits

It has been shown that the production of CD autoantibodies happens locally in the small intestinal mucosa, where they pass into to the bloodstream. However, besides being detectable in the bloodstream, these autoantibodies remain sequestered in the place where they have been produced. In untreated CD it is possible to detect tTG IgA deposits in the intestinal mucosa subepithelially and around blood vessels.[31] Interestingly, these deposits can be detected in patients with positive EMA and without villous atrophy[30,32,33] and even in patients with negative serology and Marsh type 1-3 lesions.[34-36]

In a recent series of studies on untreated CD it was demonstrated that 100% of 261 patients with villous atrophy had subepithelial IgA tTG deposits (9% had negative serum EMA), 90% had moderate to strong intensity. In contrast, 18% of the controls had deposits of minor intensity. After the gluten-free diet, there was a gradual decrease in the intensity of these deposits, which remained positive, in the long term, in 56% of the patients. The sensitivity and specificity of these deposits for CD diagnosis was of 100% and 82%, however, serology sensitivity and specificity were of 91% and 100% respectively.[36]

In a study on children with positive EMA or tTG and positive genetics (HLA-DQ2 or DQ8) but no villous atrophy, IgA tTG deposits were detected in 85% of 39 patients. Similarly, a study on another group of children revealed negative serology and Marsh type I lesions, with increased gamma/delta intraepithelial lymphocytes, allowing the detection of IgA tTG deposits in 66% of 18 patients. Instead such deposits were detected in 9% of 34 children with normal intestinal mucosa and absence of gluten sensitivity markers.[35]

4.3. Emerging Diagnostic Tools: Intraepithelial CD3+TCRγδ+ and CD3- Determination by Flow Cytometry

Flow cytometry is a powerful analytical tool for the study of intraepithelial lymphocytes (IEL) compared to immunohistochemistry. It allows fast, sensitive, reproducible and objective semi-quantitative results. Since an increase of CD3+TCRγδ+ and a decrease in CD3- IEL has been previously described as a characteristic flow cytometric pattern (FCP) of CD with atrophy,[37-39] a recent study[40] has evaluated the usefulness of this technique for diagnosing lymphocytic enteritis due to CD. In this recent study 205 patients (144 females) who underwent duodenal biopsy for clinical suspicion of CD and positive celiac genetics were evaluated. Fifty had villous atrophy, 70 lymphocytic enteritis, and 85 normal histology. Eight patients with non-celiac atrophy and 15 with lymphocytic enteritis secondary to Helicobacter pylori acted as control group. Duodenal biopsies were obtained to assess two typical flow cytometric patterns (FCP): complete CD FCP, was defined when TCRγδ+ ≥8.5% and CD3- ≤10% were detected, and incomplete CD FCP was defined when an isolated TCR γδ+ increase (≥8.5%) was detected. Moreover, anti-TG2 IgA subepithelial deposit analysis (CD IF pattern) was also assessed. Sensitivity of IF pattern, and complete and incomplete cytometric patterns for CD diagnosis in patients with positive serology (Marsh 1+3) was 92%, 85 and 97% respectively, but only the complete cytometric pattern had 100% specificity. CD cytometric pattern showed a better diagnostic performance than both IF pattern and serology for CD diagnosis in lymphocytic enteritis at baseline (95% vs 60% vs 60%, p=0.039). Thus, IEL flow cytometric pattern seems to be an accurate method for identifying CD in the initial diagnostic biopsy of patients presenting with lymphocytic enteritis, even in seronegative patients, and seems also to be better than anti-TG2 intestinal deposits.

5. Relationship between Clinical Manifestations and Degree of Histological Lesion

It was formerly thought that type 1 Marsh lesions were not associated with symptoms or signs of malabsoption.[39] However, recent studies suggest otherwise. In a multicenter study on first-degree relatives, using a diagnostic method consisting of genetic testing followed by intestinal biopsy in positive cases, we observed that a similar percentage of relatives with type 1 and 3 lesions had symptoms when compared with relatives with normal intestinal mucosa (56% and 54% vs 21%, p=0.002) (Table 4).[40] It is important to note that, in this study, relatives with lymphocytic enteropathy were diagnosed by screening within this risk group and not by their symptoms, yielding, therefore, the actual frequency of symptomatic patients in this group.

Symptoms (%)	Normal mucosa	Type 1 lesion	Type 2-3 lesion	p value
Abdominal pain	23	41	38.5	0.20
Diarrrhea	22	41	38.5	0.14
Flatulence	39	69	57	0.02
Bloating	22	56	57	0.003
Asthenia	16	47	46	0.002
Hypertransaminasemia	1.5	9	7	0.11
Osteoporosis/ Osteopenia	–	37	44	0.76

Table 4. Frequency of symptoms in first-degree relatives depending on the type of histological lesion (Modified from Esteve et al.[40]).

Another recent study compared the clinical features and analytical alterations between 1249 atrophy patients and 159 with mild enteropathy.[41] Gastrointestinal manifestations (70% vs 70%) and extraintestinal (66% vs 57%) appeared with similar frequencies in both groups.

These and similar studies have unequivocally established that patients with mild histological forms of celiac enteropathy do not suffer from a mild disease and can benefit from the GFD as well as those with atrophy.[25,42]

Although it is unknown whether individuals with lymphocytic enteropathy have the same risk of malignancy and autoimmune diseases than patients with atrophy, indirect evidence suggests that it is probably not so.[43] Therefore, the GFD is recommended for patients with lymphocytic enteropathy only if they are symptomatic (anemia, osteoporosis or both intestinal and extraintestinal bowel symptoms), mainly if the symptoms are serious and affect the quality of life. Moreover, and as already mentioned, in patients with lymphocytic enteropathy it is very important to make a correct differential diagnosis. The gluten-free diet is indicated only in symptomatic cases in which there is an unequivocal demonstration of the relationship between histological lesions and gluten intake.

6. Proposed Diagnostic Algorithm

Symptoms S	Antibodies A	Genotype G	Endoscopy/ Histology E	Score Points
Malabsorption syndrome	EmA+ and/or anti-TG2 >10xULN	×	Marsh 3b o 3c	2
Relevant CD symptoms or type 1 diabetes or first-degree relatives	Anti-TG2+ <10xULN or only anti-DGP+	Full HLA-DQ2 and/or DQ8 heterodimer	Marsh 2 or 3a or Marsh 0-1 with anti-TG2 deposits and/or an increase in lymphocytes expressing TCR gamma/delta	1
Asymptomatic	No serology available	No HLA results or only half of DQ2 (DQB1*0202)	No available histology or Marsh 0-1	0
×	All CD antibodies negative	Negative DQ2/DQ8	×	-1

Table 5. Celiac disease diagnostic algorithm: SAGE score (modified from Husby et al.[19]; the presence of gamma/delta T cells+ has been added to 0-1 Marsh histology as suggested in the literature (see corresponding section).

Recently a diagnostic algorithm has been proposed which is based on using a point scale ranging from -1 to 2 to rate symptoms, celiac antibodies, celiac genotype and suggestive endoscopic and histological changes which allows the CD diagnosis without referring to the response to the GFD (table 5).[19] The CD diagnosis becomes firm with a final score of 4 points or more. To diagnose CD when this score is lower than 4, which generally occurs in patients with negative celiac serology, it is necessary to consider the response to the GFD. In patients with suspected type 1 CD it is always necessary to assess the clinical and histological response to the GFD.

7. Difficult Cases: Overlap with Non-Celiac Gluten Hypersensitivity

Recent studies, including a placebo-controlled clinical trial have shown the existence of an entity known as non-celiac gluten-sensitivity.[44-46] This entity appears in patients who, having no duodenal histological lesion nor genetic predisposition to CD, have symptoms triggered by gluten consumption. There are still important problems in defining these patients since many authors consider that the definition encompasses those who have positive celiac disease genetics (40% of these patients are HLA-DQ2 positive) and lymphocytic duodenal infiltration. Therefore, the overlap between patients with non-celiac gluten sensitivity and celiac disease patients with type I Marsh lesion becomes evident and differential diagnosis quite difficult. It is possible that, in the future, the availability of cellular or molecular markers may help in the differential diagnosis.

8. Conclusions

In conclusion, all studies and data reviewed here demonstrate that CD diagnosis cannot rely on one single test. Collaboration between clinicians, immunologists and pathologists is essential to integrate clinical, serological, genetic and histological criteria, as well as the response to the GFD. In other words, although in many patients the presumptive diagnosis, with a high probability of success, can be performed with fewer data ("4 out of 5" rule),[13-15] it is necessary to have as much information as possible whenever possible ("5 out of 5"rule). And this is not only important for the initial diagnosis as it also is for management during the follow-up, as it is common for diagnostic doubts to arise when basal key points are not well known, and it is of relevance when there is an inadequate patient evolution. In the case of type 1 lesions, the requirement to obtain as much information as possible is even more accentuated, being necessary to frequently employ new diagnostic tools such as counting intraepithelial lymphocytes which express gamma/delta TCR or the study of IgA tTG subepithelial deposits.

References

1. Marsh MN. *Gluten, major histocompatibility complex, and the small intestine. A molecular and immunobiologic approach to the spectrum of gluten sensitivity ('celiac sprue').* Gastroenterology. 1992; 102: 330-54.

2. Oberhuber G, Granditsch G, Vogelsang H. *The histopathology of coeliac disease: time for a standardized report scheme for pathologists.* Eur J Gastroenterol Hepatol. 1999; 11: 1185-94. http://dx.doi.org/10.1097/00042737-199910000-00019

3. Corazza GR, Villanacci V. *Coeliac disease.* J Clin Pathol. 2005; 58: 573-4. http://dx.doi.org/10.1136/jcp.2004.023978

4. Ensari A. *Gluten-sensitive enteropathy (celiac disease): controversies in diagnosis and classification.* Arch Pathol Lab Med. 2010; 134: 826-36.

5. Hayat M, Cairns A, Dixon MF, O'Mahony S. *Quantitation of intraepithelial lymphocytes in human duodenum: what is normal?.* J Clin Pathol. 2002; 55: 393-5. http://dx.doi.org/10.1136/jcp.55.5.393

6. Walker MM, Murray JA, Ronkainen J, Aro P, Storskrubb T, D'Amato M, et al. *Detection of celiac disease and lymphocytic enteropathy by parallel serology and histopathology in a population-based study.* Gastroenterology. 2010; 139: 112-9. http://dx.doi.org/10.1053/j.gastro.2010.04.007

7. Walker MM, Murray JA. *An update in the diagnosis of coeliac disease.* Histopathology. 2011; 59: 166-79. http://dx.doi.org/10.1111/j.1365-2559.2010.03680.x

8. Chang F, Mahadeva U, Deere H. *Pathological and clinical significance of increased intraepithelial lymphocytes (IELs) in small bowel mucosa.* APMIS 2005; 113: 385-99. http://dx.doi.org/10.1111/j.1600-0463.2005.apm_204.x

9. Carmack SW, Lash RH, Gulizia JM, Genta RM. *Lymphocytic disorders of the gastrointestinal tract: a review for the practicing pathologist.* Adv Anat Pathol. 2009; 16: 290-306. http://dx.doi.org/10.1097/PAP.0b013e3181b5073a

10. Koot BG, ten Kate FJ, Juffrie M, Rosalina I, Taminiau JJ, Benninga MA. *Does Giardia lamblia cause villous atrophy in children?: A retrospective cohort study of the histological abnormalities in giardiasis.* J Pediatr Gastroenterol Nutr. 2009; 49: 304-8. http://dx.doi.org/10.1097/MPG.0b013e31818de3c4

11. Van de Voort JL, Murray JA, Lahr BD, Van Dyke CT, Kroning CM, Moore SB et al. *Lymphocytic duodenosis and the spectrum of celiac disease.* Am J Gastroenterol. 2009; 104: 142-8. http://dx.doi.org/10.1038/ajg.2008.7

12. Memeo L, Jhang J, Hibshoosh H, Green PH, Rotterdam H, Bhagat G. *Duodenal intraepithelial lymphocytosis with normal villous architecture: common occurrence in H. pylori gastritis.* Mod Pathol. 2005; 18: 1134-44. http://dx.doi.org/10.1038/modpathol.3800404

13. Nahon S, Patey-Mariaud De Serre N, Lejeune O, Huchet FX, Lahmek P, Lesgourgues B et al. *Duodenal intraepithelial lymphocytosis during Helicobacter pylori infection is reduced by antibiotic treatment.* Histopathology. 2006; 48: 417-23. http://dx.doi.org/10.1111/j.1365-2559.2006.02358.x

14. Kakar S, Nehra V, Murray JA, Dayharsh GA, Burgart LJ. *Significance of intraepithelial lymphocytosis in small bowel biopsy samples with normal mucosal architecture.* Am J Gastroenterol. 2003; 98: 2027-33. http://dx.doi.org/10.1111/j.1572-0241.2003.07631.x

15. Aziz I, Evans KE, Hopper AD, Smillie DM, Sanders DS. *A prospective study into the etiology of lymphocytic duodenosis.* Aliment Pharmacol Ther. 2010; 32: 1392-7. http://dx.doi.org/10.1111/j.1365-2036.2010.04477.x

16. Rosinach M, Esteve M, González C, Temiño R, Mariné M, Monzón H et al. *Lymphocytic duodenosis: aetiology and long-term response to specific treatment.* Dig Liver Dis. 2012; 44: 643-8. http://dx.doi.org/10.1016/j.dld.2012.03.006

17. Monzón H, Forné M, González C, Esteve M, Martí JM, Rosinach M et al. *Mild enteropathy as a cause of iron-deficiency anaemia of previously unknown origin.* Dig Liver Dis. 2011; 43: 448-53. http://dx.doi.org/10.1016/j.dld.2010.12.003

18. Catassi C, Fasano A. *Celiac disease diagnosis: simple rules are better than complicated algorithms.* Am J Med. 2010; 123: 691-3. http://dx.doi.org/10.1016/j.amjmed.2010.02.019

19. Husby S, Koletzko S, Korponay-Szabó IR, Mearin ML, Phillips A, Shamir R et al. *ESPGHAN Working Group on Coeliac Disease Diagnosis; ESPGHAN Gastroenterology Committee; European Society for Pediatric Gastroenterology, Hepatology and Nutrition. European Society for Pediatric Gastroenterology, Hepatology, and Nutrition guidelines for the diagnosis of coeliac disease.* J Pediatr Gastroenterol Nutr. 2012; 54: 136-60. http://dx.doi.org/10.1097/MPG.0b013e31821a23d0

20. Rostami K, Kerckhaert J, Tiemessen R, von Blomberg BM, Meijer JW, Mulder CJ. *Sensitivity of antiendomysium and antigliadin antibodies in untreated celiac disease: disappointing in clinical practice.* Am J Gastroenterol. 1999; 94: 888-94. http://dx.doi.org/10.1111/j.1572-0241.1999.983_f.x

21. Santaolalla R, Fernández-Bañares F, Rodríguez R, Alsina M, Rosinach M, Mariné M et al. *Diagnostic value of duodenal antitissue transglutaminase antibodies in gluten-sensitive enteropathy.* Aliment Pharmacol Ther. 2008; 27: 820-9. http://dx.doi.org/10.1111/j.1365-2036.2008.03652.x

22. Wahab PJ, Meijer JWR, Goerres MS, Mulder CJJ. *Coeliac disease: Changing views on gluten-sensitive enteropathy.* Scand J Gastroenterol. 2002; 37 Suppl 236: 60-5. http://dx.doi.org/10.1080/003655202320621472

23. Järvinen TT, Kaukinen K, Laurila K, Kyrönpalo S, Rasmussen M, Mäki M et al. *Intraepithelial lymphocytes in celiac disease.* Am J Gastroenterol. 2003; 98: 1332-7. http://dx.doi.org/10.1111/j.1572-0241.2003.07456.x

24. Järvinen TT, Collin P, Rasmussen M, Kyrönpalo S, Mäki M, Partanen J et al. *Villous tip intraepithelial lymphocytes as markers of early-stage coeliac disease.* Scand J Gastroenterol. 2004 May; 39(5): 428-33. http://dx.doi.org/10.1080/00365520310008773

25. Mariné M, Fernández-Bañares F, Alsina M, Farré C, Cortijo M, Santaolalla R, et al. *Impact of mass screening for gluten-sensitive enteropathy in working population.* World J Gastroenterol. 2009; 15: 1331-8. http://dx.doi.org/10.3748/wjg.15.1331

26. Haines ML, Anderson RP, Gibson PR. *Systematic review: The evidence base for long-term management of coeliac disease.* Aliment Pharmacol Ther. 2008; 28: 1042-66. http://dx.doi.org/10.1111/j.1365-2036.2008.03820.x

27. Leon F. *Flow cytometry of intestinal intraepithelial lymphocytes in celiac disease.* J Immunol Meth. 2011; 363: 177-86. http://dx.doi.org/10.1016/j.jim.2010.09.002

28. Camarero C, Eiras P, Asensio A, Leon F, Olivares F, Escobar H et al. *Intraepithelial lymphocytes and celiac disease: permanent changes in CD3-/CD7- and T cell receptor γδ subsets studied by flow cytometry.* Act Paediatr. 2000; 89: 285-90.
http://dx.doi.org/10.1111/j.1651-2227.2000.tb01330.x

29. Arranz E, Ferguson A. *Intestinal antibody pattern of celiac disease: occurrence in patients with normal jejunal biopsy histology.* Gastroenterology. 1993; 104: 1263.

30. Salmi TT, Collin P, Reunala T, Mäki M, Kaukien K. *Diagnostic methods beyond conventional histology in celiac disease diagnosis.* Dig Liver Dis. 2010; 42: 28-32.
http://dx.doi.org/10.1016/j.dld.2009.04.004

31. Korponay-Szabó IR, Halttunen T, Szalai Z, Király R, Kovács JB, Fésüs L et al. *In vivo targeting of intestinal and extraintestinal transglutaminase 2 by celiac autoantobodies.* Gut. 2004; 53: 641-8. http://dx.doi.org/10.1136/gut.2003.024836

32. Kurppa K, Ashorn M, Iltanen S, Koskinen LLE, Saavalainen P, Koskinen O et al. *Celiac disease without villous atrophy in children: A prospective study.* J Pediatr. 2010; 157: 373-80. http://dx.doi.org/10.1016/j.jpeds.2010.02.070

33. Salmi TT, Collin P, Korponay-Szabó IR, Laurila K, Partanen J, Huhtala H et al. *Endomysial antibody-negative celiac disease: clinical characteristics and intestinal autoantibody deposits.* Gut. 2006; 55: 1746-53. http://dx.doi.org/10.1136/gut.2005.071514

34. Salmi TT, Collin P, Järvinen O, Haimila K, Partanen J, Laurila K et al. *Immunoglobulin A autoantibodies against transglutaminase 2 in the small intestinal mucosa predict forthcoming celiac disease.* Aliment Pharmacol Ther. 2006; 24: 541-52.
http://dx.doi.org/10.1111/j.1365-2036.2006.02997.x

35. Tosco A, Maglio M, Paparo F, Rapacciuolo L, Sannino A, Miele E et al. *Immunoglobulin A anti-tissue transglutaminase antibody deposits in the small intestinal mucosa of children with no villous atrophy.* J Pediatr Gastroenterol Nutr. 2008; 47: 293-8.
http://dx.doi.org/10.1097/MPG.0b013e3181677067

36. Koskinen O, Collin P, Lindfords K, Laurila K, Mäki M, Kaukinen K. *Usefulness of small bowel mucosal transglutaminase-2 specific autoantibody deposits in the diagnosis and follow-up of celiac disease.* J Clin Gastroenterol. 2010; 44: 483-8.

37. Calleja S, Vivas S, Santiuste M, et al. *Dynamics of non-convencional intraepithelial lymphocytes-NK, NKT and γδ T-in celiac disease: Relationship with age, diet and histopathology.* Dig Dis Sci 2011; 56:2042-9.
http://dx.doi.org/10.1007/s10620-010-1534-5

38. Fernández-Bañares F, Carrasco A, García-Puig R, Rosinach M, González C, Alsina M, Loras C, Salas A, Viver JM, Esteve M. *Intestinal intraepithelial lymphocyte cytometric pattern is more accurate than subepithelial deposits of anti-tissue transglutaminase IgA for the diagnosis of celiac disease in lymphocytic enteritis.* Plos One 2014; 9:e101249.
http://dx.doi.org/10.1371/journal.pone.0101249

39. Ciclitira PJ. *AGA technical review on coeliac sprue.* Gastroenterology. 2001; 120: 1526-40. http://dx.doi.org/10.1053/gast.2001.24056

40. Esteve M, Rosinach M, Fernández-Bañares F, Farré C, Salas A, Alsina M et al. *Spectrum of gluten-sensitive enteropathy in first-degree relatives of patients with coeliac disease: clinical relevance of lymphocytic enteritis.* Gut. 2006; 55: 1739-45.
http://dx.doi.org/10.1136/gut.2006.095299

41. Zanini B, Caselani F, Magni A, Turini D, Ferraresi A, Lanzarotto F et al. *Celiac Disease With Mild Enteropathy Is Not Mild Disease.* Clin Gastroenterol Hepatol. 2012 Sep 27.
http://dx.doi.org/10.1016/j.cgh.2012.09.027

42. Kurppa K, Collin P, Viljamaa M, Haimila K, Saavalainen P, Partanen J et al. *Diagnosing mild enteropathy celiac disease: A randomized, controlled clinical study.* Gastroenterology. 2009; 136: 816-23. http://dx.doi.org/10.1053/j.gastro.2008.11.040

43. Esteve M, Carrasco A, Fernandēz-Bañares F. *Is a gluten-free diet necessary in Marsh I intestinal lesions in patients with HLADQ2, DQ8 genotype and withoutgastrointestinal symptoms?* Curr Opin Clin Nutr Metab Care. 2012; 15: 505-10.
http://dx.doi.org/10.1097/MCO.0b013e3283566643

44. Lundin KAE, Alaedini A. *Non-celiac gluten sensitivity.* Gastrointest Endoscopy Clin N Am. 2012; 22: 723-34. http://dx.doi.org/10.1016/j.giec.2012.07.006

45. Volta U, De Giorgio R. *New understanding of gluten sensitivity.* Nat Rev Gastroenterol Hepatol. 2012; 9: 295-9. http://dx.doi.org/10.1038/nrgastro.2012.15

46. Biesiekierski JR, Newnham ED, Irving PM, Barrett JS, Haines M, Doecke JD et al. *Gluten causes gastrointestinal symptoms in subjects without celiac disease: a double-blind randomized placebo-controlled trial.* Am J Gastroenterol. 2011; 106: 508-14.
http://dx.doi.org/10.1038/ajg.2010.487

Chapter 14

Extraintestinal Manifestations and Associated Diseases

Luis Rodrigo, Mª Eugenia Lauret-Braña, I. Pérez-Martínez

Gastroenterology Service, Asturias Central University Hospital (HUCA) and University of Oviedo, Oviedo, Spain.

lrodrigosaez@gmail.com, meugelb@hotmail.com, ipermar_79@hotmail.com

Doi: http://dx.doi.org/10.3926/oms.215

How to cite this chapter

Rodrigo L, Lauret-Braña ME, Pérez-Martínez I. *Extraintestinal Manifestations and Associated Diseases*. In Rodrigo L and Peña AS, editors. *Celiac Disease and Non-Celiac Gluten Sensitivity*. Barcelona, Spain: OmniaScience; 2014. p. 303-325.

Abstract

Celiac disease (CD) is frequently accompanied by a variety of extra-digestive manifestations, thus making it a systemic disease, rather than a disease limited to the gastrointestinal tract.

This is primarily explained by the fact that CD belongs to the autoimmune disease group, the only one with a known etiology, related to a permanent gluten intolerance. Remarkable breakthroughs have been achieved in the last decades, due to a greater interest in the diagnosis of atypical and asymptomatic patients, which are more frequent in adults. The known presence of several associated diseases provide guidance in the search of oligosymptomatic cases as well as studies performed in relatives of CD patients.

The causes for the onset and manifestation of associated diseases are diverse: some share susceptibility genes, like type 1 diabetes mellitus (T1DM); others share pathogenetic mechanisms and yet others are of an unknown nature.

General practitioners and other specialists must remember that CD may debut with extraintestinal manifestations and associated illnesses may appear both at the time of diagnosis and throughout the evolution of the disease.

The implementation of a gluten-free diet (GFD) improves the overall clinical development and the evolution of associated diseases. In some cases, such as in iron deficiency anemia, the GFD contributes to its disappearance. In other diseases, like T1DM, it helps to reduce the amount of insulin needed, thus allowing for a better control of the disease. In several other complications and/or associated diseases, an adequate adherence to a GFD may slow down their evolution, especially if it is implemented during an early stage.

1. Introduction

Celiac disease (CD) is a systemic process, autoimmune in nature, which appears in genetically predisposed individuals. Its clinical manifestations are predominantly digestive, but it is accompanied, with a certain frequency, by extradigestive manifestations that may be due to nutritional deficiencies of an autoimmune nature, of diverse types and in different locations.

Their presence speaks of a possible etiopathogenic relationship which somehow may guide diagnosis. The list of associated diseases is wide and varied, since it includes previously existing disease involvement of various organ systems, which appear simultaneously or even after the introduction of a gluten-free diet (GFD).

Sollid[1] postulates that although the CD causal antigen is a protein ingested with food, various immunopathogenic studies speak in favor of their being relevant to the development of autoimmunity. The main argument is based on genetic observations which confirm that there are multiple "loci" shared between CD and various autoimmune diseases, especially type 1 diabetes mellitus (T1DM) and rheumatoid arthritis (RA).[2] The antigenic mechanism would be effected through transglutaminase 2 (TG2).

Most of the associated diseases improve with the introduction of a GFD, although many of them also require a good substitutive or specific treatment, temporary or prolonged.

In this chapter we review a series of extraintestinal manifestations and/or diseases associated with CD, describing their frequency, possible causal relationship and recommended treatments.

2. Hematologic Manifestations (Table 1)

- Anemia:
  - Iron deficiency anemia
  - Due to folic acid and/or vitamin b12 deficiency
  - Multifactorial
  - Refractory
- Leukopenia
- Thrombopenia and Thrombocytosis
- Clotting disorders
- Venous and arterial thrombosis

Table 1. Hematological associated diseases.

2.1. Anemia

Anemia is a common finding in CD patients and it may be its most striking clinical manifestation, leading to diagnosis. Its etiology is multifactorial and its prevalence is highly variable, ranging from 12 to 70% of cases.[3-5] This anemia is usually microcytic and hypochromic, of the hypoproliferative type, reflecting a decreased intestinal absorption of iron, various vitamins and other nutrients, including folic acid and cobalamin. The presence of villous atrophy is an important factor in the reduction of iron absorption, but the former is not required for the latter to appear.

Iron deficiency anemia occurs in up to 46% of cases of subclinical CD, with higher prevalence in adults than in children and its overall frequency in patients with refractory anemia reaches up to 20% of the cases.[6-8]

In a recent study, the prevalence of CD in patients with anemia was of 5% and of up to 8.5% in those who have iron deficiency anemia.[9]

Sustained chronic iron deficiency with low levels of serum iron, transferrin saturation and ferritin is common in celiac patients, with or without associated anemia and should be an index of suspicion for possible associated CD.

It is therefore recommended that clinicians include in their daily routine iron deficiency anemia in the CD diagnosis protocol, including serological and genetic markers as well as duodenal biopsies, especially in refractory cases.[10]

The primary indicated treatment is the establishment of a GFD and iron supplements, orally or intravenously, until reserves are replenished.

2.2. Leukopenia

Fisgin et al. described the presence of leukopenia with anemia in a group of children with CD at the time of diagnosis.[11] Its prevalence in both children and in adults with celiac disease is not well understood at present.

It has been suggested that the leukopenia is primarily due to folic acid deficiency associated with copper deficiency.

Data on treatment are also very scarce. There is usually a slow improvement after establishing a GFD and it can be supplemented with oral copper sulphate supplements, should there be any deficiency of this trace element.[12,13]

2.3. Thrombocytopenia and Thrombocytosis

The decrease in platelet count has occasionally been reported in CD patients and has been postulated as of a possible autoimmune etiology. Isolated cases have been reported associated with keratoconjunctivitis and choroidopathy, suggesting again its probable autoimmune pathogenesis.

Thrombocytopenia treatment associated with CD requires the establishment of a GFD, which by itself, in some cases, can normalize the platelet counts. When this does not happen, it is advisable to resort to corticosteroid treatment for a short period until its resolution.[14,15]

Thrombocytosis may indicate the presence of increased inflammatory activity in CD patients. Carroccio et al. described the case of an elderly patient with clear-cut thrombocytosis associated with severe anemia who was diagnosed with CD. They suggested that it may also be associated with some myeloproliferative disorders and some hematologic neoplasias.[16]

Thrombocytosis can be resolved with the establishment and monitoring of a GFD.

2.4. Clotting Disorders

Untreated CD can lead to malabsorption of various nutrients, which can be manifested by a vitamin K deficiency and thus by a decrease in the presence of its dependent clotting factors. Cavallaro et al. found a decrease in the prothrombin time (PT) of up to 20% of adult celiac patients at the time of diagnosis.[17] It is unusual to find a PT decrease alongside the malabsorption of other nutrients.

Treatment involves adhering to a GFD and vitamin K deficiency correction after parenteral administration.

2.5. Venous and Arterial Thrombosis

Ramagopalan et al.[18] suggested in a study that celiac disease has an increased risk of thrombotic events than in relation to the general population. Ludvigsson et al.[19] found a greater association for venous thromboembolism in both genders, pointing out that it may even be the first clinical sign of CD suspicion. Cassela et al.[20] found that increased serum homocystinemia is relatively frequent in celiac patients and that, as is well known, it could be a causal factor for hypercoagulability.

The clinical spectrum of thromboembolism in CD patients is variable, including deep vein thrombosis, pulmonary embolism, Budd-Chiari syndrome and splenic thrombosis, as its more frequent manifestations.[21,22]

Only a few cases of arterial thrombosis have been described and the role of CD is doubtful. Similarly debatable is its influence on the development of vascular brain lesions.

3. Mucocutaneous Facial and Oral Manifestations (Table 2)

• Canker sores
• Dental enamel defects
• Sjögren's Syndrome
• Prominent forehead

Table 2. Oral, mucocutaneous and facial manifestations.

3.1. Canker Sores

The presence of recurrent oral canker sores should urge the physician to actively search for possible associated CD, since they are present in between 10% and 40% of treated celiac patients.[23] Their diagnosis is usually done by inspection and their treatment is based on the GFD, mouthwashes and local analgesics, since they are generally quite painful.

3.2. Enamel Defects

The association with enamel defects is quite characteristic. Its pathogenesis has been related to both calcium uptake defects at the time of the appearance of permanent dentition as well as with possible autoimmune effects.[23]

3.3. Sjögren's Syndrome

Eye and mouth dryness appears with relative frequency in association CD, as it happens with other autoimmune diseases. Its evolution usually does not depend on a strict adherence to a GFD.[24]

3.4. Prominent Forehead

Finizio et al. described this curious finding in 2005, first connecting it to the possible presence of CD. Currently it is considered as a rather anecdotal description, partly due to the smaller size of the lower two thirds of the face, compared with the surface of the forehead.[25]

4. Associated Neurological Diseases (Table 3)

• Polineuropathies
• Headaches/Migraines
• Depression/Anxiety
• Ataxia
• Epilepsy
• Multiple sclerosis
• Guillain-Barré syndrome
• Others

Table 3. Neurological associated diseases.

4.1. Peripheral Polyneuropathy

This is the most common neurological CD-associated involvement. Thus, in an Italian series of studies, its presence was confirmed up to 49% of the patients.[26] Its most frequent clinical manifestations include the prevalence of painful paresthesias in all four limbs, occasionally on the face, and disorders associated with sensitivity. Motor weakness is less common, affecting mainly the ankles and may appear as an abnormal gait in up to 25% of the patients.[27]

4.2. Headaches

Gabrieli et al. found, in a number of celiac patients, a migraine frequency of 4.4%, which was 10 times higher than that found in a control population (0.4%).[28] Both migraines and tension headaches occur more frequently in celiac patients than in the general population.

In a follow-up study of celiac patients, more than half of those with headaches or migraines improved significantly after the introduction of a GFD, which speaks in favor of the possible existence of a causal relationship of gluten both regarding its appearance and in its maintenance.[29]

4.3. Depression and Anxiety

In celiac patients symptoms of increased anxiety, irritability and increased fatigue appear frequently, such as those observed in depressed or anxious individuals.[30,31]

In young children most of these symptoms disappear completely after introducing the GFD, but the improvement is less noticeable in adults, who usually need pharmacological treatment for a length of time.

4.4. Cerebellar Ataxia

Gluten ataxia is the second manifestation, in order of frequency. It is defined as an idiopathic sporadic process accompanied by circulating anti-gliadin antibodies, with or without associated duodenal mucosal atrophy.[32]

Its pathogenesis is related to the existence of an autoimmune pathology and some patients improve significantly with a gluten-free diet, especially when it is administered during the first six months of its appearance but it has also been described in cases in which it makes a late appearance and may have some familial aggregation, as it occurs in CD.[33-35]

4.5. Epilepsy

Several studies clearly indicate that there is an association between CD and epilepsy, estimating it has a range of 3.3-5.5%.[36] This seems to happen more frequently in children than in adults. Control of epilepsy and the frequency and severity of its seizures improve with GFD, especially if it is initiated soon after the onset of epilepsy.[37] Gobbi's syndrome can occur both in children and in adults and it is characterized by the presence of calcifications in the parieto-occipital area; it has a low frequency.[38]

4.6. Multiple Sclerosis, Guillain-Barré Syndrome and other Processes

Demyelinating diseases of which the most characteristic example is multiple sclerosis (MS) and its variant, Optic Neuritis (ON), which have a higher association prevalence with CD and lymphocytic enteritis than in the general population, as is the case with the Guillain-Barré syndrome.[39,40]

5. Dermatological Manifestations (Table 4)

> • Dermatitis Herpetiformis (DH)
> • Psoriasis
> • Vitiligo
> • Alopecia areata
> • Chronic urticaria

Table 4. Dermatological associated diseases.

5.1. Dermatitis Herpetiformis (DH)

It is considered to be the CD of the skin and its presence is directly related to gluten hypersensitivity. It appears in 25% of celiac patients and it is characterized by vesicular and crusted lesions that appear anywhere on the body, especially in areas of physical friction. They have a symmetric distribution and are quite itchy. It is a rare lesion in children and a very common one from adolescence into adulthood. Its clinical development includes remissions and exacerbations which coincide with gluten exposure. It can be confirmed by the demonstration of granular IgA deposits at the dermo-epidermal junction. Its most effective treatment is a strict GFD. A better understanding of DH manifestations aids in the diagnosis of CD.[41]

5.2. Psoriasis

Psoriasis occurs in celiac patients with a higher prevalence than in the general population; adherence to GFD significantly improves both the evolution of skin lesions and of its associated complications.[42,43]

5.3. Alopecia Areata

It is also considered a chronic autoimmune disease. It is associated, with some frequency, with CD.[44] Unlike certain studies which described a complete resolution of alopecia after GFD, most authors agree that are not resolved by the latter.[45]

5.4. Chronic Urticaria

This type of injuries can be triggered by sudden changes in temperature (both cold and heat), being erythematous and edematous.[46] Most cases improve or disappear with GFD adherence.[47]

6. Bone Manifestations (Table 5)

- Childhood rickets
- Osteomalacia
- Osteoporosis
- Increased risk of fractures

Table 5. Bone associated diseases.

Bone demineralization is commonly associated with children at the time of diagnosis; it is estimated that one third of the children with CD have osteopenia, another third have osteoporosis and only the remaining third has normal bone mineral density (BMD)[48]; its relationship with increased prevalence of rickets and osteomalacia is well known. All these disorders improve, reverse and completely normalize with a GFD.[49]

It is also quite common in adults, its prevalence increasing with age, with an overall osteoporosis (OS) prevalence in this group estimated to be about 2 times higher than in unaffected persons within the same age range.[50]

As a result of this OS increased frequency, celiac patients generally have an increased risk of fractures, which is estimated to be 3.5 to 7 times higher when compared to the general population of the same age and sex; one in four celiac patients have a history of multiple fractures.[51,52]

In a recent Spanish study on adult CD patients, García-Manzanares et al.,[53] found that 45% of the patients had osteopenia and that in patients with villous atrophy (Marsh 3) it occurred more frequently than in those that do not have it (Marsh 1 and 2). Response to the GFD is lesser than in childhood and requires frequent calcium and vitamin D replacement therapy. Smoking also leads to a greater decrease in bone mass.

7. Associated Rheumatic Diseases (Table 6)

- Seronegative oligoarthritis
- Sacroileitis
- Polyarthritis
- Stronger association with:
  - Sjögren's syndrome
  - Systemic lupus Erythematosus (SLE)

Table 6. Rheumatogical associated diseases.

Arthritis varieties, as a group, are frequently associated in their various forms and presentations with the clinical development of CD, both in children and in adults. Thus, in a series of 200 celiac patients, it was present in 26% of the cases, a much higher frequency than that of the control population, which was of 7.5%, with a prevalence of seronegative and oligoarticular forms, as it happens in those that are associated with inflammatory bowel disease, with a slightly increased sacroileitis frequency.[54]

Reverse prevalence studies have been undertaken looking for CD by means of serological marker determination (mainly ATGT) in various rheumatic diseases, such as rheumatoid arthritis (RA), scleroderma and Sjögren's syndrome, this being where higher positive values have been found at 10%.[55]

Also, in a recent population study performed in Sweden on 29,000 patients with confirmed celiac villous atrophy, the prevalence of Lupus Erythematosus (SLE) was 3 times higher than that observed in the control population.[56]

8. Liver Manifestations (Table 7)

- Prolonged hypertransaminasemia
- Cholestatic and autoimmune hepatopathies
- Chronic hepatitis due to hepatitis C virus
- Acute fulminant hepatitis

Table 7. Liver associated diseases.

8.1. Prolonged Hypertransaminasemia

The most common change observed is fluctuating or persistent transaminase elevation, which is completely asymptomatic, present in 40% of both child and adult cases and disappears or becomes normalized with the gluten-free diet, after several years.[57]

CD comprises approximately 10% of the cases of hypertransaminasemia with an unclear origin, its presence should be investigated by serological studies and, if necessary, by means of a gastroscopy and confirmatory duodenal biopsies.[58]

8.2. Cholestatic and Autoimmune Liver Disease

Primary biliary cirrhosis (PBC), especially in its mild stages, primary sclerosing cholangitis (PSC) and some types of chronic autoimmune hepatitis (AIH) have a certain frequency of association with CD and its presence should be routinely considered as part of the diagnosis protocol. Cases of negative anti-mitochondrial antibodies (AMA) with cholestatic liver diseases have been found which turn out to be from celiac patients whose hepatopathies hence become ameliorated or, at least, stabilized with the GFD.[59]

8.3. Chronic Hepatitis C

Both diseases have been epidemiologically analyzed for a possible relation since both are relatively common and it is not exceptional that they coincide in the same patient. It is well known that antiviral treatment with interferon-alpha may unmask an associated latent CD, but routine CD screening in patients with chronic hepatitis due to HCV does not currently seem to be justified.[60]

8.4. Acute Fulminant Hepatitis

Some cases of fulminant liver failure have been described in which in a timely diagnosis of associated CD has not only improved the clinical situation but also helped to prevent a liver transplant, so an urgent systematic screening is worth making in this clinical situation due to its associated high morbidity and mortality.[61]

9. Gynecological Manifestations and Impaired Fertility (Table 8)

Menstrual disorders in women are varied and frequent, including delayed puberty, episodes of amenorrhea and early menopause. All these disorders are usually associated with iron deficiency or chronic iron deficiency anemia.[62]

Thus, in a study conducted in Italy on 62 celiac women who were compared with 186 controls, it was found that 19.4% of the former had amenorrhea versus 2.2% in the latter (OR = 33, 95% CI = 7.17-151.8 p = 0.000). It was possible to also observe an association between other menstrual disorders such as oligomenorrhea, hypomenorrhea, dysmenorrhea and metrorrhage (p < 0.05) between groups. The likelihood of complications during pregnancy is estimated to be 4 times higher in women with celiac disease (OR = 4.1, 95% CI = 2-8.6, p = 0.000). A significant correlation for CD with the threat of abortion, gestational hypertension, placental abruption, recurrent gravidarum cholestasis, premature birth and low weight pregnancies was also found (p < 0.001).[63]

- Delayed puberty
- Amenorrhea
- Menstrual disorder
- Infertility in both genders
- Repeated abortions
- Pregnancies with low fetal weight
- Premature births
- Gestational hypertension
- Pregnancy cholestasis
- Loss of libido

Table 8. Gynecological associated diseases.

All these findings clearly support the relationship between several very common gynecological disorders in celiac women, some serious, and some even grave, both for the mother and the fetus, which underscores the importance of an early CD diagnosis in women in order to improve their health and their offspring's, as the GFD normalizes and prevents most of these possible gynecological and obstetric complications. There is no consensus on the appropriateness of screening for CD in pregnant women within the routine checks carried out in their first trimester.[64-68]

In males, CD is also related to the existence of sexual disorders, manifested as decreased libido and sexual potency as well as infertility.[69,70]

10. Endocrine Diseases Associated (Table 9)

- Autoimmune Polyglandular Syndrome (APS):
  - Addison's disease
  - Primary Hypogonadism
  - Hypoparathyroidism
  - Pituitary deficiencies
- Type 1 Diabetes Mellitus
- Thyroid disorders:
  - Hashimoto's Thyroiditis
  - Hypothyroidism
  - Hyperthyroidism

Table 9. Endocrine associated diseases.

In epidemiological terms, autoimmune thyroiditis (AIT) and type 1 diabetes mellitus (T1DM), are the endocrine processes most frequently associated with CD. These diseases, apart from bronchial asthma, are the most common chronic diseases in children, and often can be associated.[71-73]

10.1. Autoimmune Polyglandular Syndrome (APS)

It includes two or more endocrine diseases associated within the same patient and which usually manifest hypofunction, excepting Graves' disease. The main processes are T1DM, AIT, adrenal insufficiency (Addison's disease), primary hypogonadism, hypoparathyroidism and some pituitary shortcomings.[74-76]

These syndromes can also be associated with other non-endocrine diseases. Four different types have been described, according to their associations.

10.2. Type 1 Diabetes Mellitus (T1DM)

Insulin-dependent diabetes and CD are commonly associated. The main reason for this is that both diseases share common susceptibility genes, HLA-II predominantly, or even some belonging to type I. Specifically, T1DM is strongly associated with the DR3-DQ2 haplotypes and also with DR4-DQ8 though less frequently than with the latter, as is the case for about 50 different diseases.[77] In all of these diseases an increase in intestinal permeability has been found, allowing the passage of different antigens, including gluten, which can trigger the appearance of these associated diseases.

About 4.5% of children and up to 6% of adults with T1DM exhibit associated CD.[78] This correlation between these two diseases is stronger as the patient's age increases. Epidemiological data vary depending on the population studied and the diagnostic criteria used. Thus in a recent study undertaken in Greece, Kakleas et al.[79] found a CD prevalence of 8.6% and the highest prevalence has been reported in Italy by Picarelli et al.,[80] reaching 13.8% for T1DM.

CD associated with T1DM, may be asymptomatic, or in most cases it manifests only mild symptoms.[81,82] Both diabetic adults and children with CD have an increased sepsis risk, especially pneumococcal, and it is recommended to vaccinate against this infectious agent.[83]

The GFD improves diabetes control and slightly reduces the insulin requirements, it improves or makes digestive discomfort disappear and normal growth weight gain are resumed in children, improving BMI.[84]

A routine annual study in T1DM patients is recommended for systematic and continuous CD screening.

10.3. Thyroid Diseases

There is a frequent association between CD and various thyroid diseases, which can occur both before and after diagnosis and thus also treated with GFD.[85-90]

Autoimmune thyroiditis occurs between 3 to 10% of celiac patients. It is characterized by the presence of circulating anti-peroxidase antibodies (anti-TPO) that may be asymptomatic with thyroid normal function, such as Hashimoto's thyroiditis, or else associated with thyroid function disorder, generally with subclinical hypothyroidism.[86,88,90,91]

In a retrospective Swedish epidemiological study, including about 14,000 patients with celiac disease diagnosed over a period of 40 years, were compared against 68,000 controls and the relative risk (RR) was compared in CD for thyroid disease, finding that, for hypothyroidism and thyroiditis, it is 4 times higher, half of which belongs to hyperthyroidism, which is only 2 times higher than in the general population.[92]

11. Autoimmune Diseases (Table 10)

- Cardiac:
  – Dilated Myocardiopathy
  – Autoimmune myocarditis
- Neurological:
  – Peripheral neuropathy
  – Cerebellous ataxia
  – Headaches
  – Epilepsy
  – Anxiety/Depression
- Liver:
  – Autoimmune hepatitis(AIH)
  – Autoimmune cholangitis(AIC)
  – Primary biliary cirrhosis (PBC)
- Endocrine:
  – Type 1 diabetes mellitus
  – Autoimmune thyroiditis
  – Addison's disease
- Rheumatic:
  – Oligoarhtritis
  – Juvenile arthritis
  – Sjögren's syndrome

Table 10. Autoimmune associated diseases.

These are much more frequent and are associated with CD, in a ratio 3 to 10 times higher than in the general population.[93-100] These diseases, of which we have spoken in their respective sections, are varied and include such diverse processes as thyroiditis, autoimmune hepatitis, cholangitis, primary biliary cirrhosis, type 1 diabetes mellitus, Sjögren's syndrome, Addison's disease, peripheral neuropathy, cardiomyopathy and psoriasis, among others.

There are several reasons for these frequent associations. The principal one is that they share the same genetic predisposition, especially with certain human leukocyte HLA system haplotypes. Another reason lies in the response to various antigenic markers such as transglutaminase-2 and the presence itself of CD, which also contributes.

The duration of exposure to gluten, determined by the age at which the CD diagnosis is made, has also been considered as an important risk factor for the development of autoimmune diseases, as they are more common in adults than in children. This underscores the need for the realization of an earlier CD diagnosis, which could have a beneficial effect on the development of associated autoimmune diseases. However, other studies have refuted this hypothesis.[101,102]

Various autoimmune diseases associated with CD improve after a strict GFD. Among these are neuropathies,[103] cardiomyopathies,[104] thyroid diseases[105] and both type 1 and type 2 diabetes mellitus.[106,107] These last usually have lymphocytic enteritis as seen in duodenal biopsies.[108]

However, in many other autoimmune diseases, their clinical evolution hardly changes after the establishment and monitoring of the GFD.

12. Inflammatory Bowel Disease

It can occur associated with CD in either of its two varieties, Crohn's disease and ulcerative colitis, with a higher frequency than in the general population.[109]

References

1. Sollid LM, Jabri B. *Celiac disease and transglutaminase 2: a model for post-translational modification of antigens and HLA association in the pathogenesis of autoimmune disorders.* Curr Opin Immunol. 2011; 23: 732-8.
   http://dx.doi.org/10.1016/j.coi.2011.08.006

2. Trynka G, Wijmenga C, van Heel DA: *A genetic perspective on coeliac disease.* Trends Mol Med. 2010; 16: 537-50. http://dx.doi.org/10.1016/j.molmed.2010.09.003

3. Bottaro G, Cataldo F, Rotolo N, Spina M, Corazza GR. *The clinical pattern of subclinical/silent celiac disease: an analysis on 1026 consecutive cases.* Am J Gastroenterol. 1999; 94: 691-6.

4. Unsworth DJ, Lock FJ, Harvey RF. *Iron-deficiency anaemia in premenopausal women.* Lancet. 1999; 353: 1100. http://dx.doi.org/10.1016/S0140-6736(05)76459-X

5. Fernández-Bañares F, Monzón H, Forné M. *A short review of malabsorption and anemia.* World J Gastroenterol. 2009; 15: 4644-52.
   http://dx.doi.org/10.3748/wjg.15.4644

6. Economu M, Karyda S, Gombakis N, Tsatra J, Athanassiou-Metaxa M. *Suclinical celiac disease in children: refractory iron deficiency as the sole presentation.* J Pediatr Hematol Oncol. 2004; 26: 153-4. http://dx.doi.org/10.1097/00043426-200403000-00001

7. Mody RJ, Brown PI, Wechsler DS. *Refractory iron deficiency anemia as the primary clinical manifestation of celiac disease.* J Pediatr Hematol Oncol. 2003; 25: 169-72.
   http://dx.doi.org/10.1097/00043426-200302000-00018

8. Carroccio A, Iannitto E, Cavataio F, Montalto G, Tumminello M, Campagna P et al. *Sideropenic anemia and celiac disease: one study, two points of view.* Dig Dis Sci. 1998; 43: 673-8. http://dx.doi.org/10.1023/A:1018896015530

9. Corazza GR, Valentini RA, Andreani ML, D'Anchino M, Leva MT, Ginaldi L et al. *Suclinical celiac disease is a frequent cause of iron-deficiency anemia.* Scand J Gastroenterol. 1995; 30: 153-6. http://dx.doi.org/10.3109/00365529509093254

10. Rodrigo L, Fuentes D, Perez I, Alvarez N, García P, de Francisco R et al. *Anemia ferropénica refractaria e intolerancia al gluten. Respuesta a una dieta sin gluten*. Rev Esp Enferm Dig. 2011; 103: 349-54.

11. Fisgin T, Yarali N, Duru F, Usta B, , Kara A. *Hematologic manifestation of childhood celiac disease.* Acta Hematol. 2004; 111: 211-4. http://dx.doi.org/10.1159/000077568

12. Pittschlier K. *Neutropenia, granulocytic hypersegmentation and coeliac disease.* Acta Paediatr. 1995; 84: 705-6.
    http://dx.doi.org/10.1111/j.1651-2227.1995.tb13737.x

13. Goyens P, Brasseur D, Cadranel S. *Copper deficiency in infants with active celiac disease.* J Peditr Gastroenterol Nutr. 1985; 4: 677-80.
    http://dx.doi.org/10.1097/00005176-198508000-00033

14. Mulder CJ, Peña AS, Jensen J, Oosterhuis JA. *Celiac disease and geographic (serpiginous) choroidopathy with occurrence of thrombocytopenic purpura.* Arch Intern Med. 1983; 143: 842. http://dx.doi.org/10.1001/archinte.1983.00350040232043

15. Eliakim R, Heyman S, Kornberg A. *Celiac disease and keratoconjunctivitis occurrence with thrombocytopenic purpura.* Arch Intern Med. 1982; 142: 1037.
    http://dx.doi.org/10.1001/archinte.1982.00340180195032

16. Carroccio A, Giannitrapani L, Di Prima L, Iannitto E, Montalto G, Notarbartolo A. *Extreme thrombocytosis as a sign of celiac disease in the elderly: Case Report.* Eur J Gastroenterol Hepatol. 2002; 14: 897-900.
http://dx.doi.org/10.1097/00042737-200208000-00017

17. Cavallaro R, Iovino P, Castiglione F, Palumbo A, Marino M, Di Bella S et al. *Prevalence and clinical associations of prolonged prothrombin time in adult untreated coeliac disease.* Eur J Gastroenterol Hepatol. 2004; 16: 219-23.
http://dx.doi.org/10.1097/00042737-200402000-00016

18. Ramagopalan SV, Wotton SV, Handel AE, Yeates D, Goldacre MJ. *Risk of venous thromboembolism in people admitted to hospital with selected immune-mediated dieases: record-linkage study.* BMC Med. 2011; 9: 1.
http://dx.doi.org/10.1186/1741-7015-9-1

19. Ludvigsson JF, Welander A, Lassila R, Ekbom A, Montgomery SM. *Risk of thromboembolism in 14,000 individuals with celiac disease.* Br J Haematol. 2007; 139: 121-7. http://dx.doi.org/10.1111/j.1365-2141.2007.06766.x

20. Cassela G, Bassotti G, Villanacci V, Di Bella C, Pagni F, Corti GL. *Is hyperhomocysteinemia relevant in patients with celiac disease?* World Jour Gastroenterol. 2011; 17: 2941-4.
http://dx.doi.org/10.3748/wjg.v17.i24.2941

21. Marteau P, Cadranel JF, Messing B, Gargot D, Valla D, Rambaud JC. *Association of hepatic vein obstruction and coeliac disease in North African subjects.* J Hepatol. 1994; 20: 650-3. http://dx.doi.org/10.1016/S0168-8278(05)80355-1

22. Zenjari T, Boruchowicz A, Desreumaux P, Laberenne E, Cortot A, Colombel JF. *Association of coeliac disease and portal venous trombosis.* Gastroenterol Clin Biol. 1995; 19: 953-4.

23. Cheng J, Malahias T, Brar P, Minaya MT, Green PH. *The association between celiac disease, dental enamel defects and aphtous ulcers in a United States cohort.* J Clin Gastroenterol. 2010; 44: 191-4.
http://dx.doi.org/10.1097/MCG.0b013e3181ac9942

24. Lidén M, Kristjánsson G, Valtýsdóttir S, Hällgren R. *Gluten sensitivity in patients with primary Sjögren´s syndrome.* Scand J Gastroenterol. 2007; 42: 962-7.
http://dx.doi.org/10.1080/00365520701195345

25. Finizio M, Quaremba G, Mazzacca G, Ciacci C. *Large forehead: a novel sign of undiagnosed coeliac disease.* Dig Liver Dis. 2005; 37: 659-64.
http://dx.doi.org/10.1016/j.dld.2005.04.014

26. Cicarelli G, Della Rocca G, Amboni M, Ciacci C, Mazzacca G, Filla A et al. *Clinical and neurological abnormalities in adult celiac disease.* Neurol Sci. 2003; 24: 311-7.
http://dx.doi.org/10.1007/s10072-003-0181-4

27. Chin RL, Sander HW, Brannagan TH, Green PH, Hays AP, Alaedini A et al. *Celiac neuropathy.* Neurology. 2003; 60: 1581-5.
http://dx.doi.org/10.1212/01.WNL.0000063307.84039.C7

28. Gabrielli M, Cremonini F, Fiore G, Addolorato G, Padalino C, Candelli M et al. *Association between migraine and Celiac disease: results from a preliminary case-control and therapeutic study.* Am J Gastroenterol. 2003; 98: 625-9.
http://dx.doi.org/10.1111/j.1572-0241.2003.07300.x

29. Zelnik N, Pacht A, Obeid R, Lerner A. *Range of neurologic disorders in patients with celiac disease.* Pediatrics. 2004; 113: 1672-6.http://dx.doi.org/10.1542/peds.113.6.1672

30. Siniscalchi M, Iovino P, Tortora R, Forestiero S, Somma A, Capuano L et al. *Fatigue in adult coeliac disease.* Aliment Pharmacol Ther. 2005; 22: 489-94.
http://dx.doi.org/10.1111/j.1365-2036.2005.02619.x

31. Carta MG, Hardoy MC, Usai P, Carpiniello B, Angst J. *Recurrent brief depression in celiac disease.* J Psychosom Res. 2003; 55: 573-4.
http://dx.doi.org/10.1016/S0022-3999(03)00547-6

32. Sapone A, Bai JC, Ciacci C, Dolinsek J, Green PH, Hadjivassiliou M et al. *Spectrum of gluten-related disorders: consensus on new nomenclature and classification.* BMC Med. 2012; 10: 13. http://dx.doi.org/10.1186/1741-7015-10-13

33. Hadjivassiliou M, Sanders DS, Woodroofe N, Williamson C, Grünewald RA. *Gluten ataxia.* Cerebellum. 2008; 7: 494-8. http://dx.doi.org/10.1007/s12311-008-0052-x

34. Ghazal FA, Singh S, Yaghi S, Keyrouz SG. *Gluten ataxia: an important treatable etiology of sporadic ataxia.* Int J Neurosci. 2012; 122: 545-6.
http://dx.doi.org/10.3109/00207454.2012.683220

35. Hernández-Lahoz C, Mauri-Capdevila G, Vega-Villar J, Rodrigo L. *Trastornos neurológicos asociados con la sensibilidad al gluten.* Rev Neurol. 2011; 53: 287-300.

36. Pengiran Tengah DS, Holmes GK, Wills AJ. *The prevalence of epilepsy in patients with celiac disease.* Epilepsia. 2004; 45: 1291-3.
http://dx.doi.org/10.1111/j.0013-9580.2004.54104.x

37. Mavroudi A, Karatza E, Papastavrou T, Panteliadis C, Spiroglou K. *Successful treatment of epilepsy and celiac disease with a gluten-free diet.* Pediatr Neurol. 2005; 33: 292-5.
http://dx.doi.org/10.1016/j.pediatrneurol.2005.05.010

38. Gobbi G, Bouquet F, Greco L, Lambertini A, Tassinari CA, Ventura A et al. *Celiac disease, epilepsy, and cerebral calcifications. The Italian Working Group on Coeliac Disease and Epilepsy.* Lancet. 1992; 340: 439-43.
http://dx.doi.org/10.1016/0140-6736(92)91766-2

39. Rodrigo L, Hernández-Lahoz C, Fuentes D, Alvarez N, López-Vázquez A, González S. *Prevalence of celiac disease in multiple sclerosis.* BMC Neurol. 2011; 11: 31.
http://dx.doi.org/10.1186/1471-2377-11-31

40. Midha V, Jain NP, Sood A, Bansal R, Puri S, Kumar V. *Landry-Guillain-Barré syndrome as presentation of celiac disease.* Indian J Gastroenterol. 2007; 26: 42-3.

41. Herrero González JE. *Guía clínica para el diagnóstico y tratamiento de la Dermatitis Herpetiforme.* Actas Dermosifiliogr. 2010; 101: 820-6.
http://dx.doi.org/10.1016/j.ad.2010.06.018

42. Ludvigsson JF, Lindelöf B, Zingone F, Ciacci C. *Psoriasis in a nationwide cohort study of patients with celiac disease.* J Invest Dermatol. 2011; 131: 2010-6.
http://dx.doi.org/10.1038/jid.2011.162

43. Michaëlsson G, Kristjánsson G, Pihl Lundin I, Hagforsen E. *Palmoplantar pustulosis and gluten sensitivity: a study of serum antibodies agianst gliadin and tissue transglutaminase, the duodenal mucosa and effects of gluten-free diet.* Br J Dermatol. 2007; 156: 659-66. http://dx.doi.org/10.1111/j.1365-2133.2006.07725.x

44. Corazza GR, Andreani ML, Venturo N, Bernardi M, Tosti A, Gasbarrini G. *Celiac disease and alopecia areata: report of a new association.* Gastroenterology. 1995; 109: 1333-7.
http://dx.doi.org/10.1016/0016-5085(95)90597-9

45. Bardella MT, Marino R, Barbareschi M, Bianchi F, Faglia G, Bianchi P. *Alopecia areata and coeliac disease: no effect of a gluten-free diet on hair growth.* Dermatology. 2000; 200: 108-10. http://dx.doi.org/10.1159/000018340

46. Pedrosa Delgado M, Martín Muñoz F, Polanco Allué I, Martín Esteban M. *Cold urticaria and celiac disease.* J Investig Allergol Clin Immunol. 2008; 18: 123-5.

47. Haussmann J, Sekar A. *Chronic urticaria: a cutaneous manifestation of celiac disease.* Can J Gastroenterol. 2006; 20: 291-3.

48. Goddard CJ, Gillet HR. *Complications of coeliac disease: are all patients at risk?* Postgrad Med. 2006; 82: 705-12. ttp://dx.doi.org/10.1136/pgmj.2006.048876

49. Kavak US, Yüce A, Koçak N, Demir H, Saltik IN, Gürakan F et al. *Bone mineral density in children with untreated and treated celiac disease.* J Pediatr Gastroenterol Nutr. 2003; 37: 434-6. http://dx.doi.org/10.1097/00005176-200310000-00007

50. Sundar N, Crimmins R, Swift G. *Clinical presentation and incidence of complications in patients with coeliac disease diagnosed by relative screening.* Postgrad Med. 2007; 83: 273-6. http://dx.doi.org/10.1136/pgmj.2006.052977

51. Walters JR, Banks LM, Butcher GP, Fowler CR. *Detection of low bone mineral density by dual energy x ray absorptiometry by unsuspected suboptimally treated coeliac disease.* Gut. 1995; 37: 220-4. http://dx.doi.org/10.1136/gut.37.2.220

52. West J, Logan RF, Card TR, Smith C, Hubbard R. *Fractures risk in people with celiac disease: a population-based cohort study.* Gastroenterology. 2003; 125: 429-36. http://dx.doi.org/10.1016/S0016-5085(03)00891-6

53. García-Manzanares A, Tenias JM, Lucendo AJ. *Bone mineral density directly correlates with duodenal Marsh stage in newly diagnosed adult celiac patients.* Scand J Gastroenterol. 2012; 8-9: 927-36.
http://dx.doi.org/10.3109/00365521.2012.688217

54. Lubrano E, Ciacci C, Ames PR, Mazzacca G, Oriente P, Scarpa R. *The arthritis of coeliac disease: prevalence and pattern in 200 adult patients.* Br J Rheumatol. 1996; 35: 1314-8.
http://dx.doi.org/10.1093/rheumatology/35.12.1314

55. Luft LM, Barr SG, Martin LO, Chan EK, Fritzler MJ. *Autoantibodies to tissue transglutaminase in Sjögren's syndrome and related rheumatic diseases.* J Rheumatol. 2003; 30: 2613-9.

56. Ludvigsson JF, Rubio-Tapia A, Chowdhary V, Murray JA, Simard JF. *Increased Risk of Systemic Lupus Erythematosus in 29,000 Patients with Biopsy-verified Celiac Disease.* J Rheumatol. 2012; 39: 1964-70. ttp://dx.doi.org/10.3899/jrheum.120493

57. Dickey W, McMillan SA, Collins JS, Watson RG, McLoughlin JC, Love AH. *Liver abnormalities associated with celiac sprue. How common are they, what is their significance, and what do we do about them?* J Clin Gastroenterol. 1995; 20: 290-2.
http://dx.doi.org/10.1097/00004836-199506000-00006

58. Volta U, De Franceschi L, Lari F, Molinaro N, Zoli M, Bianchi FB. *Coeliac disease hidden by cryptogenic hypertransaminasemia.* Lancet. 1998; 352: 26-9.
http://dx.doi.org/10.1016/S0140-6736(97)11222-3

59. Valera JM, Hurtado C, Poniachik J, Abumohor P, Brahm J. *Study of celiac disease in patients with non-alcoholic fatty liver and autoimmune hepatic diseases.* Gastroenterol Hepatol. 2008; 31: 8-11.

60. Hernandez L, Johnson TC, Naiyer AJ, Kryszak D, Ciaccio EJ, Min A et al. *Chronic hepatitis C virus and celiac disease, is there an association?* Dig Dis Sci. 2008; 53: 256-61.
http://dx.doi.org/10.1007/s10620-007-9851-z

61. Kaukinen K, Halme L, Collin P, Färkkilä M, Mäki M, Vehmanen P et al. *Celiac disease in patients with severe liver disease: gluten-free diet may reverse hepatic failure.* Gastroenterology. 2002; 122: 881-8. http://dx.doi.org/10.1053/gast.2002.32416

62. Sóñora C, Muñoz F, Del Río N, Acosta G, Montenegro C, Trucco E et al. *Celiac disease and gyneco-obstetrics complications: can serum antibodies modulate tissue transglutaminase functions and contribute to clinical pattern?* Am J Reprod Immunol. 2011; 66: 476-87. http://dx.doi.org/10.1111/j.1600-0897.2011.01020.x

63. Martinelli D, Fortunato F, Tafuri S, Germinario CA, Prato R. *Reproductive life disorders in Italian celiac women. A case-control study.* BMC Gastroenterol. 2010; 10: 89. http://dx.doi.org/10.1186/1471-230X-10-89

64. Sanders DS. *Coeliac disease and subfertility: Association is often neglected.* BMJ. 2003; 327: 1226-7. http://dx.doi.org/10.1136/bmj.327.7425.1226-e

65. EliakimR, Sherer DM. *Celiac disease: Fertility and Pregnancy.* Gynecol Obstet Invest. 2001; 51: 3-7. http://dx.doi.org/10.1159/000052881

66. Rostami K, Steegers EA, Wong WY, Braat DD, Steegers-Theunissen RP. *Coeliac disease and reproductive disorders: a neglected association.* Eur J Obstet Gynecol Reprod Biol. 2001; 96: 146-9. http://dx.doi.org/10.1016/S0301-2115(00)00457-7

67. Foschi F, Diani F, Zardini E, Zanoni G, Caramaschi P. *Celiac disease and spontaneous abortion.* Minerva Gynecol. 2002; 54: 151-9.

68. Pope R, Sheiner E. *Celiac disease during pregnancy: to screen or not to screen?* Arch Gynecol Obstet. 2009; 279: 1-3. http://dx.doi.org/10.1007/s00404-008-0803-4

69. Hogen Esch CE, Van Rijssen MJ, Roos A, Koning F, Dekker FW, Mearin ML et al. *Screening for unrecognized coeliac disease in subfertile couples.* Scand J Gastroenterol. 2011; 46: 1423-8. http://dx.doi.org/10.3109/00365521.2011.615858

70 Meloni GF, Dessole S, Vargiu N, Tomasi PA, Musumeci S. *The prevalence of coeliac disease in infertility.* Hum Reprod. 1999; 14: 2759-61.
http://dx.doi.org/10.1093/humrep/14.11.2759

71. Anderson MS. *Update in endocrine autoimmunity.* J Clin Endocrinol Metab. 2008; 93: 3663-70. http://dx.doi.org/10.1210/jc.2008-1251

72. Craig M, Hattersley A, Donaghue K. *ISPAD Clinical Practice Consensus Guidelines 200.* Ped Diabetes. 2009 (S12); 10: 3-12.
http://dx.doi.org/10.1111/j.1399-5448.2009.00568.x

73. Triolo TM, Armstrong TK, McFann K, Yu I, Rewers MJ, Klingensmith GJ et al. *Additional autoinmune disease in 33% of patients of type 1 diabetes Honest.* Diabetes Care. 2011; 34: 1211-3. http://dx.doi.org/10.2337/dc10-1756

74. Betterlre C, Delpra C, Greggio N. *Autoimmunity in isolated Addison disease and in polyglandular autoimmune diabetes type 1, 2 and 4.* Ann. Endocrinol. 2001; 62: 193.

75. Eisenbarth CS, Gottlieb PA. *Autoimmune Poliendocrine Syndromes.* New Engl J Med. 2004; 350: 2068-79. http://dx.doi.org/10.1056/NEJMra030158

76. Brook CGD, Brown RS. *Polyglandular Syndromes.* In Handbook of Clinical Pediatrics Endocrinology. Blackwell Publishing Inc. Massachussets USA. 2008; 164-71.

77. Visser J, Rozing J, Sapone A, Lammers K, Fasano A. *Tight junctions, intestinal permeability and autoimmunity: celiac disease and type 1 diabetes paradigms.* Ann NY Acad Sci. 2009; 1165: 195-205.
http://dx.doi.org/10.1111/j.1749-6632.2009.04037.x

78. Holmes GK. *Screening for coeliac disease in type 1 diabetes.* Arch Dis Child. 2002; 87: 495-8. http://dx.doi.org/10.1136/adc.87.6.495

79. Kakleas K, Sarayjanci C, Cristellis E, Papathanasiou A, Petrou V, Fotinou A et al. *The prevalence and risk factors for celiac disease among children and adolescents with type 1 diabetes mellitus.* Diab Res Clin Pract. 2010; 90: 202-8. http://dx.doi.org/10.1016/j.diabres.2010.08.005

80. Picarelli A, Sabbatella L, Di Tola M, Vetrano S, Casale C, Anania MC et al. *Anti-endomysial antibody of IgG1 isotype detection strongly increases the prevalence of coeliac disease in patients affected by type 1 diabetes mellitus.* Clin Exp Immunol. 2005; 142: 111-5. http://dx.doi.org/10.1111/j.1365-2249.2005.02866.x

81. Rami B, Sumnik Z, Schober E. *Screening detected celiac disease in children with type 1 diabetes mellitas: effect on the clinical course (a case control study).* Jour of Ped Gastroenterol and Nutr. 2005; 41: 317-21. http://dx.doi.org/10.1097/01.mpg.0000174846.67797.87

82. Telega G, Bennet TR, Werlin S. *Emerging new clinical patterns in the presentation of celiac disease.* Arch of Ped and Adolesc Med. 2008; 162: 164-8. http://dx.doi.org/10.1001/archpediatrics.2007.38

83. Ludvigsson JF, Olén O, Bell M, Ekbom A, Montgomery SM. *Coeliac disease and risk of sepsis.* Gut. 2008; 57: 1074-80. http://dx.doi.org/10.1136/gut.2007.133868

84. Narula P, Porter L, Langton J, Rao V, Davies P, Cummins C et al. *Gastrointestinal symptoms in children with type 1 diabetes screened for celiac disease.* Pediatrics. 2009; 124: 489-95. http://dx.doi.org/10.1542/peds.2008-2434

85. Valentino R, Savastano S, Tommaselli AP, Dorato M, Scarpitta MT, Gigante M et al. *Prevalence of coeliac disease in patients with thyroid autoimmunity.* Horm Res. 1999; 51: 124-7. http://dx.doi.org/10.1159/000023344

86. Ventura A, Neri E, Ughi C, Leopaldi A, Città A, Not T. *Gluten-dependent diabetes-related and thyroid-related autoantibodies in patients with celiac disease.* J Pediatr. 2000; 137: 263-5. http://dx.doi.org/10.1067/mpd.2000.107160

87. Sategna-Guidetti C, Volta U, Ciacci C, Usai P, Carlino A, De Franceschi L et al. *Prevalence of thyroid disorders in untreated adult coeliac disease patients and effect of gluten withdrawal: an Italian multicenter study.* Am J Gastroenterol. 2001; 96: 751-7. http://dx.doi.org/10.1111/j.1572-0241.2001.03617.x

88. Ansaldi N, Palmas T, Corrias A, Barbato M, D'Altiglia MR, Campanozzi A et al. *Autoimmune thyroid disease and coeliac disease in children.* J Pediatr Gastroenterol Nutr. 2003; 37: 63-6. http://dx.doi.org/10.1097/00005176-200307000-00010

89. Viljamaa M, Kaukinen K, Huhtala H, Kyronpalo S, Rasmussen M, Collin P. *Coeliac disease, autoimmune diseases and gluten exposure.* Scand J Gastroenterol. 2005; 40: 437-43. http://dx.doi.org/10.1080/00365520510012181

90. Guliter S, Yakaryilmaz F, Ozkurt Z, Ersoy R, Ucardag D, Caglayan O et al. *Prevalence of coeliac disease in patients with autoimmune thyroiditis in a Turkish population.* World J Gastroenterol. 2007; 13: 1599-601.

91. Hadithi M, de Boer H, Meijer JW, Willekens F, Kerckhaert JA, Heijmans R et al. *Coeliac disease in Dutch patients with Hashimoto's thyroiditis and vice versa.* World J Gastroenterol. 2007; 13: 1715-22.

92. Elfstrom P, Montgomery SM, Kampe O, Ekbom A, Ludvigsson JF. *Risk of thyroid disease in individuals with coeliac disease.* J Clin Endocrinol Metab. 2008; 93: 3915-21. http://dx.doi.org/10.1210/jc.2008-0798

93. Rensch MJ, Szyjkowski R, Shaffer RT, Fink S, Kopecky C, Grissmer L et al. *The prevalence of celiac disease autoantibodies in patients with systemic lupus erythematosus.* Am J Gastroenterol. 2001; 96: 1113-5.
http://dx.doi.org/10.1111/j.1572-0241.2001.03753.x

94. Sategna Guidetti C, Solerio E, Scaglione N, Aimo G, Mengozzi G. *Duration of gluten exposure in adult coeliac disease does not correlate with the risk for autoinmune disorders.* Gut. 2001; 49: 502-5. http://dx.doi.org/10.1136/gut.49.4.502

95. Dickey W, McMillan SA, Callender ME. *High prevalence of celiac sprue among patients with primary biliary cirrhosis.* J Clin Gastroenterol. 1997; 25: 328-9.
http://dx.doi.org/10.1097/00004836-199707000-00006

96. Volta U, Rodrigo L, Granito A, Petrolini N, Muratori P, Muratori L et al. *Celiac disease in autoimmune cholestatic liver disorders.* Am J Gastroenterol. 2002; 97: 2609-13.
http://dx.doi.org/10.1111/j.1572-0241.2002.06031.x

97. Iltanen S, Collin P, Korpela M, Holm K, Partanen J, Polvi A et al. *Celiac disease and markers of celiac disease latency in patients with primary Sjögren's syndrome.* Am J Gastroenterol. 1999; 94: 1042-6. http://dx.doi.org/10.1111/j.1572-0241.1999.01011.x

98. O'Leary C, Walsh CH, Wieneke P, O'Regan P, Buckley B, O'Halloran DJ et al. *Coeliac disease and autoimmune Addison´s disease: a clinical pitfall.* QJM. 2002; 95: 79-82.
http://dx.doi.org/10.1093/qjmed/95.2.79

99. Fonager K, Sørensen HT, Nørgård B, Thulstrup AM. *Cardiomyopathy in Danish patients with coeliac disease.* Lancet. 1999; 354: 1561.
http://dx.doi.org/10.1016/S0140-6736(05)76595-8

100. Frustaci A, Cuoco L, Chimenti C, Pieroni M, Fioravanti G, Gentiloni N et al. *Celiac disease associated with autoinmune myocarditis.* Circulation. 2002; 105: 2611-8.
http://dx.doi.org/10.1161/01.CIR.0000017880.86166.87

101. Ventura A, Magazù G, Gerarduzzi T, Greco L. *Coeliac disease and the risk of autoimmune disorders.* Gut. 2002; 51: 897. http://dx.doi.org/10.1136/gut.51.6.897

102. Sategna Guidetti C, Solerio E, Scaglione N, Aimo G, Mengozzi G. *Duration of gluten exposure in adult coeliac disease does not correlate with the risk for autoimmune disorders.* Got. 2001; 49: 502-5. http://dx.doi.org/10.1136/gut.49.4.502

103. Hadjivassiliou M, Kandler RH, Chattopadhyay AK, Davies-Jones AG, Jarratt JA, Sanders D S . *Dietary treatment of gluten neuropathy.* Muscle Nerve. 2006; 34: 762-6.
http://dx.doi.org/10.1002/mus.20642

104. Curione M, Barbato M, Viola F, Francia P, De Biase L, Cucchiara S. *Idiopathic dilated cardiomyopathy associated with coeliac disease: the effect of a gluten-free diet on cardiac performance.* Dig Liver Dis. 2002; 34: 866-9.
http://dx.doi.org/10.1016/S1590-8658(02)80258-4

105. Metso S, Hyytiä-Ilmonen H, Kaukinen K, Huhtala H, Jaatinen P, Salmi J et al. *Gluten-free diet and autoimmune thyroiditis in patients with celiac disease. A prospective controlled study.* Scand J Gastroenterol. 2012; 47: 43-8.
http://dx.doi.org/10.3109/00365521.2011.639084

106. Goh VL, Estrada DE, Lerer T, Balarezo F, Sylvester FA. *Effect of gluten-free diet on growth and glycemic control in children with type 1 diabetes and asymptomatic celiac disease.* J Pediatr Endocrinol Metab. 2010; 23: 1169-73.
http://dx.doi.org/10.1515/jpem.2010.183

107. Rodrigo L, Pérez-Martinez I. *Osteogenesis Imperfecta with Celiac Disease and Type II Diabetes Mellitus Associated: Improvement with a Gluten-Free Diet.* Case Report Med. 2012; 2012: 813461. http://dx.doi.org/10.1155/2012/813461

108. Kurppa K, Collin P, Viljamaa M, Haimila K, Saavalainen P, Partanen J et al. *Diagnosing mild enteropathy celiac disease: a randomized, controlled clinical study.* Gastroenterology. 2009; 136: 816-23. http://dx.doi.org/10.1053/j.gastro.2008.11.040

109. Yang A, Chen Y, Scherl E, Neugut AI, Bhagat G, Green PH. *Inflammatory bowel disease in patients with celiac disease.* Inflamm Bowel Dis. 2005; 11: 528-32. http://dx.doi.org/10.1097/01.MIB.0000161308.65951.db

Chapter 15

Bone Metabolism and Osteoporosis in Adult Celiac Disease

Alvaro García Manzanares[1], Alfredo J. Lucendo[2]

[1]Endocrinology and Nutrition. La Mancha Centro Hospital. Spain.

[2]Gastroenterology Department. Tomelloso General Hospital. Spain.

agmanzanares2010@gmail.com, alucendo@vodafone.es

Doi: http://dx.doi.org/10.3926/oms.216

How to cite this chapter

García-Manzanares A, Lucendo AJ. *Bone Metabolism and Osteoporosis in Adult Celiac Disease.* In Rodrigo L and Peña AS, editors. *Celiac Disease and Non-Celiac Gluten Sensitivity.* Barcelona, Spain: OmniaScience; 2014. p. 327-346.

Abstract

Celiac disease (CD) affects around 1-2% of the world population. Many current CD patients live with their symptoms for years before diagnosis, and are therefore exposed to the consequences of the disease, including an impaired bone mineralization. In this chapter we provide an updated discussion on the relationship between low bone mineral density (BMD), osteopenia and osteoporosis, and celiac disease. Review of the literature shows, low BMD affects up to 75% of patients with celiac disease and 40% of those diagnosed during adulthood. It can be found at any age, independently of positive serological markers and presence of digestive symptoms, contributing to deterioration in the quality of life. The prevalence of CD among osteoporotic patients is also significantly increased. Two theories try to explain the origin of low BMD: Micronutrients malabsorption (including calcium and vitamin D) determined by villous atrophy has been related to secondary hyperparathyroidism and incapacity to achieve the potential bone mass peak; chronic inflammation was also related with RANKL secretion, osteoclasts activation and increased bone reabsorption. As a consequence, CD patients have a risk for bone fractures that exceeds 40% that of matched non-affected population. Treatment of low BMD in CD comprises gluten-free diet, calcium and vitamin D supplementation, and biphosphonates, although its effects on CD have not been specifically assessed. It can be concluded that a relevant proportion of CD patients present a low BMD and a variable increase in the risk of bone fractures. Epidemiological changes in CD make bone density scans more relevant for adult celiacs.

1. Introduction

A low bone mineral density (BMD) constitutes the first diagnostic criterion for osteoporosis, a skeletal metabolic disease further defined by impaired bone microarchitecture, increased bone fragility and susceptibility to bone fractures. The availability of bone density scans as a non-invasive diagnostic technique uncovered the link between this bone disorder and celiac disease (CD) relatively few years ago.[1,2] In contrast, the association between child osteomalacia and CD has been known since the first descriptions of the latter disease, even before the origin and treatment of CD itself were known.[3] Osteomalacia is a disease characterized by low BMD, marked bone deformities and rickets, which, on rare occasions, is part of the initial presentation of CD.[4,5]

CD is a highly prevalent disease[6] that affects approximately 1% of the world population, according to serology-based screening studies.[7] While CD has been traditionally considered a predominantly childhood-onset disorder, it is now conclusively demonstrated that most patients are diagnosed when adults, as it has also been corroborated in Spain[8,9], among whom both atypical manifestations and a low suspicion index may delay the diagnosis.[10] In fact, most of those who suffer from CD are undiagnosed and women are more frequently diagnosed than men. Many current CD patients lived with their symptoms for years before diagnosis and were therefore exposed to the consequences of the disease. Furthermore, osteoporosis presents characteristics similar to those of CD in terms of frequency and underdiagnosis. It has been hypothesized that CD could explain part of the considerable "mixed bag" represented by idiopathic osteoporosis.[1,6-11] Therefore, there is a high rate of suspicion among health professionals treating both diseases (CD and osteoporosis) and using their expertise could bring many hidden cases to light, with the benefit of an accurate and early treatment.

In adult patients, changes in bone mineralization, osteopenia or osteoporosis are some of the most common CD complications and can affect up to 75% of the patients as shown in a few series of studies[1] with a prevalence among celiac sufferers that doubles that of the unaffected population in the same age range.[11] Despite this, the many studies on the subject notwithstanding, a description of how CD (a primarily digestive disorder) can affect bone metabolism has yet to be fully elucidated.

CD in itself causes significant deterioration in the quality of life[11,13], which is compounded by the presence of osteoporosis and its clinical manifestation in the form of fractures. These and other factors are the reasons why physicians adopt an interventionist stance and try to prevent its occurrence and/or mitigate its impact.

2. Osteoporosis: Definition and general concepts

Osteoporosis is the most common metabolic bone disease. It involves a reduction in bone mass and it is responsible for most fractures suffered by adults over the age of 50. It is estimated that 1 in 3 women over 50 in Europe[14] and the United States[15] will suffer an osteoporotic fracture during their lifetimes. Although BMD is considered the major determinant of osteoporosis, there are additional factors that influence bone fragility, which, in recent years, have been brought together under the term "bone quality." These include microarchitecture, bone turnover degree, build-up of lesions or microfractures and bone mineralization degree.[16]

The World Health Organization establishes different low bone mass degrees based on bone density scan measurements of any skeletal area in American Caucasoid women.[17] This strategy establishes an osteoporosis diagnosis when bone mass values are below -2.5 standard deviations (SD) of peak bone mass (i.e. the maximum BMD value reached by an adult) and an osteopenia diagnosis when those values are located between -1 SD and -2.5 SD. Severe or established osteoporosis is that presenting with a BMD less than -2.5 SD and a current or past fragility fracture.[15,18]

The results of BMD measurements are expressed as a T-score, which is the number of standard deviations by which BMD measurement differs from bone density measurement in the young population ("peak" BMD) (Table 1). Another way of expressing the results is the Z-score, which is obtained by comparing a BMD measurement with reference values for subjects of the same age and gender. It is recommended in some guidelines[22] for men and for premenopausal women.

Diagnosis	BMD criteria (T-*score*)
Normal	BMD T > -1 SD
Osteopenia or low bone density	BMD T < -1 and > -2,49 SD
Osteoporosis	BMD T < -2,49 SD
Severe osteoporosis	BMD T < -2,49 SD + fracture

T-score: comparison with the BMD value observed in the median reference population.
SD: Standard deviation; BMD: Bone mineral density.

Table 1. World Health Organization (WHO) diagnostic criteria for post-menopausal Caucasoid women.

3. Prevalence of osteoporosis among celiac disease patients

It is estimated that by the time childhood CD is diagnosed, one-third of affected children have osteoporosis, one-third have osteopenia and only the remaining third retain a normal BMD.[9] In any case, once the gluten-free diet (GFD) is instituted, most celiac children catch up to their height-weight growth curve and accelerate their rate of bone mineralization, so that most achieve normal peak bone mass by the time bone growth is completed. The main problem arises when CD is diagnosed during adulthood, once bone growth is complete and peak bone mass has been reached. Among these patients, the prevalence of osteoporosis is at least twice that of the unaffected population in the same age range.[6,20] More than half of asymptomatic celiac patients with positive serological and digestive tract markers may have bone disease at the time of diagnosis.[1,10,21-25] This also includes those without villous atrophy, that is, those who are at stages 1 and 2 of the Marsh-Oberhüber duodenal lesion classification.

Prevalence studies of bone mass loss among CD patients reveal widely variable frequencies[2,21,26-33] (Table 2); Valdimarsson *et al.* carried out a prospective study of 63 adult patients and noted a prevalence of osteoporosis of 22% in the forearm, 18% in the hip and 15% in the lumbar spine (estimated on the basis of Z-scores).[34] Bardella et al only documented low BMD among women diagnosed with CD during adulthood.[35] Meyer et al. found low BMD in the lumbar spine in 38% and in the hip in 44% of the adult celiac patients analyzed.[33] The wide variability in the frequency of low BMD in these studies may be explained by several factors, including the diagnostic criteria for osteoporosis (T or Z-score), the measurement method, the skeletal location where the measurement was obtained, patient selection and whether assessment was performed before or after a GFD was started. In any case, the available data confirm a clearly heightened prevalence of low BMD among celiac patients compared to the general population, which generally ranges around 40%.

Low BMD has been demonstrated in patients with classic symptoms[11], in sub-clinical cases[36] and even in asymptomatic patients.[26] Paradoxically, an even greater impairment has been observed among patients without digestive symptoms than among those with classic symptoms.[10] Therefore, the type of CD-related symptom does not seem to predict the presence of low BMD, which explains attempts to identify other causes.

Osteoporosis is therefore a common CD complication, which suggests that it is appropriate to consider whether or not to screen for CD in patients with idiopathic osteoporosis. Although there is no definitive consensus, the majority of opinions are in favor of this strategy[37,40], as CD frequency is 10 times higher than expected in patients with osteoporosis; in fact, a similar CD frequency among type 1 diabetics already justifies universal screening among the latter.[41] Moreover, CD screening through specific antibodies in patients with OS has led to the diagnosis of between 4[42] and 17[40] times more celiac patients.

Those studies where the results were opposed to screening for CD among osteoporosis patients can be explained due to the use of low-sensitivity antibodies; in fact, Legroux-Gerot et al. only measured anti-gliadin antibodies, while tissue anti-transglutaminase (AAtTG) was only determined in those with positive titers[43], a strategy that underdiagnoses CD. This same study established the AAtTG positivity threshold at 50 U/mL, well above the 2 U/mL threshold currently recommended for diagnosing adults.[44] Other studies suffer from similar limitations: Mather *et al.* measured antiendomysial antibodies[45], Lindh et al. antigliadin[42] and the positivity threshold for AAtTG in Laadhar's research was set at 10 U/mL .[39]

Parameter	Mean weighted value	Number of studies (number of subjects included)
Z-score, lumbar spine	-1.3	14 (490)
Z-score, hip	-1.1	7 (239)
T-*score,* lumbar spine	-1.7	1(86)
T-*score,* hip	-1.4	1 (86)
% with lumbar osteoporosis	26	6 (212)
% with hip osteoporosis	11	3 (102)
% with lumbar osteopenia	41	4 (188)
% with hiposteopenia	43	3 (102)

Table 2. Studies of BMD in adult patients with celiac disease before starting GFD (Adapted from Scott, 2000[28]).

4. Aetiology and pathogenesis of low BMD in CD

The pathogenic mechanisms underlying metabolic bone disease in patients with CD have not been fully elucidated. The origin of osteoporosis in CD has been classically associated with malabsorption of calcium and vitamin D [46] caused by intestinal villous atrophy[47], as well as by secondary hyperparathyroidism.[48] Low consumption of dairy products[51], failure to ever reach peak theoretical bone mass[26,49-50], a higher degree of duodenal injury in biopsies[51,52] and a greater diagnostic delay[20] have also been directly related to the pathogenesis of low BMD in celiac patients.

We know that vitamin D deficiency is common among patients with CD, although there are no changes in vitamin D receptor expression[53] nor is there a greater number of receptor gene mutations interfering with the metabolism of this vitamin[54] in this population. Restricted milk intake may exacerbate vitamin D deficiency; in fact, co-occurrence of lactose intolerance is common among celiac patients and it is estimated at 10%, but may increase to 50% in the presence of obvious malabsorption symptoms.[55-58] However, one must bear in mind that diet only provides 5-10% of required vitamin D[59], the rest being obtained from exposure to sunlight. Even so, studies of celiac patients have failed to establish any clear association between vitamin D levels and bone impairment. This is also the case for other intestinal diseases, such as inflammatory bowel disease.[59]

Several authors have suggested that deficits of other fat-soluble vitamins (A, K and E) and even in water-soluble vitamins (C, B_{12}, folic acid and B_6) or of minerals (such as iron, calcium, phosphorus, copper, zinc, boron, fluorine), which are required for normal bone metabolism[52,60], also result from the intestinal malabsorption exhibited by celiac patients.

Hyperparathyroidism is another implicated factor; even in patients with normal vitamin D serum levels, high PTH levels have been associated with bone mass loss.[47] Indeed, celiac patients on a

GFD frequently exhibit high serum PTH levels.[61] Reduced serum levels of IGF-1 (insulin-like growth factor-1 or somatomedin C)[62] constitute an additional hormonal factor which has been involved in patients with a lower bone mass. This was associated with decreased zinc serum levels[63], which became normal after introducing a GFD.

Despite all of the above, the malabsorption theory in and of itself has not been corroborated by some studies[52], while the complex regulation of bone turnover and the effect of the multiple nutritional factors involved, together with the discordant results of various studies, have led to the emergence of new hypotheses for the origin of osteoporosis in CD, such as the link between low BMD and chronic inflammation.[64] Indeed, a less well-known function of vitamin D is its role in the activation of the T lymphocytes that maintain the integrity of intestinal mucosal immunity, prevent infection[65] and regulate protein binding.[66] Accordingly, vitamin D deficiency has long been considered to be a trigger of autoimmune and inflammatory diseases.[67]

Chronic inflammation determines changes in bone metabolism via several proinflammatory cytokines, such as tumour necrosis factor alpha (TNF-α), interleukins (IL)-1beta, IL-6 or gamma interferon. TNF-related cytokines include the receptor activator of nuclear factor kappa-B (RANK), its ligand (RANKL), and osteopreotegerin (OPG). RANKL is a key molecule in the regulation of bone metabolism; its genetic expression is induced after activation of T lymphocytes and it is secreted by these cells. RANKL has proved to be a survival factor whose primary function is activation of osteoclasts, cells involved in bone resorption.[68] Overproduction of RANKL is implicated in a variety of degenerative diseases of bone tissue, such as rheumatoid arthritis or psoriatic arthritis, while RANKL gene inactivation in mice produces severe osteopetrosis caused by a massive osteoclast deficit.[69,70] Conversely, OPG (osteoprotegerin, for bone protection) is an osteoclastogenesis-inhibiting protein, which acts as a decoy receptor homologous to RANK, binds to its ligand RANKL, and thereby neutralizes its action.[71] OPG production is stimulated *in vivo* by oestrogens and by the anti-resorptive drug strontium ranelate.[72] IL-6 promotes the expression of both RANKL and OPG and stimulates both osteoblast formation and bone resorption.

Serum levels of RANKL and OPG are elevated in patients with CD[73] and the relative relationship established between these cytokines is therefore more important than their actual levels; hence, an imbalance in the OPG/RANKL ratio has been associated with altered bone turnover in patients with different conditions, including renal osteodystrophy[74], rheumatoid arthritis[75], Cushing's disease[76] and primary biliary cirrhosis.[77] The OPG/RANKL ratio is directly associated with IL-6 serum levels[73] and lumbar bone mass.[78] Thus, adult women with CD have OPG/RANKL ratios significantly lower than controls despite adherence to a GFD; this correlates with a lower lumbar BMD.[79] Although the role of high OPG levels in CD has not been fully elucidated, the available evidence suggests that this is a protective mechanism against other factors that cause bone damage. The mechanisms described as direct activators of osteoclastogenesis and subsequent bone mass loss[80] have recently been recognized as potential contributors to osteoporosis among patients with a range of digestive diseases. In fact, patients with CD and inflammatory bowel disease have similar profiles in terms of expression of bone metabolism regulatory cytokines.[81,83]

Finally, the aetiology of osteoporosis in CD definitely includes factors shared with the rest of the population[84] (family history, age, menopause, physical activity, smoking), as well as other specific factors such as genetic influence, the above-mentioned vitamin deficiencies, hormonal changes and the inflammatory process itself.

Years of exposure to dietary gluten before diagnosis do not seem to influence BMD significantly[26,32-33,85-86] nor does early menopause.[24] Some studies report an inverse relationship between GFD and calcium intake.[87] There is little data on the influence of patient gender on BMD, but most studies show no difference in this regard.[24,33-34,88-89] Another factor associated with poor bone condition is a low body mass index (BMI).[11,52,84,90] Patients with persistent villous atrophy despite proper adherence to the GFD (refractory CD) are particularly susceptible to osteoporosis, with a prevalence of 58% compared to 22% reported among GFD-responsive patients.[90]

5. Diagnosis of low bone mineral density in CD

All patients in whom there is clinical suspicion of osteoporosis should undergo a thorough recording of their history and a physical examination so as to identify other risk factors and/or consequences. As for imaging methods, conventional radiography has not proven to be a specific or sensitive method for assessment of changes in bone mass; therefore, osteoporosis studies should be performed using bone density scans. In the case of CD, it has been suggested that all patients diagnosed in adulthood should undergo bone densitometry[11,91] as it is a simple, non-invasive and highly accurate[92] diagnostic method (its margin of error is estimated at only 5-6%). Its greatest benefit is determining whether there is osteoporosis and the degree of impairment so that a treatment regimen can be planned. However, some studies, observing the low risk of bone fracture among celiac patients, have questioned the usefulness of routine bone density scan[28,93] as it is considered to have low cost-effectiveness. Other authors suggest using densitometry only in patients with digestive conditions[94], even though this is not a conditioning factor for greater risk.[95] In fact, celiac patients without gastrointestinal symptoms may have low BMD, which increases after start of the GFD.[10] Recent studies advocate densitometric assessment in all celiac patients diagnosed during adulthood who have villous atrophy on duodenal biopsies and/or laboratory values suggestive of malnutrition or malabsorption, regardless of their symptoms.[52]

Another issue raised in the literature concerns the optimal timing for bone density scan in celiac patients; whether at the time of CD diagnosis or after a period of adherence to the GFD. In fact, celiac children show a great bone recovery capacity after starting a GFD, so no further studies seem to be necessary until their growth period is completed. In any case, the main benefit of BMD testing would be obtained when the introduction of a different treatment rather than the GFD alone is derived from test results.

As the development of osteoporosis is determined by multiple risk factors, identifying which of these factors are most relevant, or using a score for the risk of fracture at 10 years, is highly desirable. Bone remodelling markers (such as the N-terminal telopeptide of procollagen-1, hydroxyproline, and bone alkaline phosphatase) provide additional information on the dynamics of bone turnover that is complementary to densitometry findings. In celiac patients with osteoporosis, levels of these markers are higher than in celiacs with normal BMD.[52] However, the usefulness of their determination in bone disease diagnosis is limited, so this measurement is not recommended as part of the routine evaluation of the patients with osteoporosis.

6. Bone fracture risk in CD

Due to the increased prevalence of osteoporosis, celiac patients have a high risk of fractures, estimated at between 3.5 to 7 times higher than that of the unaffected population of the same age and gender.[11] Furthermore, up to one in four adult CD patients have an established history of fractures[96], which produces significant deterioration in the quality of life.

As in other aspects of the relationship between CD and osteoporosis, quantification of fracture risk by different studies shows mixed results. These discrepancies are largely due to the way in which the data were collected; mainly from fracture reports, questionnaires, or hospital admissions. It is therefore possible that the prevalence of fractures (vertebral, hip, and overall) is underestimated in the celiac population. One of the common issues of fracture risk studies is that they lack proper morphometric assessment of the spine, which underestimates fractures at that level[2], or failure to use validated questionnaires or methods, such as the FRAX® (Fracture Risk Assessment Tool) index proposed by the World Health Organization.[97]

To date, nine published studies and one meta-analysis have estimated the incidence or prevalence of bone fractures in the adult celiac population (Table 3).[28] Their heterogeneous methodologies, use of different cut-off points for determination of osteoporosis and variable diagnostic criteria for CD translate into significant discrepancies in results. A retrospective study conducted in Argentina on 165 celiac patients determined a peripheral fracture prevalence over 3 times higher than that observed in controls.[2] The same study showed that the highest prevalence of fractures in the lumbar spine was only present in patients with CD classic symptoms.[98] A retrospective study carried out in the UK showed that 21.3% of celiac patients had a history of fractures, compared with only 2.7% of non-celiac controls, a highly significant difference quantified as a relative risk (RR) of 7.0.[102] By contrast, other studies with large sample sizes in the same geographical region found no major differences.[29] Two further studies in Europe, the first with a large number of the patients, reported a slight increase in risk of fracture: a study of approximately 13,000 patients and 65,000 controls in Sweden showed a 2.1% higher risk (95%CI: 1.8-2.4) of hip fracture and a 1.4% higher risk (95%CI: 1.3-1.5) of any type of fracture among celiacs.[31] A recent study of adult celiacs in Spain, conducted at the time of diagnosis, used the FRAX® tool to estimate the risk of fracture at 10 years. This showed a moderate risk of fracture among patients with duodenal villous atrophy (Marsh stage III), which was 3.5 times that of the patients without villous atrophy (Marsh stage I or II).[52]

Finally, the Olmos et al. meta-analysis[101], which included 21,000 celiac patients and about 100,000 controls, confirmed a 43% increase in the prevalence of fractures among celiacs (8.7% vs. 6.1%).

	Country and year	Study population	Design	Osteoporosis /fractures diagnostic methods	Fractures analyzed	Risk of fractures
Vasquez H et al [2].	Argentina, 2000	165 celiacs and 165 controls with gastrointestinal symptoms	Cross-sectional with retrospective analysis	Dual energy X-ray densitometry, spine radiography	Peripheral Lumbar spine	OR 3.5 (1.8-7.2) OR 2.8 (0.7-11.5)
Fickling WE et al [99].	UK, 2001	75 celiacs with 75 controls matched by age and sex	Cross-sectional with retrospective analysis	Dual energy X ray absorptiometry (DEXA) of lumbar spine and femoral neck	Any location	21% among celiacs, versus 3% in controls
Thomason K et al [29].	UK, 2003	244 celiacs born after 1950, 161 controls of the same age and sex	Analysis of celiac population records. Controls paired for age and sex	Lifestyle and general health questionnaire, with specific questions about history of fractures	Any location Forearm	OR 1.05 (0.68-1.62) OR 1.21 (0.66-2.25)
West J et al [96].	UK, 2003	4732 celiacs (1589 "incidents") and 23 620 controls matched by age and sex	Population cohort study from a database	Codified registry of fractures in celiacs and controls	Any location Hip Ulna, radius	HR 1.30 (1.16-1.46) HR 1.90 (1.20-3.02) HR 1.77 (1.35-2.34)
Moreno ML et al [98].	Argentina, 2004	148 celiacs and 292 controls of the same age and sex with gastrointestinal symptoms	Cross-sectional study of cases and controls	History of fracture based on interview with a predefined questionnaire	Any location	OR 5.2 (2.8-9.8) in "classic" CD. OR 1.7 (0.7-4.4) in "asymptomatic" CD.
Vestergaard P et al [31].	Denmark, 2002	1021 celiacs and 3063 controls matched by age and sex	Computerized registry of all national hospital admissions and discharges	Diagnoses of fractures in cases and controls in the same national registry	Any location Lumbar Distal radius (Colles) Neck of femur	RRI 0.7 (0.45-1.09) RRI 2.14 (0.70-6.57) RRI 2.00 (0.58-6.91) RRI 0.71 (0.27-1.89)
Davie MW et al [100]	UK, 2005	383 celiac women over 50 and 445 controls	Cross-sectional study using	Detailed questionnaire about history of fractures	Any location	OR 1.51 (1.13-1.5)
Ludvigsson JF et al [31]	Sweden, 2007	13 000 individuals with CD (4819 adults) and 65 000 controls matched by age and sex	Cross-sectional population cohort study based on hospital discharge records	Records of 1st documented fracture at any location	Any location Hip	HR 1.4 (1.3-1.5) HR 2.1 (1.8-2.4)
García-Manzanares A et al [52]	Spain, 2012	40 patients with a diagnosis of CD in adulthood	Prospective cross-sectional	Dual energy X-ray densitometry, FRAX® tool	Risk of hip fracture Risk of major osteoporotic fracture (lumbar, femoral neck, forearm and shoulder)	3.5 times greater in Marsh III on I-II. 1.34 times greater in Marsh III on I-II.

CD, celiac disease; OR, odds ratio; RRI, relative risk increase; HR: hazard ratio.

Table 3. Studies of fracture risk available in adult celiacs (Adapted from Scott, 2000[28]).

7. Treatment of low bone mineral density in patients with CD

The first-line treatment for osteoporosis in CD is the GFD itself: many studies have demonstrated its effect on bone density and calcium absorption.[21,23-24,27,32,87,90,102,105] The greatest bone mass gain described in these studies is during the first year:[24,34] The GFD leads to a 5% increase in bone mass after 1 year[1], although this is not enough for bone mass to normalize. In clinical practice conditions, the degree of adherence to the GFD also determines the recovery of bone mass, which is generally estimated at around 30%.[106,107] Furthermore, the recovery rate is higher in young celiac patients[21] than among adults,[21,34] which is largely explained by the fact that 97% of bone mass is gained in the first two decades of life and full recovery is difficult after this time.

BMD loss associated with pediatric CD responds to GFD continuously and gradually, with almost complete restoration of bone mass after about two years' treatment.[108] The earlier the age at which the GFD is started, the better and faster the response.[26] In fact, it is estimated that an increase in BMD will only take place if the GFD is started before the age of 25.[46] A proper GFD is so important for bone metabolism that lack of improvement in BMD after its introduction has been associated with persistent duodenal lesions.[11]

In addition to the GFD and in accordance with the NIH consensus statement on the treatment of osteoporosis,[15] an adequate daily intake of calcium and vitamin D should be ensured, as it is a critical factor for bone mass acquisition and maintenance. Untreated adult celiac patients have shown a 45% reduction in calcium absorption followed by an improvement of 52% after 6 months of adherence to the GFD.[109] Regarding vitamin D, at the time of diagnosis, less than 5% of Spanish adult CD patients had normal serum levels.[52] A daily intake of 1200–1500 mg calcium and 400 U vitamin D is recommended and, as in all other forms of osteoporosis, this should be supplemented with medications. Adherence to drug therapy, as to the GFD, is a crucial aspect of treatment, so patients must be kept motivated. In fact, these patients will most commonly abandon treatment with calcium and vitamin D, as it must be taken daily, while hormonal therapy and bisphosphonates (which are administered weekly) are usually adhered to correctly.[110] Drug treatment would be indicated for patients who do not achieve bone mass recovery goals and would not differ from that established for other causes of osteoporosis, with bisphosphonates being the recommended first-line therapy. However, the literature is lacking in data on the specific effect of bisphosphonates on CD-associated osteoporosis.

8. Conclusions

CD has been associated with low BMD since its very first descriptions. Osteomalacia in children with CD is now an exceptionally rare finding; unfortunately, the same cannot be said for osteoporosis and osteopenia, which occur in 40% of the patients diagnosed in adulthood and determine a variable increase in the risk of bone fracture, leading to lower quality of life. Changes in the epidemiology of CD make low BMD screening by bone density scans more relevant for adult celiacs. Subjects with villous atrophy or laboratory values suggestive of malnutrition at the time of CD diagnosis may derive greater benefit from bone density scan.

The gluten-free diet is also the basis of low BMD treatment among celiacs and it is sufficient in younger patients. In adults with low bone mass, however, it must be supplemented with calcium and vitamin D. Although specific studies are lacking, bisphosphonates might also provide an effective first line of treatment for adult celiac patients with osteoporosis.

References

1. Corazza GR, Di SM, Maurino E, Bai JC. *Bones in coeliac disease: Diagnosis and treatment. Best Pract Res Clin Gastroenterol.* 2005; 19: 453-465. http://dx.doi.org/10.1016/j.bpg.2005.01.002

2. Vasquez H, Mazure R, Gonzalez D, Flores D, Pedreira S, Niveloni S, et al. *Risk of fractures in celiac disease patients: A cross-sectional, case-control study. Am J Gastroenterol.* 2000; 95: 183-189. http://dx.doi.org/10.1111/j.1572-0241.2000.01682.x

3. Salvesen HA, Boe J. *Osteomalacia in sprue.* Acta Med Scand. 1953; 146: 290-299. http://dx.doi.org/10.1111/j.0954-6820.1953.tb10243.x

4. Basu RA, Elmer K, Babu A, Kelly CA. *Coeliac disease can still present with osteomalacia!.* Rheumatology (Oxford). 2000; 39: 335-336. http://dx.doi.org/10.1093/rheumatology/39.3.335

5. Rabelink NM, Westgeest HM, Bravenboer N, Jacobs MA, Lips P. *Bone pain and extremely low bone mineral density due to severe vitamin D deficiency in celiac disease.* Arch Osteoporos. 2011; 6: 209-213. http://dx.doi.org/10.1007/s11657-011-0059-7

6. Sundar N, Crimmins R, Swift G. *Clinical presentation and incidence of complications in patients with coeliac disease diagnosed by relative screening.* Postgrad Med J. 2007; 83: 273-276. http://dx.doi.org/10.1136/pgmj.2006.052977

7. Rodrigo-Sáez L, Fuentes-Álvarez D, Álvarez-Mieres N, Niño-García P, de Francisco García R, Riestra-Menendez S. *Enfermedad Celiaca en el 2009.* RAPD Online. 2009; 32: 339-357.

8. Reilly NR, Green PH. *Epidemiology and clinical presentations of celiac disease.* Semin Immunopathol. 2012; 34: 473-478. http://dx.doi.org/10.1007/s00281-012-0311-2

9. Goddard CJ, Gillett HR. *Complications of coeliac disease: Are all patients at risk?.* Postgrad Med J. 2006;82:705-712. http://dx.doi.org/10.1136/pgmj.2006.048876

10. Mustalahti K, Collin P, Sievanen H, Salmi J, Maki M. *Osteopenia in patients with clinically silent coeliac disease warrants screening.* Lancet. 1999; 354: 744-745. http://dx.doi.org/10.1016/S0140-6736(99)01990-X

11. Walters JR, Banks LM, Butcher GP, Fowler CR. *Detection of low bone mineral density by dual energy x ray absorptiometry in unsuspected suboptimally treated coeliac disease.* Gut. 1995; 37: 220-224. http://dx.doi.org/10.1136/gut.37.2.220

12. Dorn SD, Hernandez L, Minaya MT, Morris CB, Hu Y, Leserman J, et al. *The development and validation of a new coeliac disease quality of life survey (CD-QOL).* Aliment Pharmacol Ther. 2010; 31: 666-675. http://dx.doi.org/10.1111/j.1365-2036.2009.04220.x

13. de Lorenzo CM, Xikota JC, Wayhs MC, Nassar SM, de Souza Pires MM. *Evaluation of the quality of life of children with celiac disease and their parents: a case-control study.* Qual Life Res. 2012; 21: 77-85. http://dx.doi.org/10.1007/s11136-011-9930-7

14. Gullberg B, Johnell O, Kanis JA. *World-wide projections for hip fracture.* Osteoporos Int. 1997; 7: 407-413. http://dx.doi.org/10.1007/PL00004148

15. *Osteoporosis prevention, diagnosis, and therapy. NIH Consens Statement.* 2000; 17: 1-45.

16. Sambrook P, Cooper C. *Osteoporosis.* Lancet. 2006; 367: 2010-2018. http://dx.doi.org/10.1016/S0140-6736(06)68891-0

17. Sosa HM, Diaz CM, Diez PA, Gomez AC, Gonzalez MJ, Farrerons MJ, et al. *Guide for the prevention and treatment of glucocorticoid-induced osteoporosis of the Spanish Society of Internal Medicine.* Rev Clin Esp. 2008; 208: 33-45.
http://dx.doi.org/10.1157/13115006

18. *Consensus development conference: Diagnosis, prophylaxis, and treatment of osteoporosis.* Am J Med. 1993; 94 (6): 646-650.
http://dx.doi.org/10.1016/0002-9343(93)90218-E

19. Khan AA, Bachrach L, Brown JP, Hanley DA, Josse RG, Kendler DL, et al. *Standards and guidelines for performing central dual-energy x-ray absorptiometry in premenopausal women, men, and children.* J Clin Densitom. 2004; 7: 51-64.
http://dx.doi.org/10.1385/JCD:7:1:51

20. Younes M, Ben YH, Safer L, Fadoua H, Zrour S, Bejia I, et al. *Prevalence of bone loss in adult celiac disease and associated factors: A control case study.* Tunis Med. 2012; 90: 129-135.

21. Mora S, Weber G, Barera G, Bellini A, Pasolini D, Prinster C et al. *Effect of gluten-free diet on bone mineral content in growing patients with celiac disease.* Am J Clin Nutr. 1993; 57: 224-228.

22. Corazza GR, Valentini RA, Andreani ML, D'Anchino M, Leva MT, Ginaldi L, et al. *Subclinical coeliac disease is a frequent cause of iron-deficiency anaemia.* Scand J Gastroenterol. 1995; 30:153-156. http://dx.doi.org/10.3109/00365529509093254

23. Caraceni MP, Molteni N, Bardella MT, Ortolani S, Nogara A, Bianchi PA. *Bone and mineral metabolism in adult celiac disease.* Am J Gastroenterol. 1988; 83: 274-277.

24. McFarlane XA, Bhalla AK, Reeves DE, Morgan LM, Robertson DA. *Osteoporosis in treated adult coeliac disease.* Gut. 1995; 36: 710-714.
http://dx.doi.org/10.1136/gut.36.5.710

25. Gonzalez D, Mazure R, Mautalen C, Vazquez H, Bai J. *Body composition and bone mineral density in untreated and treated patients with celiac disease.* Bone. 1995; 16: 231-234. http://dx.doi.org/10.1016/8756-3282(94)00034-W

26. Mazure R, Vazquez H, Gonzalez D, Mautalen C, Pedreira S, Boerr L, et al. *Bone mineral affection in asymptomatic adult patients with celiac disease.* Am J Gastroenterol. 1994; 89: 2130-2134.

27. Bai JC, Gonzalez D, Mautalen C, Mazure R, Pedreira S, Vazquez H, et al. *Long-term effect of gluten restriction on bone mineral density of patients with coeliac disease.* Aliment Pharmacol Ther. 1997; 11: 157-164.
http://dx.doi.org/10.1046/j.1365-2036.1997.112283000.x

28. Scott EM, Gaywood I, Scott BB. *Guidelines for osteoporosis in coeliac disease and inflammatory bowel disease.* Gut. 2000; 46 (Suppl 1): I1-I8.
http://dx.doi.org/10.1136/gut.46.suppl_1.I1

29. Thomason K, West J, Logan RF, Coupland C, Holmes GK. *Fracture experience of patients with coeliac disease: A population based survey.* Gut. 2003; 52: 518-522.
http://dx.doi.org/10.1136/gut.52.4.518

30. Vestergaard P, Mosekilde L. *Fracture risk in patients with celiac Disease, Crohn's disease, and ulcerative colitis: a nationwide follow-up study of 16,416 patients in Denmark.* Am J Epidemiol. 2002; 156: 1-10. http://dx.doi.org/10.1093/aje/kwf007

31. Ludvigsson JF, Michaelsson K, Ekbom A, Montgomery SM. *Coeliac disease and the risk of fractures - a general population-based cohort study.* Aliment Pharmacol Ther. 2007; 25: 273-285. http://dx.doi.org/10.1111/j.1365-2036.2006.03203.x

32. Lewis NR, Scott BB. *Should patients with coeliac disease have their bone mineral density measured?*. Eur J Gastroenterol Hepatol. 2005; 17: 1065-1070.
http://dx.doi.org/10.1097/00042737-200510000-00009

33. Meyer D, Stavropolous S, Diamond B, Shane E, Green PH. *Osteoporosis in a north american adult population with celiac disease.* Am J Gastroenterol. 2001; 96: 112-119.
http://dx.doi.org/10.1111/j.1572-0241.2001.03507.x

34. Valdimarsson T, Lofman O, Toss G, Strom M. *Reversal of osteopenia with diet in adult coeliac disease.* Gut. 1996; 38: 322-327. http://dx.doi.org/10.1136/gut.38.3.322

35. Bardella MT, Fredella C, Prampolini L, Molteni N, Giunta AM, Bianchi PA. *Body composition and dietary intakes in adult celiac disease patients consuming a strict gluten-free diet.* Am J Clin Nutr. 2000; 72: 937-939.

36. Corazza GR, Di SA, Cecchetti L, Jorizzo RA, Di SM, Minguzzi L, Brusco G, et al. *Influence of pattern of clinical presentation and of gluten-free diet on bone mass and metabolism in adult coeliac disease.* Bone. 1996; 18: 525-530.
http://dx.doi.org/10.1016/8756-3282(96)00071-3

37. Drummond FJ, Annis P, O'Sullivan K, Wynne F, Daly M, Shanahan F, et al. *Screening for asymptomatic celiac disease among patients referred for bone densitometry measurement.* Bone. 2003; 33: 970-974. http://dx.doi.org/10.1016/j.bone.2003.07.002

38. Gonzalez D, Sugai E, Gomez JC, Oliveri MB, Gomez AC, Vega E, et al. *Is it necessary to screen for celiac disease in postmenopausal osteoporotic women? Calcif Tissue Int.* 2002; 71: 141-144. http://dx.doi.org/10.1007/s00223-001-1027-9

39. Laadhar L, Masmoudi S, Bahlous A, Zitouni M, Sahli H, Kallel-Sellami M et al. *Is screening for celiac disease in osteoporotic post-menopausal women necessary?* Joint Bone Spine. 2007; 74: 510-511. http://dx.doi.org/10.1016/j.jbspin.2007.01.025

40. Stenson WF, Newberry R, Lorenz R, Baldus C, Civitelli R. *Increased prevalence of celiac disease and need for routine screening among patients with osteoporosis.* Arch Intern Med. 2005; 165: 393-399. http://dx.doi.org/10.1001/archinte.165.4.393

41. *Introduction: The American Diabetes Association's (ADA) evidence-based practice guidelines, standards, and related recommendations and documents for diabetes care.* Diabetes Care. 2012; 35 (Suppl 1): S1-S2. http://dx.doi.org/10.2337/dc12-s001

42. Lindh E, Ljunghall S, Larsson K, Lavo B. *Screening for antibodies against gliadin in patients with osteoporosis.* J Intern Med. 1992; 231: 403-406.
http://dx.doi.org/10.1111/j.1365-2796.1992.tb00951.x

43. Legroux-Gerot I, Leloire O, Blanckaert F, Tonnel F, Grardel B, Ducrocq JL, et al. *Screening for celiac disease in patients with osteoporosis.* Joint Bone Spine. 2009; 76: 162-165.
http://dx.doi.org/10.1016/j.jbspin.2008.06.016

44. Santaolalla R, Fernandez-Banares F, Rodriguez R, Alsina M, Rosinach M, Marine M et al. *Diagnostic value of duodenal antitissue transglutaminase antibodies in gluten-sensitive enteropathy.* Aliment Pharmacol Ther. 2008; 27: 820-829.
http://dx.doi.org/10.1111/j.1365-2036.2008.03652.x

45. Mather KJ, Meddings JB, Beck PL, Scott RB, Hanley DA. *Prevalence of IgA-antiendomysial antibody in asymptomatic low bone mineral density.* Am J Gastroenterol. 2001; 96: 120-125. http://dx.doi.org/10.1111/j.1572-0241.2001.03461.x

46. Ciacci C, Maurelli L, Klain M, Savino G, Salvatore M, Mazzacca G, et al. *Effects of dietary treatment on bone mineral density in adults with celiac disease: Factors predicting response. Am J Gastroenterol.* 1997; 92: 992-996.

47. Selby PL, Davies M, Adams JE, Mawer EB. *Bone loss in celiac disease is related to secondary hyperparathyroidism.* J Bone Miner Res. 1999; 14: 652-657. http://dx.doi.org/10.1359/jbmr.1999.14.4.652

48. Kinsey L, Burden ST, Bannerman E. *A dietary survey to determine if patients with coeliac disease are meeting current healthy eating guidelines and how their diet compares to that of the British general population.* Eur J Clin Nutr. 2008; 62: 1333-1342. http://dx.doi.org/10.1038/sj.ejcn.1602856

49. Bernstein CN, Leslie WD. *The pathophysiology of bone disease in gastrointestinal disease.* Eur J Gastroenterol Hepatol. 2003; 15: 857-864. http://dx.doi.org/10.1097/00042737-200308000-00004

50. Fisher AA, Davis MW, Budge MM. *Should we screen adults with osteoporotic fractures for coeliac disease?* Gut. 2004; 53: 154-155. http://dx.doi.org/10.1136/gut.53.1.154-a

51. Jatla M, Zemel BS, Bierly P, Verma R. *Bone mineral content deficits of the spine and whole body in children at time of diagnosis with celiac disease.* J Pediatr Gastroenterol Nutr. 2009; 48: 175-180. http://dx.doi.org/10.1097/MPG.0b013e318177e621

52. Garcia-Manzanares A, Tenias JM, Lucendo AJ. *Bone mineral density directly correlates with duodenal Marsh stage in newly diagnosed adult celiac patients.* Scand J Gastroenterol. 2012; 8-9: 927-936. http://dx.doi.org/10.3109/00365521.2012.688217

53. Colston KW, Mackay AG, Finlayson C, Wu JC, Maxwell JD. *Localisation of vitamin D receptor in normal human duodenum and in patients with coeliac disease.* Gut. 1994; 35: 1219-1225. http://dx.doi.org/10.1136/gut.35.9.1219

54. Vogelsang H, Suk EK, Janisiw M, Stain C, Mayr WR, Panzer S. C*alcaneal ultrasound attenuation and vitamin-D-receptor genotypes in celiac disease.* Scand J Gastroenterol. 2000; 35: 172-176. http://dx.doi.org/10.1080/003655200750024344

55. Garcia-Manzanares A, Lucendo AJ. *Nutritional and dietary aspects of celiac disease.* Nutr Clin Pract. 2011; 26: 163-173. http://dx.doi.org/10.1177/0884533611399773

56. Ojetti V, Nucera G, Migneco A, Gabrielli M, Lauritano C, Danese S, et al. High prevalence of celiac disease in patients with lactose intolerance. Digestion. 2005; 71: 106-110. http://dx.doi.org/10.1159/000084526

57. Bode S, Gudmand-Hoyer E. *Incidence and clinical significance of lactose malabsorption in adult coeliac disease.* Scand J Gastroenterol. 1988; 23: 484-488. http://dx.doi.org/10.3109/00365528809093898

58. Annibale B, Severi C, Chistolini A, Antonelli G, Lahner E, Marcheggiano A, et al. *Efficacy of gluten-free diet alone on recovery from iron deficiency anemia in adult celiac patients.* Am J Gastroenterol. 2001; 96: 132-137. http://dx.doi.org/10.1111/j.1572-0241.2001.03463.x

59. Jahnsen J, Falch JA, Mowinckel P, Aadland E. *Vitamin D status, parathyroid hormone and bone mineral density in patients with inflammatory bowel disease.* Scand J Gastroenterol. 2002; 37: 192-199. http://dx.doi.org/10.1080/003655202753416876

60. Stazi AV, Trecca A, Trinti B. *Osteoporosis in celiac disease and in endocrine and reproductive disorders.* World J Gastroenterol. 2008; 14: 498-505. http://dx.doi.org/10.3748/wjg.14.498

61. Lemieux B, Boivin M, Brossard JH, Lepage R, Picard D, Rousseau L, et al. *Normal parathyroid function with decreased bone mineral density in treated celiac disease.* Can J Gastroenterol. 2001; 15: 302-307.

62. Valdimarsson T, Arnqvist HJ, Toss G, Jarnerot G, Nystrom F, Strom M. *Low circulating insulin-like growth factor I in coeliac disease and its relation to bone mineral density.* Scand J Gastroenterol. 1999; 34: 904-908. http://dx.doi.org/10.1080/003655299750025381

63. Jameson S. *Coeliac disease, insulin-like growth factor, bone mineral density, and zinc.* Scand J Gastroenterol. 2000; 35: 894-896. http://dx.doi.org/10.1080/003655200750023291

64. Bianchi ML, Bardella MT. *Bone in celiac disease.* Osteoporos Int. 2008; 19: 1705-1716. http://dx.doi.org/10.1007/s00198-008-0624-0

65. Sun J. *Vitamin D and mucosal immune function.* Curr Opin Gastroenterol. 2010; 26: 591-595. http://dx.doi.org/10.1097/MOG.0b013e32833d4b9f

66. Kong J, Zhang Z, Musch MW, Ning G, Sun J, Hart J, et al. *Novel role of the vitamin D receptor in maintaining the integrity of the intestinal mucosal barrier.* Am J Physiol Gastrointest Liver Physiol. 2008; 294: G208-G216. http://dx.doi.org/10.1152/ajpgi.00398.2007

67. Zittermann A. *Vitamin D in preventive medicine: are we ignoring the evidence?.* Br J Nutr. 2003; 89: 552-572. http://dx.doi.org/10.1079/BJN2003837

68. Buckley KA, Fraser WD. *Receptor activator for nuclear factor kappaB ligand and osteoprotegerin: regulators of bone physiology and immune responses/potential therapeutic agents and biochemical markers.* Ann Clin Biochem. 2002; 39: 551-556. http://dx.doi.org/10.1258/000456302760413324

69. McClung M. *Role of RANKL inhibition in osteoporosis.* Arthritis Res Ther. 2007; 9 (Suppl 1): S3. http://dx.doi.org/10.1186/ar2167

70. Yogo K, Ishida-Kitagawa N, Takeya T. *Negative autoregulation of RANKL and c-Src signaling in osteoclasts.* J Bone Miner Metab. 2007; 25: 205-210. http://dx.doi.org/10.1007/s00774-007-0751-2

71. Simonet WS, Lacey DL, Dunstan CR, Kelley M, Chang MS, Luthy R, et al. *Osteoprotegerin: a novel secreted protein involved in the regulation of bone density.* Cell. 1997; 89: 309-319. http://dx.doi.org/10.1016/S0092-8674(00)80209-3

72. Hofbauer LC, Khosla S, Dunstan CR, Lacey DL, Spelsberg TC, et al. *Estrogen stimulates gene expression and protein production of osteoprotegerin in human osteoblastic cells.* Endocrinology. 1999; 140: 4367-4370. http://dx.doi.org/10.1210/en.140.9.4367

73. Taranta A, Fortunati D, Longo M, Rucci N, Iacomino E, Aliberti F, et al. *Imbalance of osteoclastogenesis-regulating factors in patients with celiac disease.* J Bone Miner Res. 2004; 19: 1112-1121. http://dx.doi.org/10.1359/JBMR.040319

74. Coen G, Ballanti P, Balducci A, Calabria S, Fischer MS, Jankovic L, et al. *Serum osteoprotegerin and renal osteodystrophy.* Nephrol Dial Transplant. 2002; 17: 233-238. http://dx.doi.org/10.1093/ndt/17.2.233

75. Feuerherm AJ, Borset M, Seidel C, Sundan A, Leistad L, Ostensen M, et al. *Elevated levels of osteoprotegerin (OPG) and hepatocyte growth factor (HGF) in rheumatoid arthritis.* Scand J Rheumatol. 2001; 30: 229-234. http://dx.doi.org/10.1080/030097401316909585

76. Ueland T, Bollerslev J, Godang K, Muller F, Froland SS, Aukrust P. *Increased serum osteoprotegerin in disorders characterized by persistent immune activation or glucocorticoid excess--possible role in bone homeostasis.* Eur J Endocrinol. 2001; 145: 685-690. http://dx.doi.org/10.1530/eje.0.1450685

77. Szalay F, Hegedus D, Lakatos PL, Tornai I, Bajnok E, Dunkel K, et al. *High serum osteoprotegerin and low RANKL in primary biliary cirrhosis. J Hepatol.* 2003; 38: 395-400. http://dx.doi.org/10.1016/S0168-8278(02)00435-X

78. McCormick RK. *Osteoporosis: Integrating biomarkers and other diagnostic correlates into the management of bone fragility.* Altern Med Rev. 2007; 12: 113-145.

79. Fiore CE, Pennisi P, Ferro G, Ximenes B, Privitelli L, Mangiafico RA, et al. *Altered osteoprotegerin/RANKL ratio and low bone mineral density in celiac patients on long-term treatment with gluten-free diet.* Horm Metab Res. 2006; 38: 417-422. http://dx.doi.org/10.1055/s-2006-944548

80. Rodriguez-Bores L, Barahona-Garrido J, Yamamoto-Furusho JK. *Basic and clinical aspects of osteoporosis in inflammatory bowel disease.* World J Gastroenterol. 2007; 13: 6156-6165. http://dx.doi.org/10.3748/wjg.13.6156

81. Tilg H, Moschen AR, Kaser A, Pines A, Dotan I. *Gut, inflammation and osteoporosis: basic and clinical concepts.* Gut. 2008; 57: 684-694. http://dx.doi.org/10.1136/gut.2006.117382

82. Miheller P, Muzes G, Racz K, Blazovits A, Lakatos P, Herszenyi L, et al. *Changes of OPG and RANKL concentrations in Crohn's disease after infliximab therapy.* Inflamm Bowel Dis. 2007; 13: 1379-1384. http://dx.doi.org/10.1002/ibd.20234

83. Garcia-Manzanares A, Alvarez-Hernandez J, Pelaez N. *Soporte nutricional en la enfermedad inflamatoria intestinal.* En: Bellido Guerrero D, De Luis Román DA (Ed) Manual de nutricion y metabolismo. Editorial Diaz de Santos, S.A., 2006.

84. Di SM, Veneto G, Corrao G, Corazza GR. *Role of lifestyle factors in the pathogenesis of osteopenia in adult coeliac disease: a multivariate analysis.* Eur J Gastroenterol Hepatol. 2000; 12: 1195-1199. http://dx.doi.org/10.1097/00042737-200012110-00005

85. Mautalen C, Gonzalez D, Mazure R, Vazquez H, Lorenzetti MP, Maurino E, et al. *Effect of treatment on bone mass, mineral metabolism, and body composition in untreated celiac disease patients.* Am J Gastroenterol. 1997; 92: 313-318.

86. Di SM, Jorizzo RA, Veneto G, Cecchetti L, Gasbarrini G, Corazza GR. *Bone mass and metabolism in dermatitis herpetiformis.* Dig Dis Sci. 1999; 44: 2139-2143. http://dx.doi.org/10.1023/A:1026603309056

87. Pazianas M, Butcher GP, Subhani JM, Finch PJ, Ang L, Collins C, et al. *Calcium absorption and bone mineral density in celiacs after long term treatment with gluten-free diet and adequate calcium intake.* Osteoporos Int. 2005; 16: 56-63. http://dx.doi.org/10.1007/s00198-004-1641-2

88. Kemppainen T, Kroger H, Janatuinen E, Arnala I, Kosma VM, Pikkarainen P, et al. *Osteoporosis in adult patients with celiac disease.* Bone. 1999; 24: 249-255. http://dx.doi.org/10.1016/S8756-3282(98)00178-1

89. Sategna-Guidetti C, Grosso SB, Grosso S, Mengozzi G, Aimo G, Zaccaria T, et al. *The effects of 1-year gluten withdrawal on bone mass, bone metabolism and nutritional status in newly-diagnosed adult coeliac disease patients.* Aliment Pharmacol Ther. 2000; 14: 35-43. http://dx.doi.org/10.1046/j.1365-2036.2000.00671.x

90. Kaukinen K, Peraaho M, Lindfors K, Partanen J, Woolley N, Pikkarainen P, et al. *Persistent small bowel mucosal villous atrophy without symptoms in coeliac disease.* Aliment Pharmacol Ther. 2007; 25: 1237-1245. http://dx.doi.org/10.1111/j.1365-2036.2007.03311.x

91. American Gastroenterological Association. *American Gastroenterological Association medical position statement: Guidelines on osteoporosis in gastrointestinal diseases.* Gastroenterology. 2003; 124: 791-794. http://dx.doi.org/10.1053/gast.2003.50107

92. Svendsen OL, Hassager C, Skodt V, Christiansen C. *Impact of soft tissue on in vivo accuracy of bone mineral measurements in the spine, hip, and forearm: a human cadaver study.* J Bone Miner Res. 1995; 10: 868-873.
http://dx.doi.org/10.1002/jbmr.5650100607

93. Murray JA, Van DC, Plevak MF, Dierkhising RA, Zinsmeister AR, Melton LJ, III. *Trends in the identification and clinical features of celiac disease in a North American community, 1950-2001.* Clin Gastroenterol Hepatol. 2003; 1: 19-27.
http://dx.doi.org/10.1053/jcgh.2003.50004

94. Reyes GR, Jodar GE, Garcia MA, Romero MM, Gomez Saez JM, Luque FI, et al. *Clinical practice guidelines for evaluation and treatment of osteoporosis associated to endocrine and nutritional conditions.* Endocrinol Nutr. 2012; 59: 174-196.
http://dx.doi.org/10.1016/j.endonu.2012.01.002

95. Cellier C, Flobert C, Cormier C, Roux C, Schmitz J. *Severe osteopenia in symptom-free adults with a childhood diagnosis of coeliac disease.* Lancet. 2000; 355: 806.
http://dx.doi.org/10.1016/S0140-6736(99)04855-2

96. West J, Logan RF, Card TR, Smith C, Hubbard R. *Fracture risk in people with celiac disease: a population-based cohort study.* Gastroenterology. 2003; 125: 429-436.
http://dx.doi.org/10.1016/S0016-5085(03)00891-6

97. Kanis JA, Johnell O, Oden A, Johansson H, McCloskey E. *FRAX and the assessment of fracture probability in men and women from the UK.* Osteoporos Int. 2008; 19: 385-397.
http://dx.doi.org/10.1007/s00198-007-0543-5

98. Moreno ML, Vazquez H, Mazure R, Smecuol E, Niveloni S, Pedreira S, et al. *Stratification of bone fracture risk in patients with celiac disease.* Clin Gastroenterol Hepatol. 2004; 2: 127-134. http://dx.doi.org/10.1016/S1542-3565(03)00320-3

99. Fickling WE, McFarlane XA, Bhalla AK, Robertson DA. *The clinical impact of metabolic bone disease in coeliac disease.* Postgrad Med J. 2001; 77: 33-36.
http://dx.doi.org/10.1136/pmj.77.903.33

100. Davie MW, Gaywood I, George E, Jones PW, Masud T, Price T, et al. *Excess non-spine fractures in women over 50 years with celiac disease: a cross-sectional, questionnaire-based study.* Osteoporos Int. 2005; 16: 1150-1155.
http://dx.doi.org/10.1007/s00198-004-1822-z

101. Olmos M, Antelo M, Vazquez H, Smecuol E, Maurino E, Bai JC. *Systematic review and meta-analysis of observational studies on the prevalence of fractures in coeliac disease.* Dig Liver Dis. 2008; 40: 46-53. http://dx.doi.org/10.1016/j.dld.2007.09.006

102. Corazza GR, Di SA, Cecchetti L, Tarozzi C, Corrao G, Bernardi M, Gasbarrini G. *Bone mass and metabolism in patients with celiac disease.* Gastroenterology. 1995; 109: 122-128.
http://dx.doi.org/10.1016/0016-5085(95)90276-7

103. Valdimarsson T, Toss G, Lofman O, Strom M. *Three years' follow-up of bone density in adult coeliac disease: significance of secondary hyperparathyroidism.* Scand J Gastroenterol. 2000; 35: 274-280. http://dx.doi.org/10.1080/003655200750024146

104. McFarlane XA, Bhalla AK, Robertson DA. *Effect of a gluten free diet on osteopenia in adults with newly diagnosed coeliac disease.* Gut. 1996; 39: 180-184.
http://dx.doi.org/10.1136/gut.39.2.180

105. Molteni N, Bardella MT, Vezzoli G, Pozzoli E, Bianchi P. *Intestinal calcium absorption as shown by stable strontium test in celiac disease before and after gluten-free diet.* Am J Gastroenterol. 1995; 90: 2025-2028.

106. Green PH, Jabri B. *Coeliac disease.* Lancet. 2003; 362: 383-391.
http://dx.doi.org/10.1016/S0140-6736(03)14027-5

107. Alaedini A, Green PH. *Narrative review: Celiac disease: understanding a complex autoimmune disorder.* Ann Intern Med. 2005; 142: 289-298.
108. Mora S, Barera G, Ricotti A, Weber G, Bianchi C, Chiumello G. *Reversal of low bone density with a gluten-free diet in children and adolescents with celiac disease.* Am J Clin Nutr. 1998; 67: 477-481.
109. Ciacci C, Cirillo M, Mellone M, Basile F, Mazzacca G, De Santo NG. *Hypocalciuria in overt and subclinical celiac disease.* Am J Gastroenterol. 1995; 90: 1480-1484.
110. Rossini M, Bianchi G, Di MO, Giannini S, Minisola S, Sinigaglia L, et al. *Determinants of adherence to osteoporosis treatment in clinical practice.* Osteoporos Int. 2006; 17: 914-921. http://dx.doi.org/10.1007/s00198-006-0073-6

Chapter 16

Celiac Disease and Gastrointestinal Functional Disorders

Santos Santolaria Piedrafita

Gastroenterology and Hepatology Unit, Hospital San Jorge de Huesca, Spain.
ssantolariap@gmail.com

Doi: http://dx.doi.org/10.3926/oms.217

How to cite this chapter

Santolaria Piedrafita, S. *Celiac Disease and Gastrointestinal Functional Disorders*. In Rodrigo L and Peña AS, editors. *Celiac Disease and Non-Celiac Gluten Sensitivity*. Barcelona, Spain: OmniaScience; 2014. p. 347-362.

Abstract

Celiac disease (CD) is one of the most frequent genetic disorders diagnosed in the adult population and it may present a wide spectrum of gastrointestinal symptoms, which bear a large degree of overlap with functional dyspepsia, irritable bowel syndrome (IBS) or functional diarrhea. It has been demonstrated that CD, as diagnosed by positive serology and villous atrophy, is more frequent in patients with functional dyspepsia (1.2-6.2%) and IBS (4.7-11.4%) than in the general population. This prevalence may be higher if we consider the whole spectrum of gluten-dependent mucosal histopathological lesions, including lymphocytic enteropathy. Consequently, patients with these gastrointestinal symptoms might be misdiagnosed with a functional bowel disorder if the diagnostic approach does not include CD-specific antibody tests and duodenal biopsies. This fact might bring, as a result, a delay in CD diagnosis and treatment, with important consequences in terms of morbidity and quality of life. Non-celiac gluten sensitivity is a clinical condition characterized by symptoms that improve after gluten withdrawal, negative celiac serology and absence of enteropathy, which may be involved as a trigger in some functional bowel disorders such as IBS.

1. Introduction

The European Society of Pediatric Gastroenterology Hepatology and Nutrition (ESPGHAN) recently defined celiac disease (CD) as a systemic immune-mediated disease caused by gluten in genetically predisposed individuals, characterized by the presence of a variable combination of gluten-dependent clinical manifestations, specific antibodies, HLA-DQ2 or DQ8 haplotypes and enteropathy.[1] Classically, the CD diagnosis needed the presence of villous atrophy in duodenal biopsies, however, recent evidence shows that patients with mild forms of enteropathy (Marsh I or II lesion) may present gastrointestinal and extraintestinal symptoms with the same frequency as patients with atrophy.[2-4] The diagnosis of CD in these patients, who often have a negative serology, is not easy and requires the presence of an HLA-DQ2 or DQ8-compatible haplotype as well as the demonstrating that its symptoms and enteropathy are gluten-dependent.[5,6]

The clinical expression of CD is quite variable, ranging from very serious forms with diarrhea and dehydration to oligosymptomatic or asymptomatic forms (silent CD). In adults, its most frequent presentation is oligosymptomatic with digestive and/or extradigestive symptoms.[7] Some of the gastrointestinal symptoms, such as dyspepsia, recurrent abdominal pain or diarrhea, are very prevalent in gastroenterological practice and may be erroneously attributed to a functional gastrointestinal disorder if the diagnostic study is not completed with CD-specific antibody tests and duodenal biopsies. Since the sensitivity of serology is less than 30% in mild enteropathy, it is recommended to carry out a fuller diagnostic study with duodenal biopsies in those cases where there is a high index of clinical suspicion.[8] The use of additional immunohistochemical staining with monoclonal antibodies for CD3 lymphocytes facilitates visualization of intraepithelial lymphocytes (IELs) and thus the diagnosis of mild enteropathy forms.[9]

Functional dyspepsia, irritable bowel syndrome or functional diarrhea are some of the functional gastrointestinal disorders, which have been associated with celiac disease or non-celiac gluten sensitivity, a clinical entity of recent appearance.

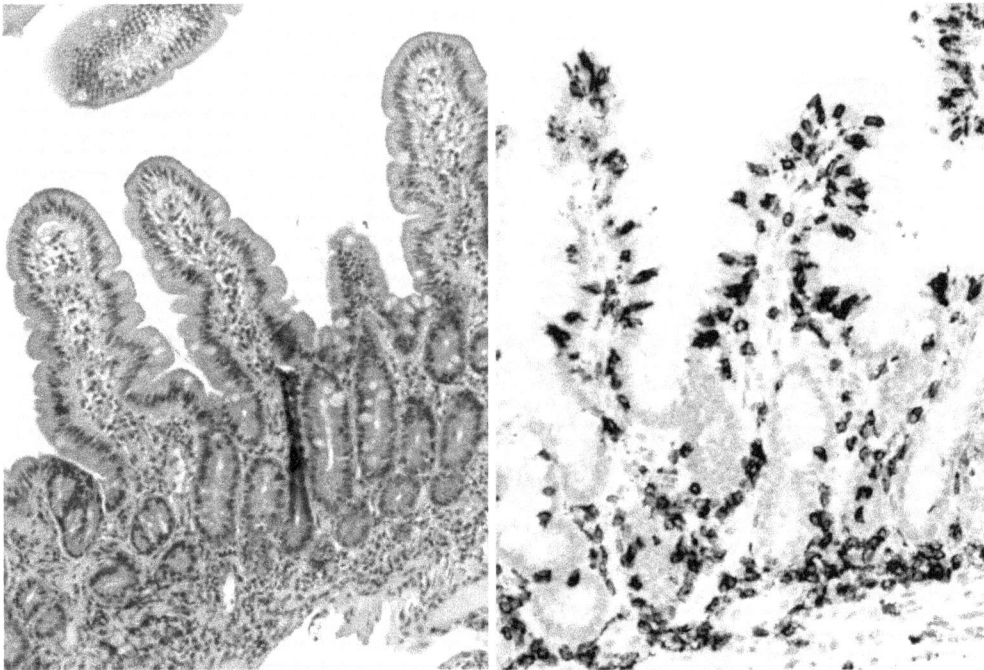

Figure 1. Immunohistochemistry with monoclonal antibodies for CD3 lymphocytes facilitates visualization of intraepithelial lymphocytes and the diagnosis of mild forms of enteropathy. Left: apparently normal villi after hematoxylin-eosin staining. Right: significant increase in intraepithelial lymphocytes after performing CD3 (+) lymphocyte immunostaining (Courtesy Dr. Vera, Department of Pathology, Hospital San Jorge, Huesca).

2. Functional Dyspepsia

Functional dyspepsia, according to the Rome III criteria, is characterized by the presence, for at least three months, of one or more of the following symptoms:

1) postprandial fullness,

2) early satiety,

3) epigastric pain,

4) epigastric burning and the absence of structural alterations in upper endoscopy that could explain these symptoms.

It could be concluded, therefore, that functional dyspepsia is a diagnosis of exclusion which is established when, in a patient with symptoms attributable to the gastroduodenal tract, there is evidence of neither structural damage (negative endoscopy) nor of biochemical damage which can explain the symptoms. This is a highly prevalent entity, which, although not serious, causes a significant impact on the quality of life of patients.[10]

Dyspepsia is also a common symptom in CD patients; it may be present in 40-60% of the cases at the time of diagnosis. Ciacci et al.,[11] in a retrospective study that analyzed 195 adult CD patients, observed how many patients presented, at the time of diagnosis, nonspecific gastrointestinal symptoms such as dyspepsia (40%), abdominal pain (35%) and meteorism (31%). Zipser et al.[12] evaluated, by means of a questionnaire, the presentation symptoms in patients diagnosed with CD between 1993 and 2001, describing how 77% of them had abdominal discomfort, 73% flatulence, and 46% nausea and/or vomiting. Esteve et al.,[2] in a study conducted in Spain in 221 first-degree relatives of 82 CD patients, observed how those relatives with enteropathy more often presented symptoms like abdominal pain (39.1% vs 23.5%), abdominal distension (52.2% vs 21.8%) and flatulence (65% vs 39%).

Several trials have evaluated the prevalence of CD in patients with dyspepsia. Although these studies are very heterogeneous in methodology and definition of dyspepsia, they show a prevalence generally superior to that of the general population, with figures ranging between 1.2% and 6.2%.[13] A meta-analysis and systematic review of these studies also shows a higher frequency of positive celiac serology (7.9% vs 3.9%) as well as of CD diagnosed by duodenal biopsy (3.2% vs 1.3%) in dyspepsia patients compared to the control population, although these differences were not statistically significant.[14]

Year	Author	Country	Study type	Patients	Diagnosis dyspepsia	Diagnosis CD	CD (%)
1999	Dickey[15]	Ireland	Case series	119	Medical criterion	Biopsy	7 (5.8)
2000	Bardella[16]	Italy	Case series	517	Medical criterion	Biopsy	6 (1.2)
2003	Vivas[17]	Spain	Cases and controls	92	Rome II	Serology + biopsy	3 (3.3)
2004	Locke[18]	USA	Population study	34	Questionnaire	Serology	2 (5.9)
2004	Cammarota[19]	Italy	Case series	396	Medical criterion	Biopsy	7 (1.7)
2005	Lima[20]	Brazil	Case series	142	Medical criterion	Biopsy	4 (1.4)
2006	Lecleire[21]	France	Cases and controls	75	Rome II	Biopsy	1 (1.3)
2007	Ozaslan[22]	Turkey	Case series	196	Rome II	Serology + biopsy	3 (1.5)
2007	Hadithi[23]	Netherlands	Case series	167	Medical criterion	Biopsy	3 (1.6)
2008	Giangreco[24]	Italy	Case series	726	Rome II	Biopsy	15 (2)
2009	Rostami-Nejad[25]	Iran	Case series	415	Medical criterion	Biopsy	28 (6.2)

Table 1. Celiac Disease prevalence studies in patients with dyspepsia.

Previous studies assess the prevalence of CD, based on positive celiac serology and the presence of villous atrophy in patients with dyspepsia. If we consider the whole spectrum of histological CD lesions, including forms of mild enteropathy, this prevalence could be even higher. A retrospective study in Spain which investigated 142 patients with dysmotility-like dyspepsia (postprandial distress) and negative duodenal endoscopy, found different histological lesion degrees in 35% of the cases. Those patients with positive tissue transglutaminase antibodies (t-TGA) (6.7%) or else HLA DQ2 and/or DQ8 haplotypes (84.1%) were invited to undergo a gluten-free diet (GFD) for a period of not less than 1 year. This strategy resulted in relief or disappearance of dyspeptic symptoms in 91.9% and in histological damage regression or improvement by 81%, establishing a final CD diagnosis in 28 of them (19.7%). It must be pointed out that the duodenal histopathological study included immunohistochemistry with CD3 lymphocyte monoclonal antibodies.[26]

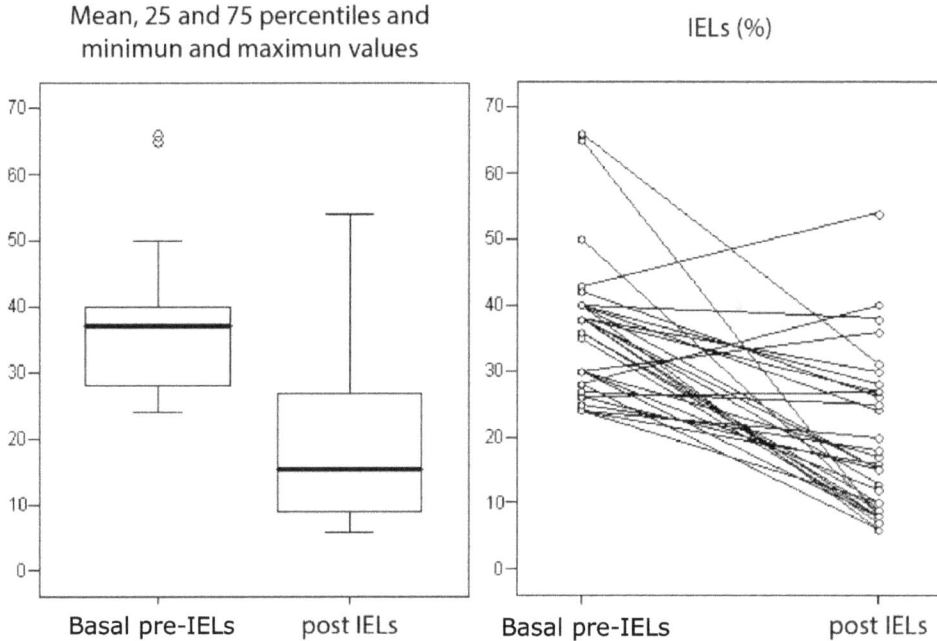

Figure 2. Intraepithelial lymphocytes (IELs) before and after starting a gluten-free diet in 32 patients with dysmotility-type dyspepsia with enteropathy in duodenal biopsies, which also had a positive serological result (t-TGA) and/or a compatible HLA-DQ2 or DQ8 genetic study.[26]

Therefore, CD can be a frequent, often unsuspected, cause of dyspepsia which could be erroneously misdiagnosed as functional dyspepsia if the diagnostic work is not completed with duodenal biopsies. The cost-effectiveness of duodenal biopsies requires well-designed studies for the purpose of excluding the presence of intestinal histological lesions that can explain the nature of the symptoms before making a functional dyspepsia diagnosis. Meanwhile, it seems reasonable to indicate duodenal biopsies in the presence of a reasonable clinical scenario and/or indicative of CD. This recommendation acquires more consistency when the patient has an HLA DQ2- or DQ8- compatible haplotype. A general analysis, including t-TGA determination, should be included as well in the initial assessment of patients with dyspepsia.[13]

3. Irritable Bowel Syndrome

Irritable bowel syndrome (IBS) is a functional gastrointestinal disorder characterized by the presence of abdominal pain or discomfort associated with changes in the frequency of and/or stool consistency. Following the Rome III recommendations, IBS is divided according to IBS stool consistency, constipation-predominant (IBS-C), diarrhea-predominant IBS (IBS-D), IBS with an alternating pattern or IBS with an undefined pattern. It is a common disorder, with a prevalence of 5-15% and, although it is not serious, it can significantly reduce the quality of life of patients. Currently the mechanisms by which IBS occurs are unknown, although it has been associated with digestive function abnormalities, especially in motility and sensitivity and there is increasing evidence supporting the existence of microinflamatory phenomena and changes in intestinal immune function.[27]

CD can frequently present with symptoms that are also characteristic of IBS, including abdominal pain (77%), bloating (73%), diarrhea (52%), constipation (7%) and an alternating bowel habit pattern (24%).[12] This means that IBS is often the initial diagnosis in many patients before the discovery of CD many years later. Other features common to both diseases include female predominance, the fact that symptoms may be precipitated by a stressful life event and the frequent concomitance of dysthymia, depression, chronic fatigue, fibromyalgia and other manifestations characteristic of functional gastrointestinal disorders, such as pyrosis and dyspepsia. Several case-control studies have evaluated the prevalence of positive celiac serology as well as CD diagnosis based on the presence of villous atrophy, in patients with IBS, demonstrating a higher prevalence (4.7-11.4%) in relation to the control population.[18,28,29]

Author	Dx	N	Serology	Biopsy	p
Sanders[28] (2001)	AGA + EMA Biopsy	Cases: 300 Controls: 300	66/300 (22%) (11 EMA+) 44/300 (15%) (2 EMA+)	14/300 (4.7%) 2/300 (0.7%)	=0.004 OR, 7 (1.7-28)
Shahbazkhain[29] (2003)	EMA Biopsy	Cases: 105 Controls:105	12/105 (11.4%) 0/105	12/105 (11.4%) 0/105 (0%)	=0.0003 OR, infinite
Locke[18] (2004)	t-TGA	Cases: 50 Controls: 78	2/50 (4%) 2/78 (2.6%)	-	NS

Table 2. Case-control studies which have evaluated the risk of celiac disease in IBS patients (AGA: antigliadin antibodies; EMA: endomysial antibodies; t-TGA: tissue transglutaminase antibodies; OR: odds ratio).

A recent systematic review and meta-analysis including 2278 patients with IBS diagnostic criteria showed they had a higher prevalence of IgA anti-gliadin antibodies (AGA) (4%; CI 95% 1.7-7.2), endomysial antibodies (EMA) or t-TGA (1.6%, CI 95% 0.7-3) as well as CD demonstrated by duodenal biopsy (4.1%, CI 95% 1.9-7). The risk of positive AGA results (OR 3.4, CI 95% 1.6-7.1), EMA or t-TGA (OR 2.9, CI 95% 1.3-6.3) and CD demonstrated by duodenal biopsy (OR 4.3, CI 95% 1.8-10.6) was also higher in IBS patients when compared to the control population.[30] However, a recent prospective study undertaken in the United States found no difference in CD prevalence as demonstrated through duodenal biopsy in 492 IBS-D patients (0.4%) and 458 asymptomatic controls (0.4%). Although statistically not significant, patients with IBS-D tested positive for celiac serology (AGA, t-TGA or EMA) in 7.3% of cases versus 4.8% in the control group.[31]

All these studies refer to patients with positive celiac serology or CD results based on the existence of villous atrophy. If we consider the whole spectrum of histological CD lesions and include all patients who have some degree of enteropathy, regardless of serological outcome, along with an HLA-DQ2 or DQ8 genetic study and gluten-dependence criteria, the prevalence of CD in IBS patients could be higher. In this sense, there is a study which evaluated the whole CD lesion spectrum in 102 patients with IBS-diarrhea and negative celiac serology (t-TGA), which showed how as much as 23% of them exhibited some degree of enteropathy and, the presence of t-TGA in the duodenal aspirate in 30%. For 26 enteropathy patients with t-TGA in the duodenal aspirate and HLA-DQ2 (+), GFD was recommended, with improvement in diarrhea and intestinal serology in all of them.[32]

Currently, the American College of Gastroenterology recommends screening for CD in patients with IBS-D and alternating pattern IBS by determining serum t-TGA. This recommendation is based on studies in which the CD diagnosis was based on finding positive celiac serology (t-TGA and EMA) and on the presence of villous atrophy in duodenal biopsies.[33] However, as previously described, patients with mild forms of enteropathy (Marsh I or II lesion) may show gastrointestinal symptoms characteristic of IBS with a frequency similar to that of patients with villous atrophy, but often, unlike the latter, the result of celiac serology is frequently negative. For this reason, duodenal biopsies in IBS patients with negative celiac serology should still be considered when there is a clinical scenario suggestive of CD, such as those patients with a family history of CD, autoimmune diseases or a previous history of growth retardation, infertility, and osteoporosis or iron deficiency anemia of unknown origin. In these cases, the HLA-DQ2 or DQ8 haplotype determination can help to reach a decision regarding the need to complete the study with duodenal biopsies.[34]

4. Functional Diarrhea

A functional diarrhea diagnosis is established in those cases in which diarrhea, often watery, is not accompanied by alarming symptoms/signs, no abnormalities in routine blood and stool tests and normal sigmoidoscopy. However, there may be different entities, such as bile acid malabsorption, disaccharide (lactose, fructose or sorbitol) malabsorption or CD, which may equally manifest an apparently functional watery diarrhea.[35]

A Spanish study prospectively evaluated the presence of CD, bile acid malabsorption and disaccharide malabsorption in 62 consecutive patients with chronic watery diarrhea and Rome II criteria for functional diarrhea or IBS-diarrhea diagnosis. The diagnostic study included the sequential performance of:

1) genetic HLA-DQ2-DQ8 study;

2) Duodenal biopsies in patients with positive HLA-DQ2 or DQ8;

3) SeHCAT test (selenium 75-tagged tauroselcholic acid scintigraphy),

4) Hydrogen breath test (lactose and fructose-sorbitol),

when all previous tests were normal or when the patient related a possible clinical sugar intolerance. According to these diagnostic test results, the patients were treated with either a gluten-free diet, the removal of dietary sugars or else with cholestyramine. With this diagnostic strategy 28 (45.2%) patients were diagnosed with bile acid malabsorption, 10 (16.1%) with CD, 10 (16.1%) with disaccharide malabsorption, 2 (3.2%) with bile acid and disaccharide malabsorption and only 12 (19.4%) patients were diagnosed with functional diarrhea. All patients diagnosed with CD had mild enteropathy and negative celiac serology (t-TGA and EMA).

It must be pointed out that the duodenal histopathological study included immunohistoche-mistry with CD3 lymphocyte monoclonal antibodies and CD diagnosis was based on clinical and histological response after the GFD.[36]

5. Non-Celiac Gluten Sensitivity

In recent years, the concept of non-celiac sensitivity to gluten (NCGS) has been introduced to refer to those patients with gluten-dependent symptoms but who do not have in serum positivity for t-TGA or EMA, with absence of enteropathy in duodenal biopsies. It has been hypothesized that unlike patients with CD, in which an adaptive immune response with antibody production is triggered, in NCGS there is only an innate response to gliadin which determines the appearance of microinflamatory changes in the intestinal mucosa reflected in increased IEL expression and the release of cytokines and other inflammation mediators.[37,38]

	Celiac disease	Non-celiac gluten sensitivity
Prevalence	Around 1%	Suspected to be around 5-6%
Pathogenesis	Adaptive immune response to gluten peptides	An innate immune response to gluten has been implied
HLA-DQ2 and/or DQ8	Present and necessary	Not necessary
Serology	T-TGA and EMA (+)	t-TGA and EMA (-). Sometimes AGA (+)
Villous atrophy	Present	Absent

Table 3. Differences between celiac disease and non-celiac gluten sensitivity (AGA: antigliadin, EMA: endomysial antibodies; t-TGA: tissue transglutaminase antibodies). Adapted from Di Sabatino.[39]

NCGS can cause gastrointestinal symptoms such as diarrhea, recurrent abdominal pain and flatulence, as well as non-gastrointestinal symptoms such as ataxia, headache, attention deficit, hyperactivity or asthenia and has been implicated as a possible cause of some functional gastrointestinal disorders. Two studies have evaluated the prevalence of NCGS in IBS patients using a double-blind methodology by comparing gluten with placebo. Biesiekierski et al.[40] evaluated a total of 34 patients with IBS in whom a CD diagnosis had been excluded and had improved clinically after performing a GFD. The patients were randomized regarding gluten (16 g/day) or placebo intake for 6 weeks. Thirteen (68%) of the 19 patients who received gluten showed poor control of digestive symptoms, compared with only 6 (40%) of 15 patients receiving placebo (p=0.0001). In a visual analog scale, patients receiving gluten presented, since the first week, worse scores in terms of overall symptoms, abdominal pain, flatulence and satisfaction with stool consistency and asthenia. No differences between the two groups were observed regarding the determination of fecal lactoferrin, serum t-TGA and AGA, high-sensitivity CRP or intestinal permeability determined by a dual lactulose-rhamnose test. Carroccio et al.[41] retrospectively evaluated 276 patients with IBS, out of a total of 920, according to the Rome II criteria, who had previously responded clinically to the withdrawal and subsequent dietary wheat overload with a double-blind placebo-controlled methodology. These patients were further classified into 2 groups: isolated wheat sensitivity (group 1, 70 patients) and wheat sensitivity associated with multiple food hypersensitivity (group 2, 206 patients). This classification was performed following a withdrawal and overload of cow's milk proteins, eggs, tomatoes and chocolate with a methodology similar to that employed with wheat. Patients in group 1 had anemia more frequently (70%), a family history of CD (14%), HLA-DQ2 or DQ8 haplotype (75%) and the presence of EMA in cultured duodenal mucosa (30%), while group 2 patients presented a more frequent coexistence of atopy (35%), IgG anti-betalactoglobin antibodies (39%), basophil activation determined by flow cytometry (80%) as well as increased eosinophils in the duodenum and colon. In relation to a control group of patients with IBS without wheat sensitivity criteria, patients in both groups had a higher frequency of anemia (24%), weight loss (35%), atopy coexistence (29%), a childhood history of food allergy (18%) as well as lymphocytic enteropathy in the duodenal mucosa (present in 96% of group 1 patients and 90% in group 2). These results, according to the authors, confirm the existence of a non-celiac wheat sensitivity and suggest that, within the same, there could be two different groups: one with features similar to CD (group 1) and one with features closer to food allergy (group 2).

These studies demonstrate the existing relationship between gluten and the occurrence of gastrointestinal symptoms in patients with a previous functional gastrointestinal disorder diagnosis such as IBS, but they also highlight the heterogeneity of NCGS. The lack of well-defined diagnostic criteria and the absence of characteristic biological and morphological parameters may turn NCGS into a "hodgepodge" in which to include all those patients with functional gastrointestinal symptoms that respond clinically to a GFD and present neither villous atrophy nor positive celiac serology.[42] It will be necessary to conduct further prospective and controlled studies to evaluate the evolution of patients with mild enteropathy, an HLA-DQ2 and/or DQ8 genetic study, but negative t-TGA to determine if these patients actually a constitute separate clinical entity or if they are part of the evolutionary spectrum of CD. The determination of subepithelial IgA deposits against tissue transglutaminase by immunofluorescence or performing an intraepithelial lymphocytes subsets characterization (IEL lymphogram) by flow cytometry could help diagnose patients who are part of the CD spectrum, but these techniques have a certain level of complexity and they are not straightforward to use routine clinical practice. [43,44]

6. Gluten and Gastrointestinal Motility Disorders

It has been shown that patients with CD may have motility disorders along their entire digestive tract, such as a decrease in lower esophageal sphincter pressure, slow small intestinal transit, delayed gallbladder emptying and accelerated colonic transit. Moreover, all these alterations tend to normalize months after starting a GFD.[45]

Motility disorders of the upper gastrointestinal tract may explain the appearance of symptoms such as postprandial fullness, bloating, flatulence, nausea, vomiting, regurgitation and pyrosis. Rocco et al.[46] evaluated gastric emptying by ultrasonography and an octanoic hydrogen test in 20 CD patients and 10 controls. They observed that CD patients showed delayed gastric emptying (252 ± 101 minutes) compared with control patients (89 ± 16 minutes) and that it became normal one year after starting a GFD (97 ± 14 minutes). Bassoti et al.[47] studied antroduodenojejunal motility using manometry in 11 patients with untreated CD, 12 CD patients treated with GFD for at least one year and 33 control patients. They found that CD patients showed interdigestive (fasting) and postprandial motility disorders relative to control patients. In the fasting period a decrease in the interdigestive migrating motor complex frequency was observed, with phase I and phase II shortening, and a lower phase III propagation velocity. These changes improved once the GFD was begun although they failed to disappear completely, a fact, which the authors attributed to the persistence of mild enteropathy signs in some patients.

The pathophysiology of these motor alterations in CD is not well known and it has been explained by the existence of complex interactions between the malabsorption of certain nutrients, the existence of an autonomic nervous system dysfunction and, finally, changes in the secretion of certain gastrointestinal hormones.[45] The presence of unabsorbed fats in the small intestine may favor a delay in gastric emptying and slowing of orocecal transit time. On the other hand, the immune response generated by gluten in the intestinal mucosa, along with the increase of inflammatory cells in the lamina propria and the secretion of various cytokines and inflammatory mediators could affect the nerve cells of the intestinal nerve plexus and cause an extrinsic autonomic neuropathy with subsequent gastrointestinal dysmotility.[48] Finally, alterations have been described in the gastrointestinal secretion of certain hormones, which (among other functions) may alter gastrointestinal motility. Several studies have demonstrated the existence of a decrease in postprandial cholecystokinin secretion and an increase in plasma levels of neurotensin, peptide YY and somatostatin.[49-51] As is the case with gastrointestinal motility changes, the secretion of these gastrointestinal peptides tend towards normalization once a GFD is initiated.[45]

On the other hand, it has been shown that gluten, especially gliadin, may have a direct toxic effect on the intestinal mucosa which is not mediated by an adaptive immune response and which, therefore, does not require the HLA-DQ2 and DQ8 heterodimers. This direct action of gluten on intestinal epithelium, along with the activation of an innate immune response, has been implicated in the production of gastrointestinal and extraintestinal symptoms in patients diagnosed with NCGS.[37] The pathogenic mechanisms involved in the direct response to gliadin include increased intestinal permeability secondary to zonulin release, apoptosis induction, increased oxidative stress and cholinergic nervous system stimulation by opioid receptor activation.[37,52] The activation of an innate immune response with IL-15 release and IEL stimulation can also lead to a microinflamatory response and involvement of the nerve cells of the enteric nerve plexus, resulting in gastrointestinal dysmotility.[53] Finally, fructans present in cereals and fermentation of gluten peptides by sulfate-reducing bacteria increase the production of ammonia and hydrogen sulfide, gases which can also cause gastrointestinal and non-gastrointestinal symptoms such as asthenia.[54]

7. Summary and Conclusions

CD is one of the most frequent genetic disorders diagnoses in population, which is increasingly being diagnosed with more frequency in adults. Its clinical presentation often being including gastrointestinal symptoms that may overlap with those described in functional dyspepsia, IBS or functional diarrhea.

A higher frequency of CD, based on positive serology results and villous atrophy, has been shown in patients with functional dyspepsia and IBS compared to the general population. If we consider the whole spectrum of histological CD lesions, including milder forms such as lymphocytic enteropathy, this frequency could be even greater.

The diagnosis of mild enteropathy form is not easy since often the result of celiac serology is negative. In these cases it is necessary to demonstrate the presence of an HLA-DQ2 or DQ8 compatible haplotype and confirm that the symptoms and enteropathy are gluten-dependent. The determination of subepithelial IgA deposits against tissular transglutaminase or the performance of an IEL lymphogram could help diagnose patients who are part of the CD spectrum but these techniques are not straightforward to use in routine clinical practice.

Patients with gluten-dependent digestive symptoms, negative celiac serology and absent or mild enteropathy have been included in a new clinical entity called non-celiac gluten sensitivity. At present, there are no well-defined diagnostic criteria for this condition and some of these patients could be part of the evolutionary spectrum of CD.

The existence of alterations in motility in the upper gastrointestinal tract, such as delayed gastric emptying or abnormal motor activity, could explain the appearance of symptoms such as postprandial fullness, bloating, flatulence, nausea, vomiting, regurgitation and pyrosis. Characteristic IBS symptoms in CD patients may be caused by effects on the digestive function derived from direct toxic gluten effect on the intestinal epithelium and the activation of an innate immune response.

CD could be a frequent, often unsuspected, cause of very prevalent symptoms, such as dyspepsia, IBS or seemingly "functional" diarrhea. Patients with these symptoms may be erroneously diagnosed with functional gastrointestinal disorder study if the diagnostic study is not completed with CD-specific antibody tests and the performance of duodenal biopsies. This fact might bring, as a result, a delay in CD diagnosis and treatment, with important consequences in terms of morbidity and of the patient's quality of life.

It will be necessary to conduct well-designed prospective studies evaluating the cost-effectiveness relationship of duodenal biopsies in patients with dyspepsia, IBS and functional diarrhea. Meanwhile it seems reasonable to include a t-TGA determination in these patients' initial assessment and to indicate duodenal biopsy when there is a clinical scenario suggestive of CD (including HLA-DQ2 and DQ8 genetic testing).

References

1. Husby S, Koletzko S, Korponay-Szabo IR, Mearin ML, Phillips A, Shamir R. *European Society for Pediatric Gastroenterology, Hepatology, and Nutrition guidelines for the diagnosis of coeliac disease.* J. Pediatr. Gastroenterol. Nutr. 2012; 54: 136-60. http://dx.doi.org/10.1097/MPG.0b013e31821a23d0

2. Esteve M, Rosinach M, Fernandez-Bañares F, Farre C, Salas A, Alsina M, et al. *Spectrum of gluten-sensitive enteropathy in first-degree relatives of patients with coeliac disease: clinical relevance of lymphocytic enteritis.* Gut 2006; 55: 1739-45. http://dx.doi.org/10.1136/gut.2006.095299

3. Tursi A, Brandimarte G. *The symptomatic and histologic response to a gluten-free diet in patients with borderline enteropathy.* J Clin Gastroenterol 2003; 3613-7. http://dx.doi.org/10.1097/00004836-200301000-00006

4. Kurppa K, Collin P, Viljamaa M, Haimila K, Saavalainen P, Partanen J, et al. *Diagnosing Mild Enteropathy Celiac Disease: A Randomized, Controlled Clinical Study.* Gastroenterology 2009; 136: 816-823. http://dx.doi.org/10.1053/j.gastro.2008.11.040

5. Catassi C, Fasano A. *Celiac disease diagnosis: simple rules are better than complicated algorithms.* Am J Med 2010; 123: 691-3. http://dx.doi.org/10.1016/j.amjmed.2010.02.019

6. Esteve M, Carrasco A, Fernandez-Bañares F. *Is a gluten-free diet necessary in Marsh I intestinal lesions in patients with HLADQ2, DQ8 genotype and without gastrointestinal symptoms?* Current Opinion in Clinical Nutrition & Metabolic Care 2012; 15: 505-10. http://dx.doi.org/10.1097/MCO.0b013e3283566643

7. Vivas S, Ruiz de Morales JM, Fernandez M, Hernando M, Herrero B, Casqueiro J, et al. *Age-related clinical, serological, and histopathological features of celiac disease.* Am J Gastroenterol. 2008; 103: 2360-5. http://dx.doi.org/10.1111/j.1572-0241.2008.01977.x

8. Vivas S, Santolaria S. Enfermedad Celíaca. In: Ponce J, Castells A, Gomollon F, eds. *Tratamiento de las Enfermedades Gastroenterológicas.* 3ª ed. Barcelona: Asociación Española de Gastroenterología. 2010: 265-278.

9. Mino M, Lauwers GY. *Role of lymphocytic immunophenotyping in the diagnosis of gluten-sensitive enteropathy with preserved villous architecture.* Am J Surg Pathol. 2003; 27: 1237-42. http://dx.doi.org/10.1097/00000478-200309000-00007

10. Grupo de trabajo de la guía de práctica clínica sobre dispepsia. Manejo del paciente con dispepsia. *Guía de practica clínica.* Asociación Española de Gastroenterologia, Sociedad Española de Medicina de Familia y Comunitaria y Centro Cochrane Iberoamericano, 2012.

11. Ciacci C, Cirillo M, Sollazzo R, Savino G, Sabbatini F, Mazzacca G. *Gender and clinical presentation in adult celiac disease.* Scand J Gastroenterol. 1995; 30: 1077-81. http://dx.doi.org/10.3109/00365529509101610

12. Zipser RD, Patel S, Yahya KZ, Baisch DW, Monarch E. *Presentations of adult celiac disease in a nationwide patient support group.* Dig Dis Sci. 2003; 48: 761-4. http://dx.doi.org/10.1023/A:1022897028030

13. Santolaria Piedrafita S, Fernandez Banares F. *[Gluten-sensitive enteropathy and functional dyspepsia].* Gastroenterol Hepatol. 2012; 35: 78-88. http://dx.doi.org/10.1016/j.gastrohep.2011.10.006

14. Ford AC, Ching E, Moayyedi P. *Meta-analysis: yield of diagnostic tests for coeliac disease in dyspepsia.* Aliment Pharmacol Ther. 2009; 30: 28-36.
http://dx.doi.org/10.1111/j.1365-2036.2009.04008.x

15. Dickey W. *Diagnosis of coeliac disease at open-access endoscopy.* Scand J Gastroenterol. 1998; 33: 612-5. http://dx.doi.org/10.1080/00365529850171882

16. Bardella MT, Minoli G, Ravizza D, Radaelli F, Velio P, Quatrini M, et al. *Increased prevalence of celiac disease in patients with dyspepsia.* Arch Intern Med. 2000; 160: 1489-91. http://dx.doi.org/10.1001/archinte.160.10.1489

17. Vivas S, Ruiz de Morales JM, Martinez J, González MC, Martín S, Martín J, et al. *Human recombinant anti-transglutaminase antibody testing is useful in the diagnosis of silent coeliac disease in a selected group of at-risk patients.* Eur J Gastroenterol Hepatol. 2003; 15: 479-83. http://dx.doi.org/10.1097/01.meg.0000059104.41030.1c

18. Locke GR, 3rd, Murray JA, Zinsmeister AR, Melton LJ, 3rd, Talley NJ. *Celiac disease serology in irritable bowel syndrome and dyspepsia: a population-based case-control study.* Mayo Clin Proc. 2004; 79: 476-82. http://dx.doi.org/10.4065/79.4.476

19. Cammarota G, Pirozzi GA, Martino A, Zuccala G, Cianci R, Cuoco L, et al. *Reliability of the "immersion technique" during routine upper endoscopy for detection of abnormalities of duodenal villi in patients with dyspepsia.* Gastrointest Endosc. 2004; 60: 223-8. http://dx.doi.org/10.1016/S0016-5107(04)01553-6

20. Lima VM, Gandolfi L, Pires JA, Pratesi R. *Prevalence of celiac disease in dyspeptic patients.* Arq Gastroenterol. 2005; 42: 153-6.
http://dx.doi.org/10.1590/S0004-28032005000300005

21. Lecleire S, Di Fiore F, Antonietti M, Savoye G, Lemoine F, Le Pessot F, et al. *Endoscopic markers of villous atrophy are not useful for the detection of celiac disease in patients with dyspeptic symptoms.* Endoscopy 2006; 38: 696-701.
http://dx.doi.org/10.1055/s-2006-925373

22. Ozaslan E, Akkorlu S, Eskioglu E, Kayhan B. *Prevalence of silent celiac disease in patients with dyspepsia.* Dig Dis Sci. 2007; 52: 692-7.
http://dx.doi.org/10.1007/s10620-006-9453-1

23. Hadithi M, von Blomberg BM, Crusius JB, Bloemena E, Kostense PJ, Meijer JW, et al. *Accuracy of serologic tests and HLA-DQ typing for diagnosing celiac disease.* Ann Intern Med. 2007; 147: 294-302.
http://dx.doi.org/10.7326/0003-4819-147-5-200709040-00003

24. Giangreco E, D'Agate C, Barbera C, Puzzo L, Aprile G, Naso P, et al. *Prevalence of celiac disease in adult patients with refractory functional dyspepsia: value of routine duodenal biopsy.* World J Gastroenterol. 2008; 14: 6948-53.
http://dx.doi.org/10.3748/wjg.14.6948

25. Rostami-Nejad M, Villanacci V, Mashayakhi R, Molaei M, Bassotti G, Zojaji H, et al. *Celiac disease and Hp infection association in Iran.* Rev Esp Enferm Dig. 2009; 101: 850-4.
http://dx.doi.org/10.4321/S1130-01082009001200004

26. Santolaria S, Alcedo J, Cuartero B, Díez I, Abascal M, García Prats M, et al. *Spectrum of gluten-sensitive enteropathy in patients with dysmotility-like dyspepsia.* Gastroenterol Hepatol 2013; 36: 11-20. http://dx.doi.org/10.1016/j.gastrohep.2012.07.011

27. Grupo de trabajo de la guía de práctica clínica sobre el síndrome del intestino irritable. *Manejo del paciente con síndrome del intestino irritable.* Asociación Española de Gastroenterología, Sociedad Española de Familia y Comunitaria y Centro Cochrane Iberoamericano., 2005.

28. Sanders DS, Carter MJ, Hurlstone DP, Pearce A, Ward AM, McAlindon ME, et al. *Association of adult coeliac disease with irritable bowel syndrome: a case-control study in patients fulfilling ROME II criteria referred to secondary care.* Lancet 2001; 358: 1504-8. http://dx.doi.org/10.1016/S0140-6736(01)06581-3

29. Shahbazkhani B, Forootan M, Merat S, Akbari MR, Nasserimoghadam S, Vahedi H, et al. *Coeliac disease presenting with symptoms of irritable bowel syndrome.* Aliment Pharmacol Ther 2003; 18: 231-5. http://dx.doi.org/10.1046/j.1365-2036.2003.01666.x

30. Ford AC, Chey WD, Talley NJ, Malhotra A, Spiegel BMR, Moayyedi P. *Yield of Diagnostic Tests for Celiac Disease in Individuals With Symptoms Suggestive of Irritable Bowel Syndrome Systematic Review and Meta-analysis.* Archives of Internal Medicine 2009; 169: 651-658. http://dx.doi.org/10.1001/archinternmed.2009.22

31. Cash BD, Rubenstein JH, Young PE, Gentry A, Nojkov B, Lee D, et al. *The prevalence of celiac disease among patients with nonconstipated irritable bowel syndrome is similar to controls.* Gastroenterology 2011; 141: 1187-93.
 http://dx.doi.org/10.1053/j.gastro.2011.06.084

32. Wahnschaffe U, Ullrich R, Riecken EO, Schulzke JD. *Celiac disease-like abnormalities in a subgroup of patients with irritable bowel syndrome.* Gastroenterology 2001; 121: 1329-38.

33. Spiegel BM, Farid M, Esrailian E, Talley J, Chang L. *Is irritable bowel syndrome a diagnosis of exclusion?: a survey of primary care providers, gastroenterologists, and IBS experts.* Am J Gastroenterol. 2010; 105: 848-58. http://dx.doi.org/10.1038/ajg.2010.47

34. Mearin F, Montoro M. Síndrome de intestino irritable. In: Montoro M, García Pagan J, eds. *Gastroenterologia y Hepatología: Problemas comunes en la práctica clínica.* Barcelona: Jarpyo, 2011: 523-568.

35. Fine KD, Schiller LR. *AGA technical review on the evaluation and management of chronic diarrhea.* Gastroenterology 1999; 116: 1464-86.
 http://dx.doi.org/10.1016/S0016-5085(99)70513-5

36. Fernandez-Bañares F, Esteve M, Salas A, Alsina M, Farre C, Gonzalez C, et al. *Systematic evaluation of the causes of chronic watery diarrhea with functional characteristics.* Am J Gastroenterol. 2007; 102: 2520-8.
 http://dx.doi.org/10.1111/j.1572-0241.2007.01438.x

37. Verdu EF, Armstrong D, Murray JA. *Between Celiac Disease and Irritable Bowel Syndrome: The "No Man's Land" of Gluten Sensitivity.* Am J Gastroenterol 2009; 104: 1587-1594. http://dx.doi.org/10.1038/ajg.2009.188

38. Troncone R, Jabri B. *Coeliac disease and gluten sensitivity.* J Intern Med 2011; 269: 582-90. http://dx.doi.org/10.1111/j.1365-2796.2011.02385.x

39. Di Sabatino A, Corazza GR. *Nonceliac gluten sensitivity: sense or sensibility?* Ann Intern Med 2012; 156: 309-11.
 http://dx.doi.org/10.1059/0003-4819-156-4-201202210-00010

40. Biesiekierski JR, Newnham ED, Irving PM, Barrett JS, Haines M, Doecke JD, et al. *Gluten causes gastrointestinal symptoms in subjects without celiac disease: a double-blind randomized placebo-controlled trial.* Am J Gastroenterol. 2011; 106: 508-14.
 http://dx.doi.org/10.1038/ajg.2010.487

41. Carroccio A, Mansueto P, Iacono G, Soresi M, D'Alcamo A, Cavataio F, et al. *Non-Celiac Wheat Sensitivity Diagnosed by Double-Blind Placebo-Controlled Challenge: Exploring a New Clinical Entity.* Am J Gastroenterol. 2012. http://dx.doi.org/10.1038/ajg.2012.236

42. Ferch CC, Chey WD. *Irritable bowel syndrome and gluten sensitivity without celiac disease: separating the wheat from the chaff.* Gastroenterology 2012; 142: 664-6. http://dx.doi.org/10.1053/j.gastro.2012.01.020

43. Korponay-Szabo IR, Halttunen T, Szalai Z, Laurila K, Kiraly R, Kovacs JB, et al. *In vivo targeting of intestinal and extraintestinal transglutaminase 2 by coeliac autoantibodies.* Gut. 2004; 53: 641-8. http://dx.doi.org/10.1136/gut.2003.024836

44. Jarvinen TT, Kaukinen K, Laurila K, Kyronpalo S, Rasmussen M, Maki M, et al. *Intraepithelial lymphocytes in celiac disease.* Am J Gastroenterol. 2003; 98: 1332-1337. http://dx.doi.org/10.1111/j.1572-0241.2003.07456.x

45. Tursi A. *Gastrointestinal motility disturbances in celiac disease.* J Clin Gastroenterol 2004; 38: 642-5. http://dx.doi.org/10.1097/01.mcg.0000118792.58123.c1

46. Rocco A, Sarnelli G, Compare D, De Colibus P, Micheli P, Somma P, et al. *Tissue ghrelin level and gastric emptying rate in adult patients with celiac disease.* Neurogastroenterology and Motility 2008; 20: 884-890. http://dx.doi.org/10.1111/j.1365-2982.2008.01130.x

47. Bassotti G, Villanacci V, Mazzocchi A, Mariano M, Incardona P, Clerici C, et al. *Antroduodenojejunal motor activity in untreated and treated celiac disease patients.* Journal of Gastroenterology and Hepatology 2008; 23: E23-E28. http://dx.doi.org/10.1111/j.1440-1746.2007.04868.x

48. Usai P, Usai Satta P, Lai M, Corda MG, Piras E, Calcara C, et al. *Autonomic dysfunction and upper digestive functional disorders in untreated adult coeliac disease.* Eur J Clin Invest. 1997; 27: 1009-15. http://dx.doi.org/10.1046/j.1365-2362.1997.2340781.x

49. Hopman WP, Rosenbusch G, Hectors MP, Jansen JB. *Effect of predigested fat on intestinal stimulation of plasma cholecystokinin and gall bladder motility in coeliac disease.* Gut. 1995; 36: 17-21. http://dx.doi.org/10.1136/gut.36.1.17

50. Bardella MT, Fraquelli M, Peracchi M, Cesana BM, Bianchi PA, Conte D. *Gastric emptying and plasma neurotensin levels in untreated celiac patients.* Scand J Gastroenterol. 2000; 35: 269-73. http://dx.doi.org/10.1080/003655200750024137

51. Wahab PJ, Hopman WP, Jansen JB. *Basal and fat-stimulated plasma peptide YY levels in celiac disease.* Dig Dis Sci. 2001; 46: 2504-9. http://dx.doi.org/10.1023/A:1012344424300

52. Arranz E, Garrote JA. *Novel mechanisms of gliadin immunotoxicity?* Gut. 2010; 59: 286-7. http://dx.doi.org/10.1136/gut.2009.189332

53. Bernardo D, Garrote JA, Allegretti Y, Leon A, Gomez E, Bermejo-Martin JF, et al. *Higher constitutive IL15R alpha expression and lower IL-15 response threshold in coeliac disease patients.* Clin Exp Immunol. 2008; 154: 64-73. http://dx.doi.org/10.1111/j.1365-2249.2008.03743.x

54. Bernardo D, Garrote JA, Arranz E. *Are non-celiac disease gluten-intolerant patients innate immunity responders to gluten?* Am J Gastroenterol. 2011; 106: 2201; author reply 2201-2. http://dx.doi.org/10.1038/ajg.2011.297

Chapter 17

Refractory Celiac Disease

Luis Vaquero, Laura Arias, Santiago Vivas

Gastroenterology Service, University Hospital of León, Biomedicine Institute, León University, Spain.

luisvaqueroayala@gmail.com, lariasrodriguez@hotmail.com, svivasa@gmail.com

Doi: http://dx.doi.org/10.3926/oms.218

How to cite this chapter

Vaquero L, Arias L, Vivas S. *Refractory Celiac Disease.* In Rodrigo L and Peña AS, editors. *Celiac Disease and Non-Celiac Gluten Sensitivity*. Barcelona, Spain: OmniaScience; 2014. p.363-376.

Abstract

The main cause of failure to respond to a gluten-free diet (GFD) is persistent gluten ingestion, generally unnoticed. The refractory celiac disease (RCD) diagnosis is established after excluding other diseases, given the persistence of malabsorption and villous atrophy. This situation may appear initially after the disease diagnosis (primary) or after the initial response, when symptoms relapse despite strict adherence to a GFD (secondary).

RCD comprises a heterogeneous group of patients, usually in adults, which share a fortunately uncommon cause of non-responsiveness to the GFD (<5% of the celiac population). The detection changes in the intraepithelial lymphocyte population of the duodenal mucosa is of fundamental importance. When these lymphocytes appear in a population that does not express the surface T-cell receptor (CD3 and CD8), this is a potentially aggressive form of CD with a higher percentage of progression towards lymphoma (type II RCD).

Therapy is based on an adequate nutritional support and the use of corticosteroids or immunosuppressants (azathioprine and infliximab). The high risk of progression towards T cell lymphoma in type II RCD demands the use of different therapeutic regimens. Although currently no treatment has clearly shown to be effective in the long term, cladribine, immunotherapy with anti-CD52 (or similar treatments) and autologous stem cell transplantation are options to consider in the management of type II RCD. Antibodies that block interleukin-15 epithelial secretion, which is a key molecule in the pathogenesis, may have potential as new therapies.

1. Introduction

Removal of gluten in celiac disease (CD) is associated with clinical and histological recovery in most patients. Days or weeks after starting the GFD, a significant clinical improvement is observed, while histological lesions recover more slowly and, mostly in adults, they may persist for several months or even, in the absence of symptoms, for years in more than a third of the cases.[1,2]

However, a small percentage of celiac patients does not respond to a strict gluten-free diet; their intestinal villous atrophy persists, constituting the thus named[3] refractory celiac disease (RCD). RCD is a relatively rare entity, which appears in the adult form of CD and may progress with high morbidity and mortality. In recent years there has been an important advance in the understanding of its pathogenesis and various treatment options have emerged.[4] Since it appears in adult celiac disease, the rest of this chapter focuses only on adult disease forms.

2. Initial Management of the Lack of Response to the Gluten-Free Diet

The first step before reaching the RCD diagnosis is the initial management of the patients who do not respond to gluten withdrawal from the diet. This can happen in up to 20 % of the patients once the diagnosis is made.[2] Furthermore, in CD diagnosed in adulthood, over 30 % of the patients fail to recover from atrophy of the duodenal mucosa.[2] In cases of lack of clinical response, with or without mucosal recovery, after an initial diagnosis review many causes of lack of response to diet and of intestinal damage must be discarded (Table 1).

Continuous gluten intake, usually inadvertent and regular, is the leading cause of symptom persistence. Other drugs or substances containing gluten as an excipient must be ruled out. The persistence of high antibody titers (transglutaminase and endomysium) is a good indicator of ongoing contact with gluten.[5,6] However, the possibility has been put forward that these antibodies could lose the sensitivity to detect minor dietary transgressions in both children and in adults.[6,7] Overall, a thorough interrogation should be performed in conjunction with a dietary log and the help of a dietitian or nutritionist should be enlisted.

Intolerance to other foods, especially carbohydrates, is generally associated with CD, especially at the beginning.[8,9] Conducting tests based on breath hydrogen measuring may be useful for carbohydrate malabsorption evaluation, and in turn, to rule out intestinal bacterial overgrowth. Both carbohydrate intolerance and bacterial overgrowth may be responsible for the persistence of symptoms after excluding gluten from the diet.[10]

Exocrine pancreatic insufficiency may occur associated with villous atrophy, both in children and in adults.[9,11] Fecal chymotrypsin and elastase determination can help diagnose and establish the indication for initiating enzyme supplements. These patients should receive special attention in order to determine if pancreatic insufficiency reverses after initiating the GFD or if it otherwise remains as a primary insufficiency. A recent epidemiological study made in Sweden has found that patients with CD have a risk of developing chronic pancreatitis three times greater than the general population, and that they have five times the risk of needing pancreatic enzymes.[12]

Lack of adherence to diet (latent o unknown)
Intolerance to other foods (lactose, fructose)
Bacterial overgrowth
Pancreatic insufficiency
Microscopic or collagenous colitis
Inflammatory bowel disease
Collagenous sprue
Giardiasis
Ulcerative jejunitis
Infectious diarrhea
Autoimmune enteropathy
Common variable immunodeficiency syndrome
Intestinal lymphoma
Other tumors
Refractory celiac disease

Table 1. Causes of non-responsiveness to the gluten-free diet.

Microscopic colitis is an entity that shares CD's HLA genetic predisposition, which favors the association between these two diseases.[13,14] This occurs more frequently in females and when symptoms are primarily associated with persistent diarrhea.[14] In these cases, the performance of a colonoscopy with colon biopsies and proper treatment are imperative. A higher prevalence of inflammatory bowel disease among celiac disease patients than among the general population has been described[15] as well as a possible association of shared risk genes among CD, ulcerative colitis and Crohn's disease.[16] Therefore, the association between these diseases should be investigated when there is no response to the GFD.

CD is frequently associated with autoimmune conditions.[17] Thus it is that ulcerative jejunitis[18] or autoimmune enteropathy[19] can be observed as a cause of persistent symptoms. The common variable immunodeficiency syndrome may also occur in CD patients or else generate CD-like cases with villous atrophy but no response to the gluten-free diet, which require specific management.[20]

As always, malignancies should be ruled out, especially intestinal T-cell lymphoma, as a complication of CD. Weight loss, abdominal pain and night sweats are common symptoms when this kind of tumor is present.[21] Video capsule endoscopy[22,23] and double-balloon enteroscopy[24] are the two current techniques that have proven to be of great help for locating these tumors.

3. Definition and Epidemiology of Refractory Celiac Disease

Finally, once these causes have been ruled out, RCD will be diagnosed by exclusion. RCD was originally described in 1978 by Trier et al.[25] to define patients with villous atrophy and persistent diarrhea, unresponsive to GFD for at least 6 months. The American Gastroenterological Association (AGA),[26] has recently defined it as the persistence of villous atrophy and clinical malabsorption, unresponsive to the GFD. This situation may initially appear without actually responding to the GFD from its (primary) diagnosis or in patients already diagnosed with CD who, after a variable period, cease to respond to the GFD (secondary).[27] For some authors, the lack of initial response to gluten would lead to suspect that it is not really CD and therefore call it *non-celiac refractory sprue*.[28] Generally speaking, when there is no initial response to the GFD, the CD diagnosis should be revised. The existence of compatible data such as typical serology, HLA-DQ2 (+) or a family history support the RCD diagnosis. The absence of any of these parameters forces us to make a differential diagnosis with other pathologies.

Its frequency is of less than 5% of all CD patients. A Boston CD referral center recently reported an RCD prevalence of 4%.[29] In other studies, however, the prevalence does not exceed 1 % of the adult celiac population.[30] Its appearance in ages below 30 years is exceptional and most cases occur over the age of 50, with a higher prevalence in females.[31]

4. Pathogenesis and Classification

In recent years, knowledge of the pathogenic mechanisms involved in CD development has progressed. The adaptive immune response to the gluten level in the lamina propria has been well described. The lamina propria lymphocytes react to gliadin peptides once deaminated by the enzyme tissue transglutaminase. The presentation of these peptides is mediated by DQ2 and DQ8. Once the gliadin peptides have been recognized by these T lymphocytes (CD4+), they become active and secrete interferon-γ, which triggers the inflammatory response and is directly related to villous atrophy.[32]

However, less progress has been made in explaining the intraepithelial lymphocyte (IEL) increase since these already appear in the early stages of the disease and do not decrease after the GFD.[33] These T cells differ phenotypically from those present in the lamina propria, as these are mostly CD8+ with an increased expression of the γδ-type antigen receptor.[34] They are currently being the subject of special attention for their involvement in major CD complications: RCD and intestinal type T-cell lymphoma.[35,36] Interleukin 15 (IL-15) produced by enterocytes, in close contact with these IELs, appears to play a key role in the homeostasis of this lymphocyte population and in their potential transformation in RCD and lymphoma development.[37,38] An increase in the monocytic and enterocytic IL-15 transcriptional regulation appears to be the basis for the development of RCD and especially for type II RCD.[39]

In healthy subjects and uncomplicated celiac patients, IELs express the CD103 surface marker, which differentiates them from the lamina propria lymphocytes. Furthermore, they mostly have a lymphocyte T CD3+ CD8+ phenotype which can express the αβ or γδ T cell receptor (TCR).[34] Depending on the characteristics of this IEL population, two types of RCD can be differentiated, with different therapeutic approaches and prognosis.[35,39]

- Type I RCD: Here the IEL population presents phenotype surface markers similar to those of patients with active CD who have not started the GFD. Furthermore when, by means of molecular biology techniques, the T cell receptor gene arrangement is analyzed, it is seen to be polyclonal.

- Type II RCD: In this case the IEL phenotype is altered, constituting an "aberrant" population. This lymphocyte population has lost surface markers (CD3, CD8 and TCR), retaining the CD103 which characterizes it as intraepithelial, as well as CD3 intracytoplasmic expression. Furthermore, this population exhibits an oligo- or monoclonal TCR rearrangement. Due to these characteristics, type II RCD is also called *T cell cryptic intestinal lymphoma*, and considered to be a latent T lymphoma.[40]

5. Symptoms and Diagnosis

Clinical malabsorption associated with diarrhea is common to both RCD types. The type I usually appears in younger patients and its symptoms are less marked. Other autoimmune disorders, infections or thromboembolic phenomena can often be associated[41] with RCD. In type II, the average age is higher (50-60 years) and symptoms are usually more marked, with severe malabsorption and weight loss. Some patients may experience skin lesions mainly in limbs, similar to gangrenous pyoderma, as well as infections or fever with no known cause.[35] Weight loss and persistent diarrhea caused by malabsorption occur in up to 80 % of the cases and require discarding RCD in celiac patients.[29]

Endoscopy allows the observation of duodenal fold atrophy as well as of ulcerations which can lead to suspect ulcerative jejunitis. These ulcers, can also be seen in the stomach and the colon in RCD-II.[42] In order to view the entire small intestine and rule out the presence of lesions at different levels, capsule endoscopy can be helpful.[23] Lesions visualized by the capsule can be categorized by a biopsy taken by means of a push or a double balloon enteroscopy (it reaches distal sections with greater ease).[43]

Radiological tests, especially Computerized Axial Tomography (CAT) help rule out the presence of tumors, particularly intestinal lymphoma. Sometimes it is possible to observe an increase in the size and number of the mesenteric ganglia without a lymphoma or a diffuse thickening of the intestinal wall.[44]

The histology of duodenal mucosa exhibits an increased villous atrophy similar to those found in CD cases that have not yet started a GFD. Standard staining cannot differentiate between the both RCD types, being necessary to perform immunohistochemical staining on CD3 and CD8. As it can be seen in Figure 1, in both RCD types there is an IEL increase which are stained with CD3 (at a cytoplasmic level). But the first datum that steers us towards type II RCD is that, unlike type I and non-refractory celiac disease, these IELs cannot be stained with CD8.[45]

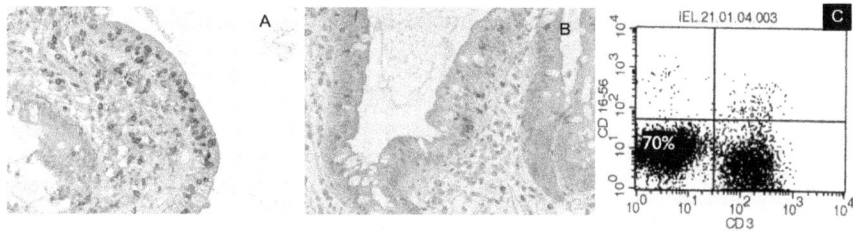

Figure 1. Aberrant lymphocyte population in type II RCD. (A) Immunohistochemistry of duodenal biopsy, where an increase in intraepithelial lymphocytes, whose cytoplasm is stained with CD3 marker, can be observed. However, this population is not stained with the CD8 marker (B). In panel C, by means of flow cytometry, it is confirmed that this aberrant population does not express surface CD3 in nearly 70% of intraepithelial lymphocytes.

More useful and informative is performing flow cytometry on biopsy samples, not only to categorize lymphocyte populations, but also to quantify this IEL "aberrant population" (Figure 1c). Thus RCD-II is identified in a population that mostly expresses surface CD103 (typical of IELs and unlike lamina propria lymphocytes), but that expresses neither surface CD3 (it does express intracytoplasmatic CD3 which can be observed in immunohistochemistry) nor surface CD8.[46]

When faced with type II RCD, a possible clonal TCR rearrangement must be sought by means of molecular techniques. The presence of oligo- or monoclonality is usually associated with RCD-II, but it is not essential for diagnosis.[41]

The aberrant RCD-II lymphocyte population can be found not only in duodenal biopsies, but also in those from the stomach, colon and peripheral blood.[42] This suggests that RCD-II is a disease that is not limited to the small intestine, but that it expands to the whole gastrointestinal tract and can spread through the blood. A datum of a high aberrant cell percentage (>80%) together with a clonal TCR rearrangement is highly predictive of developing an enteropathy-associated intestinal T lymphoma (EATL).[47,48]

Figure 2 offers an approach to celiac patients unresponsive to the gluten-free diet. This approach groups, on one hand, the initial focus on the lack of response to the diet and, on the other, diagnosis and management of suspected RCD.

CD with persistence of symptoms and/or atrophy while on a gluten-free diet

↓

Check diagnosis
Confirm diet compliance
Perform lactose and fructose tolerance test and SBI
Colonoscopy and biopsies: Microscopic colitis and IBD
Discard exocrine pancreatic insufficiency

↓

| Intensify GFD Dietary counselling | ← Positive — | **Serology** |

Negative ↓

| Rule out other causes of villous atrophy | ← Negative — | HLA DQ2/DQ8 |

Positive ↓

Suspicion of refractory celiac disease

↓

Duodenal biopsy: Immunohistochemistry
Flow cytometry
Nutritional support
Endoscopic capsule and TC

↓

| Rule out other causes of non-responsiveness to GFD | ← No — | Villous atrophy |

Marsh IIIa-c and aberrant T lymphocytes < 20%

Marsh IIIa-c and aberrant T lymphocytes > 20%

Type I refractory CD

Type II refractory CD

| Clinical follow-up and biopsy 3-6 afterwards | ← | Corticosteroids Azathioprine Infliximab |

Management coordinated with hematology
Alemtuzumab/cladribine
Autologous marrow transplant
Rule out intestinal lymphoma

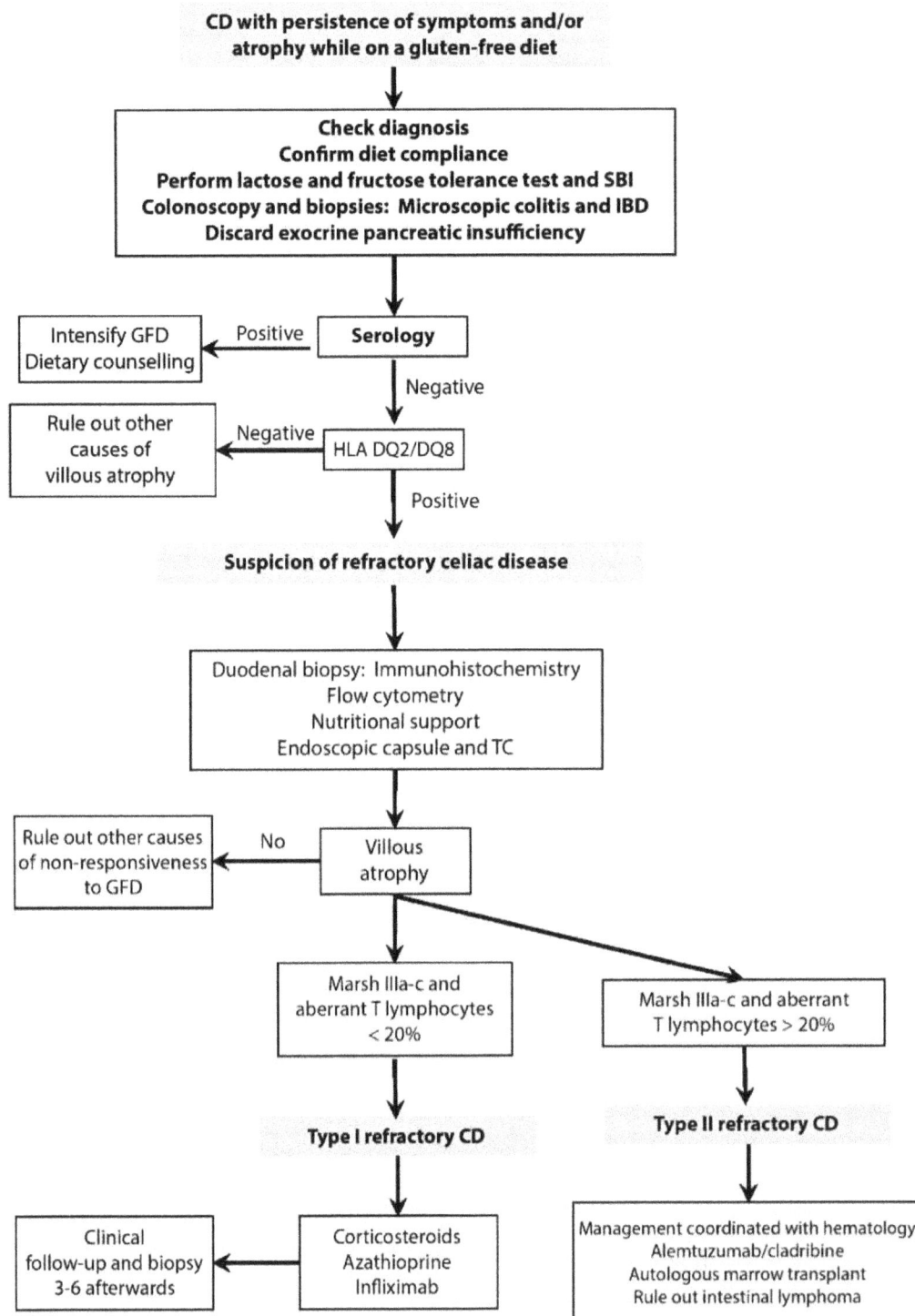

Figure 2. Approach for celiac patients unresponsive to the gluten-free diet.

6. Evolution and Prognosis

In general, RCD has a poor prognosis, with less than a 50% survival rate 5 years after diagnosis, for type II.[31,49] Although RCD is a heterogeneous group of entities, RCD-I may be an earlier stage of the disease than RCD-II, with a possibly less aggressive progression. The prognosis is linked to the presence and size of the population of aberrant IELs, which influences the risk of developing intestinal lymphoma.[50]

The presence of TCR clonality observed in RCD-II is also observed in intestinal lymphoma samples. This suggests a transformation of the aberrant lymphocytic cells we see in RCD in a high degree T lymphoma.[36]

It is currently not clear how to monitor patients with RCD in order to make an early lymphoma detection. Capsule endoscopy may reveal the presence of early tumor lesions in the small intestine. Positron Emission Tomography (PET) could also differentiate between RCD and an already developed lymphoma.[51] In general, a close clinical monitoring should be undertaken to search for the appearance of neoplasias upon deterioration of the patient or the appearance of alarming symptoms. Biopsies for histological, immunohistochemical and flow cytometry studies should be performed at least every 6 months until refractoriness is resolved. Faced with a type II RCD, we should identify biopsies and shorten the interval for monitoring the aberrant lymphocyte population, for an early detection of a progression towards a lymphoma[48] (Figure 2).

7. Treatment

The first step is a mainly nutritional support treatment, parenterally if necessary. Hydroelectrolytic disorders and mineral (iron, zinc, magnesium and calcium) and vitamin (B12, folic acid, K and D) deficiencies must be corrected. Of course, a strict gluten-free diet must be followed.

Current evidence regarding treatment is based on case series and expert opinions, without the benefit of controlled clinical trials. This is due to the low prevalence of this complication and to the differentiation of both RCD types.[4]

7.1. Treatment of Type I RCD

Besides the usual nutritional support, an elemental diet, based on amino acids, has been tested on these patients. The results showed clinical and histological improvements, coupled with a mucous interleukin 15 and interferon-γ secretion decrease in an RCD-I group of the patients.[52] The results observed using the elemental diet are short-term; it is necessary to progress further in the therapeutic scale.

Although there are no randomized studies, the most commonly used drugs are corticosteroids.[41] These are used intravenously or orally, depending on the clinical severity, a prednisone or prednisolone dose of 1 mg/kg. Local-action corticosteroids like budesonide have also been employed, with a similar clinical efficacy.[53] Overall clinical response to corticosteroids is good on the short term, although histological improvement is not observed in a large percentage of cases. Furthermore, clinical recurrence is common upon their suspension.[41]

Cases with relapse after corticosteroid suspension or those in clinical remission who have had RCD-I, could be candidates for long-term immunosuppressive therapy. Azathioprine, has been the most tested drug, with a high rate of clinical and histological response.[54] Treatment dose and duration are not well established and it is generally recommended to follow the same guidelines as in inMammatory bowel disease.

Cyclosporine A, *inpihig am*, tacrolimus and methotrexate have obtained variable results in isolated clinical cases.[55] Perhaps *inpihig am* has been the most evaluated and it is the one with the best results in several cases. Its use could be reserved for situations involving azathioprine intolerance or lacfl of response to it.

7.2. Treating Type II RCD

There is no established treatment for this aggressive RCD form. It is recognized however, that in an aberrant and clonal lymphocyte population, the therapeutic approach should be more aggressive.[56] Here corticosteroids or *inpihig am* may favor a transient clinical improvement, but with no ekect on clonal proliferation. Immunosuppressants such as azathioprine may even promote lymphoma progression and its use is not recommended.[56] Recombinant human interleuflin-10 (IL10-hr), has been employed to inhibit Th1 immune response to gliadin. However, it has not proved ekective in reported a series of 10 RCD-II cases.[57]

Antineoplastic agents used in the management of leuflemias and lymphomas, have been recently tested. Cladribine (2-clorodeoxyadenosine) is a synthetic purine analog, used in hairy cell leuflemia (a rare *F lyg 1bog a* type). Its use in a number of RCD-II cases caused clinical and histological improvement but with aberrant lymphocyte population persistence and progression to lymphoma in 40% of the cases.[58]

Aleg tuTug am is an anti-CD52 monoclonal antibody used in the treatment of chronic lymphocytic leuflemia. Its use in an RCD-II case resulted in a clinical and histological improvement, together with a progressive decline in the aberrant clonal lymphocyte population of clonal and remission maintenance for more than 36 months.[50] The response has been variable in other cases, perhaps associated with dikerent stages of disease.

Autologous bone marrow transplantation, after intensive chemotherapy, has been used in both in an established lymphoma[59] as well as in an RCD-II series, with good clinical and histological outcomes and reduced clonal lymphocyte populations.[60]

Nevertheless, there is no current ideal treatment for this RCD-II clonal population, which is the reason why novel therapies that act more speciffcally are being sought. In this regard, interleuflin-15 blocflage may be a promising approach. The production of these cytoflines is increased by the epithelium of RCD-II patients.[38] Additionally it has been described that, when overexpressed, it can induce lymphoma in transgenic mice[61] and that it directs Ij L expansion and activity in relation to enterocytes.[37,38,62,63] Thus, blocfling its activity, the elimination of the aberrant Ij L population can not only be achieved, but also the prevention of epithelial destruction.

References

1. Murray JA, Watson T, Clearman B, et al. *Effect of a gluten-free diet on gastrointestinal symptoms in celiac disease.* Am J Clin Nutr. 2004; 79: 669-73.

2. Rubio-Tapia A, Rahim MW, See JA, et al. *Mucosal recovery and mortality in adults with celiac disease after treatment with a gluten-free diet.* Am J Gastroenterol. 2010; 105: 1412-20. http://dx.doi.org/10.1038/ajg.2010.10

3. Vivas S, Ruiz de Morales JM. *Refractory celiac disease.* Gastroenterol Hepatol. 2008; 31: 310-6.

4. Rubio-Tapia A, Murray JA. *Classification and management of refractory coeliac disease.* Gut. 2010; 59: 547-57. http://dx.doi.org/10.1136/gut.2009.195131

5. Bazzigaluppi E, Roggero P, Parma B, et al. *Antibodies to recombinant human tissue-transglutaminase in coeliac disease: diagnostic effectiveness and decline pattern after gluten-free diet.* Dig Liver Dis. 2006; 38: 98-102. http://dx.doi.org/10.1016/j.dld.2005.10.020

6. Vahedi K, Mascart F, Mary JY, et al. *Reliability of antitransglutaminase antibodies as predictors of gluten-free diet compliance in adult celiac disease.* Am J Gastroenterol. 2003; 98: 1079-87. http://dx.doi.org/10.1111/j.1572-0241.2003.07284.x

7. Troncone R, Mayer M, Spagnuolo F, et al. *Endomysial antibodies as unreliable markers for slight dietary transgressions in adolescents with celiac disease.* J Pediatr Gastroenterol Nutr. 1995; 21: 69-72. http://dx.doi.org/10.1097/00005176-199507000-00012

8. Murphy MS, Sood M, Johnson T. *Use of the lactose H2 breath test to monitor mucosal healing in coeliac disease.* Acta Paediatr. 2002; 91: 141-4. http://dx.doi.org/10.1080/080352502317285117

9. Fine KD, Meyer RL, Lee EL. T*he prevalence and causes of chronic diarrhea in patients with celiac sprue treated with a gluten-free diet.* Gastroenterology. 1997; 112: 1830-8. http://dx.doi.org/10.1053/gast.1997.v112.pm9178673

10. Abdulkarim AS, Burgart LJ, See J, et al. Etiology of nonresponsive celiac disease: results of a systematic approach. Am J Gastroenterol. 2002; 97: 2016-21. http://dx.doi.org/10.1111/j.1572-0241.2002.05917.x

11. Tursi A, Brandimarte G, Giorgetti G. *High prevalence of small intestinal bacterial overgrowth in celiac patients with persistence of gastrointestinal symptoms after gluten withdrawal.* Am J Gastroenterol. 2003; 98: 839-43. http://dx.doi.org/10.1111/j.1572-0241.2003.07379.x

12. Carroccio A, Iacono G, Montalto G, et al. *Pancreatic enzyme therapy in childhood celiac disease. A double-blind prospective randomized study.* Dig Dis Sci. 1995; 40: 2555-60. http://dx.doi.org/10.1007/BF02220441

13. Sadr-Azodi O, Sanders DS, Murray JA, et al. *Patients With Celiac Disease Have an Increased Risk for Pancreatitis.* Clin Gastroenterol Hepatol. 2012; 10: 1136-42. http://dx.doi.org/10.1016/j.cgh.2012.06.023

14. Fine KD, Do K, Schulte K, et al. *High prevalence of celiac sprue-like HLA-DQ genes and enteropathy in patients with the microscopic colitis syndrome.* Am J Gastroenterol. 2000; 95: 1974-82. http://dx.doi.org/10.1111/j.1572-0241.2000.02255.x

15. Stewart M, Andrews CN, Urbanski S, et al. *The association of coeliac disease and microscopic colitis: a large population-based study.* Aliment Pharmacol Ther. 2011; 33: 1340-9. http://dx.doi.org/10.1111/j.1365-2036.2011.04666.x

16. Yang A, Chen Y, Scherl E, et al. *Inflammatory bowel disease in patients with celiac disease*. Inflamm Bowel Dis. 2005; 11: 528-32.
    http://dx.doi.org/10.1097/01.MIB.0000161308.65951.db

17. Parmar AS, Lappalainen M, Paavola-Sakki P, et al. *Association of celiac disease genes with inflammatory bowel disease in Finnish and Swedish patients*. Genes Immun. 2012; 13: 474-80. http://dx.doi.org/10.1038/gene.2012.21

18. Ventura A, Magazzu G, Greco L. *Duration of exposure to gluten and risk for autoimmune disorders in patients with celiac disease*. SIGEP Study Group for Autoimmune Disorders in Celiac Disease. Gastroenterology. 1999; 117: 297-303.
    http://dx.doi.org/10.1053/gast.1999.0029900297

19. De Tomas J, Munoz Calero A, Gonzalez Lara V, et al. *Ulcerative jejunitis: a complication of celiac disease*. Rev Esp Enferm Dig. 1994; 86: 761-3.

20. Corazza GR, Biagi F, Volta U, et al. *Autoimmune enteropathy and villous atrophy in adults*. Lancet. 1997; 350: 106-9. http://dx.doi.org/10.1016/S0140-6736(97)01042-8

21. Diez R, Garcia MJ, Vivas S, et al. *Gastrointestinal manifestations in patients with primary immunodeficiencies causing antibody deficiency*. Gastroenterol Hepatol. 2010; 33: 347-51. http://dx.doi.org/10.1016/j.gastrohep.2009.12.012

22. Halfdanarson TR, Litzow MR, Murray JA. *Hematologic manifestations of celiac disease*. Blood. 2007; 109: 412-21. http://dx.doi.org/10.1182/blood-2006-07-031104

23. Krauss N, Schuppan D. *Monitoring nonresponsive patients who have celiac disease*. Gastrointest Endosc Clin N Am. 2006; 16: 317-27.
    http://dx.doi.org/10.1016/j.giec.2006.03.005

24. Green PH, Rubin M. *Capsule endoscopy in celiac disease: diagnosis and management*. Gastrointest Endosc Clin N Am. 2006; 16: 307-16.
    http://dx.doi.org/10.1016/j.giec.2006.03.003

25. Heine GD, Hadithi M, Groenen MJ, et al. *Double-balloon enteroscopy: indications, diagnostic yield, and complications in a series of 275 patients with suspected small-bowel disease*. Endoscopy. 2006; 38: 42-8. http://dx.doi.org/10.1055/s-2005-921188

26. Trier JS, Falchuk ZM, Carey MC, et al. *Celiac sprue and refractory sprue*. Gastroenterology. 1978; 75: 307-16.

27. Rostom A, Murray JA, Kagnoff MF. *American Gastroenterological Association (AGA) Institute technical review on the diagnosis and management of celiac disease*. Gastroenterology. 2006; 131: 1981-2002.
    http://dx.doi.org/10.1053/j.gastro.2006.10.004

28. Trier JS. *Celiac sprue*. N Engl J Med. 1991; 325: 1709-19.
    http://dx.doi.org/10.1056/NEJM199112123252406

29. Biagi F, Corazza GR. *Defining gluten refractory enteropathy*. Eur J Gastroenterol Hepatol 2001; 13:561-5,Leffler DA, Dennis M, Hyett B, et al. *Etiologies and predictors of diagnosis in nonresponsive celiac disease*. Clin Gastroenterol Hepatol. 2007; 5: 445-50.
    http://dx.doi.org/10.1016/j.cgh.2006.12.006

30. Roshan B, Leffler DA, Jamma S, et al. *The incidence and clinical spectrum of refractory celiac disease in a north american referral center*. Am J Gastroenterol. 2011; 106: 923-8.
    http://dx.doi.org/10.1038/ajg.2011.104

31. West J. *Celiac disease and its complications: a time traveller's perspective*. Gastroenterology. 2009; 136: 32-4. http://dx.doi.org/10.1053/j.gastro.2008.11.026

32. Malamut G, Afchain P, Verkarre V, et al. *Presentation and long-term follow-up of refractory celiac disease: comparison of type I with type II*. Gastroenterology. 2009; 136: 81-90. http://dx.doi.org/10.1053/j.gastro.2008.09.069

33. Sollid LM. Coeliac disease: dissecting a complex inflammatory disorder. Nat Rev Immunol. 2002; 2: 647-55. http://dx.doi.org/10.1038/nri885

34. Marsh MN. *Gluten, major histocompatibility complex, and the small intestine. A molecular and immunobiologic approach to the spectrum of gluten sensitivity ('celiac sprue').* Gastroenterology. 1992; 102: 330-54.

35. Collin P, Wahab PJ, Murray JA. *Intraepithelial lymphocytes and coeliac disease.* Best Pract Res Clin Gastroenterol. 2005; 19: 341-50.
http://dx.doi.org/10.1016/j.bpg.2005.01.005

36. Cellier C, Delabesse E, Helmer C, et al. *Refractory sprue, coeliac disease, and enteropathy-associated T-cell lymphoma. French Coeliac Disease Study Group.* Lancet 2000; 356: 203-8. http://dx.doi.org/10.1016/S0140-6736(00)02481-8

37. Daum S, Weiss D, Hummel M, et al. *Frequency of clonal intraepithelial T lymphocyte proliferations in enteropathy-type intestinal T cell lymphoma, coeliac disease, and refractory sprue.* Gut. 2001; 49: 804-12. http://dx.doi.org/10.1136/gut.49.6.804

38. Di Sabatino A, Ciccocioppo R, Cupelli F, et al. *Epithelium derived interleukin 15 regulates intraepithelial lymphocyte Th1 cytokine production, cytotoxicity, and survival in coeliac disease.* Gut. 2006; 55: 469-77. http://dx.doi.org/10.1136/gut.2005.068684

39. Mention JJ, Ben Ahmed M, Begue B, et al. *Interleukin 15: a key to disrupted intraepithelial lymphocyte homeostasis and lymphomagenesis in celiac disease.* Gastroenterology. 2003; 125: 730-45.
http://dx.doi.org/10.1016/S0016-5085(03)01047-3

40. Malamut G, Meresse B, Cellier C, et al. *Refractory celiac disease: from bench to bedside.* Semin Immunopathol. 2012; 34: 601-13. http://dx.doi.org/10.1007/s00281-012-0322-z

41. Isaacson PG. *Relation between cryptic intestinal lymphoma and refractory sprue.* Lancet 2000; 356: 178-9. http://dx.doi.org/10.1016/S0140-6736(00)02472-7

42. Daum S, Cellier C, Mulder CJ. *Refractory coeliac disease.* Best Pract Res Clin Gastroenterol. 2005; 19: 413-24. http://dx.doi.org/10.1016/j.bpg.2005.02.001

43. Verkarre V, Asnafi V, Lecomte T, et al. *Refractory coeliac sprue is a diffuse gastrointestinal disease.* Gut. 2003; 52: 205-11. http://dx.doi.org/10.1136/gut.52.2.205

44. Gay G, Delvaux M, Fassler I. *Outcome of capsule endoscopy in determining indication and route for push-and-pull enteroscopy.* Endoscopy. 2006; 38: 49-58.
http://dx.doi.org/10.1055/s-2005-921176

45. Mallant M, Hadithi M, Al-Toma AB, et al. *Abdominal computed tomography in refractory coeliac disease and enteropathy associated T-cell lymphoma.* World J Gastroenterol. 2007; 13: 1696-700. http://dx.doi.org/10.1016/j.gastrohep.2009.12.012

46. Patey-Mariaud De Serre N, Cellier C, Jabri B, et al. *Distinction between coeliac disease and refractory sprue: a simple immunohistochemical method.* Histopathology. 2000; 37: 70-7. http://dx.doi.org/10.1046/j.1365-2559.2000.00926.x

47. Cellier C, Patey N, Mauvieux L, et al. *Abnormal intestinal intraepithelial lymphocytes in refractory sprue.* Gastroenterology. 1998; 114: 471-81.
http://dx.doi.org/10.1016/S0016-5085(98)70530-X

48. de Mascarel A, Belleannee G, Stanislas S, et al. *Mucosal intraepithelial T-lymphocytes in refractory celiac disease: a neoplastic population with a variable CD8 phenotype.* Am J Surg Pathol. 2008; 32: 744-51. http://dx.doi.org/10.1097/PAS.0b013e318159b478

49. Liu H, Brais R, Lavergne-Slove A, et al. *Continual monitoring of intraepithelial lymphocyte immunophenotype and clonality is more important than snapshot analysis in the surveillance of refractory coeliac disease.* Gut. 2010; 59: 452-60.

http://dx.doi.org/10.1136/gut.2009.186007

50. Rubio-Tapia A, Kelly DG, Lahr BD, et al. *Clinical staging and survival in refractory celiac disease: a single center experience*. Gastroenterology. 2009; 136: 99-107; quiz 352-3.

51. Vivas S, Ruiz de Morales JM, Ramos F, Suarez-Vilela D. *Alemtuzumab for refractory celiac disease in a patient at risk for enteropathy-associated T-cell lymphoma*. N Engl J Med. 2006; 354: 2514-5. http://dx.doi.org/10.1056/NEJMc053129

52. Hoffmann M, Vogelsang H, Kletter K, et al. *18F-fluoro-deoxy-glucose positron emission tomography (18F-FDG-PET) for assessment of enteropathy-type T cell lymphoma*. Gut. 2003; 52: 347-51. http://dx.doi.org/10.1136/gut.52.3.347

53. Olaussen RW, Lovik A, Tollefsen S, et al. *Effect of elemental diet on mucosal immunopathology and clinical symptoms in type 1 refractory celiac disease*. Clin Gastroenterol Hepatol. 2005; 3: 875-85.
http://dx.doi.org/10.1016/S1542-3565(05)00295-8

54. Daum S, Ipczynski R, Heine B, et al. *Therapy with budesonide in patients with refractory sprue*. Digestion. 2006; 73: 60-8. http://dx.doi.org/10.1159/000092639

55. Goerres MS, Meijer JW, Wahab PJ, et al. *Azathioprine and prednisone combination therapy in refractory coeliac disease*. Aliment Pharmacol Ther 2003; 18:487-94.
http://dx.doi.org/10.1046/j.1365-2036.2003.01687.x

56. Gillett HR, Arnott ID, McIntyre M, et al. *Successful infliximab treatment for steroid-refractory celiac disease: a case report*. Gastroenterology. 2002; 122: 800-5.
http://dx.doi.org/10.1053/gast.2002.31874

57. Cellier C, Cerf-Bensussan N. T*reatment of clonal refractory celiac disease or cryptic intraepithelial lymphoma: A long road from bench to bedside*. Clin Gastroenterol Hepatol. 2006; 4: 1320-1. http://dx.doi.org/10.1016/j.cgh.2006.09.011

58. Mulder CJ, Wahab PJ, Meijer JW, et al. *A pilot study of recombinant human interleukin-10 in adults with refractory coeliac disease*. Eur J Gastroenterol Hepatol. 2001;13: 1183-8. http://dx.doi.org/10.1097/00042737-200110000-00010

59. Al-Toma A, Goerres MS, Meijer JW, et al. *Cladribine therapy in refractory celiac disease with aberrant T cells*. Clin Gastroenterol Hepatol. 2006; 4: 1322-7; quiz 1300.
http://dx.doi.org/10.1016/j.cgh.2006.07.007

60. Rongey C, Micallef I, Smyrk T, et al. *Successful treatment of enteropathy-associated T cell lymphoma with autologous stem cell transplant*. Dig Dis Sci. 2006; 51: 1082-6.
http://dx.doi.org/10.1007/s10620-006-8013-z

61. Al-Toma A, Visser OJ, van Roessel HM, et al. *Autologous hematopoietic stem cell transplantation in refractory celiac disease with aberrant T cells*. Blood. 2007; 109: 2243-9. http://dx.doi.org/10.1182/blood-2006-08-042820

62. Fehniger TA, Suzuki K, Ponnappan A, et al. *Fatal leukemia in interleukin 15 transgenic mice follows early expansions in natural killer and memory phenotype CD8+ T cells*. J Exp Med. 2001; 193: 219-31. http://dx.doi.org/10.1084/jem.193.2.219

63. van Heel DA. *Interleukin 15: its role in intestinal inflammation*. Gut. 2006; 55: 444-5.
http://dx.doi.org/10.1136/gut.2005.079335

Chapter 18

Medical Follow-up of Celiac Patients

Alberto Rubio-Tapia

Associated Consultant and Assistant Professor of Medicine, Gastroenterology and Hepatology Division. Mayo Clinic, Rochester, Minnesota, U.S.A.

rubiotapia.alberto@mayo.edu

Doi: http://dx.doi.org/10.3926/oms.219

How to cite this chapter

Rubio-Tapia A. *Medical Follow-up of Celiac Patients.* In Rodrigo L and Peña AS, editors. *Celiac Disease and Non-celiac Gluten Sensitivity*. Barcelona, Spain: OmniaScience; 2014. p. 377-387.

Abstract

This chapter presents practical recommendations for the medical follow-up of patients with celiac disease. The gluten-free diet is currently the only available treatment for celiac disease. Patients with celiac disease require lifelong adherence to the gluten-free diet and medical follow-up. The benefits of strict adherence to the gluten-free diet including control of symptoms, seroconversion, and mucosal healing are discussed in detail. Despite extensive evidence of the benefits of the strict adherence to the gluten-free diet, rates of compliance and medical follow-up in clinical practice are less than optimal. The advantages and limitations of the four methods currently available for assessment of compliance to gluten-free diet (detailed dietary history, serology, histology and structured questionnaires) are summarized. Expert opinion and guidelines endorsed by several Medical Societies agree on the necessity of a medical follow-up; however, there is no universal consensus about how to perform said medical follow-up in daily practice. An algorithm for the medical follow-up of celiac disease patients is suggested based on available evidence and the author's institutional experience, which includes regular medical follow-up, annual serology measurement, evaluation of a detailed dietary history, assessment of clinical response and correction of nutritional deficiencies.

1. Initial Considerations

- The gluten-free diet is the only available treatment for celiac disease.

- Celiac patients require lifelong medical monitoring.

- There is no consensus regarding the most effective way to implement this medical monitoring.

- The basic objectives of medical monitoring are to facilitate adherence to the gluten-free diet and keep track of clinical response to treatment.

2. Introduction

The only currently available treatment for celiac disease is a strict adherence to the gluten-free diet, which involves removing all foods that contain wheat, barley and rye.[1] The benefits of a strict adherence to the gluten-free diet in celiac patients are considerable and include symptom control and prevention of complications.[2]

The percentage of people who achieve strict adherence to treatments involving a change in eating habits (59% on average) is among the lowest compared with other medical treatment modalities.[3] *Compliance with medical treatment has a direct and objective influence in patient prognosis.* The basic goals of medical celiac disease follow-up are to facilitate monitoring the gluten-free diet and to monitor patient response to the treatment.[4] Unfortunately, medical monitoring is deficient in most celiac patients and, in many cases, nonexistent.[5] Therefore, it is not surprising that the percentage of adherence to the gluten-free diet is variable (42-91%).[2] Celiac patients require a medical monitoring plan and it is evident that establishing or confirming the diagnosis should not be the ultimate end of consultation with the gastroenterologist.[6]

Celiac disease is a chronic condition and, as such, requires lifelong medical follow-up.[7] Although most experts recommend medical follow-up, there is no consensus on how and who should carry out medical monitoring in daily practice.[8] There are few quality studies, based on evidence, on how to establish monitoring rules.

The objectives of this chapter are 1) to summarize the evidence on the benefits of strict adherence to a gluten-free diet and 2) to propose practical recommendations for the health monitoring of celiac disease patients based on available expertise and the author's institutional experience.

3. Benefits of Adherence to the Gluten-Free Diet

The gluten-free diet is a safe and effective treatment for controlling celiac disease symptoms and it may also decrease the risk of complications.[9] A notable improvement in diarrhea may be observed as early as 7 days into the diet; it also improves in most of the patients (80%) within 60 days of strict adherence to the gluten-free diet.[10]

A strict gluten-free diet adherence is associated with a decrease in the absolute value of basal titers of anti-tissue transglutaminase antibodies (and other specific antibodies), which can be observed as early as 3 months into the gluten-free diet and tends to become more pronounced within the first year.[11] Antibody seroconversion (change of a test result from positive to negative) in relation to tissue transglutaminase was observed in 93% of the patients who submitted to an annual monitoring.[12]

Intestinal villi recovery is often incomplete and requires several years of strict adherence to the gluten-free diet in patients diagnosed as adults.[13,16] In our experience, the recovery of intestinal villi in adult celiac patients was of 34% after 2 years and of 66% after 5 years of adhering to the gluten-free diet.[14] On the other hand, the recovery of intestinal villi in children appears to happen much earlier, occurring in 95% of the cases within the first 2 years after starting the gluten-free diet, although the evidence is limited.[15]

Strict adherence to a gluten-free diet for at least 5 years appears to decrease the risk of developing lymphoma (relative risk was of 78% in patients without adherence to the diet and of 17% in patients who complied with the gluten-free diet).[17] The risk of lymphoproliferative disease was null in celiac patients without villous atrophy[18], which suggests that the good adhesion to the gluten-free diet with subsequent normalization of histology may be an aim to consider in medical monitoring.

4. Adherence Monitoring Methods

There are four methods available to verify proper compliance with the gluten-free diet, such as: 1) Consultation with a dietitian, 2) Tracking of serology evolution, 3) Monitoring of bowel biopsy changes and 4) Use of structured questionnaires to assess adherence to the gluten-free diet.[8,19]

Consultation with a dietitian is the "gold standard" to control adherence to the gluten-free diet.[1]

Tissular anti-transglutaminase and anti-endomysium antibody titers greatly diminish and/or become normal in patients with good adherence to the gluten-free diet.[11,20,21] In patients with a strict adherence to the gluten-free diet and who achieve seroconversion, anti-tissue transglutaminase and anti-endomysium antibodies rise when a gluten challenge test is performed.[20] These data suggest that the presence of positive anti-transglutaminase (or anti-endomysium) antibodies in the symptomatic patient after one year of follow-up requires further evaluation in order to detect the presence of accidental or intentional gluten contamination.[22] Furthermore, negative antibodies can be observed in symptomatic patients who are exposed to accidental contamination with small amounts of gluten and in those who, while remaining asymptomatic, have follow-up biopsies with persistent atrophy.[14] The absence of serum antibodies in symptomatic patients (usually severe), with a strict adherence to a gluten-free diet is a feature of refractory celiac disease.[23]

Intestinal biopsy is the only currently available method to definitively assess the recovery of the intestinal mucosa. The need for intestinal biopsy during follow-up is a highly controversial topic.[24] The video capsule is a new technique able to detect lesions suggesting intestinal mucosal atrophy (fissures, lack of folds, paving pattern) at the moment of clinical diagnosis and mucosal response after starting a gluten-free diet[25]; however, it has not been systematically evaluated as a clinical follow-up method.

Finally, the use of a structured questionnaires to evaluate adherence to the gluten-free diet has been proposed.[1,9,26,27] Generally, these questionnaires seem to correlate with the antibody level and/or the results of follow-up intestinal biopsies. The information obtained using the questionnaire developed in Boston (CDAT) appears to be superior to monitoring through the determination of tissular anti-transglutaminase antibodies.[19] The questionnaire validated in Italy has the advantage that it can be administered by persons without any experience and that the average time for its completion is of one minute.[27] A limitation for the implementation of structured questionnaires in daily clinical practice is the need for their validation in clinical contexts and languages different from the one used where the questionnaire was initially created.

5. Medical Follow-up Recommendations

All medical societies and the opinion of international experts agree on the usefulness of performing a medical follow-up, but there is no unanimous consensus about what is the best way to do this.[28] The medical follow-up that patients obtain is generally based on local and/or personal practices.

The recommendations proposed by medical societies or expert opinions for monitoring are quite diverse.[4,8,29] Most recommend periodic monitoring of symptoms, serology (anti-transglutaminase antibodies), consultation with an expert dietician and joining a local and/or regional support group. No consensus exists on the type of general laboratory studies needed to control the celiac patient's routine, on the need of regular bone densitometry tests and on intestinal biopsies during the follow-up.[28] The cost of follow-up visits can vary significantly according to the protocol used.[28] No study suggests that, regarding a long-term prognosis, one follow-up protocol is better than the other. The American Gastroenterological Association (AGA) recommends performing the following general laboratory studies in follow-up visits: complete blood count, folate, ferritin, calcium and alkaline phosphatase.[4] By contrast, the North American Society of Pediatric Gastroenterology, Hepatology and Nutrition (NASPGHAN) recommends no routine general laboratory studies in celiac children during follow-up visits.[29]

In the authors' clinical practice clinical monitoring of children and adults is performed 3-6 months into the gluten-free diet and then once every year (Figure 1).

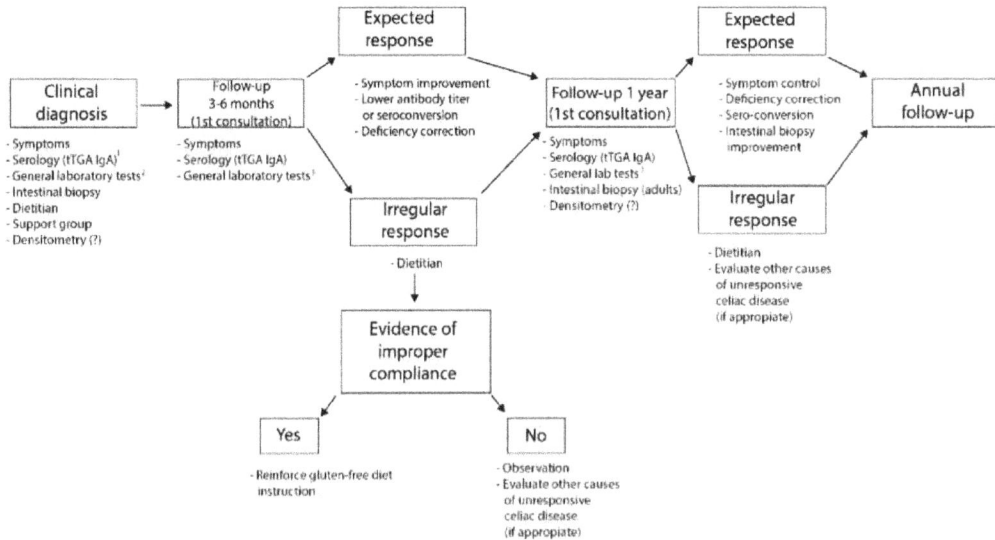

Figure 1. Clinical follow-up diagram for children and adults. [1] tTGA IgA (anti-tissue transglutaminase IgA antibody) is the serology of choice for the diagnosis and management of celiac patients. [2] General laboratory diagnoses include complete blood count, alanine aminotransferase (ALT), vitamins (A, D, E, and B12), copper, zinc, carotenoids, folate, ferritin, iron. [3] General laboratory monitoring will only include only those studies that were abnormal at the time of diagnosis to verify their proper correction with the specific treatment.

The objectives of follow-up visits include:

- Documenting the improvement/disappearance of symptoms.

- Monitoring adherence to the gluten-free diet and to identify barriers to its successful implementation.

- Weight and height measurement (in children, complete growth assessment).

- Evaluating the response (titer decrease) of specific antibodies, relative to the baseline (the same antibody that was positive at diagnosis must be used and ideally, at the same laboratory).

- Confirming the correction of all nutritional deficiencies identified at diagnosis (for which monitoring laboratory tests should be individualized).

In the authors' institution consultation with the dietitian is performed at diagnosis and during the follow-up visit conducted within one year of initiating the gluten-free diet. Subsequent consultations with a nutrition specialist are evaluated in each individual case, taking into account the results obtained after the initial instruction and the presence of persistent or recurrent symptoms.[30] In routine clinical practice, consultation with the dietitian whenever possible is favored, although the authors' admit they work in a center specialized in celiac disease management. A group of British celiac patients who answered a survey stated that their preferred follow-up method was consulting with a dietitian and having a doctor available if necessary.[31] A common problem is that some centers lack access to dietitians experienced in gluten-free diet management. Additionally, no study shows that consulting with both a dietitian and a physician is better, in terms of prognosis, than consulting with only one of them. A Finnish study suggests that a high percentage of dietary adherence (>80%) can be achieved with a medical follow-up carried out in by the primary care physician.[32]

3 to 6 months after the initial visit, the next one will take place one year after starting treatment with the following objectives:

- Documenting the total monitoring of symptoms.

- Checking anti-transglutaminase antibody seroconversion.

- Confirming the correction of general laboratory tests that were altered at the time of diagnosis.

There is sufficient evidence to indicate that regular monitoring including annual serology (anti-tissue transglutaminase) promotes adherence to the gluten-free diet.[12] Although it may seem questionable, the authors' include in their daily clinical practice an indication for repeat endoscopy with intestinal biopsies in the monitoring of adults in order to check histological response to treatment (usually after 1-2 years of proper adherence to gluten-free diet). The follow-up biopsy is particularly useful to evaluate histological response to the gluten-free diet in those patients who were diagnosed in the context of a specific negative serology and whose initial biopsy showed villous atrophy (in the authors' experience, 15-20% of the patients).[33] Intestinal biopsy monitoring is not considered necessary in children with good clinical response and anti-transglutaminase antibody seroconversion.

In all patients the authors' assess bone mineral density by densitometry at diagnosis or within one year of initiating a gluten-free diet, although this recommendation may seem questionable.

It is the authors' practice to recommend to all their patients to join a local and/or regional celiac patient support group. Participation in a support group or patients' association is one of the factors consistently associated with better adherence to the gluten-free diet.[34]

In patients with good clinical response, subsequent follow-up visits are made each year (sometimes every 2 years) and include assessment of adherence to the gluten-free diet and serology. In a study conducted in Italy, which included a systematic and determined yearly anti-tissue transglutaminase antibodies for 5 years in a series of 2245 patients, it was demonstrated that 69% of the patients achieved permanent seroconversion; 1% did not achieve seroconversion and, in 30% of the cases, the results of serology monitoring oscillated between positive and negative values.

The goals of long-term medical follow-up of celiac disease patients in remission are to strengthen instruction on adherence to the gluten-free diet and avoid or facilitate early detection of associated diseases and/or complications.

6. Conclusions

Celiac patients require medical monitoring for life. There is no consensus on how to carry out monitoring. Generally, available recommendations are based on expert opinion. There is sufficient evidence to ensure that strict adherence to a gluten-free diet generates a positive impact in the short-to-long-term in celiac disease patients.

Acknowledgments

This work was made possible by support provided by the American College of Gastroenterology Junior Faculty Development Award.

References

1. See J, Murray JA. *Gluten-free diet: the medical and nutrition management of celiac disease*. Nutr Clin Pract. 2006; 21: 1-15.
    http://dx.doi.org/10.1177/011542650602100101
2. Hall NJ, Rubin G, Charnock A. *Systematic review: adherence to a gluten-free diet in adult patients with coeliac disease*. Aliment Pharmacol. Ther. 2009; 30: 315-30.
    http://dx.doi.org/10.1111/j.1365-2036.2009.04053.x
3. DiMatteo MR. *Variations in patients' adherence to medical recommendations: a quantitative review of 50 years of research*. Med. Care. 2004; 42: 200-9.
    http://dx.doi.org/10.1097/01.mlr.0000114908.90348.f9
4. Rostom A, Murray JA, Kagnoff MF. *American Gastroenterological Association (AGA) Institute technical review on the diagnosis and management of celiac disease*. Gastroenterology. 2006; 131: 1981-2002.
    http://dx.doi.org/10.1053/j.gastro.2006.10.004
5. Herman ML, Rubio-Tapia A, Lahr BD, Larson JJ, Van Dyke CT, Murray JA. *Patients with celiac disease are not followed up adequately*. Clin Gastroenterol Hepatol. 2012; 10: 893-899 e1. http://dx.doi.org/10.1016/j.cgh.2012.05.007
6. Gibson PR, Shepherd SJ, Tye-Din JA. *For celiac disease, diagnosis is not enough. Clin. Gastroenterol*. Hepatol. 2012; 10: 900-1. http://dx.doi.org/10.1016/j.cgh.2012.03.020
7. Di Sabatino A, Corazza GR. *Coeliac disease*. Lancet. 2009; 373: 1480-93.
    http://dx.doi.org/10.1016/S0140-6736(09)60254-3
8. Pietzak MM. *Follow-up of patients with celiac disease: achieving compliance with treatment*. Gastroenterology. 2005; 128: S135-41.
    http://dx.doi.org/10.1053/j.gastro.2005.02.025
9. Haines ML, Anderson RP, Gibson PR. *Systematic review: The evidence base for long-term management of coeliac disease*. Aliment Pharmacol Ther. 2008; 28: 1042-66.
    http://dx.doi.org/10.1111/j.1365-2036.2008.03820.x
10. Murray JA, Watson T, Clearman B, Mitros F. *Effect of a gluten-free diet on gastrointestinal symptoms in celiac disease*. Am J Clin Nutr. 2004; 79: 669-73.
11. Nachman F, Sugai E, Vazquez H, Gonzalez A, Andrenacci P, Niveloni S, et al. *Serological tests for celiac disease as indicators of long-term compliance with the gluten-free diet*. Eur J Gastroenterol Hepatol. 2011; 23: 473-80.
    http://dx.doi.org/10.1097/MEG.0b013e328346e0f1
12. Zanini B, Lanzarotto F, Mora A, Bertolazzi S, Turini D, Cesana B, et al. *Five year time course of celiac disease serology during gluten free diet: Results of a community based "CD-Watch" program*. Dig Liver Dis. 2010; 42: 865-70.
    http://dx.doi.org/10.1016/j.dld.2010.05.009
13. Lanzini A, Lanzarotto F, Villanacci V, Mora A, Bertolazzi S, Turini D, et al. *Complete recovery of intestinal mucosa occurs very rarely in adult coeliac patients despite adherence to gluten-free diet*. Aliment Pharmacol Ther. 2009; 29: 1299-308.
    http://dx.doi.org/10.1111/j.1365-2036.2009.03992.x
14. Rubio-Tapia A, Rahim MW, See JA, Lahr BD, Wu TT, Murray JA. *Mucosal Recovery and Mortality in Adults With Celiac Disease After Treatment With a Gluten-Free Diet*. Am. J. Gastroenterol. 2010; 105: 1412-20. http://dx.doi.org/10.1038/ajg.2010.10

15. Wahab PJ, Meijer JW, Mulder CJ. *Histologic follow-up of people with celiac disease on a gluten-free diet: Slow and incomplete recovery*. Am J Clin Pathol. 2002; 118: 459-63. http://dx.doi.org/10.1309/EVXT-851X-WHLC-RLX9

16. Macdonald WC, Brandborg LL, Flick AL, Trier JS, Rubin CE. *Studies of Celiac Sprue. Iv. The Response of the Whole Length of the Small Bowel to a Gluten-Free Diet*. Gastroenterology. 1964; 47: 573-89.

17. Holmes GK, Prior P, Lane MR, Pope D, Allan RN. *Malignancy in coeliac disease --effect of a gluten free diet*. Gut. 1989; 30: 333-8. http://dx.doi.org/10.1136/gut.30.3.333

18. Elfstrom P, Granath F, Ekstrom Smedby K, Montgomery SM, Askling J, Ekbom A, et al. *Risk of lymphoproliferative malignancy in relation to small intestinal histopathology among patients with celiac disease*. J. Natl. Cancer Inst. 2011; 103: 436-44. http://dx.doi.org/10.1093/jnci/djq564

19. Leffler DA, Dennis M, Edwards George JB, Jamma S, Magge S, Cook EF, et al. *A simple validated gluten-free diet adherence survey for adults with celiac disease.* Clin Gastroenterol Hepatol. 2009; 7: 530-6, 536 e1-2. http://dx.doi.org/10.1016/j.cgh.2008.12.032

20. Burgin-Wolff A, Dahlbom I, Hadziselimovic F, Petersson CJ. *Antibodies against human tissue transglutaminase and endomysium in diagnosing and monitoring coeliac disease*. Scand J Gastroenterol. 2002; 37: 685-91. http://dx.doi.org/10.1080/00365520212496

21. Koop I, Ilchmann R, Izzi L, Adragna A, Koop H, Barthelmes H. *Detection of autoantibodies against tissue transglutaminase in patients with celiac disease and dermatitis herpetiformis*. Am J Gastroenterol. 2000; 95: 2009-14. http://dx.doi.org/10.1111/j.1572-0241.2000.02086.x

22. Green PH, Cellier C. *Celiac disease*. N Engl J Med. 2007; 357: 1731-43. http://dx.doi.org/10.1056/NEJMra071600

23. Rubio-Tapia A, Murray JA. C*lassification and management of refractory coeliac disease. Gut.* 2010; 59: 547-57. http://dx.doi.org/10.1136/gut.2009.195131

24. Harris LA, Park JY, Voltaggio L, Lam-Himlin D. C*eliac disease: clinical, endoscopic, and histopathologic review.* Gastrointest. Endosc. 2012; 76: 625-40. http://dx.doi.org/10.1016/j.gie.2012.04.473

25. Murray JA, Rubio-Tapia A, Van Dyke CT, Brogan DL, Knipschield MA, Lahr B, et al. *Mucosal atrophy in celiac disease: extent of involvement, correlation with clinical presentation, and response to treatment*. Clin. Gastroenterol. Hepatol. 2008; 6: 186- 93; quiz 125. http://dx.doi.org/10.1016/j.cgh.2007.10.012

26. Biagi F, Andrealli A, Bianchi PI, Marchese A, Klersy C, Corazza GR. *A gluten-free diet score to evaluate dietary compliance in patients with coeliac disease*. Br. J. Nutr. 2009; 102: 882-7. http://dx.doi.org/10.1017/S0007114509301579

27. Biagi F, Bianchi PI, Marchese A, Trotta L, Vattiato C, Balduzzi D, et al. *A score that verifies adherence to a gluten-free diet: a cross-sectional, multicentre validation in real clinical life.* Br. J. Nutr. 2012; 28(108): 1884-8.

28. Silvester JA, Rashid M. *Long-term follow-up of individuals with celiac disease: an evaluation of current practice guidelines.* Can J Gastroenterol. 2007; 21: 557-64.

29. Hill ID, Dirks MH, Liptak GS, Colletti RB, Fasano A, Guandalini S, et al. *Guideline for the diagnosis and treatment of celiac disease in children: recommendations of the North American Society for Pediatric Gastroenterology, Hepatology and Nutrition.* J Pediatr Gastroenterol Nutr. 2005; 40: 1-19. http://dx.doi.org/10.1097/00005176-200501000-00001

30. Rubio-Tapia A, Barton SH, Murray JA. *Celiac disease and persistent symptoms*. Clin Gastroenterol Hepatol. 2011; 9: 13-7; quiz e8.
http://dx.doi.org/10.1016/j.cgh.2010.07.014

31. Bebb JR, Lawson A, Knight T, Long RG. *Long-term follow-up of coeliac disease-what do coeliac patients want?* Aliment Pharmacol Ther. 2006; 23: 827-31.
http://dx.doi.org/10.1111/j.1365-2036.2006.02824.x

32. Kurppa K, Lauronen O, Collin P, Ukkola A, Laurila K, Huhtala H, Maki M, Kaukinen K. *Factors Associated with Dietary Adherence in Celiac Disease: A Nationwide Study*. Digestion. 2012; 86: 309-14. http://dx.doi.org/10.1159/000341416

33. Rashtak S, Ettore MW, Homburger HA, Murray JA. *Combination testing for antibodies in the diagnosis of coeliac disease: comparison of multiplex immunoassay and ELISA methods*. Aliment Pharmacol Ther. 2008; 28: 805-13.
http://dx.doi.org/10.1111/j.1365-2036.2008.03797.x

34. Leffler DA, Edwards-George J, Dennis M, Schuppan D, Cook F, Franko DL, et al. *Factors that influence adherence to a gluten-free diet in adults with celiac disease*. Dig Dis Sci. 2008; 53: 1573-81. http://dx.doi.org/10.1007/s10620-007-0055-3

Chapter 19

Quality of Life and Psychological Distress in Celiac Disease

Cristina Sfoggia, Gabriela Longarini, Florencia Costa, Horacio Vázquez, Eduardo Mauriño, Julio C. Bai

Small Intestine Section, Clinical Unit, Department of Medicine; Dr. Bonorino Udaondo Gastroenterological Hospital. Buenos Aires, Argentina.

csfoggia@hotmail.com, gabilongarini@hotmail.com, floppycosta@gmail.com, hvazquez@intramed.net, eduardomaurino@speedy.com.ar, jbai@intramed.net

Doi: http://dx.doi.org/10.3926.oms.220

How to cite this chapter

Sfoggia C, Longarini G, Costa F, Vázquez H, Mauriño E, Bai JC. *Quality of Life and Psychological Distress in Celiac Disease*. In Rodrigo L and Peña AS, editors. *Celiac Disease and Non-Celiac Gluten Sensitivity*. Barcelona, Spain: OmniaScience; 2014. p. 389-406.

C. Sfoggia, G. Longarini, F. Costa, H. Vázquez, E. Mauriño, JC Bai

Abstract

Both the quality of life and the psychological status of celiac disease patients have been explored in recent research. This chapter aims to review the reported evidence on the psychological aspects of celiac disease and the patients' perception of the disorder. Nevertheless, studies show controversial and contradictory results. When evaluated prior to diagnosis, patients with a symptomatic clinical presentation had an evident decrease in their quality of life. The gluten-free diet improves such perception. On the other hand, evidence on the quality of life in patients with subclinical disease is not so clear. Depression is the most commonly referred and studied mental disorder. Depression has been reported to be more prevalent and severe in celiac patients than in the general population. The interaction between physiological and environmental factors, seems to be responsible for the disturbance. Anxiety disorders have also been reported, but with less clear results. Currently, it seems accurate to consider them to be forms reactive to diagnosis or to be associated with difficulties in following the diet and its impact on social life. In this sense, the evidence seems to suggest that these could be considered as adjustment disorders with an anxiety state. Regarding the effects of treatment on these symptoms, there is currently no agreement since improvements have been reported in some studies but not in others. Importantly, depression may affect the adherence to treatment, disease evolution and perception of quality of life and, therefore, its presence ought to be investigated upon diagnosis.

1. Introduction

Celiac disease (CD) is an autoimmune chronic T cell-mediated enteropathy, precipitated by gluten ingestion, that appears in genetically predisposed individuals affecting, affecting around 1% of the general population.[1] The gluten-free diet (GFD) is the only treatment that effectively relieves its symptoms, normalizes biochemical changes and the disease's intestinal mucosal damage.[1] Lifelong compliance with the GFD can be challenging for the patients due to its high economic cost, social restrictions and difficulties in complying with it.[2] For these reasons, in recent years, there has been growing interest in evaluating a number of issues such as: whether the disease affects the patients' Quality of Life (QoL), if this is related to clinical presentation characteristics, if the treatment has a positive impact on these parameters or if mood disturbances, such as depression or anxiety, could influence the QoL and compliance with the GFD.[3-6]

Given the evidence of an extremely wide variability range of CD symptoms, recent efforts have sought to clarify and unify clinical criteria.[2] Thus, clinical CD presentations have been classified into: Symptomatic (with intestinal and extraintestinal symptoms, also called classical CD) and subclinical (patients with or without the characteristic signs that occur below the threshold of clinical detection).[2] It is to be expected, as confirmed by research, that clinical differences correlate with psychological aspects and QoL, both before diagnosis and after starting the GFD.[7]

This chapter will explore existing scientific knowledge about the relationship between CD and QoL, psychological distress, depression and anxiety, as well as the implications and consequences entailed by a treatment based on the GFD.

2. Quality of Life

Health Related Quality of Life (HRQoL) expresses health status as perceived by the individual, in relation to the disease itself and the effects that treatments have on the recipient; it is quite clear that this concept focuses on the patient's subjective aspect. HRQoL measurement is a quantitative assessment of the health status and it includes not only physical but also emotional and social aspects. Such measurement has become mandatory in the analysis of the effectiveness of the treatments employed and the evolution of specific conditions, especially in chronic diseases. HRQoL analysis is based on a multidimensional concept, which includes assessment of the patient's psychological well-being, emotional state, physical and social functioning and general health perception.[3-6] Regarding gastrointestinal diseases, the most important aspects include the perception of gastrointestinal symptoms relief and the benefits it may bring to the functional status and general well-being.[4] HRQoL can be measured by a variety of instruments, both general and disease-specific questionnaires. General questionnaires cover a wide spectrum of domains and allow comparison between different diseases and populations, whereas disease-specific questionnaires for each focus on particular aspects of it and its treatment and are more sensitive in detecting small changes in the QoL.[6] Most studies assessing QoL in CD patients used general questionnaires that focus on generic items developed for chronic diseases. The most frequently used are: *Short Form Health Survey* (*SF-36*), the *Psychological General Well-being* (*PGWB*) index, *EuroQuol-5D* questionnaire (*EQ*) and the *Gastrointestinal Quality of Life Index* (*GIQLI*).[3-6] The SF-36 measures functional status and well-being and it includes eight items divided into three categories: physical health status, mental status, and a combination of both which includes vitality and general health.[4,9,11] GIQLI is a self-administered questionnaire designed to assess QoL in patients with gastrointestinal diseases.[5] EQ is a self-administered questionnaire with a descriptive profile along with a QoL index. It covers five areas: mobility, self-care, daily activities, pain and anxiety-depression.[5,7,9] PGWB is a validated and reliable questionnaire which allows evaluating the patient's distress and mental state.[10] In recent years CD-specific questionnaires have been introduced both for pediatric and adults populations but, unfortunately, evidence for their efficacy is still limited.[3,5,6]

2.1. Quality of Life in Celiac Disease Patients: Importance of Clinical Presentation and Effect of the Gluten-Free Diet

Since the beginning, the investigations focused on the analysis of CD patients' QoL, it was believed that QoL was significantly reduced before diagnosis. Later studies with an adequate clinical characterization, revealed and confirmed the impression that, before diagnosis, patients with active disease and classical gastrointestinal symptoms show a marked decrease in QoL when compared with the general population.[4,7,9] In this context, prospective studies have shown that symptomatic celiac patients submitted QoL diagnostic scores similar to those of patients with chronic disabling disorders such as those cerebrovascular accidents.[7]

A limited number of studies have shown that individuals diagnosed with CD as a consequence of screening in populations at high risk for the disease have a better QoL than patients diagnosed on the basis of symptoms[8,12-15] (Figure 1). It is noteworthy that the vast majority of those surveyed who turned out to have CD, corresponded to the subclinical group. The longitudinal study made by Nachman et al[12], with a four-year follow-up after diagnosis, showed that surveyed patients had QoL scores similar to those of the general population without significant changes from the baseline. A recent study by Rosén et al.[17] evaluated QoL in adolescents diagnosed by screening in a high-risk population. In this study, it was observed that, despite the fact that this population was characterized as subclinical, not all patients saw themselves as healthy and that the CD diagnosis, along with its treatment, represented a benefit to their health. However, a subgroup saw the illness as a stigma that limited their daily lives which, especially in the social field, was more pronounced in the female gender.

In general, these studies suggest that the onset of the GFD implies an improvement in the QoL which, for some authors, produces similar long-term scores to those of the general population.[8] However, other authors suggest that QoL improvement due to the GFD does not come close to the general population's perception.[6,11] A quick assessment of these disparities regarding response to the GFD suggests it could be due to cultural differences between the populations involved; however, the most notable differences seem to lie in the type of research design. Thus, most of the research studies use a crossover design which evaluates different populations both at the time of diagnosis and after treatment; this methodological aspect diminishes the conclusions' value. The few studies which had a prospective and longitudinal design suggest that GFD has a significant impact on the QoL of patients. Moreover, some studies reported a positive GFD impact regarding the QoL, both in its classical and subclinical forms. Thus Ciacci et al.[27] found that 84% of the patients improved their QoL perception after initiating the GFD. Casellas et al.,[5] who evaluated the QoL using the GIQLI and EQ questionnaires before treatment and after the GFD, found that diminished values in both pre-treatment questionnaires improved significantly after GFD and that they were similar to those of the general population. Finally,

Nachman et al.[8] confirmed these observations and showed that the positive impact of the GFD was more significant in the first three months after starting specific treatment (Figure 1). The QoL scores after one year of GFD were comparable to those of the general population, regardless of clinical severity of the diagnosis or the degree GFD compliance (Figure 1). Interestingly, the continuation of this longitudinal study showed a deterioration in the SF-36 items after 4 years of treatment (Figure 2). The most remarkable point regarding this observation is that patients who adhered strictly to the GFD had a similar QoL to that of controls. Conversely, partially compliant patients had a significant deterioration of the QoL (Figure 3).[12] An interesting finding of this study was that patients with less severe symptoms at the time of diagnosis had a decrease in QoL indexes after four years of GFD regardless of the degree of compliance to the latter. The authors postulate that this effect might be due to the burden such a restrictive diet would imply in relation to low disease perception.[12]

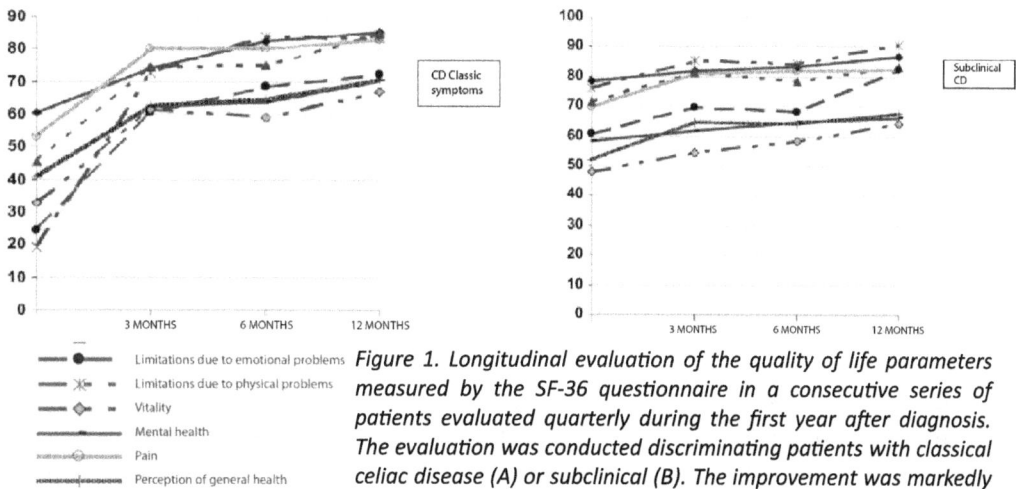

Figure 1. Longitudinal evaluation of the quality of life parameters measured by the SF-36 questionnaire in a consecutive series of patients evaluated quarterly during the first year after diagnosis. The evaluation was conducted discriminating patients with classical celiac disease (A) or subclinical (B). The improvement was markedly significant after 3 months of treatment.[6]

Most observations suggest that female CD patients often have greater QoL impairment than men, both at the time of diagnosis and after treatment, even with strict GFD compliance. These findings are mainly observed in the different mental domains of the questionnaires.[3,5,6,9,11] It has been proposed that this phenomenon may be due to the higher prevalence of anxiety in women.[6] The presence of clinical symptoms and a decrease in the QoL could be related to the existence of a second undetected disorder, often irritable bowel syndrome, pancreatic insufficiency, bacterial overgrowth or microscopic colitis.[6,14]

SF-36

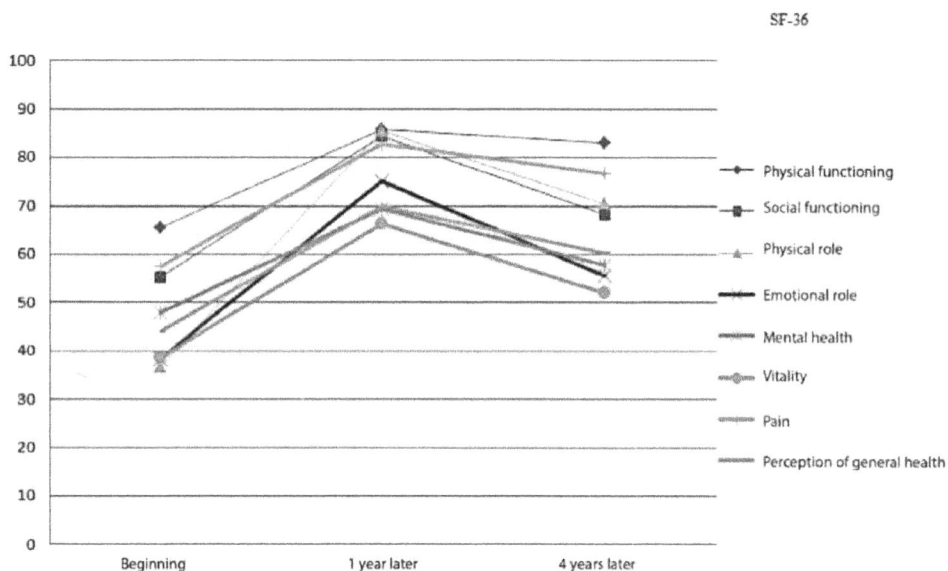

Figure 2. Quality of life reported by SF-36 questionnaires in a general population of celiac disease patients evaluated at the time of diagnosis, at one and at four years after starting treatment. The score increase after one year means an improvement in the evaluated parameters. A deterioration is observed in most parameters after four years. [12]

Summing up this section, patients with CD have a lower QoL than the general population. Evidence suggests that this involvement is important in symptomatic patients, especially those with classic symptoms. By contrast, the few studies on (usually subclinical) patients diagnosed by screening concur on the fact that these patients have no QoL decline. The GFD produces rapid improvement of all QoL aspects in symptomatic CD patients. The response of subclinical patients to treatment would seem to be of little significance.

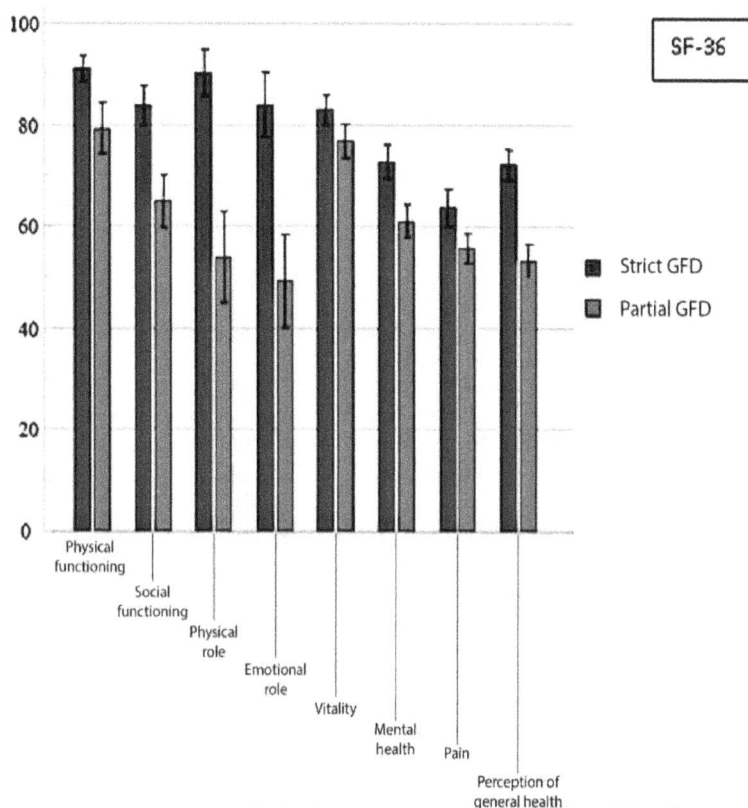

Figure 3. Quality of life after four years of follow-up according to the degree of compliance with the gluten-free diet: Strict (blue bars) or partial (red bars). Patients with strict adherence scores have significantly better QoL than those with partial compliance.[12]

3. Celiac Disease and Psychological Disorders

Addressing the issue of psychological distress in CD is, at first glance, very interesting but often difficult to understand. A multiplicity of studies have focused on its evaluation, especially during the last decade, with dissimilar and even contradictory results. Since the first descriptions of the disease, references were made to psychological symptoms and disorders, albeit in a vague fashion which was not consistent with a specific condition. Thus, for example, these descriptions spoke of a "weariness" which was considered to be psychic in origin, since it which persisted even when the patient had improved clinically.[18] Behavior characterized by "tantrums, irritability and a negative attitude" was described, in 1950, in a group of children who changed dramatically immediately after starting the GFD, while, in adults, a "syndrome of insomnia, depression and headache" was described.[19]

Throughout the disease's short history, celiac patients have been characterized as mentally peculiar, nervous, unstable, depressed and even as schizophrenic.[20,21] By 1970, D. Goldberg[22] performed the first standardized assessment of a series of a group of patients on a GFD and found a high prevalence of depressive traits that showed no relation either with gastrointestinal symptoms or nutritional status. After one-year follow-up, the same author found no schizophrenic patients among those evaluated (a disease that had been previously reported by Dohan[21]) and noted that those individuals who remained sick often had a family history of psychiatric illness. He concluded that signs of depression, common in celiac patients, were possibly related to genetic factors. Subsequently, other authors also found a higher prevalence of psychiatric history prior to CD diagnosis, depression being the most frequently associated psychic disorder.[23] Furthermore, anxiety disorders (diagnostic reactive anxiety state, social phobia and panic disorder) have also been associated with CD but, in this case, without conclusive evidence.

4. Anxiety

While high levels of nonspecific anxiety have been reported in celiac patients, this does not appear to be a stable personality trait, but a state reactive to diagnosis or secondary to symptoms. A study by Addolorato et al.[24] seems to suggest this. These authors assessed anxiety and depression using the *Hamilton State-Trait Anxiety* scale and the *Zung Self-Rating Depression Scale*, respectively. They found that anxiety reversed in the following year. A significantly higher number of patients with panic disorder and depression has also been reported but generally associated with a third very common CD medical condition, autoimmune thyroiditis. Therefore, the authors propose a possible causal association.[25]

Social phobia, another anxiety disorder, has been associated with CD, as well as specific or generalized forms, present both in newly diagnosed patients and in those who were already complying with the GFD.[26] As expected, a significantly higher percentage of associated depression was also observed. This could be considered to be consistent with the findings of C. Ciacci et al.,[27] who described more problems in social life and anxiety related to feeling different from the general population in patients diagnosed after the age of 20, even in cases with good diet compliance. Interestingly, this cross-sectional study of unrelated populations detected no differences between newly diagnosed patients compared with those who were complying with the GFD.[27] Unlike previous evidence, a study performed in Germany suggested an increased risk of a probable anxiety disorder (but not depression) restricted to celiac women complying with GFD when compared to the general population.[28] It is striking, in this study, that the risk was lower among patients who lived alone. Again, we face the question of the weight of social factors and it could be thought that, for some women with celiac disease who adhere to the GFD, the social environment may be experienced more as a burden than as helpful. A 10-year follow-up study by Hallert et al.,[29] which evaluated the burden of the disease in terms of concerns, restrictions and personal balance, showed that women expressed more concern about its impact on relationships with friends and about having to abstain from the "important things" in life. Finally, a recent meta-analysis based on a review of 11 selected studies which evaluated the strength of the association between anxiety and CD, concluded that adults with celiac disease do not differ, in terms of anxiety levels, from the general population or from people with other chronic diseases.[30]

To sum up, anxiety seems to be present in CD patients, not as a characteristic of the disease itself, but possibly as reaction to the diagnosis or the difficulties associated with complying with the diet and its social impact. In this sense, we believe that the diagnosis of an adjustment disorder with an anxiety state, should be considered at least in a group of patients.

5. Depression

Depression is the psychic disorder to which earliest reference is made and the most studied in relation to CD. Here the term is used in its broadest sense without discriminating its different clinical forms, as published studies have used a variety of assessment tools, which do not allow an accurate transposition of their results. In 1982, Hallert and Derefeldt[23] reported similar findings in an area of Sweden with a high prevalence of CD, they reported that 21% of the patients had received psychiatric care prior to diagnosis, depression being the most common finding. In a subsequent study, Hallert and Aström[31] found significantly higher levels in scale 2 of the *Depression Minnesota Multiphasic Personality Inventory-2* compared with a control group of surgical patients. Interestingly, this result did not correlate significantly with abdominal symptoms and these authors described a characteristic depressive mood in patients, different from other medical conditions, such as colitis. This led them to consider depressive psychopathology as a feature of adults with CD, suggesting that this is possibly a consequence of malabsorption, a hypothesis which will be discussed later. In a study by Vaitl and Stouthamer-Geisel, who evaluated a cohort of 182 CD patients using a self-administered questionnaire (*Symptom Check List Revised (SCL 90-R)*), observed that a significant proportion of the patients had a history of psychological symptoms for which they had received drug treatment (32%) and/or psychotherapy (14%). These authors concluded that celiac patients had a "psycho-vegetative" state of exhaustion with a distinct depressive component.[32]

Research studies carried out in Italy in 1998 transversely evaluated depression in adult CD patients compared with healthy individuals and patients with persistent chronic hepatitis.[33] Using a modified version of the *Zung Self-Rating Depression Scale,* they concluded that depressive symptoms are characteristic of celiac patients, independently of the time of diagnosis and GFD compliance. Despite these limitations in establishing these new conclusions, these authors identified three main characteristics associated with CD: reactivity, pessimism, asthenia and anhedonia. Also Addolorato et al.[24] found that a large number of patients had depression, and that this was maintained without significant changes after one year with a GFD. The authors proposed that this depression may be related to a reduction in QoL. Recently, two longitudinal and prospective studies by Nachman et al.[8,12] which evaluated QoL and depression at the time of diagnosis and after four years' follow-up, showed high percentages of initial depression, especially in patients with classic symptomatic clinical course (gastrointestinal symptoms). This condition improved dramatically after a year with the GFD, and deteriorated slightly during the four-year evaluation, without reverting to the initial pathological levels (Figure 4). The authors found an inverse relationship between depressive symptoms and adherence to the diet (Figure 5). Similarly, Finnish authors detected an initial improvement in QoL in a group with a GFD after a year of treatment; however, QoL evaluated eight years after diagnosis worsened in relation to the control group. Despite differences in research regarding the populations involved materials, the methodology applied to the investigations and results that preclude comparison between studies, we can say that there is enough consensus in that depression occurs with greater frequency and severity among celiac patients than in the general population. Additionally, a very large population study in Sweden found a statistically significant association between CD and depression, which seems to leave no room for doubt[34]. Finally, a recent meta-analysis published by Smith and Gerdes[30] came to a similar conclusion reviewing 18 different published studies. These authors concluded that more than 8,000 new negative reports would be required for the association if these results were to be denied. However, there is no agreement in the literature regarding the effects that the GFD has on these symptoms, having reported improvements in some studies[8,12,36,37] but not in others.[24,33]

Summing up, depression is demonstrably associated with CD and its evaluation should be part of the diagnosis. It is important to consider that depression can adversely affect the course of the disease by decreasing the motivation and energy to comply with the diet, having a negative impact on interpersonal relationships including the doctor-patient relationship and inducing a negative evaluation of treatment outcomes by the patient.[51] Depressed people are three times more likely not to comply with treatment than those who are not.[52] Regarding the effects the GFD has on depression, it is still premature to draw conclusions given the differences shown by this research. Surely the assessment of advantages and disadvantages of treatment is one of the future lines of enquiry. Finally, an interesting field arises today regarding absorption-related factors and immune processes, especially inflammatory processes related to the gut-brain connection.[32]

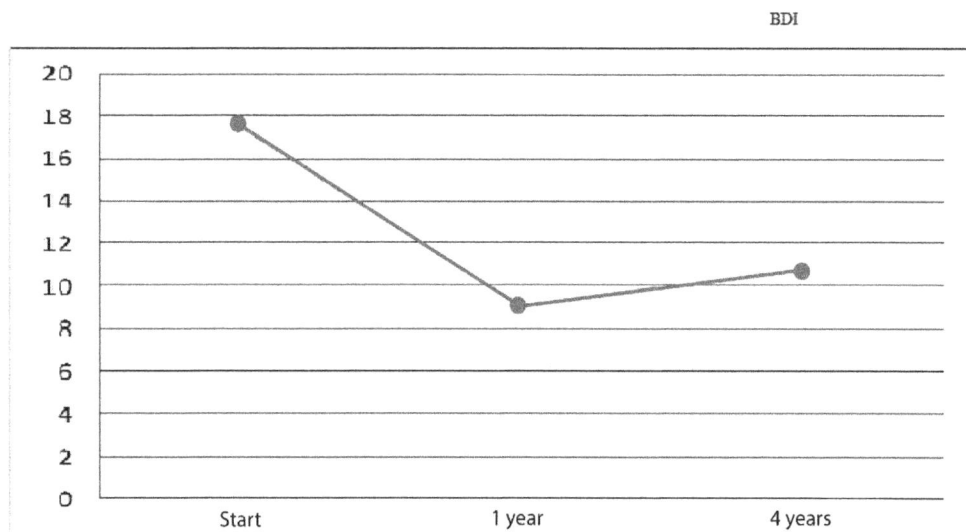

Figure 4. Depression level progression at the time of diagnosis and during long-term monitoring (one to four years) as measured by the Beck Depression Index (BDI) in a series of CD patients.[12]

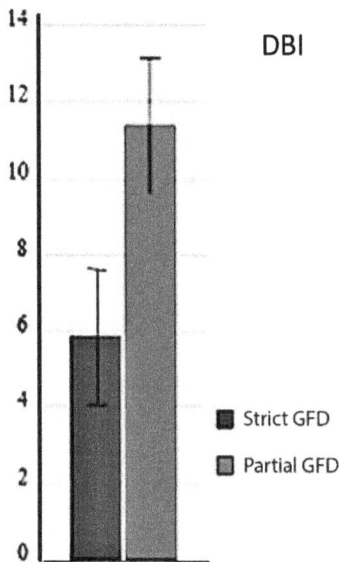

Figure 5. Depression levels four years after diagnosis as measured by the Beck Depression Inventory (DBI) index in a series of celiac disease patients categorized according to the degree of compliance with the gluten-free diet (blue bar: Strict compliance, red bar: Partial compliance).[12]

5.1. Research on the Pathophysiology of Depression

From the pathophysiological point of view, depression is a complex and multifactorial condition generated by several kinds of factors, including, among others: Biological, such as nutritional (linked to malabsorption and its consequences), genetic, immunological and endocrinological.[25,43] In addition, one must consider the psychological and environmental factors since CD is a chronic disease[51] where suffering can be generated by the symptoms and the inconvenience of having to follow a lifelong restrictive diet. Nutrient malabsorption could be the mediating mechanism between CD and depression by interfering with the production of key neurotransmitters for mood regulation, in particular, deficiencies relative to tryptophan malabsorption, necessary for the production of serotonin, a key neurotransmitter for mood regulation.[35] Hallert et al.[36] determined metabolite concentrations of the three major monoamines in cerebrospinal fluid in a short series of patients and found a significant reduction in the levels of 5-hydroxy-indole acetic, homovanillic acid and 3-methoxy-4-hydroxy feniletilenglicol (MOPEG), all of them indicative of a reduction in the central metabolism of the three monoamines (serotonin, dopamine and norepinephrine). Their concentrations, particularly those of MOPEG, inversely correlated with depressive symptoms. In a subsequent study, the same authors explored monoamine concentrations in patients treated with a GFD.[37] This study suggested that the low level of the same could be related to poor intestinal absorption. Monoamine synthesis is regulated, among other dietary components, by vitamin B6, which is generally malabsorbed by celiac patients. The same Scandinavian group followed up celiac patients diagnosed with depression who had not improved after one year despite the GFD having normalized their mucosal intestinal damage.[38] When they were reassessed three years later and after receiving vitamin B6 orally (80 mg/day of pyridoxine), they observed a significant decrease in depressive symptoms. In a multicenter, double-blind study on patients who followed a strict GFD and took daily vitamin B supplementation, normalization of plasma homocysteine levels (marker of B vitamin status) was demonstrated, which correlated with the improvement of the general welfare and significant decrease in anxiety and depression.[39] Other malabsorption effects can cause symptoms that are confused with and/or overlap with depression. Folic acid deficiency can cause fatigue, apathy, and impaired memory. Iron deficiency, with or without anemia, can cause tiredness and easy fatigue. In this regard, an Italian study more recently assessed the prevalence, characteristics and associations of chronic fatigue and depression.[40] The results showed that fatigue is a feature of CD which improves little with the GFD. These authors suggested that fatigue may have a cognitive and affective origin and that it would tend to decrease in treated patients, while depression would remain or even worsened.

CD is associated with other autoimmune endocrine diseases such as type I diabetes mellitus and Hashimoto's thyroiditis, both with increased risk of depression.[41,42] Carta et al.[25] found a high prevalence of panic and depression disorders in those celiac patients with positive antithyroid antibodies. They suggested that the association with subclinical thyroiditis could represent a significant risk factor for these psychiatric disorders. Garud et al.[43] studied the prevalence of psychiatric and autoimmune disorders in CD, finding that the risk of depression was the same as that of the general population, but that it became higher when associated with DM1, doubling the percentage of patients with clinical depression.

6. Celiac Disease and the Emotional Realm

The psycho-emotional component of CD cannot be dismissed given that psychological distress and social and emotional adaptation to the disease and its treatment surely play an important role. Depression can develop as a result of the discomfort produced by symptoms of the disease, even in the very frequent cases in which the patient doesn't receive an initial diagnosis and wanders from one doctor to another for years, without finding an answer to his or her condition. Again we find some contradictory results, since at least in two studies depression did not correlate with the presence of somatic symptoms.[11,28] However, Nachman et al.[8] while evaluating a cohort of patients at the time of diagnosis using the Beck Depression Inventory (BDI), found a high prevalence of moderate and/or severe depression in patients with symptomatic classical clinical presentation, but with values equal to the general population in subclinical cases. In a recent epidemiological study conducted in Canada, the annual prevalence of major depressive disorders in people with one or more diseases was 9.2% compared with 4.0% in those who reported no other condition.[44] In this study, major depression in people with bowel disorders, Crohn's disease and colitis was of 16.4%, findings similar to those of other investigations.[45,46] All chronic diseases have a strong impact on the QoL. One of the major changes, perhaps generating further deterioration, is the emotional aspect, since the person is necessarily forced to undergo a rapid adaptation process, which passes through different stages, which evoke a range of usually negative emotions (fear, anger, anxiety). In the case of CD, it may appear that the balance of the necessary dietary changes with a view to their intended is highly positive. In this sense, it should not be very difficult to accept the disease and certainly benefits, this happens often. However, adaptation to GFD is more difficult than it seems upon first impression. Patients must make permanent changes to important aspects of their life and regarding self-control, for which they need knowledge, skills and discipline. Considering these difficulties, it is not surprising that a significant number of patients develop psychosocial problems. Linking all these factors, an Italian study evaluated the impact of a chronic disease in relation to CD's psychiatric symptoms, the degree of acceptance of the disease and the impact that the diet has on QoL.[4] The results showed significantly high anxiety levels and depression in the celiac group and in the diabetic group compared with healthy controls. Furthermore, the duration of the gluten restriction correlated with significantly depression higher levels in newly diagnosed patients. The authors concluded that frequent affective disorders in celiac patients are linked to the fact that it is a chronic disease and to difficulties in adjusting to the diet, and should not be considered disease traits in themselves.

Diet restrictions have a bigger influence on the style of life of celiac patients than what it was previously thought since they strongly interfere in daily activities and social life. A survey of celiac patients (74% women) showed several areas where maintaining a GFD has a negative impact in situations such as eating out with the family, travelling and at work.[48] An interesting Swedish study dealt with situations which often lead to confusion and discomfort in relation to the disease causing conflicts (dilemmas) to celiac people with a GFD.[49] The results indicated that they affect different areas: the emotional area, interpersonal relationships and celiac patient's daily activities in different settings: at work, shopping, travelling, and eating out and at home. The predominant feelings were: isolation, shame, fear of gluten contamination and concern over being troublesome. In interpersonal relationships, situations like being forgotten or neglected, not wanting to draw attention because of the disease and to avoid talking about the subject or lowering their guard so as to avoid being exposed. Finally, daily life complications are related to the lesser availability of gluten-free products, increased effort and to being constantly vigilant and alert. However, despite the above, many patients with chronic diseases do not show high levels of distress, which raises the question of which may be the protective factors. Many studies have shown the importance of considering the individual characteristics and coping skills of patients as central factors. The way in which a patient responds to problems can be become a favorable or negative point for our physical and mental wellbeing. In this regard, the presence of a specific celiac psychological profile has been suggested.[50] Its main characteristics would be high irritability accompanied by high psychophysiological reactivity and a kind of conformity that reflects both the difficulty in expressing feelings as much as the desire to have a good image in front of others. The authors proposed that this increased psychophysiological reactivity could be related to the worry and the weight of shouldering a chronic disease, as well as with hyper vigilance in relation to food. The trend towards a conforming behavior may be related to avoidance of situations with greater exposure consistent with a lifestyle limited by the presence of a chronic disease.

7. Conclusions and Recommendations

In recent years, the QoL concept in relation to CD has become relevant. Classic CD patients prior to diagnosis showed a low QoL, which experience a significant improvement by the GFD. In contrast, the situation in patients with subclinical CD is not as clear. Depression is more prevalent and more severe in celiac patients than in the general population. We do not know if there is a major etiopathogenic factor that accounts for it; however, it is more appropriate to think in the synergy of several factors that possibly interact in varying proportions. On the other hand, there is no such certainty regarding anxiety disorders. In any case, it is necessary to take into account the need to assess the presence of both disorders at the time of diagnosis, especially depression. This recommendation is related to the proven association that this mental disorder has on the development, adherence and response to treatments, as has been observed in various chronic diseases. Its evaluation during primary care consultations can be done by means of simple questions and from there it can be decided whether the case is suitable for psychiatric or psychological referral.

References

1. Green PH, Cellier C. *Celiac disease.* N Engl J Med. 2007; 357: 1731-43.
    http://dx.doi.org/10.1056/NEJMra071600

2. Ludvigsson JF, Leffler DA, Bai JC, Biagi F, Fasano A, Green PH et al. *The Oslo definitions for coeliac disease and related terms.* Gut. 2013; 62: 43-52.
    http://dx.doi.org/10.1136/gutjnl-2011-301346

3. Hallert C, Lohiniemi S. *Quality of life of celiac patients living on a gluten-free diet.* Nutrition. 1999; 15: 795-7. http://dx.doi.org/10.1016/S0899-9007(99)00162-8

4. Fera T, Cascio B, Angelini G, Martini S, Guidetti CS. *Affective disorders and quality of life in adult coeliac disease patients on a gluten-free diet.* Eur J Gastroenterol Hepatol. 2003; 15: 1287-92. http://dx.doi.org/10.1097/00042737-200312000-00006

5. Casellas F, Rodrigo L, Vivancos JL, Riestra S, Pantiga C, Baudet JS et al. *Factors that impact health-related quality of life in adults with celiac disease: a multicenter study.* World J Gastroenterol. 2008; 7(14): 46-52. http://dx.doi.org/10.3748/wjg.14.46

6. Kurppa K, Collin P, Mäki M, et al. *Celiac disease and health-related quality of life.* Expert Rev Gastroenterol Hepatol. 2011; 5: 83-90. http://dx.doi.org/10.1586/egh.10.81

7. Gray AM, Papanicolas IN. *Impact of symptoms on quality of life before and after diagnosis of coeliac disease: results from a UK population survey.* BMC Health Serv Res. 2010; 27(10): 105. http://dx.doi.org/10.1186/1472-6963-10-105

8. Nachman F, Mauriño E, Vázquez H et al. *Quality of life in celiac disease patients: prospective analysis on the importance of clinical severity at diagnosis and the impact of treatment.* Dig Liver Dis. 2009; 41: 15-25. http://dx.doi.org/10.1016/j.dld.2008.05.011

9. Norström F, Lindholm L, Sandström O, Nordyke K, Ivarsson A. *Delay to celiac disease diagnosis and its implications for health-related quality of life.* BMC Gastroenterol. 2011; 7(11): 118. http://dx.doi.org/10.1186/1471-230X-11-118

10. Roos S, Kärner A, Hallert C. *Psychological well-being of adult coeliac patients treated for 10 years.* Dig Liver Dis. 2006; 38: 177-80. http://dx.doi.org/10.1016/j.dld.2006.01.004

11. Hallert C, Grännö C, Grant C, Hultén S, Midhagen G, Ström M et al. *Quality of life of adult coeliac patients treated for 10 years.* Scand J Gastroenterol. 1998; 33: 933-8. http://dx.doi.org/10.1080/003655298750026949

12. Nachman F, del Campo MP, González A et al. *Long-term deterioration of quality of life in adult patients with celiac disease is associated with treatment noncompliance.* Dig Liver Dis. 2010; 42: 685-91. http://dx.doi.org/10.1016/j.dld.2010.03.004

13. Mustalahti K, Lohiniemi S, Collin P, Vuolteenaho N, Mäki M. *Gluten-free diet and quality of life in patients with screen detected celiac disease.* Effect Clin Pract. 2002; 5: 105-13.

14. Johnston SD, Rodgers C, Watson RG. *Quality of life in screen-detected and typical coeliac disease and the effect of excluding dietary gluten.* Eur J Gastroenterol Hepatol. 2004; 16: 1281-6. http://dx.doi.org/10.1097/00042737-200412000-00008

15. Paavola A, Kurppa K, Ukkola A, et al. *Gastrointestinal symptoms and quality of life in screen-detected celiac disease.* Dig Liver Dis. 2012; 44: 814-8.
    http://dx.doi.org/10.1016/j.dld.2012.04.019

16. Zarkadas M, Cranney A, Case S et al. *The impact of a gluten-free diet on adults with coeliac disease: results of a national survey.* J Hum Nutr Diet. 2006; 19: 41-9.
    http://dx.doi.org/10.1111/j.1365-277X.2006.00659.x

17. Rosén A, Ivarsson A, Nordyke K, Karlsson E, Carlsson A, Danielsson L et al. *Balancing health benefits and social sacrifices: a qualitative study of how screening-detected celiac disease impacts adolescents' quality of life.* BMC Pediatr. 2011; 10(11): 32. http://dx.doi.org/10.1186/1471-2431-11-32
18. Hess Thaysen HE. *Non-tropical Sprue.* Munksgaard, Copenhagen. 1932.
19. Daynes G. *Bread and tears - naughtiness, depression and fits due to wheat sensitivity.* Proc Royal Soc Med. 1956; 49: 391-94.
20. Paulley JW. *Emotion and personality in the etiology of steatorrhea.* American J Dig Dis. 1959; 4: 352-60. http://dx.doi.org/10.1007/BF02231167
21. Dohan FC. *Cereals and schizophrenia: data and hypothesis.* Acta Psychiatr Scand. 1966; 42: 125-32. http://dx.doi.org/10.1111/j.1600-0447.1966.tb01920.x
22. Goldberg D. *A psychiatric study of patients with diseases of the small intestine.* Gut. 1970; 11: 459-65. http://dx.doi.org/10.1136/gut.11.6.459
23. Hallert C, Derefeldt T. *Psychic disturbances in adult coeliac disease. I. Clinical observations.* Scand J Gastroenterol. 1982; 17: 17-9. http://dx.doi.org/10.3109/00365528209181037
24. Addolorato G, Capristo E, Chittoni C et al. *Anxiety but not depression decreases in coeliac patients after one-year gluten-free diet: a longitudinal study.* Scand J Gastroenterol. 2001; 36: 502-06. http://dx.doi.org/10.1080/00365520119754
25. Carta MG, Hardoy MC, Boi MF et al. *Association between panic disorder, major depressive disorder and celiac disease: a possible role of thyroid autoimmunity.* J Psychosom. 2002; 53: 789-93. http://dx.doi.org/10.1016/S0022-3999(02)00328-8
26. Addolorato G, Mirijello A, Dangelo C et al. *Social phobia in celiac disease.* Scand J Gastroenterol. 2008; 43: 410-5. http://dx.doi.org/10.1080/00365520701768802
27. Ciacci C, D'Agate C, De Rosa A et al. *Self-rated quality of life in celiac disease.* Dig Dis Sci. 2003; 48: 2216-20. http://dx.doi.org/10.1023/B:DDAS.0000004530.11738.a2
28. Hauser W, Janke KH, Klump B, Gregor M, Hinz A. *Anxiety and depression in adult patients with celiac disease on a gluten-free diet.* World J Gastroenterol. 2010; 16: 2780-7. http://dx.doi.org/10.3748/wjg.v16.i22.2780
29. Hallert C, Grännö C, Hultén S, Midhagen G, Ström M et al. *Living with celiac disease: controlled study of the burden of illness.* Scand J Gastroenterol. 2002; 37: 39-42. http://dx.doi.org/10.1080/003655202753387338
30. Smith DF, Gerdes LU. *Meta-analysis on anxiety and depression in adult celiac disease.* Acta Psychiatr Scand. 2012; 125: 189-93. http://dx.doi.org/10.1111/j.1600-0447.2011.01795.x
31. Hallert C, Aström J. *Psychic disturbances in adult coeliac disease. II. Psychological findings.* Scand J Gastroenterol. 1982; 17: 21-24. http://dx.doi.org/10.3109/00365528209181038
32. D. Vaitl, F. *Stouthamer-Geisel. Die Zöliakie - eine psychosomatisch fehleingeschätzte Störung.* Publiziert MMW. 1992; 134.
33. Ciacci C, Iavarone A, Mazzacca G, De Rosa A. *Depressive symptoms in adult coeliac disease.* Scand J Gastroenterol. 1998; 33: 247-50. http://dx.doi.org/10.1080/00365529850170801
34. Ludvigsson JF, Reutfors J, Osby U, Ekbom A, Montgomery SM. *Coeliac disease and risk of mood disorders–a general population-based cohort study.* J Affect Disord. 2007; 99: 117-26. http://dx.doi.org/10.1016/j.jad.2006.08.032

35. Russo S, Kema I, Fokkema M, Boon CJ, Willemse HBP, Elisabeth Ge et al. *Tryptophan as a link between psychopathology and somatic states.* Psychosomatic Medicine. 2003; 65: 665-71. http://dx.doi.org/10.1097/01.PSY.0000078188.74020.CC

36. Hallert C, Aström J, Sedvall G. *Psychic disturbances in adult coeliac disease. III. Reduced central monoamine metabolism and signs of depression.* Scand J Gastroenterol. 1982; 17: 25-8. http://dx.doi.org/10.3109/00365528209181039

37. Hallert C, Sedvall G. *Improvement in central monoamine metabolism in adult coeliac patient starting a gluten-free diet.* Psychol Med. 1983; 13: 267-71. http://dx.doi.org/10.1017/S003329170005087X

38. Hallert C, Aström J, Walan A. *Reversal of psychopathology in adult coeliac disease with the aid of pyridoxine (vitamin B6).* Scand J Gastroenterol. 1983; 18: 299-304. http://dx.doi.org/10.3109/00365528309181597

39. Hallert C, Svensson M, Tholstrup J *et al. Clinical trial: B vitamins improve health in patients with celiac disease living on a gluten-free diet.* Aliment Pharm Ther. 2009; 29: 811-6. http://dx.doi.org/10.1111/j.1365-2036.2009.03945.x

40. Siniscalchi M, Iovino P, Tortora R, Forestiero S, Somma A, Capuano L et al. *Fatigue in adult coeliac disease.* Aliment Pharmacol Ther. 2005; 22: 489-94. http://dx.doi.org/10.1111/j.1365-2036.2005.02619.x

41. Anderson RJ, Freedland KE, Clouse RE, Lustman PJ. *The prevalence of comorbid depression in adults with diabetes: a meta- analysis.* Diabetes Care. 2001; 24: 1069-78. http://dx.doi.org/10.2337/diacare.24.6.1069

42. Björntorp P. *Epidemiology of the relationship between depression and physical illness.* Physical Consequences of Depression. 2001: 67-85.

43. Garud S, Leffler D, Dennis M et al. *Interaction between psychiatric and autoimmune disorders in coeliac disease patients in the Northeastern United States.* Aliment Pharmacol Ther. 2009; 29: 898-905. http://dx.doi.org/10.1111/j.1365-2036.2009.03942.x

44. Gagnon L, Patten SB. *Major depression and its association with long-term medical conditions.* Can J Psychiatry. 2002; 47: 149-52.

45. Patten SB, Beck CA, Kassam A, Williams JV, Barbui C, Metz LM. *Long-term medical conditions and major depression: strength of association for specific conditions in the general population.* Can J Psyquiatry. 2005; 50: 195-202.

46. Bernklev T, Jahnsen J, Lygren I, Jahnsen J, Moum B et al. *Health-related quality of life in patients with inflammatory bowel disease measured with the short form-36: psychometric assessments and a comparison with general population norms.* Inflamm Bowel Dis. 2005; 11: 909-18. http://dx.doi.org/10.1097/01.mib.0000179467.01748.99

47. Addolorato G, Marsigli L, Capristo E et al. *Anxiety and depression: a common feature of health care seeking patients with irritable bowel syndrome and food allergy.* Hepatogastroenterology. 1998; 45: 1559-64.

48. Lee A, Newman JM. *Celiac diet: its impact on quality of life.* J. Am Diet Assoc. 2003; 103: 1533-35. http://dx.doi.org/10.1016/j.jada.2003.08.027

49. Sverker A, Hensing G, Hallert C. *Controlled by food-lived experiences of coeliac disease.* J Hum Nutr Dietet. 2005; 18: 171-80. http://dx.doi.org/10.1111/j.1365-277X.2005.00591.x

50. Ciacci C, Troncone A, Vacca M, De Rosa A. *Characteristics and quality of illness behaviour in celiac disease.* Psychosomatics, 2004; 45: 336-42. http://dx.doi.org/10.1176/appi.psy.45.4.336

51. Katon WJ. *Clinical and health services relationships between major depression, depressive symptoms, and general medical illness.* Biological Psychiatry. 2003: 54: 216-26. http://dx.doi.org/10.1016/S0006-3223(03)00273-7

52. DiMatteo MR, Lepper HS, Croghan TW. *Depression is a risk factor for noncompliance with medical treatment: meta-Analysis of the effects of anxiety and depression on patient adherence.* Arch Inter Med. 2000; 160: 2101-7.
http://dx.doi.org/10.1001/archinte.160.14.2101

Chapter 20

Acceptability Analysis, Cultural Aspects and Personal Impact of Diagnosis

Eduardo Cueto Rúa[1], Luciana Guzmán[1], Cecilia Zubiri[1], Gabriela Inés Nanfito[1], María Inés Urrutia[2], Leopoldo Mancinelli[3]

[1]Pediatric Gastroenterology. Division of Gastroenterology, Hospital Sor María Ludovica, La Plata, Argentina.

[2]Scientific Calculist, Gastroenterology Division, Hospital Sor María Ludovica, La Plata, Argentina.

[3]Clinical Psychology Gastroenterology Division, Hospital Sor María Ludovica, La Plata, Argentina.

cuetorua.eduardo@gmail.com, guzman_155@hotmail.com, cecizubiri03@hotmail.com, gnanfito@hotmail.com, urrutia@isis.unlp.edu.ar, leopoldomancinelli@gmail.com

Doi: http://dx.doi.org/10.3926/oms.225

How to cite this chapter

Cueto-Rúa E, Guzmán L, Zubiri C, Nanfito GI, Urrutia MI, Mancinelli L. *Acceptability Analysis, Cultural Aspects and Personal Impact of Diagnosis.* In Rodrigo L and Peña AS, editors. *Celiac Disease and Non-Celiac Gluten Sensitivity.* Barcelona, Spain: OmniaScience; 2014. p. 407-434.

E. Cueto Rúa, L. Guzmán, C. Zubiri, G.I. Nanfito, M.I. Urrutia, L. Mancinelli

Abstract

The authors have performed 1500 surveys on the subject of *acceptability of the celiac condition*, based on a questionnaire on the frequency of various claims by the celiac community. The questionnaire design resulted from previous meetings in which the authors participated as guest experts. The authors intended to characterize the subjective reactions of the attendants to said meetings. With that in mind, an investigation was made on the age, gender, educational level, number of celiac relatives, time and degree of adherence to the gluten-free diet, clinical features at the beginning of treatment, what issues patients find to be troublesome in every-day life, their wishes when confronted with this peculiar condition, their fantasies and their realistic expectations.

It was found that most of the participants were female and that educational level has a positive impact regarding a complete adherence to the diet. The number of persons with CD in the same family conspires against diet adherence and the most important social issue was not having restaurants with a gluten-free menu.

It was also discovered that the attendants' hoped-for solution was a cure and that their realistic expectation was to have safe, palatable and affordable food throughout the whole country as well as a law that took notice of their condition. When the 1306 surveys on the *Impact of Diagnosis* were analyzed, it was found that the exact words used by the physician and the patient's level of education do not play a key role in the time it takes to accept the celiac condition. In addition, it became clear that the words used by the physician have different effects when first heard by an adult with celiac disease and when first heard by a mother of children with celiac disease. These words, according to the authors' analyses, contribute to heighten emotions in patient support groups but definitely hinder the acceptance process.

1. Introduction

As pediatricians, the authors have always held that the concept of celiac disease is composed of words and gestures. For this reason, the physicians' attitude, at the time of diagnosing a patient and during the rest of the clinical management, must be carefully restrained. The purpose of this is to have a positive impact in the perception of this ailment, which will impose a lifestyle on young patients.

A sense of caring towards the patient must be taught to the patient's parents and family. If a two year-old patient is constantly addressed using words that denote compassion or pain and if it is suggested, through expressions and gestures, that these feelings are harbored for him or her, it will be hardly possible to expect this person to feel fully confident during his or her future development. Unknowingly, the authors have acted according to Pedro Lain Entralgo's (1908-2001) postulates which state that "A physician must be able to walk in his patient's shoes in order to feel what his patient feels and finally to help the patient overcome his difficulties".

The fact of thus conceiving the problem and the implications of intolerance to a foodstuff which, in Western culture, has symbolic and even (occasionally) religious associations led the authors to found, in 1978, the *Argentinian Celiac Disease Association*, the first one in America and the second one world-wide.[1]

Inspired by the teachings of Dr. Horacio Toccalino (1931-1977) and having more than 40 years of history, the authors' group has investigated celiac disease and many of its different aspects, among which it is possible to highlight the establishment of a precise and objective mathematical relation to the degree of enteropathy according to the villus-crypt ratio, which has been efficiently used for over 30 years without modifications[2]; the discovery, in 1985, of the auto anti-smooth muscle antibody values[3], of their variability in the challenge test[4] and also (according to diet compliance) using them since that date in screening asymptomatic family members.[5] The authors also underline the fact that they have employed a clinical and laboratory scoring system which has allowed to efficiently estimate the probability of suffering from celiac disease.[6,7] In addition, the Argentinian Ministry of Health has proposed that it be used[8] and that it be available online at no cost. Lastly, the social situation of the celiac disease patient has been taken into account. The authors have helped elaborate the current laws regarding the subject and have deeply studied and analyzed the patients' subjective reactions, needs and demands.[9]

Due to the abeve, the authors were invited to contribute this chapter.

Between March 2008 and December 2009, 1500 surveys of celiac disease patients were performed among those who attended the meetings of the Argentine Celiac Disease Association, trying to assess a number of social and cultural aspects. Between August 2011 and December 2012, another survey to evaluate the impact of diagnosis was performed.

It must be stated that Argentina has a high Celiac Disease (CD) prevalence, quite similar to that found in European countries. This country, especially the large cities along the Atlantic Coast and Río de la Plata and its tributary streams, has been the host of massive immigrations from Europe, especially from Spain and Italy. Additionally, Argentina is a great wheat producer, exporter and consumer, baseline conditions favorable for the development of the disease. Regarding CD prevalence, a study by Dr. JC Gómez et al., carried out in couples that underwent the prenuptial testing between 1999 and 2000, revealed a CD ratio of 1/167.[10] On the other hand, a multi-centric test performed by Dr. M. Mora and collaborators on children who were subjected to pre-surgical tests for scheduled surgery, or from emergency cases or else for physical aptitude tests, revealed a prevalence of 1/79.[11] In the Gastroenterology Service at the Interzone Hospital, specialized in Pediatrics in the city of La Plata, after reviewing the data base, the authors found that, from January 1st, 2000 to December 31st, 2010, 852 patients with a male/female ratio of 2/1 had been diagnosed.

2. Acceptability

In the first survey, named *acceptability*, the following subjects are discussed:

1) Age.

2) Gender.

3) Number of celiac disease patients at home.

4) Order of birth of the celiac patient (firstborn, middle child, last child or only child). The authors added one more parameter: whether a child is born separated by six or more years from the preceding sibling, who in turn is classified as last-only child.

5) Number of years of compliance with the gluten-free diet.

6) Clinical presentation at the time of diagnosis.

7) The patient's educational level.

8) The patient's parents' educational level, whether the former is a child or an adult.

9) Dietary transgressions.

10) Frequency of transgressions.

11) Location where said transgressions occur.

12) Whether they happen while alone or with company.

13) What kind of unsuitable food the patient desires to consume.

14) What product prompted the transgression.

15) Other incitements.

16) Whether the patient seeks help from support groups.

17) Whether the patient finds support or if he feels ill-treated in support groups or by his family.

18) What the patient dislikes about CD.

19) The patient's fantasies regarding the disease.

20) The patient's expectations regarding this clinical entity.

21) The patient's province of residence.

In order to achieve its goal, the survey was carried out at the meetings of the Argentinian Celiac Disease Association and in its different branches throughout the country as well as by means of other NGO's that support celiac disease patients and their families.

This project was undertaken in eleven Argentinian provinces and yielded the following distribution:

- Province of Buenos Aires: 57.8%
- City of Buenos Aires: 13.1%
- Santa Fe: 7.6%
- San Luis: 4.9%
- Córdoba: 4%
- Tierra del Fuego: 3.3%
- Neuquén: 2.9%
- Salta: 1.8%
- Other provinces: 4.3%.

It is noteworthy that when the authors, as health care professionals, participated in the meetings, the attendance was twice or even thrice than what would have been expected without their attendance.

To assess diet compliance after the surveys were done, the authors established a score ranging from 1 to 10. A score of 10 was given to those patients who rigorously complied with diet consuming only suitable products. A score of 7 was given to those who transgressed the diet about once a year. A score of 3 was obtained by those who committed transgressions on a monthly basis. A score of 2 was given to those who committed transgressions weekly and finally, a score of 1 was given to those who consumed gluten daily. This allowed to grade the level of diet compliance in each province. The ones analyzed were those in which more than 25 people were surveyed.

The results were as follows:

- Córdoba, with 60 participants who scored an average of 8.71%.
- Santa Fe: 114/8.62%.
- City of Buenos Aires: 196/8.6%.
- Province of Buenos Aires: 866/8.08%.
- Tierra del Fuego: 50/8.04%.
- Salta: 27/7.81%.
- Neuquén: 43/6.04%.

Age groups were used to classify the people surveyed:

- Earliest infancy (1 to 5 years old).
- Second infancy (6 to 12 years old).
- Adolescents (13 to 17 years old).
- Young adults (18 to 40 years old).
- Adults (41 to 60 years old).
- Older adults (over 61 years old).

This afforded a singular understanding of the celiac disease situation.

So far, it is clear that Celiac Disease is a permanent gluten intolerance, but it is necessary to remember that the protein itself comes from a foodstuff with an enormous cultural symbolism and that it is legally added to a vast number of industrialized products. This toxic protein, which generates celiac disease in the patient, is found in wheat, oats, barley and rye, a fact that became known through the scientific research of Dicke, Weijers and Van de Kamer[12,13] (worthy of a posthumous nobel prize).

The main issues to be addressed were: What happens during and after the moment when the physician diagnoses a patient? What impact does it have on the patient's life? How does this affect the patient-physician relation? Is the diet properly adhered to? If any, which are the reasons for giving up and transgressing the diet? The authors were also interested in determining whether the patient's educational level (and that of the patient's parents) somehow influenced diet compliance.

The concept of Celiac Disease is something that has to be constructed, and the first brick of this structure is placed by the physician at the time of the diagnosis.

The words used, the facial expression, the poise shown, the fact of having arrived to a positive and final diagnosis with implication of having solved one problem and not witnessing the beginning of another are indispensable for the patient to feel that this is the start of a better life and not the starting point of a series of adversities and sufferings.

Once the patient has been diagnosed, it is important thing to control his or her food, which must be based on a diet without wheat, oats, barley and rye. A physician takes 7 seconds to prescribe a diet that the celiac disease patient will have to follow for the next 70 years. Out of the thousands of foodstuffs humans have at their disposal, only four are prohibited (wheat, oat, barley and rye). One of them, barley, is currently being studied, with conflicting results.[14,15] As Real and collaborators demonstrated, "these results suggest that the oats have a wide variation range of their immunotoxic potential, which could be due to the differences in the immunogenicity degree in its sequences".[16]

The wide usage of gluten-bearing cereals in the West makes diet compliance challenging. This diet, which seems theoretically simple to follow, becomes, in practice, a trial for the patients who must follow it[17] and for the physicians and dieticians who must collaborate with and guide the patient.

Gluten consumption, for the celiac disease patient, voluntary or not, carries the potential risk of associated diseases, which is why the patient must be warned of this risk.[18]

After having thoroughly analyzed the survey variables, some observations come to mind. The global acceptability percentage for the Gluten Free Diet (GFD) among people who attend to support group meetings hovers around 70%, probably being for this reason slightly higher than in the reviewed bibliography[19]; however there are countries with a strong celiac disease culture in which diet compliance is stronger.[20]

The adolescent population represents a challenge. Many publications echo this view.[21,22] Adolescence constitutes a period in which the gluten-free diet is frequently abandoned. For this reason, regular medical examination is imperative, as are serum antibody determination and testing for signs and symptoms that can reveal nutritional deficiencies and other autoimmune diseases.

Regarding the situation of celiac disease patients living in the same house, it would seem that when only one family member is afflicted, GFD compliance is very effective and it would seem that the family actually plays a protective role. When several family members suffer from celiac disease, the transgression of one can trigger a domino effect in the rest of the affected family members. It is here where the greatest failure rate is seen: There seems to be a permissive attitude among family members. Even if some patients, after transgressing the diet, show symptoms like headaches, vomiting or abdominal pain, it is also true that there are many who remain asymptomatic. It should be pointed out that in those families with more than one celiac disease patient, these last were identified through family screening, which is the reason why these patients have never felt ill and the reason why their transgressions did not have any clinical manifestations.

When analyzing how the birth order is related to compliance with the GFD, it is reasonable to conclude that single children are better in adhering to the treatment. These children have a family that focuses exclusively on them. In the case of last-only children, those whose preceding sibling is at least six years older, families have a different behavior since they might have been the outcome of an unexpected pregnancy, a fact that has strong connotations for the mother. Generally, these children are pampered, probably because of the sense of responsibility felt by the parents. It is not by chance that, the last-only child, is worse in adhering to the diet, has more cavities (excessive consumption of sweets) is more often constipated (low fiber consumption and high dairy product consumption).[23-24]

This survey showed that earlier diagnoses correlate with a higher transgression percentage, as other authors have observed.[25]

This would seem to be related to the lack of clinical expression of these transgressions and, therefore, since the patient does not feel ill, he or she continues to indulge in them.[26,27]

As for the CD presentation form, it has been observed that it determines the degree of gluten-free diet compliance, but, contrary to expectations, those who exhibited the most severe initial symptoms do not adhere to the diet as thoroughly as those who have monosymptomatic diseases or those who were diagnosed through associated diseases. Furthermore, those who have lower adherence to the diet are those who are found through family screening. These patients, generally asymptomatic, do not perceive the disease and are unable see any benefit in following the diet.

In terms of the relation between educational level and the GFD, it seemed reasonable to conclude that patients with a higher educational level have greater access to information and to health services and, therefore, also possess the means to indulge in an expensive diet.[28] Another significant, noteworthy fact was that children or adults whose mothers had dropped out of university reached the highest percentage in diet compliance. Nevertheless, this peculiarity lacked a significant statistic value. It is not being suggested here that these studies be abandoned but, rather, that further care ought to be exercised in a similar situation (Graph 1A).

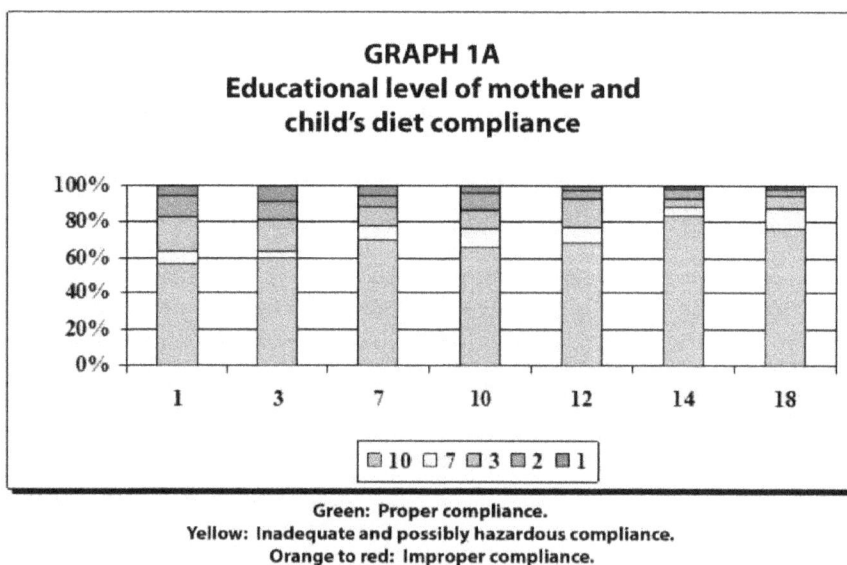

GRAPH 1A
Educational level of mother and child's diet compliance

Green: Proper compliance.
Yellow: Inadequate and possibly hazardous compliance.
Orange to red: Improper compliance.

Graph 1A. Level of diet compliance and educational levels reached by the child's mother. When the first groups are compared (illiterate or incomplete primary school) with the last two groups (incomplete university or graduate) there is a significant difference. p = 0.00001.

Even though there is still a lot of controverted data to analyze, during the last decade a significant number of published articles have shown weighty evidence on the long-term efficacy of the GFD to prevent complications and undesirable associations.[29]

However, despite the benefits of the GFD, a percentage of patients decides not to adhere to it or else they do, but not strictly.[30] Ideally, celiac disease patients should monitored regularly by a team that includes physicians, dieticians and psychologists. Nonetheless, the strongest support comes from celiac patients' associations who can empathize with the problem since they already experience it first-hand in their daily lives.

Finally, these surveys revealed that the celiac disease patient's longed-for solution is a cure for the disease through some scientific discovery; realistically, celiac disease patients desire safe and affordable foodstuffs available throughout the whole country and a law that truly takes into account the social problems generated by celiac disease.

2.1. Conclusions about Acceptability

Briefly, the conclusions of the acceptability study were as follows:

a) GFD compliance was of 70%.

b) GFD compliance is the same for each gender, whether in children or in adults.

c) The worst score was seen in adolescents (Graph 2A).

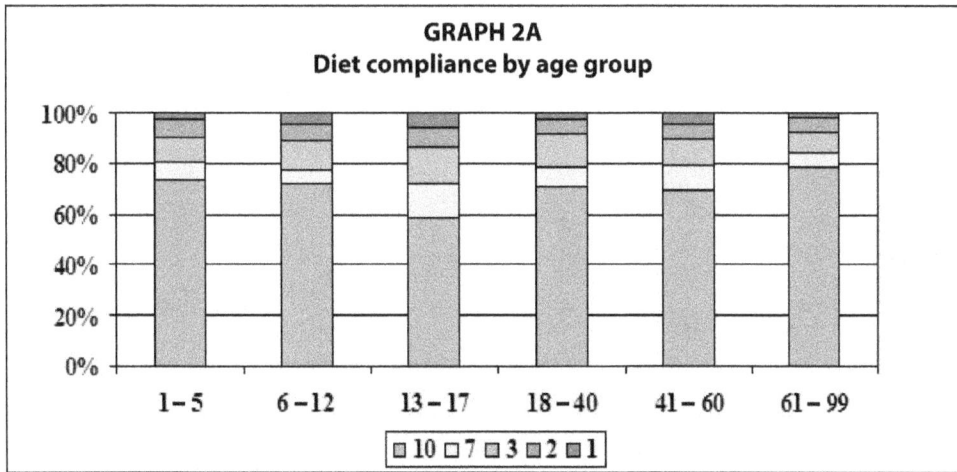

Green: Proper compliance.
Yellow: Inadequate and possibly hazardous compliance.
Orange to red: Improper compliance.
Graph 2A. Diet compliance level by age group. Highest diet compliance level is achieved by the 61 year-old or more group. Second is the group of 1-5 year-old children under the care of their mothers; the group with the worst compliance were the adolescents (13 to 17 years old).

d) GFD compliance diminished as the number of family members with CD increased (Graph 3A).

e) GFD compliance deteriorated as years elapsed from the time of diagnosis (Graph 4A).

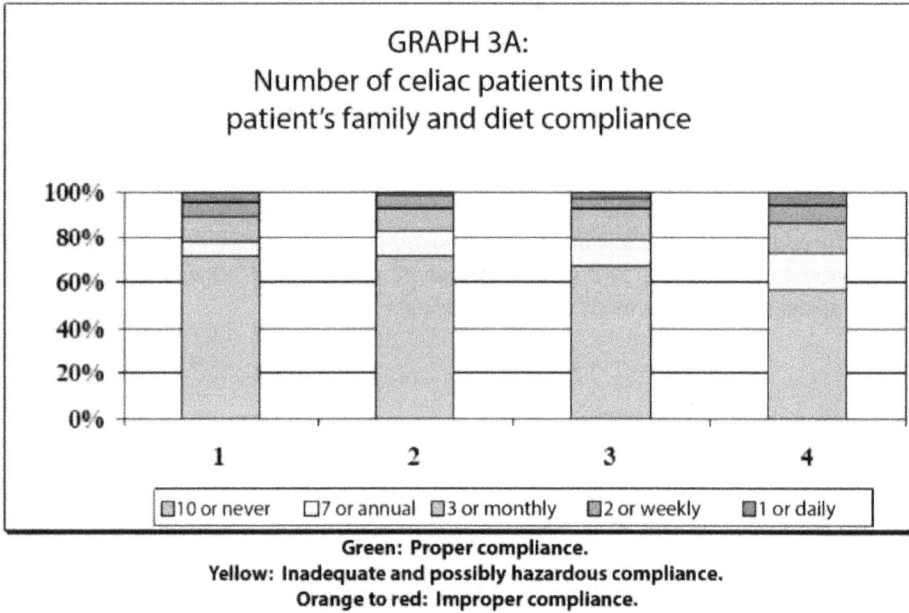

Graph 3A. GFD compliance level revealing a decline according to the number of members in the family. Statistically, this observation was significant. p= 0.04.

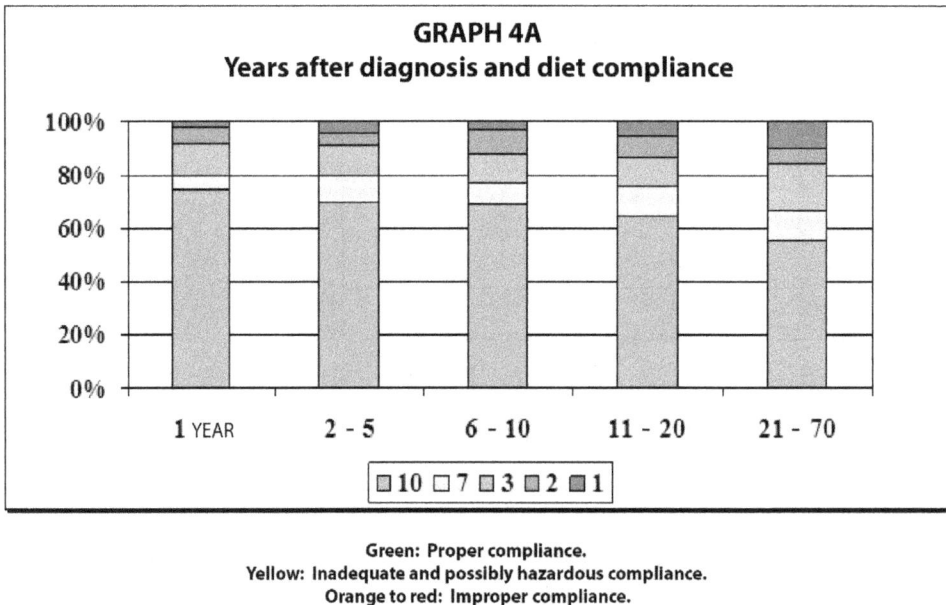

Graph 4A. Gradual lack of diet compliance as years elapse. Increasing amounts of years are grouped; analysis of this phenomenon yields a highly significant value of p=0.001.

f) In general, Gluten-Free Diet compliance level is better when educational level is higher. Nevertheless, this did not yield a significant statistical value.

g) Best GFD compliance level was seen in single children, while the worst case was seen in last-single children.

h) Highest treatment adherence was seen in the cases where the patient was diagnosed by finding monosymptomatic forms of celiac disease, the worst treatment adherence occurred in patients diagnosed through family screening.

i) Most transgressions were committed at home.

j) Products like bread, pastry and sandwiches were highly desired.

k) Easily accessible and smaller products like candies and cookies proved to be an irresistible temptation.

l) The four issues that are most troublesome for the patient are: (Graph 5A).

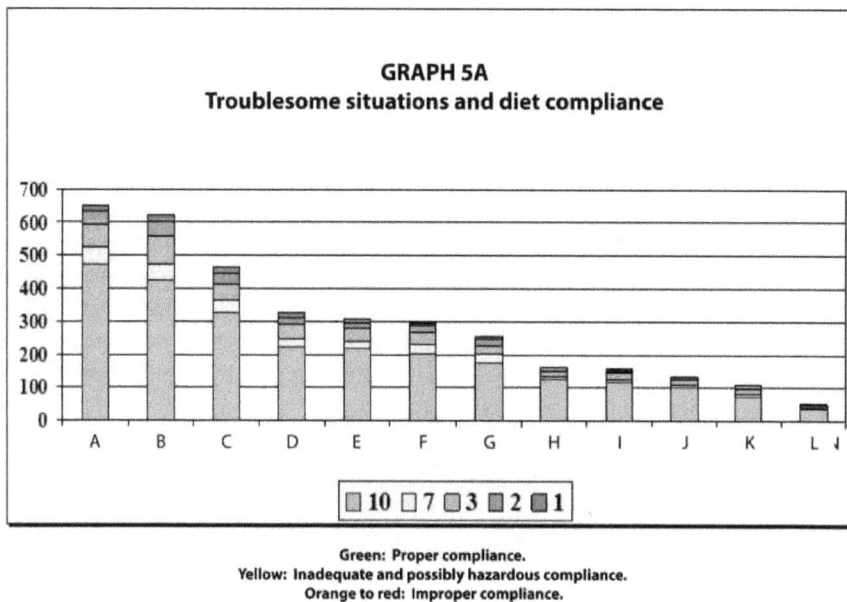

GRAPH 5A
Troublesome situations and diet compliance

Green: Proper compliance.
Yellow: Inadequate and possibly hazardous compliance.
Orange to red: Improper compliance.

Graph 5A. A decreasing scale of the most bothersome situations for a celiac disease patient:
A: Restaurants without a GFD menu; B: Being forced to carry their own food; C: Not finding gluten-free products in 24-hr stores; D: Being asked inappropriate CD-related questions; E: Not being taken into account by the private health system; F: Not receiving social benefits for their condition; G: Being made to feel different; H: Feeling a burden to the family; I : The lack of seriousness given to the subject by teachers; J : When a professional states that small amounts of gluten will not do any harm; K : When a professional states that there may be a cure; L: Patients has no complaints.

1) Restaurants without a GFD menu.

2) Having to carry their own food.

3) Not finding gluten-free products in 24hr. stores.

4) Being asked inappropriate CD-related questions.

m) The celiac disease patient's fantasy: a definitive cure.

n) A desired, plausible reality: a law that fully contemplates the Celiac Disease condition.

o) In general terms, diet compliance is satisfactory.

3. Second Survey: Sociocultural Aspects. Impact of Diagnosis; Terms Used by the Physician; the Patient's Emotions; the Patient's Educational Level and the Time Needed to Accept the Celiac Disease Condition

3.1. Introduction

Human relationships are diverse in nature; some are superficial, others are profound and some are of a singular complexity, such as the one between physician and patient. As Dr. Moreno Rodríguez stated, "the physician-patient relationship has been, is and will always be the most sensitive and human aspect of medicine".[31] As pediatricians, making lifelong diagnoses has led the authors to consider the appropriate way to do this, to measure and analyze the words used, to try empathize with the patient and to reinforce what is said with the appropriate gestures and attitude, exhibiting a considerate but firm attitude. When the patient is advised that he or she must strive to make things happen because they won't happen by themselves, the moment when the diagnosis is made must also be considered.

The precepts for medical practice are found in the Hippocratic Oath, "...I will direct the diet with a view to the patients' recovery, according to my strength and judgment...", "...I direct my patients' recovery according to my strength and judgement".[32]

The physician's characteristics in this relationship were summarized by Hippocrates more than 2000 years ago when he stated that the former must possess four main qualities: knowledge, wisdom, humanity and integrity. These qualities are well reflected in the three parameters established by Pedro Laín Entralgo: 1) To empathize with the patient, 2) To feel what the patient feels, 3) To be willing to help the patient when he or she faces difficulties.[33]

In order to achieve these parameters, the physician must thoroughly know the etiopathogeny of celiac disease, its different presentation forms, how to reach diagnosis, its treatment and its complications; but the patients' feelings can only be known by listening to them and allowing them to express themselves. This is why the authors have undertaken different surveys and, from these premises, dedicated themselves to the study of the impact of the diagnosis and to evaluate the physician's responsibility in it.

4. Analysis of diagnostic impact

In order to continue with the diagnostic impact analysis, a second stage was undertaken surveying 1306 people in support groups' meetings recognized in Argentina or at their branches.

To this end, three identical surveys were designed for: 1) Adults with celiac disease, 2) The patient's relatives and 3) Children with celiac disease who could answer it by themselves or with their parents' help.

The survey was anonymous and it included:

1. Age.

2. Gender.

3. Number of celiac disease patients in the house.

4. Years of following the diet.

5. Patient's educational level or his or her mother's:
    a. 1 to 7: grade school
    b. 8 to 12: high school
    c. 14: incomplete university
    d. 18: university graduate

6. Reaction to diagnosis, with the following possibilities:
    6.1. Happiness.
    6.2. Tranquility.
    6.3. Resignation.
    6.4. Upset.
    6.5. Sadness.
    6.6. Annoyance.
    6.7. Anguish.
    6.8. Anger.
    6.9. Fear.

7. How long did it take for the patient to accept the celiac disease condition?

8. Diet transgressions:
    a. No transgressions.
    b. Once a year.
    c. Monthly.
    d. Weekly.
    e. Daily.

9. How does the patient feel in the support group
    9.1. Very good.
    9.2. Good.
    9.3. Neutral.
    9.4. Used.
    9.5. Hurt.
    9.6. Out of place.

10. Where does the patient want to find or buy gluten-free products?
    10.1. Neighborhood stores.
    10.2. Supermarkets.
    10.3. Health-food stores.
    10.4. Pharmacies or drug stores.

11. City where the patient lives.

12. Province where the patient lives.

13. Words used by the physician when diagnosing (does the patient remember any of the following?):
    a. A severe disease/misfortune.
    b. A true disease.
    c. Celiac Disease.
    d. Food intolerance.
    e. A diet solves the problem.

The surveyed patients' ages ranged from 1 to 84 years old. In the cases of those patients who were unable to answer, their parents provided the data. Percentages by province surveyed:

a. Buenos Aires: 44.1%   g. Santa Cruz: 3.1%
b. Córdoba: 12.3%   h. Río Negro: 1.6%
c. City of Buenos Aires: 11.2%   i. Jujuy: 1.5%
d. Chubut: 10.9%   j. San Luis: 1.3%
e. Entre Ríos: 7.0%   k. La Pampa: 1.2%
f. Corrientes: 3.1%   l. All other provinces: 2.6%

People from 164 different cities participated in this survey.

1) Age, gender and number of celiac disease patients in the family were analyzed, making distinctions between adults, patients' relatives and children with celiac disease (Table 1).

2) Patients were grouped according to the number of years of adherence to the diet and their distribution was analyzed percentually, which yielded six groups, among which those who participated the most were those patients who have been following the diet for 2 to 5 years (Table 2).

	Celiac adults 58.6%	Celiac relatives 36.4%	Celiac children 5%
Number 1306 Gender	765 F 79.2% M 18.8%	476 F 67.4% M 32.6%	65 F 68.8% M 31.2%
Mean age DS	42.5 years +/- 14.04		11.3 years +/- 3.00
Educational level Mean DS Median Mode	13.4 +/- 3.64 14 12		7.2 +/- 3.13 8 8

F: female, M: male

Table 1. General data on the surveyed population. The celiac patients' relatives category is variegated since its members included both genders and all age groups, thus a mean cannot be found for neither their ages nor their educational levels.

1306 cases	Celiac adults 48.6 %	Celiac relatives 36.4%	Celiac children 5%
0 years	13.7 %	11.9 %	12.5 %
1 year	17.4 %	19.9 %	20.3 %
2 a 5 years	37.9 %	39.0 %	40.6 %
6 a 10 years	17.9 %	20.3 %	20.3 %
11 a 20 years	8.3 %	8.1 %	6.3 %
21 years or more	4.7 %	0.8 %	0.0 %

Table 2. Distribution according to years of following the diet. The group with the highest meeting attendance is the group which has 2 to 5 years of adhering to the diet. If we add the following group, 6 to 10 years adhering to the diet, between them both account for more than 50% of the attendance.

3) As for reaction to diagnosis, there is a dependence between this variable between being an adult or a relative of a celiac child, with a significant difference (p= 0.001). It can be seen that emotions like anguish and tranquility have higher percentages. When exclusively analyzing these last two survey percentages, it becomes noteworthy that, when relatives of celiac patients answer (mostly mothers), the answer is anguish. In contrast, in adults and children, the larger percentage expresses tranquility (Table 3, Graph 6).

Reaction to diagnosis 1306 cases	Celiac adults 58.6%	Celiac relatives 36.4%	Celiac children 5%
1-Joy	7.9%	3.7%	9.8%
2-Tranquility	24.6%	24.6%	29.5%
3-Resignation	14.3%	8.9%	6.6%
6-Annoyed/upset	8.0%	9.3%	8.2%
7-Anguish/sadness	26.2%	34.6%	21.3%
8-Anger/fury	8.6%	5.4%	14.8%
9-Fear	10.4%	13.6%	9.8%

Table 3. Reactions to diagnosis. The prevailing emotions are anguish and tranquility in all three groups. In the children's group, tranquility prevails; in the other two, anguish prevails.

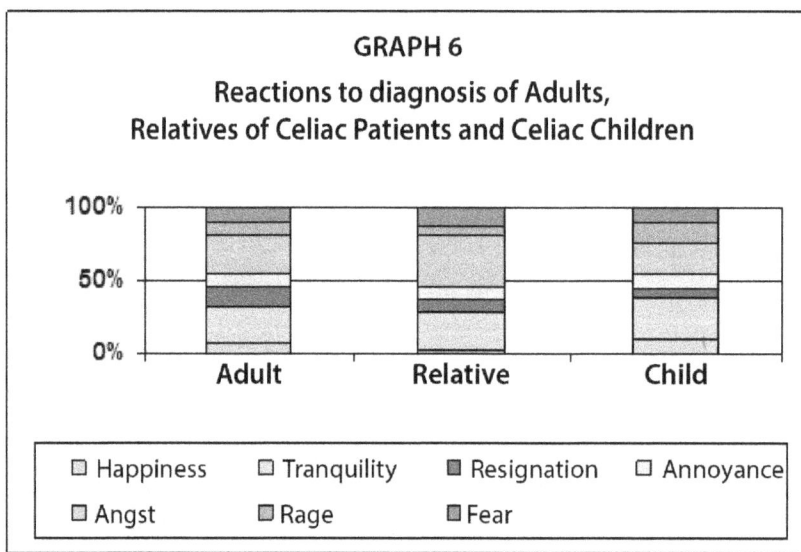

Cool tones: Positive response.
Warm tones: Negative response.

Graph 6. Diagnosis impact. Although they have similar reactions, the patients' relatives group is slightly ahead of the rest in terms of annoyance, anguish, anger and fear.

4) Regarding the time required to accept celiac disease, it can be seen that children are the fastest to accept their new condition. When analysis was made considering acceptance during the first six months, the percentage difference seen in adults was statistically significant (p=0.023).

Time it takes to accept CD 1306 cases	Celiac adults %	Celiac relatives %	Celiac children %
1 week	42.6	43.4	53.8
1 month	18.5	24.7	16.9
6 months	10.5	7.4	15.4
1 year	9.6	11.3	4.6
Several years	7.2	5.4	4.6
Never	11.6	7.8	4.6

Table 4. Time elapsed before celiac disease acceptance. Acceptance is of over 60% among all three groups in a span of a month or less.

However, in the first month, the children's acceptance reached 70.7% while adults' stayed at 61.1% (Table 4).

5) If we analyze the words expressed (or those the patient thinks he or she remembers at the time of diagnosis), "misfortune" is the one found to be most significant for relatives (mother). On the other hand, regarding the term "Celiac Disease", mothers remember (or believe they remember) that the diagnosis was communicated or perceived as "disease", while adults and children related it mostly to the word "celiac".

Furthermore, comparing the mothers' perception percentages to those of adults, the difference is highly significant (p= 0.000) (Table 5, Graph 7).

Terms used or recalled	Adults with CD %	Celiac relatives %	Celiac children %
"Misfortune"	6.9	13.9	4.2
"Disease"	11.5	34.3	25.0
"Celiac"	55.4	24.1	41.7
"Intolerance"	13.7	8.8	4.2
"Diet"	12.4	19.0	25.0

Table 5. Words used or remembered by the patient or patient's relative when receiving the diagnosis.

Another noteworthy point was that the words used by the physician, or their interpretation by the patient, did not significantly influence the time it takes to accept the disease. It can be also said that the only advantage of term "misfortune" is that it has the highest compliance percentage but also the disadvantage of having the highest percentage of lack of acceptance of the disease.

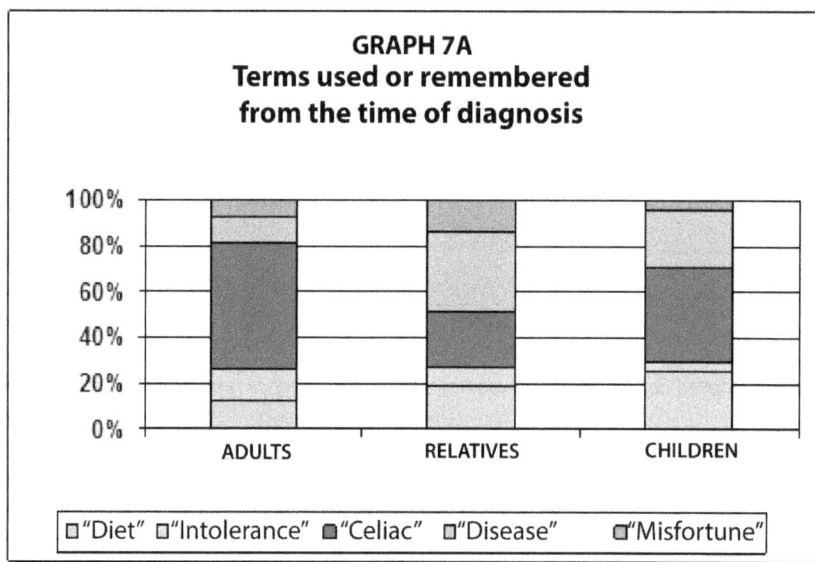

Cool tones: Positive response.
Warm tones: Negative response.

Graph 7. Impact. This graph shows that, among the words used by the physician, or as recalled by the mother or relatives, the word "disease" is the most important. Conversely, adults and children remember the word "celiac". "Misfortune" has a greater impact on the patient's relatives.

6) Comparison between groups with elementary and higher education, regarding acceptance in a span of one week or not at all, was not significant. Acceptance time, in this survey, seems to be more related to personal history or patient's background than to educational level. The same thing happens when comparing the words remembered to have been used by the physician at the time of diagnosis, where educational level plays no role.

7) Generally speaking, the words used by physicians at the time of diagnosis and the level of diet compliance demonstrate that persons who thought to have a severe disease or remembered the diagnosis as a "misfortune", actually adhered better to the diet than those with whom the term "intolerance" was used, with a highly significant high difference (p= 0.008) (Table 6, Graph 8).

Words used / frequency of transgressions	Misfortune %	Celiac disease %	Celiac %	Intolerance %	Diet %
Never	84.2	83.6	73.0	70.7	83.0
Yearly	5.3	3.4	8.7	14.6	8.0
Monthly	3.5	6.0	12.8	7.3	4.0
Weekly	5.3	6.0	4.1	3.7	4.0
Daily	1.8	0.9	1.4	3.7	1.0

Table 6. Relation between the words uttered by the physician and different transgression levels.

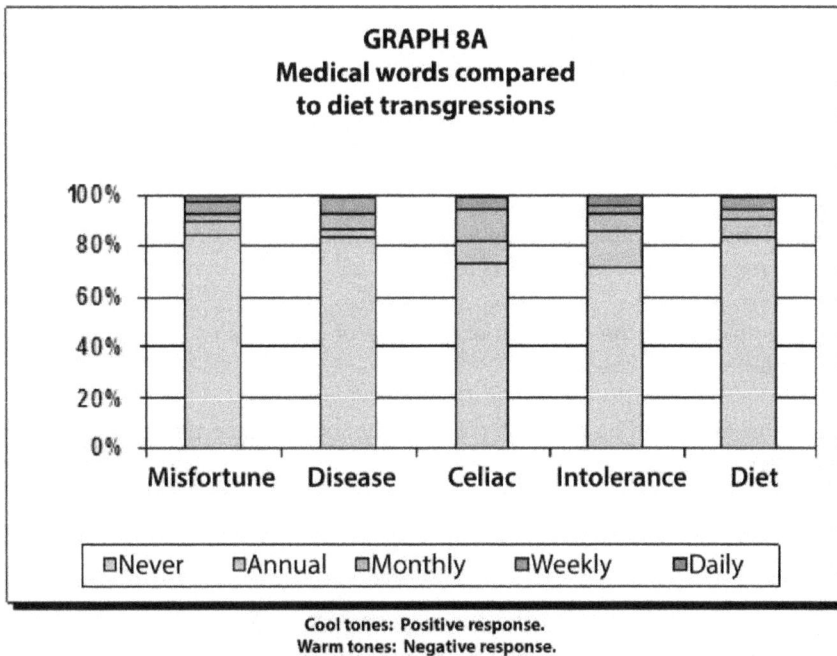

Cool tones: Positive response.
Warm tones: Negative response.

Graph 8. Impact. The words "misfortune" and "disease" have a satisfactory impact on diet compliance, as opposed to the word "intolerance", which exhibits correlation with poorer diet compliance.

8) Regarding the way patients felt at self-help group meetings, the well-being index rose to 92%.

9) Regarding the locations where celiac disease patients were most interested in acquiring their food, the results were:

Supermarkets/stores:	51.2 %	Health food stores/supermarkets:	41.6 %
Stores/health food stores:	3.8 %	Supermarkets/pharmacies:	2.4 %
Stores/pharmacies:	0.5 %	Health food stores/pharmacies:	0.5 %

Supermarkets alone had a total of 95.2%, local stores 55.5%, health food stores 45.9% and pharmacies only 3.4%.

Briefly, the conclusions of the impact survey are:

1. Reaction to diagnosis was different in relation to the group to which they belonged. Patients, adults or children with celiac disease react differently from the patient's relatives (mothers).

2. The emotion prevalent among adults with celiac disease and patients' relatives (mother) was "anguish", while in children with celiac disease the main one was "tranquility".

3. Even though most celiac disease patients rapidly accept their condition, children stood out significantly regarding their promptness to do so.

4. The terms employed by the physician at the time of diagnosis have a significant impact on the mother but not so in children.

5. The The terms employed by the physician also do not influence the time it takes to accept their condition.

6. The patient's educational level does not affect or modify the result of the variables analyzed here.

7. The urgency with which the physician states the diagnosis encourages the patient's relatives to have a better adherence to the diet and to have a positive experience in support groups. Exactly the opposite happens when the seriousness of the matter is depreciated, which correlates with the patients usually not feeling well in support groups.

8. The urgency with which the physician states the diagnosis does not have any impact on diet compliance among adult celiac disease patients.

9. The urgency with which the physician makes the diagnosis does not make adult patients accept their celiac disease condition in spite of adhering to the diet.

10. People mostly choose to buy their products at supermarkets; neighborhood stores are in a distant second place, followed by health food stores and, more distantly, drug stores.

It could be inferred from this last point that the celiac disease patient wants to live with his or her condition in a normal fashion and not associated with the health care system.

5. Celiac Disease: A Systemic Overview

Diagnosing a person with celiac disease generates a series of structural changes and readjustments within the family, which usually last a long time.

After receiving the news, nothing will be as it used to be within the family group: its functioning immediately abandons its habitual spontaneity and the simplest and most casual movements become burdened by a layer of complexity. What previously were simple outings and trips must now be the subject of a much more detailed attention and a series of preparations and often the plans must be aborted.

On the other hand, it is possible that the family group will divide itself into two clearly differentiated subsystems: one will be formed by the patient and the person who will provide him or her with logistic support (the mother if it is a child or an adolescent; the wife or husband if it is an adult). The other subsystem will be formed by the rest of the family.

The difference between these two subgroups obeys the change produced in interpersonal relationships since the moment the diagnosis is given, since the patient and his support have established a closer link, attend to medical consultation together, receive hygiene and diet advice and have begun to participate in support groups which discuss celiac disease.

Meanwhile, even if the rest of the family becomes acquainted with the new dietary and culinary rules, it could express lack enthusiasm regarding the treatment. So, it can be said, without fear of exaggeration, that the rest of the family may prefer to act unconcernedly rather than shouldering such a complex situation.

This difference between both subsystems, which does not necessary occur in all cases, but quite often, is triggered mainly by interpersonal due to the fact that not all family members empathize with the problem, even though it is clearly serious. These differences among family members generate discomfort.

5.1. Level of Adherence and Family Balance

Adherence to treatment depends in keeping an attitude of continuous alert to avoid eating food which cannot be tolerated by the celiac patient. In order to sustain this regimen through time, it is necessary that both subsystems start working as a team, involving the family as a whole in the treatment adherence. Thus, everyone should show interest in the details regarding the diet and culinary resources.

A family which adheres to the treatment would try by all means to encourage and keep adherence, and so cancelling the gap that initially separated both subsystems.

When this is not possible, the gap between both subsystems will only widen, conflicts will increase and the system tries to save itself by sacrificing its weaker link: treatment adherence. The diet is interrupted and the family prefers to ignore the situation.

5.2. Treatment Adherence and Adolescence

As it occurs with chronic pathologies and organ transplantations, adolescent celiac disease patients may exhibit attitudes of resistance, rebelliousness and diet neglect. This is caused by the hostile emotions generated by being compelled to follow a strict diet, barred from the enjoyment which others have with no limitations; the adolescent must also face the conflicts and discomforts of a stage in his or her life when he or she feels willing to confront and defy his or her elders. An obvious and infallible way to achieve this by not following the GFD.

The adults, who by now are getting used to the rigors of the treatment, now see themselves forced to face another source of conflict: the celiac patient's adolescence. In the ensuing tug-of-war between adults and adolescents, the latter can pressure the adults by threatening to abandon the treatment supported by allies external to the family, such as their group of friends or peers.

In spite of having assurance of their parents' affection, adolescents have a strong necessity to be part of a group and to earn its approval. Therefore, an adolescent will not hesitate to act in a way that pleases their peers, even when this may be disagreeable to his or her parents. The lack of treatment adherence in this phase can be furthered by a lack of parental skill.

5.3. Extended family and treatment adherence

The extended family can exert an important influence regarding the way treatment is faced, which will vary depending on the type of relationship previously established between the celiac patient's family and its relatives, as well as on the degree of proximity between them. It often happens that certain gaps in treatment adherence may have been provoked by messages from older adults who disbelieve the diagnosis and who consider the prohibition to consume bread, a foodstuff traditionally held to be beneficial and which has religious associations, to be illogical. Fortunately, situations like these are greatly decreasing in Argentina.

It must be taken into account that some suggestions offered by older, trustworthy relatives, which are repeated with regularity, can exert great influence, above all if they are compounded by the enjoyment implied by abandoning the diet. The advice or suggestions offered such relatives, which stems from their personal experience, can be well received by the younger relative, who may react favorably to an excuse to satisfy his or her oral desire.

Thus it is important to take into account the opinions of all the family members in order to avoid well-meant but counterproductive messages.

5.4. Treatment Adherence and Mass Media

An important adjuvant to treatment adherence comes from the TV programming which contain, culinary and kitchen hygiene suggestions and methods, as well as testimonials from celiac patients and stories which awaken the audience's interest, whether they tolerate gluten or not, and demonstrate a diet which will be palatable for all and which will cast aside the idea of a bland, elemental diet. Thus, the gap between tolerant and intolerant patients starts to narrow in such a way that the former may feel tempted to try the latter's diet.

Media coverage of the constant testimonies of a large number celiac patients, be they famous or anonymous, show us a full and pleasant life with total treatment adherence and allows an amelioration of the negative aspects of the celiac disease condition. It must be admitted that, in celiac disease, there is a series of systems that reciprocally influence each other and the most powerful of these, mass media, exerts a decisive influence on the pathology and in the way it is perceived. Through them, gluten intolerance is shown to mass audiences and given a widespread character, legitimacy and prestige.

5.5. Promoting adherence to treatment

Since adherence to the gluten-free diet is the treatment's cornerstone, efforts to that end start since the very first medical consultation, when diagnosis and treatment conditions are expounded and maintained. These injunctions are directed to the celiac patient but they must equally reach all the members of his or her family system since all of them must be bearers of the physician's message and therefore they need to collaborate in this continuous and prolonged effort to adhere to the physicians' prescriptions. It must be borne in mind that this intolerance is expressed against a ubiquitous substance which is found almost all edible products and which is not easily detectable, which is the reason why the patient, besides having a firm conviction regarding the diet, must be alert in all situations involving the consumption of food.

Adherence to treatment can sometimes falter due to periods of anxiety, frustration and anger triggered by painful circumstances or by psychological conditions reactive to stressing environmental factors. The patient appeals to food as a safety valve against stress. Under these circumstances, the family system, which by now is acquainted with this kind of reaction must rush for a medical consultation to prevent the patient's reaction from becoming a habitual pattern.

5.6. Gluten and Tobacco: Celiac Culture and other People's Consideration

Intolerance to gluten and tobacco smoke exhibits, from a systemic point of view, some coincidences. Until the middle of the last century, non-smokers who wanted to travel, eat, or rest in open smoke-free spaces, had to explicitly require it and then they were directed towards separate locations. Now, the situation is inverted. Smokers must be confined to separate areas if they desire to eat and smoke in a restaurant and totally abstain from it while using public transportation or while travelling by airplane.

Nowadays, the situation of celiac patients in public areas resembles to that of the non-smokers of past decades. When they arrive in cities where celiac disease is barely known, or even unknown, they must somehow think of a way to gather the ingredients of a reasonable meal. It is also probable that in restaurants which offer gluten-free dishes are not fully conscious of the special care needed when handling kitchen utensils and which may not have appropriate experience regarding this kind of food.

Nevertheless, the situation is changing and gluten-free dishes seem more appetizing. The social media is full of advertisements and offers and it is foreseeable that in a not too distant future celiac patients will be able to enjoy the same comforts as non-smokers do today.

5.7. Acceptance of the disease

When we talk about the acceptance of this disease, the patient supposedly has gone through an assimilation, a sudden and clarifying confirmation about his or her situation, which radically changes his or her attitude towards treatment. This may be an idealized view of what actually is a process composed of advances and retreats negotiated with relevant persons in their environment. For this reason, due to the lack of a definitive conviction, the patient must always be motivated and monitored so that he or she will be kept on the lookout regarding his or her adherence to the treatment's prescriptions.

There are many daily circumstances that place the celiac patient in a difficult situation, making him or her complain about these restrictions, above all those that generate exclusion and set him or her aside from his or her peers. When attending a social gathering carrying his or her own food, the patient may feel that this situation sets him or her aside and that it brands him or her with an unwanted distinction.

It can be argued, logically, that after several years of following a gluten-free diet, the patient achieves such identification with his complex dietary routine that his social interaction occurs smoothly. In spite of this, it is probable that some personal problem or a minimal logistic inconvenience may prevent him or her from having access to the food he or she needs at the appropriate moment, which may trigger an outburst of anguish or rage against his or her gluten-intolerant condition.

It must be admitted that true acceptance of the celiac disease condition will only occur when gluten-free products become as accessible, affordable and appetizing as other mass-consumption products. The lack of these or difficulty in obtaining them hurts the patient's self-esteem and casts him or her in the position of a second-class citizen. As the great national poem of Argentina wisely states: "The heart of he who must beg bleeds copiously" (Martín Fierro).[34]

Conclusions about the impact of diagnosis on celiac patients and on their social environment demonstrates clearly the need to identify the persons involved in this process. The answer to the announcement of a chronic condition is processed differently both in mothers' and in the childrens' mind. While the former worries because she understands the term "chronicity", for the latter it is no more than a short- or very short-term matter. This is the reason for the child's serene behavior and for the mother's anguish and alarm. The child can quickly accept his or her condition since the matter will be completely handled by his or her parents or some other significant adult or trusted person in the family.

It is necessary to establish a communication protocol with the medical team, so as to fine-tune, each time more accurately, its influence in the management of the therapeutic process' course, of a better and fuller acceptance of the celiac condition and on a prompter and firmer acceptance of said condition.

The commercial outlet choice where to purchase or consume suitable dietary products, has a connotation which is completely concordant with the celiac condition, that is to say, with the need to be a part of the community, to be able to meet neighbors and friends at the supermarket, of erasing, even if only symbolically, the barriers that separate the patient from those who tolerate gluten. Purchasing food at a drug store suggests, for the celiac condition, a condition of discrimination.

It can be concluded that this kind of surveys are necessary and useful since they may afford a deeper understanding of celiac disease and of its social and emotional aspects.

References

1. Cueto-Rúa EA, Pecotche G. *La Enfermedad celíaca y su entorno. Creación del Club de Madres.* En: XI Congreso Argentino de Pediatría. Argentina, Mar del Plata. Sesión Temas Libres. Coordinador R. Maggi. 1981.

2. Drut R, Cueto-Rúa EA. *Análisis cuantitativo e inmunohistoquímico de la mucosa yeyunal de niños con enfermedad celíaca y con dieta libre de gluten.* Arch Argen Pediatr. 1985; 83: 20-4.

3. Comité de Gastroenterología de la Sociedad Argentina de Pediatría. *Conclusiones de la Jornada de Diagnóstico de Intestino Delgado.* Hospital de Niños de La Plata. Arch Arg Pediatr. 1986; 84: 38-9.

4. Cueto-Rúa EA, Menna ME, Morales V, Pecotche G. *Enfermedad celíaca y anticuerpos anti músculo liso.* Arch Arg Pediatr. 1986; 84: 269-73.

5. Cueto-Rúa EA, Menna ME, Morales V, Drut R. *Anticuerpos antimúsculo liso en la detección y seguimiento del enfermo celíaco.* Acta Gastroent Latinoamer. 1987; 3: 227-34.

6. Cueto-Rúa EA. *Enfermedad Celíaca.* Programa Nacional de Actualización Pediátrica 2004; 1: 13-30.

7. Cueto-Rúa EA, Gómez JC, Crivelli A, Guzmán L. *Guías, criterios y score de Diagnóstico.* Ministerio de Salud de la Povincia de Buenos Aires Disponible en: http://www.ms.gba.gov.ar/EducacionSalud/celiaquia/celiaquia.html

8. Programa de Enfermedad Celíaca. Ministerio de Salud de la Nación. Argentina. Disponible en: http://www.msal.gov.ar/celiacos/w-criterios-biopsia.html

9. Guzmán L, Cueto-Rúa EA. *Enfermedad celíaca.* Factores que influyen en la adherencia al tratamiento. Revista Ludovica Pediátrica 2011; 5: 166-74.

10. Gomez JC, Selvaggio GS, Viola M et al. *Prevalence of celiac disease in Argentina: screening of an adult population in the La Plata area.* Am J Gastroenterol. 2001; 96: 2700-04. http://dx.doi.org/10.1111/j.1572-0241.2001.04124.x

11. Mora M, Litwin N, Tocca MDC. *Prevalencia de enfermedad celíaca: estudio multicéntrico en población pediátrica en cinco distritos urbanos de Argentina.* Rev Argent Salud Pública. 2010; 1(4): 26-31. Disponible en http://bit.ly/11iSAvB

12. Dicke WK. *Coeliac disease. Investigation of harmfull effects of certain types of cereal on patients with coeliac disease.* MD Thesis Univ Utrecht.

13. Dicke WK, Weijers HA, Van de Kamer JH. *Coeliac disease presence in weath of a factors faving feleteriuseffects in cases of coeliac diseas.* Acta Paediat. 1953; 42: 34-42. http://dx.doi.org/10.1111/j.1651-2227.1953.tb05563.x

14. Janatuinen EK, Pikkarainen PH, Kemppainen TA, et al. *A comparison of diets with and without oats in adults with celiac disease.* N Engl J Med. 1995; 333: 1033-7. http://dx.doi.org/10.1056/NEJM199510193331602

15. Comino I, Real A, de Lorenzo L, Cornell H, López-Casado MÁ, Barro F, et al. *Diversity in oat potential immunogenicity: basis for the selection of oat varieties with no toxicity in coeliac disease.* Gut. 2011; 60: 915-22. http://dx.doi.org/10.1136/gut.2010.225268

16. Real A, Comino I, de Lorenzo L, Merchaán F, Gil-Humanes J, Giménez MJ, et al. *Molecular and immunological characterization of gluten proteins isolated from oat cultivars that differ in toxicity for celiac disease.* PLoS One. 2012; 7(12): e48365. http://dx.doi.org/10.1371/journal.pone.0048365

17. Edwards G, Leffler DA, Dennis MD, Franko DL, Blom-Hoffman J, et al. *Psychological correlates of gluten-free diet adherence in adults with celiac disease*. J Clin Gastroenterol. 2009; 43: 301-6. http://dx.doi.org/10.1097/MCG.0b013e31816a8c9b

18. Ruiz A, Polanco I. *Exposición al gluten y aparición de enfermedades autoinmunes en la enfermedad celíaca.* Pediátrika. 2002; 22: 311-9.

19. Hall NJ, Rubin G, Charnock A. *Source school of applied sciences, University of Sunderland, Sunderland, UK. Systematic review: adherence to a gluten-free diet in adult patients with coeliac disease.* Aliment Pharmacol Ther. 2009; 30: 315-30. http://dx.doi.org/10.1111/j.1365-2036.2009.04053.x

20. Kurppa K, Lauronen O, Collin P, et al. *Factors Associated with Dietary Adherence in Celiac Disease: A Nationwide Study.* Digestion. 2012; 86: 309-14. http://dx.doi.org/10.1159/000341416

21. Roma E, Roubani A, Kolia E, Panayiotou J, Zellos A, Syriopoulou VP. *Dietary compliance and life style of children with coeliac disease.* J Hum Nutr Diet. 2010; 23: 176-82. http://dx.doi.org/10.1111/j.1365-277X.2009.01036.x

22. Olsson C, Hörnell A, Ivarsson A, Sydner YM. *The everyday life of adolescent coeliacs: issues of importance for compliance with the gluten-free diet.* J Hum Nutr Diet. 2008; 21: 359-67. http://dx.doi.org/10.1111/j.1365-277X.2008.00867.x

23. Cueto-Rúa EA. *Estreñimiento. Una epidemia programada.* Revista Gastrohnup. 2011; 13: 58-65.

24. Cueto-Rúa EA, Miculán S. *Constipación y encopresis.* Ludovica Pediátrica. 2008; 2: 71-3.

25. Black JL, Orfila C. *Impact of coeliac disease on dietary habits and quality of life.* J Hum Nutr Diet. 2011; 24(6): 582-7. http://dx.doi.org/10.1111/j.1365-277X.2011.01170.x

26. Leffler DA, Edwards-George J, Dennis M, Schuppan D, Cook F, Franko DL, et al. *Factors that influence adherence to a gluten-free diet in adults with celiac disease.* Dig Dis Sci. 2008; 53: 1573-81. http://dx.doi.org/10.1007/s10620-007-0055-3

27. Errichiello S, Esposito O, Di Mase R Camarca ME, Natale C, Limongelli MG, et al. *Celiac disease: predictors of compliance with a gluten-free diet in adolescents and young adults.* J Pediatr Gastroenterol Nutr. 2010; 50: 54-60. http://dx.doi.org/10.1097/MPG.0b013e31819de82a

28. Samaşca G, Iancu M, Pop T, Butnariu A, Andreica M, Cristea V, et al. *Importance of the educational environment in the evolution of celiac disease.* Labmedicine. 2011; 42: 497-501. http://dx.doi.org/10.1309/LM1HFQPSN56ZQYLJ

29. Hopman EG, Koopman HM, Wit JM, Mearin ML. *Dietary compliance and health-related quality of life in patients with coeliac disease.* Eur J Gastroenterol Hepatol. 2009; 21: 1056-61. http://dx.doi.org/10.1097/MEG.0b013e3283267941

30. Rosén A, Ivarsson A, Nordyke K, Karlsson E, Carlsson A, Danielsson L, et al. *Balancing health benefits and social sacrifices: A qualitative study of how screening-detected celiac disease impacts adolescents' quality of life.* BMC Pediatrics. 2011; 11: 32. http://dx.doi.org/10.1186/1471-2431-11-32

31. Moreno Rodríguez MA. *El arte y la ciencia del diagnóstico médico. Principios seculares y problemas actuales.* La Habana: Editorial. Científico-Técnica; 2001. P. 59.

32. Rancich AM, Gelpi RJ. *Análisis de los principios éticos en Juramentos Médicos utilizados en las Facultades de Medicina de la Argentina en relación al Hipocrático.* Medicina Buenos Aires. 1998; 58: 147-52.

33. Lain Entralgo P. *La relación médico enfermo.* Madrid: Revista de Occidente; 1964.

34. Hernández J. *Consejos de Martín Fierro y el viejo Vizcacha.* Disponible en: http://www.redargentina.com/refranes/consejosferro.asp

Chapter 21

Immunotoxic Gluten Fraction Detection: Applications in Food Safety

Isabel Comino, Ana Real, María de Lourdes Moreno, Carolina Sousa

Department of Microbiology and Parasitology. Faculty of Pharmacy. University of Sevilla, Spain.

icomino@us.es, arc@us.es, lmoreno@us.es, csoumar@us.es

Doi: http://dx.doi.org/10.3926/oms.59

How to cite this chapter

Comino I, Real A, Moreno ML, Sousa C. *Immunotoxic Gluten Fraction Detection: Applications in Food Safety*. In Rodrigo L and Peña AS, editors. *Celiac Disease and Non-Celiac Gluten Sensitivity*. Barcelona, Spain: OmniaScience; 2014. p. 435-446.

I.Comino, A.Real, M.D.Moreno, C.Sousa

Abstract

The only currently available therapy for celiac patients is a life-long strict gluten-free diet, however, it generates numerous social and economic repercussions. Various studies have suggested that failure to comply with the diet is frequent in celiac patients. For this reason, and because of the currently recognized importance of nutrition in the management of CD, the development of new strategies for monitoring the gluten-free diet is essential. The toxicity of cereals such as oats is questioned. Studies have shown that oat's immunogenicity depends on interindividual sensitivity and the cultivar used. The incorporation of harmless oat varieties in food products may improve the nutritional quality of the gluten-free diet. Additionally in the search for a less-toxic barley, it has been demonstrated that cultivated varieties contain lower levels of immunogenic gluten than the wild ones. This fact is important in breeding programs of cultivated species and in the preparation of certain foods and beverages derived from toxic cereals.

1. Introduction

Currently, the only existing treatment for patients with celiac disease (CD) is to follow a strict life-long gluten-free diet (GFD) by excluding toxic dietary wheat proteins (gliadin and glutenin), and their counterparts in barley (hordeins), rye (secalins), and oats (avenins), as well as in hybrids of these grains (such as kamut and triticale) and derivatives thereof (starch, flour, etc.)[1].

In most celiac patients, strict compliance with a GFD leads, in a few months, to the rapid and complete recovery of the normal architecture and function of the small intestinal mucosa, as well as to symptom remission and normalization of serological tests[2]. However, maintaining a GFD is not easy, not only due to the high cost involved, but there are also situations that favor involuntary gluten intake, such as its presence in a high proportion of manufactured products. Approximately, more than half of the commercial food contains gluten from wheat, barley, rye or oats, including those in which it only acts as a thickening agent or binder. The risk posed by these foodstuffs for celiac patients makes it convenient to carry out a rigorous gluten content control.

In European legislation, the acceptable gluten amount in food which seeks to be labeled "gluten-free" is of 20 parts per million (ppm or mg/kg). Another category has also been provided, food with "very low gluten content" which is used for products made with wheat, rye, barley, oats or their crossbred varieties, but which have been specially treated to eliminate gluten. Food labelled as "very low gluten content" may not exceed 100 ppm (REGULATION (CD) Number 41/2009 concerning the composition and labeling of foodstuffs suitable for people intolerant to gluten, http://bit.ly/RdEqVI). Therefore, control of gluten-free products requires the use of quantitative methods with highly specificity and sensibility. The use of inadequate control methods exposes celiac patients to important health problems. This also leads to severe economic losses and legal problems associated with questionable identification of gluten-free products. At industrial level, rigorous control of the raw materials used and the final marketed product must be excercised.

To certify suitable food, no product is exempt from analysis. Inadvertent contamination and adulteration seriously compromise the health and quality of life these patients. The industrial use of wheat flour and/or derived components (starch, gluten) used to increase water retention capacity, improve texture, preserve structure and quality attributes, leads to the presence of toxic proteins. Furthermore, during the production process, foods are subjected to heat treatments and other processes able to modify their gluten content. This product modification is a problem in order to quantify the gluten immunotoxic fractions.

Due to the complexity of the system being analyzed, the only way to provide a safe diet for celiac patients is the use of highly sensitive and specific tests. The techniques for gluten analysis are mass spectrometry, immunological methods based on monoclonal antibodies (MAbs) or PCR techniques.

Mass spectrometry is based on the determination of the characteristic mass spectra of different gluten fractions. Furthermore, through these techniques the peptides contained in different types of food can be characterized[3]. They require complex instrumentation and equipment calibration, expensive equipment, extensive facilities and a complex process of developing spectral profile libraries.

The most frequently used method in food analysis are MAbs produced specifically against gluten. These antibodies recognize gluten repetitive regions[4,5] or have been designed from toxic regions in the gluten protein sequences[6-9]. Some of these antibodies have been incorporated into various ELISAs to be used in food gluten content analysis[8-10]. These methods are the most convenient and widely used as they unite simplicity, sensitivity and economy, in addition to being able to directly detect proteins toxic to celiac patients.

Another option, used primarily as a complement to the above mentioned ones, is based on PCR techniques using primers that encode prolamine repetitive sequences[11,12]. Unlike ELISA, PCR is an indirect technique for detecting gluten protein which does not quantify the presence of these proteins, but that of the DNA which encodes them.

2. Suitability of Oats in the GFD

The introduction of oats in the GFD has been a topic subject to debate in recent years[13,14]. Adherence to a strict GFD may sometimes be difficult due to the narrow range of permitted ingredients and any dietary restrictions, such as oat consumption, can be a relief for celiac patients. Nutritionally wise, oatmeal is an important source of protein, fat, vitamins, minerals and fibers, and therefore, could be beneficial for people with CD. In addition, the palatability of oats and their wide availability may contribute to greater acceptance in a diet free of wheat, barley and rye.

Oats differs from other cereals in their prolamin content, which is of 10-20% of the total protein, in contrast to wheat prolamins, which can be between 40-50%. Furthermore, various cereal prolamins differ in molecular size and amino acid content. In avenin, the proline and glutamine proportion (amino acids rich in toxic regions) is lower than in other toxic cereals (Figure 1).

Janatuinen et al.[17] lconducted the first controlled study on the toxicity of oats in CD. Since then, several studies have evaluated the safety of oat consumption for celiac patients. Some researchers claim that celiac patients tolerate oats with no sign of intestinal inflammation[14,17,18], in fact, many countries allow the use of oats in "gluten-free" food, for example Gluten-Free Oats®. On the other hand, there are studies that confirm the toxicity of certain types of oats for celiac patients and the impossibility of regular oats consumption. Arentz-Hansen et al.[15] described the intestinal damage suffered by some patients after consuming oats and a GFD. In these patients an immune response against avenins may be triggered similar to that produced by gluten from wheat, rye or barley. A study led by Dr. Knut Lundin[19] with 19 celiac patients who were consuming 50 grams of oats/day for 12 weeks showed that one of the celiac patients proved to be oat sensitive. This suggests the need to distinguish groups of celiac patients according to their sensitivity to cereals, and to identify the immunogenicity source in avenin peptides.

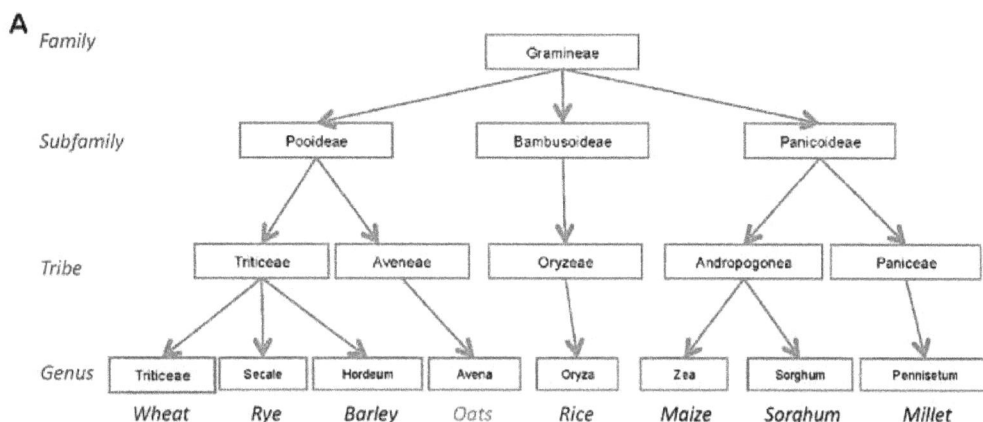

A

Family

Gramineae

Subfamily

Pooideae   Bambusoideae   Panicoideae

Tribe

Triticeae   Aveneae   Oryzeae   Andropogonea   Paniceae

Genus

Triticeae	Secale	Hordeum	Avena	Oryza	Zea	Sorghum	Pennisetum
Wheat	*Rye*	*Barley*	*Oats*	*Rice*	*Maize*	*Sorghum*	*Millet*

B

Basic prolamin characteristics	Wheat	Oats	Rice
Number of genes	>100	8-25	34 (21 transcribed)
Size	20-40 kDa	19-31 kDa	10-16 kDa
aas prevalence	Gln (35%) Pro (25%)	Gln (30%) Pro (10%)	Gln (22%) Pro (<other cereals)
Prolamins based on total proteins in grain	40-50%	10-20%	25%

Figure 1. Taxonomic and molecular relationship of oats to other food cereals in the context of CD. A. Taxonomy of oats in the grass family in relation to cereals toxic for celiac patients, such as wheat, barley and rye, and non-toxic cereals such as rice, maize, sorghum and millet. B. Molecular characteristics of the prolamins from wheat, oats and rice. Modified according to Kagnoff.[16]

Silano et al.[20,21] conducted a series of *in vitro* tests with different varieties of oats and found that all varieties tested were toxic to celiac patients, with differences in the levels of toxicity. Therefore, it is critical to qualitatively and/or quantitatively determine the immunotoxic potential of oats due to the clinical implications for celiac patients.

2.1. Diversity in the Potential Immunogenicity of Different Oat Varieties

The differences in the type of oats used, the oat purity and the study design did not allow a clear answer on whether or not oats are safe for all celiac patients. Besides, "pure" (uncontaminated) oats are considered gluten-free according to CD regulation No. 41/ 2009. However, a study by our research group explains the apparent contradictions found in previous research related to the safety of oats for celiac patients[21]. We demonstrated that oat immunogenicity varies depending on the cultivar used.

Nine oat varieties from various Australian and Spanish commercial sources were used. The purity of the oat material was carefully controlled and shown to be free of contamination. The analysis of DNA amplification products confirmed that the oat samples were not contaminated with wheat, barley, rye or mixtures of these grains. The toxicity of the different oat varieties was evaluated by MAb G12 immunoassay, an antibody obtained from one of the most toxic peptides described for CD, the α-2 gliadin 33-mer peptide. Three varieties of oats were distinguished based on their MAb G12 reactivity: a group with high reactivity, a group which showed an intermediate reactivity and another without detectable reaction (Figure 2). The potential immunotoxicity of three oat types was evaluated by cell proliferation and interferon-γ release (IFN-γ), using peripheral blood T lymphocytes from celiac patients. Thus, it was demonstrated that mAb G12 reactivity against the storage proteins of different oat varieties correlated with immunological studies of samples from celiac patients[21].

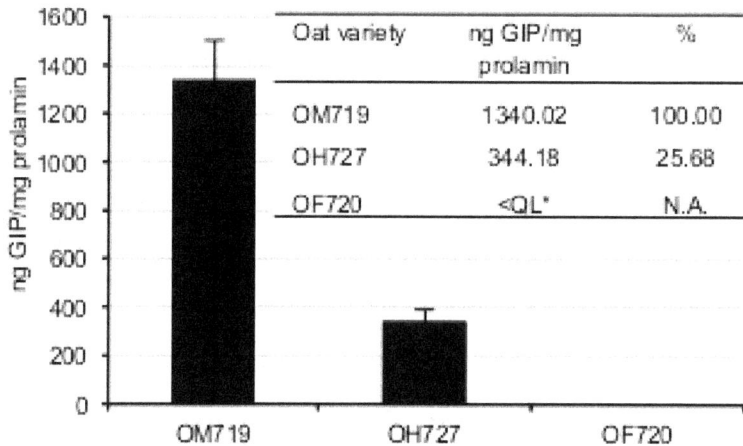

Figure 2. GIP concentration in different oat varieties. The GIP concentration is determined by competitive ELISA using G12-HRP. OM719, OH727, OF720: oat varieties. (GIP: Gluten Immunogenic Peptides)
%: Percentage of GIP in each variety in relation to the more reactive, OM719.
*GIP concentration below the assay's quantification limit (5.4 ng/mL).
N.A.: Not applicable. Modified according to Comino et al.[21]

In comparison with wheat gliadins, the avenins have been little studied, and the number of full avenin genes present at the moment in the databases is limited and from few genotypes, so that the variability of avenin genes in oats is not well represented. It has recent been known that, like wheat, oat grains have both monomeric and polymeric avenins[22]. A direct correlation between the immunogenicity of the different varieties of oats and the presence of the specific peptides with a higher/lower potential immunotoxicity has been found, that could explain why certain varieties of oats are toxic for celiac patients and other not[22,23].

The addition of some oat varieties to gluten-free food could not only improve the patient's nutritional status but it may also provide some benefits in the treatment of some diseases related to cholesterol, diabetes or intestinal transit problems. These studies provides new insights into the dilemma of oats in CD and suggests practical methods for selecting those varieties tolerable by celiac patients.

Given the importance of the source of oats used, this topic should be taken into account in food safety regulations, in the labeling of gluten-free products that may contain oats, as well as in the design of clinical trials on the effect of oats in celiac patients.

3. Natural Immunotoxicity Variation in Cultivated and Wild Barley Varieties

Compliance with GFD present difficulties due to inadvertent ingestions or voluntary transgressions. Consequently, different strategies have been proposed to develop new therapies for CD[24-27]. A possible alternative is based on the identification of new cereal varieties with low toxicity profiles, which could contribute to improving the quality and variety of foods destined to the celiac community. In the case of oats, immunological studies revealed that certain varieties had no toxicity for celiac patient[21]. Different studies have investigated the possible immunogenicity of wheat varieties by means of antibodies to immunogenic wheat peptides and T cell reactivity from celiac individuals[6]. It is unknown whether all barley varieties are equally toxic to celiac patients. In this sense, our research group has studied the toxicity of different barley lines, investigating *Hordeum vulgare*, a cultivable barley variety, and *Hordeum chilense*, a wild barley variety, used for the development of new cultivable cereals.

Barley is an important cereal crop, mainly used for food, obtaining malt, making beer and distilled spirits. In recent years, the use of barley has been increased, largely due to its high nutritional value. Barley seeds provide complex carbohydrates (mainly starch), minerals, vitamins, and fiber, which provide benefits in helping reduce blood cholesterol. In addition, its high fiber and other components have a satiating effect, which can positively affect weight control as well as improved intestinal transit[28,29].

In our study we first compared the differences in toxicity levels between different varieties of barley[30]. Rigorous control of sample purity both by visual examination as well as by PCR techniques was executed, afterwards, the hordein banding pattern was analyzed by MALDI-TOF MS. Our results showed there was a greater number of hordein bands for wild varieties. These mass spectrum differences may be related both to the seed's functional properties as well as the toxicity in connection with CD. The results obtained by G12 immunological techniques showed large differences between the *H. vulgare* and *H. chilense* lines, the wild barley lines being more immunogenic. Also, differences in immunotoxic potential were found between varieties of a same barley species (Figure 3). The stimulatory capacity of these barley varieties was evaluated by peripheral blood cell proliferation and IFN-γ release and from the intestinal mucosa of active celiac patients. All barley varieties were able to stimulate IFN-γ secretion, at both in peripheral blood and in the intestinal mucosa. However, one of the wild varieties was the one that showed stronger activity in relation to the pathogenesis of CD.

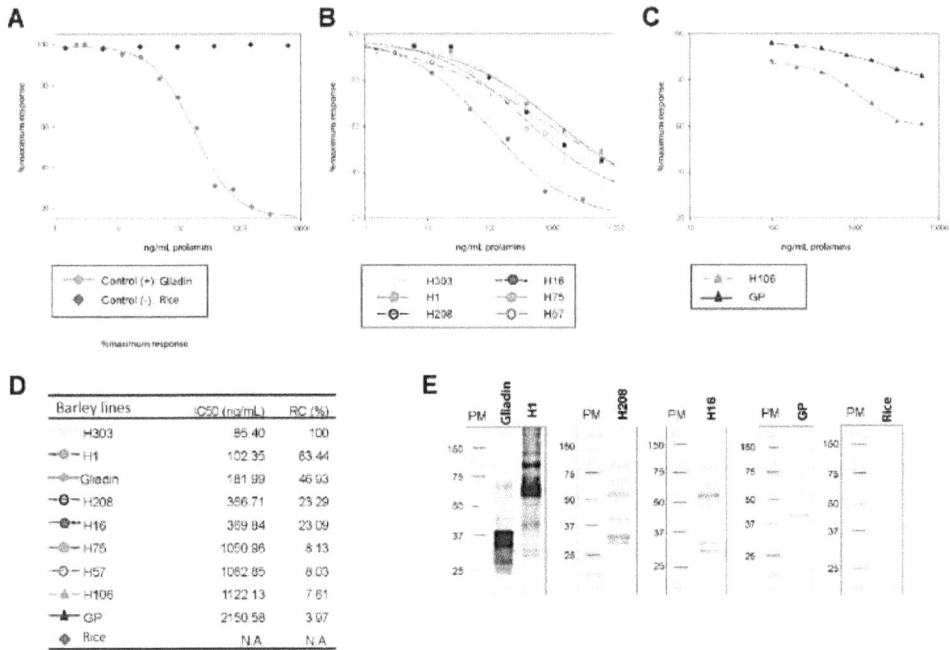

Figure 3. Relative affinity of anti-gliadin 33-mer G12 mAb against different barley lines.
(A, B, C and D) G12 competitive ELISA to determine the relative antibody affinity to the various barley lines. Gliadin and rice were used as positive and negative controls, respectively.
(E) G12 Western blot prolamins of different barley lines. The membranes were revealed with mAb G12. MW, molecular weight (kDa).
IC50: antigen concentration of which a 50% reduction of the maximum signal is obtained.
CR: Cross-reactivity. Modified according to Comino et al.[28]

A correlation between the type of barley used and immunotoxicity for celiac patients has established. It has been shown that cultivated barley varieties exhibit lower levels of toxic gluten than wild ones. These findings could help develop new lines with low gluten levels, which may be intended for the manufacture of food and beverages with gluten amounts below the threshold allowed for celiac patients[31]. Thus, for example, during the brewing process the initial quantity of toxic peptides can be lowered a thousand times in the different extraction and fermentation processes[32]. Barley varieties with reduced immunotoxicity[30] could be included in genetic breeding aimed at developing varieties that could serve as raw material for the production of toxic peptide-free beers.

The incorporation of wild germplasm in breeding programs is a common practice to increase the genetic base of cultivated species. However, care must be exercised not to increase the toxicity of cultivated varieties, as in the case of barley, because, according to the results obtained by Comino et al.[30], wild varieties may contain higher levels of toxic gluten than cultivated varieties.

4. Conclusions

The GFD is currently the only treatment for celiac patients, therefore, the characterization and quantification of the toxic gluten fraction in food and raw materials for the celiac patients is essential. There is a wide variability in the immunotoxic potential of different cereal varieties. It has been demonstrated that there is no strict correlation between gluten content and immunotoxic potential, due to the fact that some gluten epitopes may be less immunogenic than others.

Immunogenicity of oats varies depending on the cultivar used, there being varieties which could be safe for celiac patients and be enrich the GFD. Likewise, it has been shown that cultivated barley varieties, although there are differences between them, exhibit lower levels of toxic gluten compared to wild ones. This fact is important for breeding programs of cultivated species and for the preparation of certain foods and/or beverages derived from toxic cereals.

References

1. Kupper C. *Dietary guidelines and implementation for celiac disease.* Gastroenterol. 2005; 128: S121-7. http://dx.doi.org/10.1053/j.gastro.2005.02.024
2. Green PH, Jabri B. *Coeliac disease*. Lancet. 2003; 362: 383-91. http://dx.doi.org/10.1016/S0140-6736(03)14027-5
3. Camafeita E, Alfonso P, Mothes T, Méndez E. *Matrix-assisted laser desorption/ionization time-of-flight mass spectrometric micro-analysis: The first non-immunological alternative attempt to quantify gluten gliadins in food samples.* J. Mass Spectrom. 1997; 32: 940-47. http://dx.doi.org/10.1002/(SICI)1096-9888(199709)32:9<940::AID-JMS550>3.0.CO;2-2
4. Osman AA, Uhlig HH, Valdes I, Amin M, Méndez E, Mothes T. *A monoclonal antibody that recognizes a potential coeliac-toxic repetitive pentapeptide epitope in gliadins*. Eur. J. Gastroenterol. Hepatol. 2001; 13: 1189-93. http://dx.doi.org/10.1097/00042737-200110000-00011
5. Doña V, Urrutia M, Bayardo M, Alzogaray V, Goldbaum FA, Chirdo FG. *Single domain antibodies are specially suited for quantitative determination of gliadins under denaturing conditions.* J. Agric. Food Chem. 2010; 58: 918-26. http://dx.doi.org/10.1021/jf902973c
6. Spaenij-Dekking EH, Kooy-Winkelaar EM, Nieuwenhuizen WF, Drijfhout JW, Koning F. *A novel and sensitive method for the detection of T cell stimulatory epitopes of alpha/beta- and gamma-gliadin.* Gut. 2004; 53: 1267-73. http://dx.doi.org/10.1136/gut.2003.037952
7. Mitea C, Kooy-Winkelaar Y, van Veelen P, de Ru A, Drijfhout JW, Koning F *et al. Fine specificity of monoclonal antibodies against celiac disease-inducing peptides in the gluteome.* Am. J. Clin. Nutr. 2008; 88: 1057-66.
8. Morón,B, Bethune MT, Comino I, Manyani H, Ferragud M, López MC *et al. Toward the assessment of food toxicity for celiac patients: characterization of monoclonal antibodies to a main immunogenic gluten peptide.* PLoS One. 2008; 3: e2294. http://dx.doi.org/10.1371/journal.pone.0002294
9. Morón B, Cebolla A, Manyani H, Alvarez-Maqueda M, Megías M, Thomas MC, *et al. Sensitive detection of cereal fractions that are toxic to celiac disease patients by using monoclonal antibodies to a main immunogenic wheat peptide.* Am. J. Clin. Nutr. 2008; 87: 405-14.
10. Méndez E, Vela C, Immer U, Janssen FW. *Report of a collaborative trial to investigate the performance of the R5 enzyme linked immunoassay to determine gliadin in gluten-free food.* Eur. J. Gastroenterol. Hepatol. 2005; 17: 1053-63. http://dx.doi.org/10.1097/00042737-200510000-00008
11. Henterich N, Osman AA, Méndez E, Mothes T. *Assay of gliadin by real-time immunopolymerase chain reaction.* Nahrung. 2003; 47: 345-48. http://dx.doi.org/10.1002/food.200390079
12. Hernández M, Esteve T, Pla M. *Real-time polymerase chain reaction based assays for quantitative detection of barley, rice, sunflower, and wheat.* J. Agric. Food Chem. 2005; 53: 7003-9. http://dx.doi.org/10.1021/jf050797j

13. Koskinen O, Villanen M, Korponay-Szabo I, Lindfors K, Mäki M, Kaukinen K. *Oats not induce systematic or mucosal autoantibody response in children with coeliac disease.* J. Pediatric Gastroeneterol. Nutr. 2009; 48: 559-65.
http://dx.doi.org/10.1097/MPG.0b013e3181668635

14. Pulido OM, Gillespie Z, Zarkadas M, Dubois S, Vavasour E, Rashid M, Switzer C *et al. Introduction of oats in the diet of individuals with celiac disease: a systematic review.* Adv. Food Nutr. Res. 2009; 57: 235-85.
http://dx.doi.org/10.1016/S1043-4526(09)57006-4

15. Arentz-Hansen H, Fleckenstein B, Molberg Ø, Scott H, Koning F, Jung G *et al. The molecular basis for oat intolerance in patients with celiac disease.* PLoS Medic. 2004; 1: 84-92. http://dx.doi.org/10.1371/journal.pmed.0010001

16. Kagnoff MF. *Overview and pathogenesis of celiac disease.* Gastroenterol. 2005; 128: S10-18. http://dx.doi.org/10.1053/j.gastro.2005.02.008

17. Janatuinen EK, Pikkarainen PH, Kemppainen TA, Kosma VM, Järvinen RM, Uusitupa MI *et al. A comparison of diets with and without oats in adults with celiac disease.* N. Engl. J. Med. 1995; 333: 1033-37. http://dx.doi.org/10.1056/NEJM199510193331602

18. Thompson T. *Oats and the gluten-free diet.* J Am Diet Assoc. 2003; 103:376-9.
http://dx.doi.org/10.1053/jada.2003.50044

19. Lundin KE, Nilsen EM, Scott HG, Løberg EM, Gjøen A, Bratlie J *et al. Oats induced villous atrophy in coeliac disease.* Gut. 2003; 52: 1649-52.
http://dx.doi.org/10.1136/gut.52.11.1649

20. Silano M, Di Benedetto R, Maialetti F, De Vincenzi A, Calcaterra R, Cornell HJ *et al. Avenins from different cultivars of oats elicit response by coeliac peripheral lymphocytes.* Scand. J. Gastroenterol. 2007; 42: 1302-5.
http://dx.doi.org/10.1080/00365520701420750

21. Comino I, Real A, de Lorenzo L, Cornell H, López-Casado MÁ, Barro F *et al. Diversity in oat potential immunogenicity: Basis for the selection of oat varieties with no toxicity in coeliac disease.* Gut. 2011; 60: 915-20. http://dx.doi.org/10.1136/gut.2010.225268

22. Sollid LM, Khosla C. *Novel therapies for coeliac disease.* J. Intern. Med. 2011; 269: 604-13. http://dx.doi.org/10.1111/j.1365-2796.2011.02376.x

23. Tripathi A, Lammers KM, Goldblum S, Shea-Donohue T, Netzel-Arnett S, Buzza MS *et al. Identification of human zonulin, a physiological modulator of tight junctions, as prehaptoglobin-2.* Proc. Natl. Acad. Sci. U.S.A. 2009; 106: 16799-804.
http://dx.doi.org/10.1073/pnas.0906773106

24. Gil-Humanes J, Pistón F, Tollefsen S, Sollid LM, Barro F. *Effective shutdown in the expression of celiac disease-related wheat gliadin T-cell epitopes by RNA interference.* Proc. Natl. Acad. Sci. U.S.A. 2010; 107: 17023-28.
http://dx.doi.org/10.1073/pnas.1007773107

25. Daveson AJ, Jones DM, Gaze S, McSorley H, Clouston A, Pascoe A, *et al. Effect of hookworm infection on wheat challenge in celiac disease-a randomised double-blinded placebo controlled trial.* PLoS One. 2011; 6: e17366.
http://dx.doi.org/10.1371/journal.pone.0017366

26. Baik BK, Ullrich SE. *Barley for food: characteristics, improvement, and renewed interest.* J. Cereal Science. 2008; 48: 304-18. http://dx.doi.org/10.1016/j.jcs.2008.02.002

27. Finnie C, Svensson B. *Barley seed proteomics from spots to structures.* J. Proteomics. 2009; 72: 315-24. http://dx.doi.org/10.1016/j.jprot.2008.12.001

28. Comino I, Real A, Gil-Humanes J, Pistón F, de Lorenzo L, Moreno ML, *et al. Significant differences in potential immunotoxicity of barley varieties for celiac disease*. Molecular Nutrition and Food Research. 2012; 56: 1697-707.
    http://dx.doi.org/10.1002/mnfr.201200358
29. Dostálek P, Hochel I, Méndez E, Hernando A, Gabrovská D. *Immunochemical determination of gluten in malts and beers.* Food Add. Contam. 2006; 11: 1074-78.
    http://dx.doi.org/10.1080/02652030600740637

Chapter 22

Cereal-Derived Gluten-Free Foods

Cristina M. Rosell

Institute of Agrochemistry and Food Technology (IATA-CSIC). Spain

crosell@iata.csic.es

Doi: http://dx.doi.org/10.3926/oms.221

How to cite this chapter

Rosell C.M. *Cereal-Derived Gluten-Free Foods.* In Rodrigo L and Peña AS, editors. *Celiac Disease and Non-Celiac Gluten Sensitivity.* Barcelona, Spain: OmniaScience; 2014. p.447-461.

Abstract

During the last decades, the demand for gluten-free products has escalated due to the increased number of diagnosed celiac patients. The celiac patient population seeks gluten-free products resembling gluten-containing products, even with similar nutritional quality.

The present chapter aims to provide information about the design and development of cereal-based gluten-free products as well as on their technological, nutritional and sensory characteristics. During the last decade there has been an exponential increase in the number of gluten-free products in the market. Initially, the development of these products focused on making economically viable and palatable products. However the current awareness of a healthy diet also applies to gluten-free foods.

Gluten-free foods derived from grains are rich in carbohydrates and fats but deficient regarding some macronutrients and micronutrients. It is for this reason that gluten-free diets can generate unbalanced, long-term diets deficient in some nutrients. The addition of other ingredients/nutrients like omega-3 oils, specific proteins, fibers, probiotics and prebiotics is seen as an option to improve the nutritional composition of gluten-free foods.

1. Introduction

Cereals are the staple food for most of the world's population and occupy an undisputed place at the base of the various recommended food pyramid nutritional guidelines. However, despite the benefits of eating these grains, they are able to cause allergies and food intolerances, gluten intolerance, celiac disease being of special interest. The term "gluten" designates a protein fraction from wheat, rye, barley, oats or their crossbred varieties and derivatives thereof, to which some persons are intolerant and which is insoluble in water and in 0.5 M NaCl.[1]

Gluten is present in cereal grains such as wheat *(Triticum aestivum),* rye *(Secale cereale),* spelt *(Triticum spelta), kamut (Triticum turgidum),* triticale *(Triticum spp x Secale cereale)* and some oat varieties *(Avena sativa).*[2]

Currently the celiac patients' community has, as sole treatment, a nutritional therapy that restricts their food to gluten-free products; therefore, the consumption of cereals such as wheat, rye, barley and foods containing these grains is excluded. Specifically, the CD N 41/2009[1] Regulation defines "food products for gluten intolerant people" as those foodstuffs intended for particular diet which are processed, treated or specially prepared to meet the special dietary needs of gluten-intolerant people.

The limits on the composition and labeling of gluten-free foods set by CD Regulation No. 41/2009[1] are:

- Foodstuffs for gluten-intolerant people, consisting of one or more ingredients from wheat, rye, barley, oats or their crossbred varieties, which have been especially processed to reduce gluten, must not contain a gluten level exceeding 100 mg/kg in the food as sold to the final consumer. The labeling, advertising and presentation of the abovementioned products will bear the term "very low gluten content". They may bear the term "gluten-free" if their gluten content does not exceed 20 mg/kg in the food as sold to the final consumer.

- Oats contained in foodstuffs for gluten-intolerant people must be produced, prepared or treated specially to avoid contamination by wheat, rye, barley or their crossbred varieties and the gluten content must not exceed 20 mg/kg.

- Foodstuffs for gluten-intolerant people, consisting of one or more ingredients which substitute wheat, rye, barley, oats or their crossbred varieties shall not contain a level of gluten exceeding 20 mg/kg in the food as sold to the final consumer. The labeling, presentation and advertising of these products must be labeled as "gluten-free".

The food categories most affected by this limitation are wheat-based bread and bakery products. Therefore, this chapter focuses primarily on this type of food and on the various technological alternatives that have been developed to mimic the function of gluten in baked goods. Other foods may contain "invisible gluten", namely wheat or gluten derivatives that may be included among the ingredients used as thickener or protective film. Hamburgers, sauces, powdered soups, processed cheese, etc., are included in this group.

In general, gluten-free products are of lower quality than their gluten-bearing counterparts since their structure disintegrates easily and they have a very dry texture.

2. Ingredients for Manufacturing Food Derived from Gluten-Free Cereals

Gluten accounts for nearly 80% of the proteins found in wheat, it confers its elastic properties to flour and provides bread with consistency and viscoelastic crumb. The composition of gluten, composed mostly by proteins formed by glutenin and gliadin, explains its cohesiveness and viscoelastic properties. The gliadin fraction contributes to the viscous properties and extensibility of the bread dough while glutenin confers elasticity and strength. The relative proportions between gliadins and glutenins affect the functional properties of bread dough.

The elimination of gluten, especially in bread recipes, results in liquid batters which generate breads with crumbly texture and other quality defects associated with color and flavor. Therefore, the manufacture of gluten-free bread requires the use of polymeric ingredients that mimic the function of gluten during the baking process.

2.1. Cereals and Other Grains Gluten-free

Gluten-free grains available for gluten-free bread production are rice, maize, buckwheat, teff and kamut®. There has been a notable increase in the use of rice flour in the formula of gluten-free products due to its organoleptic characteristics and hypoallergenicity,[3] although the use of a hydrocolloid emulsifier, enzyme or protein is necessary to give it viscoelastic properties.[4] Several studies have focused on gluten-free bread-like products made with rice flour, in which the impact of wholemeal rice flour has been analized,[5] as have the effects of hydrocolloids[6] and of mixtures with other flours and starches[7-10] or with other proteins.[11-12] These studies confirm the importance of flour characteristics, of the other ingredients and of the process in the instrumental and sensory characteristics of the end products.

Brites et al.[13] described the bread baking process based on *broa* (traditional Portuguese bread) production technology. The production of sorghum bread has also been described.[14-15] Grain flours, including rice and other grains such as unconventional legumes, musaceans, roots and tubers are perceived as potential ingredients in the development of numerous products worldwide; there are even many traditional products in several countries which could be used for this end.

Pseudocereals such as sorghum, millet, quinoa, amaranth and buckwheat are also being introduced as ingredients in the formula of gluten-free products. In North America, several breads based on amaranth can be found, with which it is possible to improve nutritional composition since it has a larger amount of protein, fiber and minerals.[16] Flour obtained from buckwheat and millet are richer in protein and minerals and, therefore, have been proposed for the development of nutritionally richer alternative products.

2.2. Other Ingredients, Additives and Processing Aids

Other ingredients typically present in the manufacture of gluten-free breads are starch, dairy, eggs, soy protein and hydrocolloids. The presence of a certain amount of starch significantly improves the quality of gluten-free breads. Rice, potato or tapioca starches are preferable for this purpose.

Hydrocolloids

Hydrocolloids are essential additives in gluten-free bread production since they mimic, to some extent, the function of gluten through the granting of viscosity or viscoelastic properties. In the baking industry these compounds contribute to improving the food's texture, water holding capacity, aging delay and increase overall product quality during storage.[17]

Hydrocolloids, such as locust bean gum, guar gum, xanthan gum and agar are used as substitutes for gluten in the development of rice flour breads targeting the celiac or gluten-intolerant population.[6,18-19] The specific volume of these breads increased in the presence of hydrocolloids, excepting xanthan gum. However, Gambus et al.[20] obtained the largest volume in gluten-free bread using xanthan, which also decreased the crumb hardness of fresh bread fresh and 72-hour storage. Furthermore, these authors concluded that the combination of xanthan gum, pectin and guar gum allowed for products of a better quality.

The crumb characteristics are also modified by the presence of hydrocolloids, in particular, greater porosity has been obtained in the presence of 1% carboxymethylcellulose (CMC) and β-glucans or 2% pectin. Among the cellulose derivatives, hydroxypropylmethylcellulose (HPMC) is a suitable structuring agent and thus a gluten substitute, with good ability to retain gas.[21] Xanthan gum and HPMC have been highlighted as good gluten replacements that improve quality[22] (Figure 1). Regarding the effective mechanism, it has been described that the addition of HPMC to rice flour significantly increases the viscoelastic properties of dough, the overall effect being a strengthening of the rice dough mass.[21]

Combinations of additives and/or technological processing aids to obtain palatable gluten-free products are generally sought.

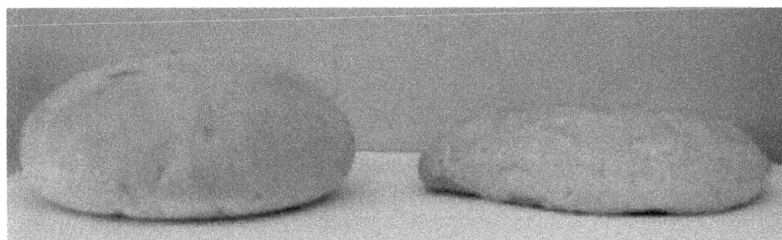

Figure 1. Effect of HPMC on rice bread volume (Photo: C. Marco).

Proteins

Gluten-free breads are generally protein-deficient when compared with their wheat flour counterparts. Several strategies have been proposed to increase the protein content of breads and other gluten-free cereal products. The enrichment of rice flour crackers with soy flour (25%) increases protein with reduced cost and also improves palatability.[23] Marco and Rosell[24] described that the resulting mixture of rice flour mix with 13 g/100 g of soy protein isolate and 4 g/100 g of HPMC results in gluten-free bread with an energy intake of 220.31 kcal/100 g whose composition (42.38% carbohydrates, 10.56% protein and 0.95% fat) is similar to that of gluten-bearing bread products. The addition of milk solids, inulin and fish surimi has been proposed as an alternative to increase dietary fiber content and protein in gluten-free breads.[25] The use of leguminous flours in the composition of gluten-free products is increasing due to their high protein content. With this objective in mind pea, lentil, bean and chickpea flours have been used.[26]

Dietary Fiber

The enrichment of gluten-free bakery products with dietary fiber confers texture, gelling capacity, thickening, emulsifying and stabilizing their properties. Among the fibers that have been proposed for the enrichment of gluten-free breads are wheat, maize, oats and barley.[27] The addition of these fibers to 6 g/100 g improves the product's nutritional profile without significantly altering its palatability. When amounts of 9 g/100 g are added, products with a 218% higher fiber content than that of the reference bread are achieved, but with significantly impaired palatability.

Stojceska et al.[28] increased the total dietary fiber content in gluten-free products using extrusion and incorporating different fruits and vegetables such as apples, beets, carrots, cranberries and teff flour. These authors incorporated up to 30% to a gluten-free formula consisting of rice flour, potato starch, maize starch, powdered milk and soy flour. By optimizing the extrusion conditions it was possible to obtain gluten-free products enriched in dietary fiber.

Enzymes

Another option for improving the quality of gluten-free breads is to use enzymes or technological aids.[29] Enzymes like amylase, protease, hemicellulase, lipase, oxidase, transglutaminase and oxidase have been used to improve the quality of bakery products. Some of these enzymes have been used as technological adjuvants to improve the quality of gluten-free breads. Among the various available enzymes, transglutaminase and glucose oxidase have allowed improvements in the texture of gluten-free bread, although the effect depends greatly on the flour used in the formula.[30-31] Both enzymes form intra- and intermolecular bonds between rice proteins generating a protein network. However, the protein network generated by these enzymes does not completely mimic gluten functions and the presence of a hydrocolloid is necessary.[30-31] The action of transglutaminase can also be enhanced by the addition of other proteins that increase the number of lysine residues which limit the enzyme crosslinking action. Moore et al.[32] studied transglutaminase impact on gluten-free breads containing soy protein, milk or egg. The most striking effect was a reduction in bread volume of due to protein polymerization.

Sourdoughs

Sourdoughs are a very attractive alternative to improve the quality of gluten-free breads. Sourdough is a natural fermentation starter which has been used to ferment numerous types of food. These doughs are obtained by mixing flour, water and other ingredients and allowing them to be fermented by naturally present lactic acid bacteria and yeasts. These microorganisms proceed mainly from the flour and the environment, but the microbiota specific to each sourdough depends on exogenous factors such as temperature and fermentation time. The use of sourdough in bread making is a widespread practice due to its positive effects on the quality of bakery products. Among them, improved texture, aroma and flavor, increased nutritional value and longer half-life should be emphasized. Therefore, its use has spread to gluten-free baked goods. There is little information on the use of sourdough in the formulas for baked gluten-free products. Crowley et al.[33] conducted a comparative study on the sourdough influence of various lactic acid bacteria on the texture of gluten-free products. In recent years, several patents have been published which are focused on the use of various lactic acid bacteria for gluten-free bakery products manufacture aimed at improving quality and reducing any potential residual toxicity.[34-35]

3. Preparation Processes of Gluten-Free Cereal Products

Food production of gluten-free grain-derived food faces many technological difficulties associated with the absence of the functionality of gluten. This absence has forced to adapt the formulas or recipes and manufacturing processes for the production of bread, cakes, cakes, pizzas, pastas and other grain products with sensory characteristics as similar as possible to those of their gluten counterparts.

3.1. Manufacturing Process of Gluten-Free Breads

The production of gluten-free breads differ significantly from traditional wheat bread making, in which the solid ingredients are kneaded with water, followed by bulk fermentation, division, rounding, fermentation and baking. These formulas are generally very complex and consist of mixtures of the aforementioned ingredients and of various additives (Table 1). Most gluten-free breads are made with high water content and the dough masses they generate are very fluid. Furthermore, they require very short kneading and fermentation times. Regarding the formulas, in numerous occasions the response surface methodology has been used to optimize the concentration of each ingredient.[21] The search for parameters characteristic of each one of the gluten-free doughs, which will allow to predict the quality of gluten-free baked products, is an important issue.

Matos and Rosell[36] described statistically significant correlations between dough consistency when subjected to heating and cooling and crumb hardness, so that these parameters could be used to predict final product quality.

Bread type	Qualitative Composition
Pan Bread	Maize starch, water, sugar, eggs, vegetable margarine, acidifier, preservative, yeast, thickener, salt, leavening agents, antioxidants
Rustic Bread	Maize starch, water, vegetable margarine, acidifier, preservative, antioxidants, aromas, colorants, eggs, sugar, yeast, emulsifier, dextrose, humectants, stabilizers, salt
Carré Bread	Maize starch, water, vegetable margarine, acidifier, preservative, antioxidants, aromas, colorants, eggs, sugar, yeast, emulsifier, dextrose, humectant, stabilizer, salt
Round Bread buns	Potato starch, Maize starch, water, caseinates, sugar, vegetable oil, maize flour, yeast, soy protein, stabilizers, salt, preservatives
Brioches	Maize starch, water, sugar, eggs, vegetable margarine, acidifier, preservative, aromas, colorant, thickener, yeast, emulsifier, salt, leavening agents, aniseed, cinnamon, antioxidants
Carré Bread	Maize starch, rice starch, water, vegetable oil, sugar, thickener, lupin protein, yeast, salt, vegetable fiber, aromas, emulsifier
Pan Bread	Maize starch, water, sugar, eggs, vegetable margarine, acidifier, preservative, aromas, colorant, yeast, thickener, emulsifier, salt, leavening agents, antioxidant
Precooked Baguette	Maize starch, water, sugar, yeast, thickeners, salt, leavening agents, acidifier, preservative, aroma, colorant
Precooked Baguette	Maize starch, water, sugar, thickener, emulsifier, salt, yeast, preservative, leavening agents, antioxidant
Bread loaf	Maize starch, vegetable margarine, salt, sugar, emulsifier, leavening agents, antioxidant, thickener, preservative and yeast
Pan Bread	Maize starch, vegetable margarine, salt, sugar, emulsifier, leavening agents, antioxidant, thickener, preservative and yeast

Table 1. Ingredients and additives in the commercial gluten-free breads formulas

3.2. Manufacturing Process of Gluten-Free Cookies

The manufacture of gluten-free cookies involves no such problems since their gluten network develops minimally and the essential ingredients this type of products are starch and sugar. The manufacture of gluten-free cookies uses maize, millet, buckwheat, rice and potato starches combined with fat (palm oil, microencapsulated fat, low-fat content milk solids). Combinations of rice, maize, potato and soybean with microencapsulated fat originates gluten-free cookies of a quality comparable to those obtained with wheat flour.[37] Cookies also have been obtained by substituting wheat flour by rice flour. An optimized formula for these products includes rice flour (70%), soybean meal (10%), maize starch (10%) and potato starch (10%).[37]

3.3. Manufacturing Process of Gluten-Free Cakes

Cake is obtained by mixing and cooking from masses prepared with flour starches. In cakes, the gluten network is not required and starch is the most important constituent, which determines cake structure. Numerous formulas have been proposed for the manufacture of gluten-free cookies. Gularte and Pallarés[38] compared the characteristics of gluten-free cakes (made with rice flour) with those of gluten-bearing cakes. Both cakes exhibited no significant differences in color, texture and chewiness. Protein-enriched gluten-free cakes have even been made enriched adding leguminous flours[26] or else fibers diverse dietary fibers.[39]

3.4. Gluten-Free Pasta and Extruded Products

Pasta production includes the preparation of dough obtained by mixing hard wheat flour (semolina) with water and then extruding it to obtain the desired shape and size. In gluten-free pasta, the absence of gluten can be countered with the mixture of pregelatinized starch and maize flour before adding water or else pregelatinizing the starch during the mixing or extrusion. The use of high or ultra-high temperature during the pasta drying process to denature proteins and maintain its integrity during cooking is another option. Pseudo-cereals have also been used in gluten-free pasta formula. The combination of buckwheat, amaranth and quinoa with egg albumin, emulsifiers and enzymes has yielded gluten-free noodles with adequate quality features.[40] Buckwheat produces better quality noodles with adequate firmness. Maize and quinoa mixtures, or else quinoa and rice flour mixtures have also been used to obtain gluten-free spaghetti.[41]

4. Gluten-Free Bakery Products

4.1. Baking Gluten-Free Quality Products

Traditionally, products aimed at celiac patients were designed solely focusing on the absence of allergens, using polymer mixtures that could generate products with similar sensory characteristics gluten than those of their gluten-bearing counterparts. In recent years, the celiac community has attracted the attention of food companies and food technologists and a wide variety of gluten-free products has been developed. In the case of baked goods, the variety of commercial products is mainly due to the introduction of numerous formats and presentations rather than to the design of new products with different sensory and/or nutritional properties. Available gluten-free bakery products are characterized by being composed of starch and gluten-free cereal flour mixtures. The quality and characteristics of gluten-free breads depend mainly on the ingredients used to make them (Figure 2). Thus, maize breads have an intense aroma and flavor. In 2002, Arendt et al.[42] reviewed commercial gluten-free bread quality, detecting low quality due to their rapid aging, dry, crumbly texture and intense, unpleasant aroma. Gluten-free breads tend to age rapidly, due to the high amount of starch in the formulas. Furthermore, due to the absence of gluten there is more water available which originates soft crusts rapid crumb hardening. In recent years there have been many studies which seek to improve the quality of these products adding sourdoughs, hydrocolloids, enzymes, emulsifiers and proteins.

Since quality is a completely subjective term, there have been some researches which seek to establish relationships between sensory attributes and certain technological parameters determined by means of analytical instrumentation. Matos and Rosell[36] have established some correlations between the gluten-free bread crumb hydration properties and crumb cohesiveness and resilience.

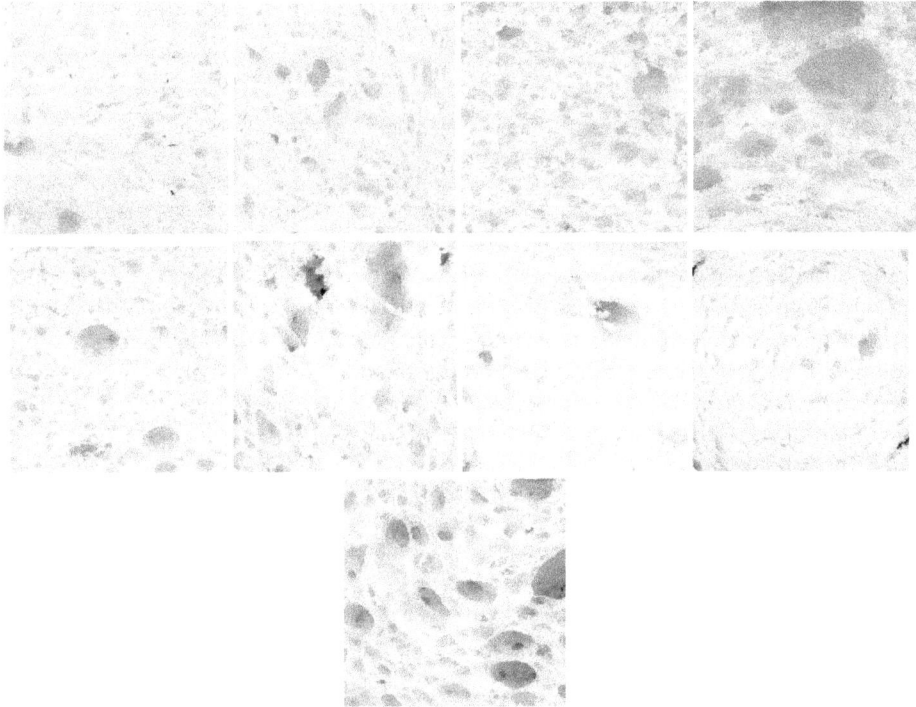

Figure 2. Digital images of different commercial gluten-free breadcrumbs (30x30 mm) (Photo: ME Matos).

4.2. Nutritional Aspects of Gluten-Free Products

Gluten-free products are generally not enriched or fortified and are often obtained from refined flours or starches. Consequently these products do not have the same amount of nutrients as their gluten-bearing counterparts. In a study by Matos and Rosell[43], 11 different types of gluten-free bread commercial available in Spanish supermarkets were evaluated in nutritional terms. The nutritional composition of commercial gluten-free breads had variations of 40-62% in carbohydrates, 0-8% in proteins, 1-11% in fat and highly variable fiber contents (0-6%) (Table 2). This profile differs significantly from the gluten-bearing bakery products which, in spite of their various existing formats, share a very similar nutritional composition which varies between 41-56% for carbohydrates, 8.0-13.0% for protein and 2.0-4.0% for fat, among its major constituents. These data indicate that nutritional differences in continuous gluten-free bread ingestion may arise if the ingestion of other types of food is not modified.

These differences in the nutritional profile of gluten-free products and their gluten counterparts have led to reformulate gluten-free products seeking to obtain nutritionally balanced products which will provide the necessary nutrients for people who are forced to follow these treatment guidelines. Thus, gluten-free breads enriched with calcium and inulin have been designed to combat calcium deficiency and provide a greater fiber intake.[44]

Product	Moisture content (%)	Protein (%)	Fat (%)	Minerals (%)	Total carbohydrates (%)
1	29.63	3.16	8.51	2.12	86.21
2	31.63	6.94	16.91	1.10	75.05
3	29.50	7.31	16.56	1.66	74.47
4	27.17	15.05	7.33	1.85	75.76
5	26.27	5.13	10.64	2.01	82.22
6	41.66	4.92	4.86	2.03	88.18
7	33.60	3.96	8.28	4.53	83.22
8	21.10	1.01	2.00	4.03	92.96
9	31.33	0.91	2.03	5.43	91.63
10	36.13	1.91	26.10	3.57	68.42
11	42.03	2.80	18.32	3.98	74.91
Average	31.82	4.83	11.05	2.94	81.18

Table 2. Chemical composition, expressed in dry g/100 g of 11 commercial types of gluten-free breads.[43]

Acknowledgements

We gratefully acknowledge the funding received from the Higher Council for Scientific Research (CSIC) and the Generalitat Valenciana to Scientific Excellence Groups (Prometeo Project 2012/064), as well as the Celiac Association of Madrid (Spain).

References

1. Reglamento (CE) nº 41/2009 de la Comisión, de 20 de enero de 2009, sobre la composición y etiquetado de productos alimenticios apropiados para personas con intolerancia al gluten. Diario Oficial n° L 016 de 21/01/2009 pp. 0003-5.

2. Comino I, Real A, de Lorenzo L, Cornell H, López-Casado MA, Barro F et al. *Diversity in oat potential immunogenicity: basis for the selection of oat varieties with no toxicity in coeliac disease.* Gut. 2011; 60: 915-22. http://dx.doi.org/10.1136/gut.2010.225268

3. Rosell CM, Gómez M. *Rice.* In: Bakery products: Science and Technology. Ed Y.H. Hui. Blackwell Publishing, Ames, Iowa. USA. ISBN: 978-0-81-380187-2. 2006. pp. 123-133. http://dx.doi.org/10.1002/9780470277553.ch6

4. Rosell CM, Marco C. *Rice.* In: Gluten free cereal products and beverages. Ed E.K. Arendt, F. dal Bello. Elsevier Science, UK. ISBN: 978-0-12-373739-7. 2008. pp. 81-100. http://dx.doi.org/10.1016/B978-012373739-7.50006-X

5. Kadan RS, Robinson MG, Thibodeux DP, Pepperman AB. *Texture and other physiochemical properties of whole rice bread.* Journal Food Science. 2001; 66: 940-4. http://dx.doi.org/10.1111/j.1365-2621.2001.tb08216.x

6. Lazaridou A, Duta D, Papageorgiou M, Belc N, Biliaderis CG. *Effects of hydrocolloids on dough rheology and bread quality parameters in gluten-free formulations.* Journal of Food Engineering. 2007; 79: 1033-47. http://dx.doi.org/10.1016/j.jfoodeng.2006.03.032

7. Pruska-Kędzior A, Kędzior Z, Gorący M, Pietrowska K, Przybylska A, Spychalska K. *Comparison of rheological, fermentative and baking properties of gluten-free dough formulations.* European Food Research Technology. 2008. 227: 1523-36. http://dx.doi.org/10.1007/s00217-008-0875-1

8. Sciarini LS, Ribotta PD, León AE, Pérez GT. *Influence of gluten-free flours and their mixtures on batter properties and bread quality.* Food Bioprocess Technology. 2010; 3: 577-85. http://dx.doi.org/10.1007/s11947-008-0098-2

9. Matos ME, Rosell CM. *Quality indicators of rice based gluten-free bread-like products: relationships between dough rheology and quality characteristics.* Food Bioprocess Technology. 2012. http://dx.doi.org/10.1007/s11947-012-0903-9

10. Demirkesen I, Mert B, Sumnu G, Sahin S. *Rheological properties of gluten-free bread formulations.* Journal of Food Engineering. 2010. 96: 295-303. http://dx.doi.org/10.1016/j.jfoodeng.2009.08.004

11. Marco C, Rosell CM. *Functional and rheological properties of protein enriched gluten free composite flours.* Journal of Food Engineering. 2008; 88(1): 94-103. http://dx.doi.org/10.1016/j.jfoodeng.2008.01.018

12. Marco C, Rosell CM. *Effect of different protein isolates and transglutaminase on rice flour properties.* Journal of Food Engineering. 2008; 84(1): 132-9. http://dx.doi.org/10.1016/j.jfoodeng.2007.05.003

13. Brites C, Trigo MJ, Santos C, Collar C, Rosell CM. *Maize based gluten free bread: influence of production parameters on sensory and instrumental quality.* Food Bioprocess Technology: An International Journal. 2010; 3(5): 707-15. http://dx.doi.org/10.1007/s11947-008-0108-4

14. Taylor JRN, Dewar J. *Developments in sorghum food technologies.* In: Taylor, S. Ed. Advances in Food and Nutrition Research, 43. San Diego, CA. Academic Press, 2001. pp. 217-64. http://dx.doi.org/10.10186/S1043-4526(01)43006-3

15. Taylor JRN, Schober T, Bean SR. *Non-traditional uses of sorghum and pearl millet.* Journal of Cereal Science. 2006; 44: 252-71.
http://dx.doi.org/10.1016/j.jcs.2006.06.009

16. Gambus H, Gambus F, Sabat R. *The research on quality improvement of gluten-free bread by Amaranthus flour addition.* Zywnosc. 2002. 9: 99-112.

17. Molina-Rosell C. *Hidrocoloides en panadería.* Molinería y Panadería. 2011; 16-23.

18. Kang MY, Choi YH, Choi HC. *Interrelation between physicochemical properties of milled rice and retrogradation of rice bread during cold storage.* Journal Korean Society Food Science Technology. 1997; 26: 886-91.

19. Cato L, Gan JJ, Rafael LGB, Small DM. *Gluten free breads using rice flour and hydrocolloid gums.* Food Australia. 2004. 56: 75-8.

20. Gambus H, Sikora M, Ziobro R. *The effect of composition of hydrocolloids on properties of gluten-free bread.* Acta Scientiarum Polonorum-Technologia Alimentaria. 2007; 6: 61-74.

21. Gujral HS, Guardiola I, Carbonell JV, Rosell CM. *Effect of cyclodextrinase on dough rheology and bread quality from rice flour.* Journal of Agricultural and Food Chemistry. 2003; 51(13): 3814-8. http://dx.doi.org/10.1021/jf034112w

22. Anton AA, Artfield SD. *Hydrocolloids in gluten-free breads: a review.* International Journal of Food Sciences and Nutrition. 2008. 59: 11-23.
http://dx.doi.org/10.1080/09637480701625630

23. Jaekel LZ, Schons PF, Rodrigues RS, Silva LH. *Caracterização físico-química e avaliação sensorial de biscoito tipo "cookies" com grãos de soja.* En: Congresso de Iniciação Científica, 8. Anais CD Rom. Pelotas: UFPel. 2004.

24. Marco C, Rosell CM. *Breadmaking performance of protein enriched, gluten-free breads.* European Food Research and Technology. 2008; 227(4): 1205-13.
http://dx.doi.org/10.1007/s00217-008-0838-6

25. Gallagher E, Gormley TR, Arendt EK. *Recent Advances in the Formulation of Gluten-free Cereal-based Products.* Trends Food Science Technology. 2004; 15: 143-52.
http://dx.doi.org/10.1016/j.tifs.2003.09.012

26. Gularte MA, Gómez, M. Rosell CM. *Impact of legume flours on quality and in vitro digestibility of starch and protein from gluten-free cakes.* Food Bioprocess Technology: An International Journal. 2012; 5: 3142-50.
http://dx.doi.org/10.1007/s11947-011-0642-3

27. Sabanis D, Lebesi D, Tzia C. *Effect of dietary fibre enrichment on selected properties of gluten-free bread.* LWT-Food Science and Technology. 2009; 42: 1380-89.
http://dx.doi.org/10.1016/j.lwt.2009.03.010

28. Stojceska V, Ainsworth P, Plunkett A, Ibanolu S. *The advantage of using extrusion processing for increasing dietary fibre level in gluten-free products.* Food Chemistry. 2010; 121: 156-64. http://dx.doi.org/10.1016/j.foodchem.2009.12.024

29. Rosell CM, Collar C. *Effect of various enzymes on dough rheology and bread quality.* In: Recent Research Developments in Food Biotechnology. Enzymes as Additives or Processing Aids. Ed R. Porta, P. Di Pierro and L. Mariniello. Research Signpost, Kerala, India. ISBN: 978-8-13-080228-2. 2008. pp. 165-83.

30. Gujral HS, Rosell CM. *Functionality of rice flour modified with a microbial transglutaminase.* Journal of Cereal Science. 2004; 39(2): 225-30. http://dx.doi.org/10.1016/j.jcs.2003.10.004

31. Gujral H, Rosell CM. *Improvement of the breadmaking quality of rice flour by glucose oxidase.* Food Research International. 2004; 37(1): 75-81. http://dx.doi.org/10.1016/j.foodres.2003.08.001

32. Moore MM, Heinbockel M, Dockery P, Ulmer HM, Arendt EK. *Network formation in gluten-free bread with application of transglutaminase.* Cereal Chemistry. 2006. 83: 28-36. http://dx.doi.org/10.1094/CC-83-0028

33. Crowley P, Schober T, Clarke C, Arendt E. *The effect of storage time on textural and crumb grain characteristics of sourdough wheat bread.* European Food Research and Technology. 2002; 214: 489-96. http://dx.doi.org/10.1007/s00217-002-0500-7

34. Gallo G, De Angelis M, McSweeney PLH, Corbo MR, Gobetti M. *Partial purification and characterization of an X-prolyl dipeptidyl aminopeptidase from Lactobacillus sanfranciscensis CB1.* Food Chemistry. 2005; 9: 535-44. http://dx.doi.org/10.1016/j.foodchem.2004.08.047

35. Sikken D, Lousche K. *Starter preparation for producing bakery products.* European Patent EP13611796. 2003.

36. Matos ME, Rosell CM. *Relationship between instrumental parameters and sensory characteristics in gluten-free breads.* European Food Research Technology. 2012; 235: 107-17. http://dx.doi.org/10.1007/s00217-012-1736-5

37. Schober TJ, O'Brien CM, McCarthy D, Darnedde A, Arendt EK. *Influence of gluten free flour mixes and fat powders on the quality of gluten free biscuits.* European Food Research and Technology, 2003; 216: 369-76. http://dx.doi.org/10.1007/s00217-003-0694-3

38. Gularte MA, Pallares MG. *Reología y características físicas de bizcochos de harina de arroz.* En: Simposio Latino Americano de Ciencia de Alimentos, 5. Anais CD Rom. Montevidéo: Suctal. 2003.

39. Gularte MA, de la Hera E, Gómez M, Rosell CM. *Effect of different fibers on batter and gluten-free layer cake properties.* LWT-Food Science and Technology. 2012; 48: 209-14. http://dx.doi.org/10.1016/j.lwt.2012.03.015

40. Schoenlechner R, Jurackova K, Berghofer E. *Pasta production from the pseudo-cereals amaranth, quinoa and buckwheat.* Proceedings of the 12th ICC Cereal and Bread Congress, 2004. Harrogate, UK.

41. Ramírez JL, Silva Borges JT, Euzebio do Nascimento R, Ramirez Ascheri DP. *Functional properties of precooked macaroni of raw quinoa flour (Chenopodium quinoa Wild) and rice flour (Oryza sativa L).* Alimentaria. 2003; 342: 71-5.

42. Arendt EK, O'Brien CM, Schober TJ, Gallagher E, Gormley TR. *Development of gluten free cereal products.* Farm Food. 2002; 21-7.

43. Matos Segura ME, Rosell CM. *Chemical composition and starch digestibility of different gluten-free breads.* Plant Foods for Human Nutrition. 2011; 66(3): 224-30. http://dx.doi.org/10.1007/s11130-011-0244-2

44. Krupa U, Rosell CM, Sadowska J, Soral-Smietana M. *Bean starch as ingredient for gluten-free bread.* Journal of Food Processing and Preservation. 2010; 34(Suppl. 2): 501-18. http://dx.doi.org/10.1111/j.1745-4549.2009.00366.x

Chapter 23

Wheat Varieties Suitable for Celiac Patients

María J. Giménez[1], Javier Gil-Humanes[2], Carmen Victoria Ozuna[1], Francisco Barro[1]

[1]Institute for Sustainable Agriculture, CSIC, 14080 Córdoba, Spain.
[2]Department of Genetics, Cell Biology and Development and Center for Genome Engineering, University of Minnesota, Minneapolis, Minnesota, USA.

mjga06@ias.csic.es, javigil@ias.csic.es, cvozuna@ias.csic.es, fbarro@ias.csic.es

Doi: http://dx.doi.org/10.3926/oms.224

How to cite this chapter

Giménez MJ, Gil-Humanes J, Ozuna CV, Barro F. *Wheat Varieties Suitable for Celiac Patients.* In Rodrigo L and Peña AS, editors. *Celiac Disease and Non-Celiac Gluten Sensitivity.* Barcelona, Spain: OmniaScience; 2014. p. 461-475.

M.J. Giménez, J. Gil-Humanes, C.V. Ozuna, F. Barro

Abstract

Domesticated wheat is very complex genetically due to its origins in an ancestral diploid species, which underwent a process of natural hybridization and subsequent polyploidization. All cultivated wheat varieties and their wild relatives contain epitopes, which are toxic in relation to celiac disease (CD). RNAi is an excellent tool for silencing single genes or groups of them. Combining this technology with genetic manipulation the authors have down-regulated the toxic epitopes present in ω-, γ-, and α-gliadins of bread wheat. Monoclonal antibodies showed a decrease of almost 98% in the presence of toxic gluten. Protein extracts from those lines were assayed using specific T lymphocytes for DQ2 and DQ8 epitopes, showing that the new wheat lines were 100 times less reactive than their parental genotypes. These results represent a major breakthrough in achieving wheat types suitable for CD patients. The silencing of gliadins is a new breeding trait and can be transferred by crossbreeding with elite wheat varieties. A daily intake between 10 and 50 mg of gluten could be safe for most CD patients, suggesting that the transgenic lines reported here could be used in foodstuffs tolerated by many CD patients. Moreover, these lines could serve as a basis for treating other gluten pathologies such as wheat-dependent exercise-induced anaphylaxis and gluten sensitivity.

1. Introduction

Although celiac disease (CD) has been known since ancient times, the first references relating it to the intake of certain foods do not appear until the late nineteenth century. During the first half of the twentieth century the pernicious effect of bread in celiac patients was already known, but it was not until after World War II that Dicke, Weijers and Van De Kamer[1] observed that certain cereal grains, especially wheat and rye, were detrimental to children with CD, demonstrating the role of gluten as the agent responsible for triggering the disease. Since then, the gluten-free diet has been the only effective therapy for treating it and, during this time, great strides have been made in identifying the elements within gluten responsible for gluten enteropathy. At first glance, it might appear that, once known, toxic epitopes could be easily removed by plant breeding techniques and thus obtain varieties suitable for consumption by celiac patients. In fact, a similar process has taken place since the beginning of agriculture with other grains, whose domesticated varieties do not produce toxic substances (or do so to a lesser extent) which wild species often do have as, for example, antinutrients in legumes and glucosinolates in cabbages and more recently, erucic acid in rapeseed. In the case of wheat, the main gluten-bearing cereal, this is not a simple task due to the complexity of its genetics and of the proteins of which it is composed.

2. Wheat

The term "wheat" refers to the group of cereals, both domesticated and wild, belonging to the botanical genus *Triticum*, of the *Triticeae* tribe, belonging to the *Poiideae* subfamily of the grass family. Barley and rye are included in the same tribe as wheat, while oats belong to another tribe of the same subfamily. Other important grasses are maize and rice, which, along with wheat, are humanity's main cereal staples.[2]

Wheat grain is used to make flour, wheat meal, beer and a wide variety of food products, each world region making use of certain wheat types for specific ends. After the thousands of years elapsed since the beginning of its cultivation, each culture has developed characteristic habits and customs regarding wheat consumption.

From a genetic point of view, domesticated wheat is quite complex due to its origin in an ancestral diploid species, which has gone through natural hybridization processes and subsequent polyploidization. The main two species of agriculturally important wheat, durum (for pasta) and bread wheat (90% of all wheat produced in the world) are, respectively, tetraploid (two genomes, AABB) and hexaploid (three genomes, AABBDD) (Figure 1). The first originated naturally through the spontaneous hybridization of two diploid species between 0.5 and 2 million years ago, each one the donor of A and B genomes. Bread wheat (AABBDD) originated in the cultivated fields around 8,000 years ago, through spontaneous hybridization between durum wheat (AABB) and *A. tauschii*, a diploid species that donated the D genome (Figure 1). All wheat species have chromosome numbers in multiples of seven, including the diploid, tetraploid and hexaploid species with 14, 28 and 42 chromosomes, respectively. Wheat chromosomes are named using a number and a letter indicating from which genome it proceeds. Because of the close relationship between the donor species of the A, B and D genomes, for each pair of homologous chromosomes from one of the genomes present in bread wheat, there is a pair of similar chromosomes (homeologous) in the other genomes. In practice, polyploid wheat composition implies that each one of its genes is encoded two (durum wheat) or three times (bread wheat), so that changing a character through genetic improvement implies more effort than that which would have to be performed for a diploid species.

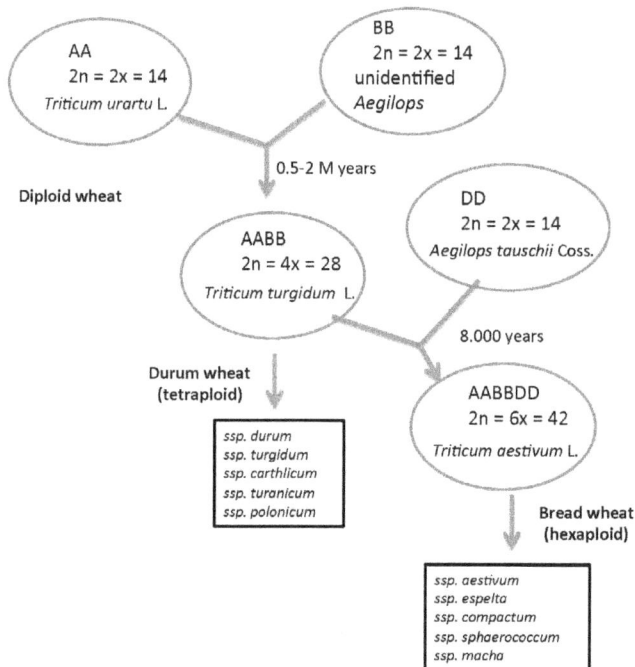

Figure 1. Origin of bread wheat (hexaploid) and pasta wheat (tetraploid) from diploid ancestors and subsequent polyploidization. Bread wheat, which comprises 90% of the wheat grown in the world, has a very recent origin.

3. Wheat Protein

Wheat grain is composed of proteins with a structural or metabolic function and by storage proteins (gluten).[3] The latter have the function of providing nutrients, such as amino acids, to the seedling in its early stages of development. According to Osborne's original classification[4] based on wheat grain protein solubility differences, these would be composed of albumins, globulins, prolamins (gliadin) and glutelins (glutenins). Gluten represents 80% of total grain protein and consists of gliadins and glutenins (Figure 2), which have different physicochemical properties due to their different ability to form polymers. While gliadins are monomeric, glutenins are assembled into polymers, stabilized by disulfide bonds, which remain physically, linked together, forming large aggregates of variable size. These proteins are the largest known in nature.

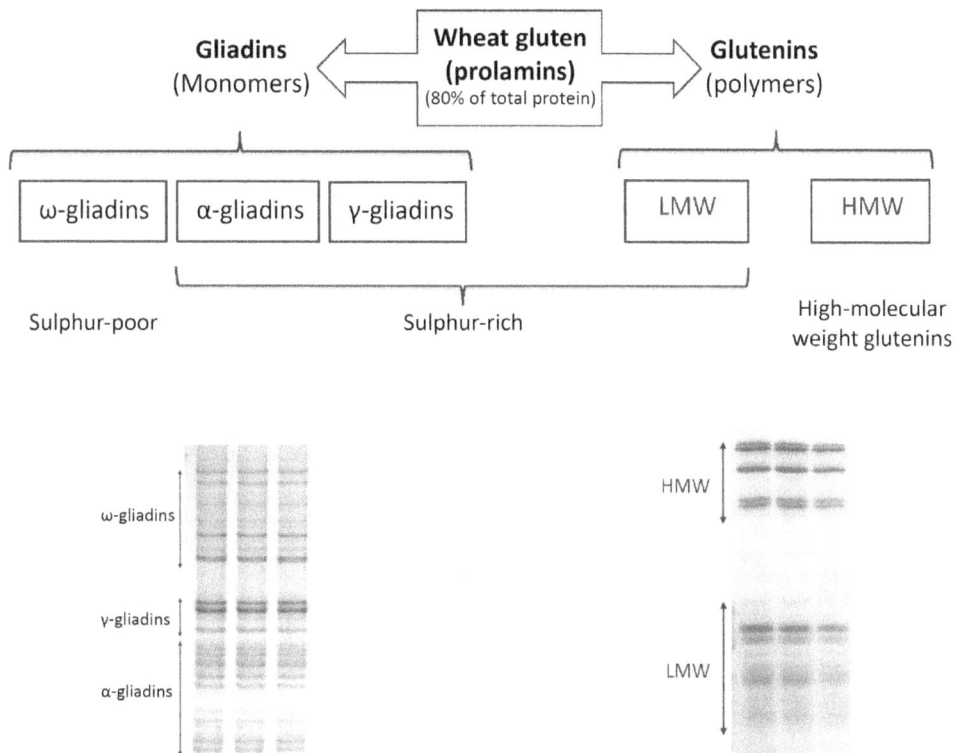

Figure 2. Wheat gluten composition. Gluten is a complex mixture of proteins belonging to two groups: glutenins and gliadins. While glutenin forms polymers, gliadin remains a monomer. Proteins in each group may be extracted and separated on SDS-PAGE gels (glutenin) and A-PAGE gels (Gliadins). Glutenin are divided into high (HMW) and low (LMW) molecular weight glutenins. Gliadins are formed by three structural groups: ω-, γ- and α-gliadins.

The classification of gluten proteins based on solubility has been offset today thanks to knowledge of their nature and genetics, so that the glutenins must also be considered to be prolamins since they are soluble in aqueous ethanol following interchain disulfide bonds reduction and since; in addition, they are closely related to gliadins in an evolutionary sense.[5] Within glutenins, two fractions are distinguished according to their separation by electrophoresis using polyacrylamide gels containing sodium dodecyl sulfate (SDS PAGE): low and high molecular weight glutenins (LMW and HMW, respectively), whereas gliadins are classified into three structural groups: ω-, γ- and α-gliadin according to their mobility in polyacrylamide gels with an acid pH (A-PAGE) (Figure 2).

Gluten is, therefore, a complex of proteins whose genetic regulation is also intricate. Diploid wheat species contain two closely linked HMW glutenin genes encoded in the *Glu-1* locus on the long arm of chromosome 1, and a group of LMW glutenin genes, also closely linked, encoded by the *Glu-3* locus in short arm of chromosome 1. Gliadins occur in groups of linked genes (blocks) located on the short arm of chromosomes 1 and 6 (Figure 3). Most γ- and ω-gliadins are located in the *Gli-1* locus on the short arm of chromosome 1, near the *Glu-3* locus (LMW glutenin subunits), while the α-gliadins are controlled by the *Gli-2* locus on the short arm of chromosome 6. Other minor loci on the short arm of chromosome 1 regulate some gliadin and LMW glutenin. Each block includes a variable number of genes that are inherited as a locus, making it very difficult to separate one gliadin gene from another, within the same block, by genetic recombination. Since bread wheat possesses three genomes, its complement is three times larger: several hundred different proteins whose genes are inherited in blocks, most of them being gliadins and LMW glutenins.

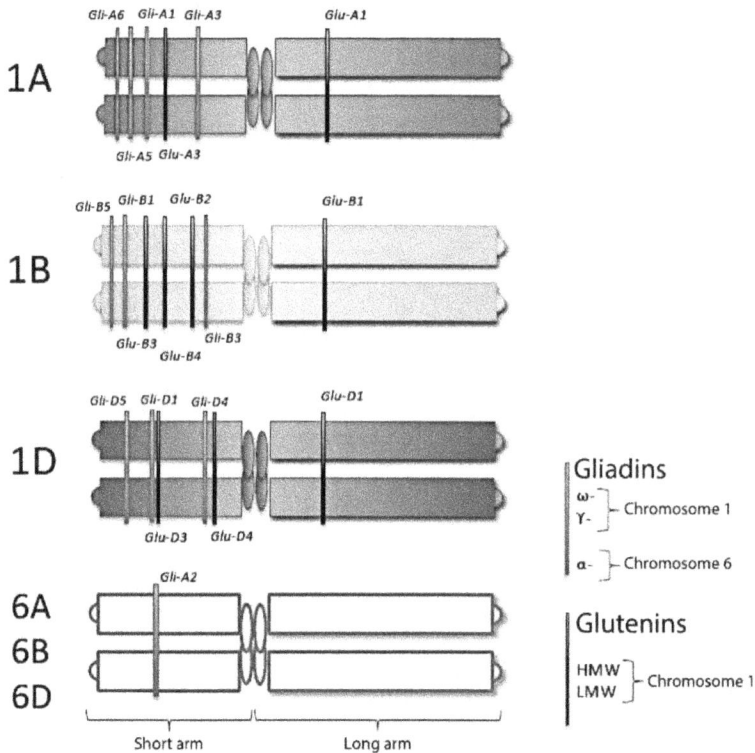

Figure 3. Chromosomal location of glutenin and gliadin loci in hexaploid wheat. The high molecular weight glutenins are located on the long arm of chromosome 1 group. ω- and γ-gliadins are located at various loci on the short arm of chromosome 1 group while the α-gliadins are located on chromosome 6. Low molecular weight glutenins are also located on the short arm of chromosome 1 group, closely linked to the gliadin loci.

4. The Gluten Toxic Fraction

The food codex standard on foodstuffs for special dietary destined for gluten-intolerant persons (CODEX STAN 118-1979) defines gluten as "a protein fraction from wheat, rye, barley, and oats or their crossbred varieties and derivatives the same, to which some people are intolerant and which is insoluble in water and 0.5 M NaCl." Moreover, the same codex defines "prolamins" equating them with "gliadins"; despite this last having been pointed out as incorrect, it had not been corrected in the latest revision of 2008. These definitions of gluten and prolamins can lead to confusion so it is important to make it clear that not all gluten proteins are toxic, and that all those which are toxic are not so to the same extent. The term *gluten* will be used in this chapter to refer to the entire prolamin fraction, not to be confused with the gluten related to food for celiac patients, which actually refers to the toxic portion thereof. The latter will be referred to as *toxic gluten*.

Wheat gluten proteins are rich in the amino acids proline (15%) and glutamine (30%) and have unusually low aspartic and glutamic acid content. The high proline amount is the cause that gluten proteins are digested by gastrointestinal proteases with great difficulty, resulting in relatively large peptides that accumulate in the small intestine.[6] These peptides are the perfect substrate for the glutamine residues deamidation in glutamate mediated by transglutaminase 2 (TG2), fundamental for the creation of the T lymphocyte-stimulating epitopes involved in CD.[7,8]

Gliadins are indubitably the main toxic component in gluten, especially α and γ-gliadins since most (DQ2 or DQ8)-specific CD4+ T lymphocytes[9-11] obtained from small intestinal biopsies from celiac patients seem to recognize this fraction. In recent years, based on their T-lymphocyte stimulation ability, immunotoxic epitopes have been identified in wheat gluten proteins and in other grasses. At the time of the writing of this chapter, and only taking into account bread wheat, in the IEDB epitope database (http://www.iedb.org/) 190 T-lymphocytes stimulating epitopes related to CD can be found. Of these, 94 are caused by α-gliadin molecules, 74 by γ-gliadin, 12 by ω-gliadin, 8 in LMW glutenin and 2 in HMW glutenin. Therefore, the gluten gliadin fraction is by far largely responsible for CD. Since immunogenic epitopes induce the autoimmune response that generates CD, the type and number of epitopes determine the toxicity of each gluten protein variant. A particular peptide, α-gliadin 33-mer (residues 57-89), which is highly resistant to proteolysis, contains 6 epitopes recognized by T lymphocytes, which makes it a major contributor to the gluten immunotoxicity.[12]

5. Are There any Non-Toxic Wheat Varieties?

Gluten confers unique viscoelastic properties to wheat dough, hence the huge variety of foods that can be made. Humankind, in the wheat-domestication process, has been selecting for this trait and at no time has there been a process of genetic selection considering toxicity in relation to CD. However, inside gluten, there is some variability regarding the relative content of each of the prolamin fractions: glutenin and gliadin, specifically, as well as within the species.[13-15] This variability is the reason why 129 different α-gliadin sequences can be found in the GenBank protein database (http://www.ncbi.nlm.nih.gov/genbank/). Seventy-one of these variants were added in 2012. Great efforts are made to find non-toxic or low toxicity variants in wheat as well as in related wild species tracing the presence of T lymphocyte-stimulating epitopes in gliadin gene sequences from different wheat species.[16] Gliadin gene sequence analysis has shown that simple changes in certain amino acids in the peptide toxins would be enough to make them lose their T lymphocyte-stimulatory nature and, since there are non-toxic natural variants of these peptides,[16] genetic selection has been suggested as a tool for obtaining varieties containing non-toxic epitopes.[17] However, due to the close linkage of the genes found in them, recombination within a locus is unlikely, and so far it seems doubtful that by crossbreeding and recombination non-toxic wheat varieties can be obtained. These studies have also found that *Aegilops tauschi* prolamin sequences, donor of one of the three bread wheat genomes (D genome) are richer in immunotoxic epitopes than those of other related species.[18] This could be one of the reasons why bread wheat is more toxic than the durum wheat: the latter lacks the D genome. However, when the gluten content in durum and bread wheat varieties are examined, even though there are differences between varieties,[19] these values are well above the maximum limit allowed for celiac patients (Figure 4). Consequently, gluten toxicity has become more a quantitative than a qualitative issue and the solution is to apply modern biotechnology techniques to develop less toxic wheat varieties, which can be tolerated by celiac patients.

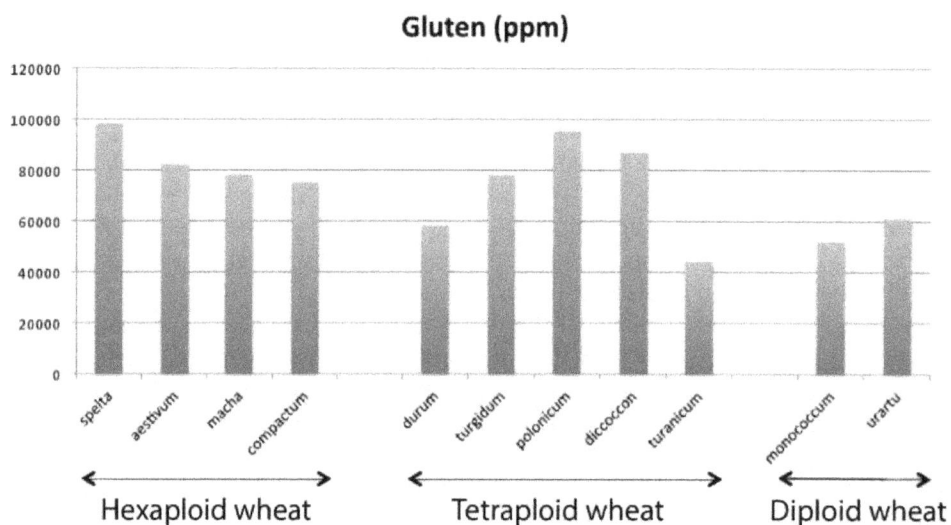

Figure 4. Gluten content in hexaploid, tetraploid and diploid genotypes. Gluten content was determined by ELISA assays with R5 antibodies. The values shown represent the mean of seven lines within each genotype.

6. Development of Wheat Varieties Suitable for Celiac Patients

The low toxic gluten content character is, as we have seen, extremely complex and its genetic regulation is insufficiently known. Biotechnological techniques based on specific gene silencing by RNA interference (RNAi) are the option which, to date, has been better explored. This technique involves a very specific post-transcriptional gene silencing mechanism by which small RNA molecules complementary to messenger RNA (mRNA) lead to its degradation, thereby preventing its translation into proteins.[20,21] The discovery of its mechanism earned researchers Andrew Fire and Craig Mello the Medicine Nobel prize in 2006, and they have already noted the potential this technique would have in medicine, since any gene whose sequence is known may be the target of a tailor-made interfering RNA and therefore, it can be turned off, thereby ending whatever adverse effect it may have.

In principle, the most direct approach is to specifically eliminate gliadin where toxic epitopes have been described, so that new varieties retain their properties for bread making. The use of this specific gliadin silencing technology in wheat grain implies a very precise knowledge of the synthesis of this protein group of in the grain[22] and the use of very specific promoters[22,23] which operate only in the grain, so that the silencing fragment may be successfully synchronized with the gliadin synthesis to be silenced. Thus, the α-gliadins in the "Florida" variety[24] and γ-gliadins in the "Bobwhite" variety (Figure 5)[25] have been successfully silenced. However, the reduction in the content of a specific group of gliadins has not led to varieties with toxicity levels that may be considered suitable for celiac patients (Figure 5B). One of the reasons for this lack of toxicity level reduction may be a prolamin synthesis offset[26] so that the decrease of a specific gliadin group is compensated with proteins from another gliadin group, which also contain toxic epitopes. However, wheat varieties with reduced levels of various toxic fractions could contribute to reducing the gluten burden for the entire population if introduced as parents in breeding programs seeking to obtain "less toxic" varieties by means of crossbreeding, genetic recombination and the selection of genotypes that contains the appropriate silencing.

To prevent this compensatory effect and obtain a more effective toxicity reduction in new wheat varieties, the best option is the use of chimeric RNA interference capable of silencing the genes of the three groups: ω-, γ- and α-gliadin. The construction of an RNAi chimeric fragment involves identifying highly conserved zones in the genes of each of the three gliadin groups and combining said sequences in a single silencing fragment. Gene silencing may be enhanced by using the same silencing fragment and a combination of promoters specific to the grain, but with different expression patterns. This strategy would allow the silencing fragment to run for longer stages of grain development.

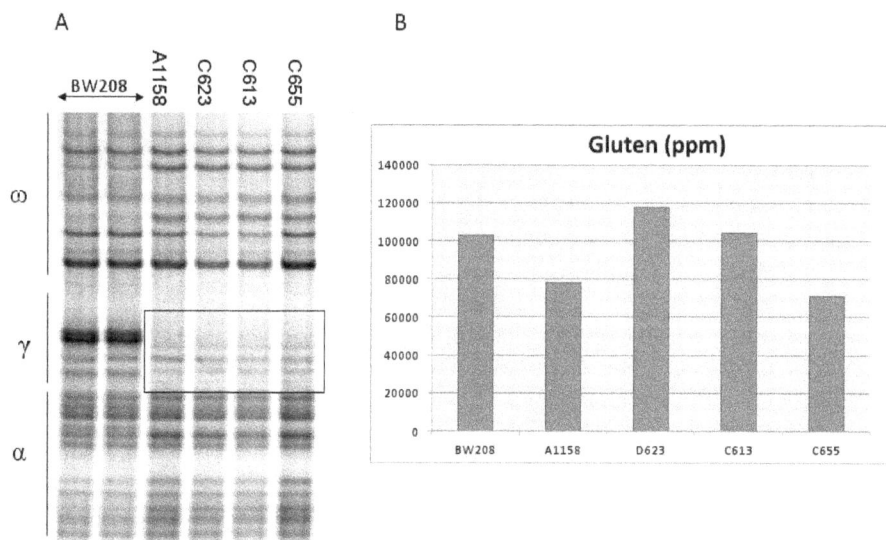

Figure 5. Specific silencing of γ-gliadins in wheat grain. A. The silencing vector expression is highly specific and only reduces γ-gliadin. B. Gluten content, as determined by ELISA R5, in several lines with γ-gliadin silenced.

With this technique we have produced a collection of more than 50 wheat lines of different varieties and, therefore, bearing different gliadin patterns. As shown in Figure 6A, the chimeric fragment used was effective in silencing genes belonging to the three gliadin groups. The use of different promoters apparently enhances the silencing effect and the two promoters used were equally effective in silencing the gliadins.[27] In addition, the chimeric RNAi fragment was also very effective in silencing gliadins from different wheat varieties.[24] The specificity of the RNAi fragment is shown in Figure 6B, showing silencing in the gliadin fraction but not in albumins and globulins. However, the specific gliadin silencing causes a compensating effect on other proteins such as glutenins[27,28] and also on the albumin and globulin fraction[28] so that there are no great differences in the total protein content between the gliadin-free and their respective gliadin-bearing controls.[27] ELISA sandwich quantification using R5 antibodies has shown that in some lines the gluten percentage has decreased by about 98%. Those tested with specific T lymphocytes specific to some particular highly stimulatory epitopes corroborated this data. The results of the quantification of the proliferation of T lymphocytes specific to the DQ2-α-II, DQ8-α-, DQ2-γ-VII and DQ8-γ-I epitopes in response to gluten from silenced lines, digested with pepsin and trypsin, were actually very large.[27] For some of these lines, the protein amounts required were a hundred times greater than those of their respective controls in order to obtain a response in the activation of T lymphocytes that recognize the DQ2-α-II[24] epitope situated in 33 mer, one of most immunotoxic peptides known.[13] The T lymphocyte clones specific for other epitopes (DQ2-γ-VII, DQ8-α-I and DQ8-γ-I) located in γ- and α-gliadins did not exceed the detection level for the highest evaluated protein extract concentrations.[27] Similar results were found with T lymphocyte clones that recognize the highly stimulatory epitopes present in ω-gliadins[29] which showed a very small proliferative response when compared to gliadin-bearing controls.[27]

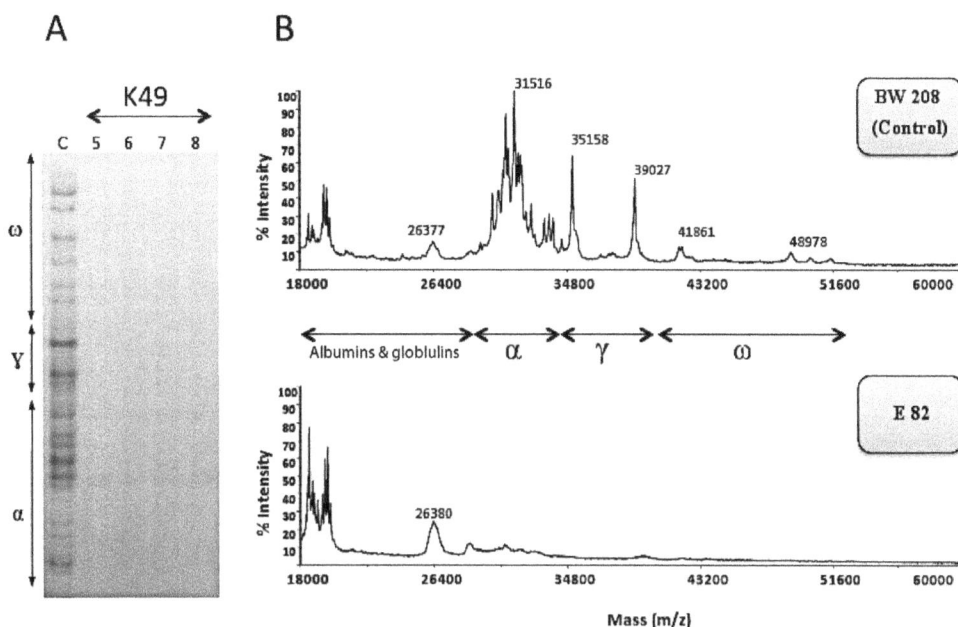

C, control line with gliadins.

Figure 6. RNAi gene silencing in the three gliadin groups. A. A-PAGE gel which shows that the expression of a chimeric RNAi containing highly conserved sequences for the three gliadin groups causes an effective silencing of all gliadins in the grains of bread wheat. B. MALDI-TOF, which shows that silencing is specific for gliadin, while other fractions (such as albumins and globulins) are not reduced.

The wheat varieties described show a reduction in the three gliadin fractions, so that they might be suitable for other gluten related pathologies. For example, exercise-dependent anaphylaxis, which occurs in susceptible individuals after practicing sports, is triggered by genes encoded on the short arm of chromosome 1B of durum and bread wheat genes, ω-5-gliadins. [30,31] In the lines described, this protein fraction is highly reduced, so these flours could help to combat this grave pathology. Gluten sensitivity, a new gluten intolerance disease, which excludes celiac disease and allergy, affects 6% of the U.S. population[32] (whose treatment is a gluten-free diet) and could also benefit from the new varieties described this work.

An important issue is to conserve flour and baking quality in the new varieties without toxic gluten. Ideally, they could be widely used to produce bread and other food products for celiac patients and other gluten intolerances so that their organoleptic properties should be as close to normal wheat bread as possible.

HMW glutenin subunits are functionally very important, as they are the main determinants of gluten elasticity, a property that correlates directly with the baking qualities of flour. The baking quality of the lines was assessed using the SDS sedimentation test, since the obtained sedimentation volumes are correlated to the bread-making qualities. [33] Most of the gliadin-free lines showed SDS sedimentation values comparable to the control lines and only five lines had significantly lower values than the control lines.[24] However, SDS sedimentation values of these five lines are still comparable to those of medium quality bread wheat varieties.

7. Conclusions

To date, various studies indicate that all varieties of cultivated wheat and their wild relatives are toxic and although there are differences between them, they are well above the limit tolerated by celiac patients. RNAi is an excellent tool for the specific silencing of T-cell stimulating-epitopes present in the three gliadin groups. These results are a major breakthrough in achieving wheat varieties suitable for most celiac patients. Moreover, these lines could serve as a basis for treating other gluten related pathologies such as exercise-dependent anaphylaxis and non-celiac gluten sensitivity. The "silencing" can be transferred by crossbreeding with other wheat varieties thus allowing the availability of enough genetic variability for the selection even less toxic lines than those already produced. In the case of the toxicity described for some glutenins, especially those of high molecular weight, varieties that carry nontoxic alleles could easily be selected and be used as parents in breeding programs.

References

1. Dicke WK, Weijers HA, Van De Kamer JH. *Coeliac disease. II. The presence in wheat of a factor having a deleterious effect in cases of coeliac disease.* Acta Paediatr. 1953; 42(1): 34-42. http://dx.doi.org/10.1111/j.1651-2227.1953.tb05563.x

2. FAOSTAT. Enero de 2013. http://faostat.fao.org/site/339/default.aspx

3. Shewry PR, Halford NG. *Cereal seed storage proteins: structures, properties and role in grain utilization.* J Exp Bot. 2002; 53(370): 947-58.
   http://dx.doi.org/10.1093/jexbot/53.370.947

4. Osborne TB. *The proteins of the wheat kernel.* Carnegie institution of Washington, 1907.

5. Shewry PR, Tatham AS, Forde J, Kreis M, Miflin BJ. *The classification and nomenclature of wheat gluten proteins: A reassessment.* J Cereal Sci. 1986; 4(2): 97-106.
   http://dx.doi.org/10.1016/S0733-5210(86)80012-1

6. Wieser H. *The precipitating factor in coeliac disease.* Baillière's Clin Gastroenterology. 1995; 9(2): 191-207. http://dx.doi.org/10.1016/0950-3528(95)90027-6

7. Wal Y van de, Kooy Y, Veelen P van, Peña S, Mearin L, Papadopoulos G, et al. *Cutting Edge: Selective deamidation by tissue transglutaminase strongly enhances gliadin-specific T cell reactivity.* J Immunol. 1998; 161(4): 1585-88.

8. Molberg O, Mcadam SN, Körner R, Quarsten H, Kristiansen C, Madsen L, et al. *Tissue transglutaminase selectively modifies gliadin peptides that are recognized by gut-derived T cells in celiac disease.* Nat Med. 1998; 4(6): 713-17.
   http://dx.doi.org/10.1038/nm0698-713

9. Lundin, KE, Scott H, Hansen T, Paulsen G, Halstensen TS, Fausa O, et al. *Gliadin-specific, HLA-DQ(alpha 1*0501,beta 1*0201) restricted T cells isolated from the small intestinal mucosa of celiac disease patients.* J Exp Med. 1993; 178(1): 187-96.
   http://dx.doi.org/10.1084/jem.178.1.187

10. Lundin KE, Scott H, Fausa O, Thorsby E, Sollid LM. *T cells from the small intestinal mucosa of a DR4, DQ7/DR4, DQ8 celiac disease patient preferentially recognize gliadin when presented by DQ8.* Hum Immunol. 1994; 41(4): 285-91.
    http://dx.doi.org/10.1016/0198-8859(94)90047-7

11. Arentz-Hansen H, Mcadam SN, Molberg Øyvind, Fleckenstein B, Lundin KEA, Jørgensen TJD, et al. *Celiac lesion T cells recognize epitopes that cluster in regions of gliadins rich in proline residues.* Gastroenterology. 2002; 123(3): 803-9.
    http://dx.doi.org/10.1053/gast.2002.35381

12. Shan L, Molberg O, Parrot I, Hausch F, Filiz F, Gray GM, et al. *Structural basis for gluten intolerance in celiac sprue.* Science. 2002; 297(5590): 2275-9.
    http://dx.doi.org/10.1126/science.1074129

13. Wieser H. *Comparative investigations of gluten proteins from different wheat species I. Qualitative and quantitative composition of gluten protein types.* Eur Food Res Technol. 2000; 211(4): 262-8. http://dx.doi.org/10.1007/s002170000165

14. Wieser H, Koehler P. *Is the calculation of the gluten content by multiplying the prolamin content by a factor of 2 valid?* Eur Food Res Technol. 2009; 229(1): 9-13.
    http://dx.doi.org/10.1007/s00217-009-1020-5

15. Žilić S, Barać M, Pešić M, Dodig D, Ignjatović-Micić D. *Characterization of proteins from grain of different bread and durum wheat genotypes.* Int J Mol Sci. 2011; 12(9): 5878-94. http://dx.doi.org/10.3390/ijms12095878

16. Spaenij-Dekking L, Kooy-Winkelaar Y, Van Veelen P, Wouter Drijfhout J, Jonker H, Van Soest L, et al. *Natural variation in toxicity of wheat: potential for selection of nontoxic varieties for celiac disease patients.* Gastroenterology. 2005; 129(3): 797-806. http://dx.doi.org/10.1053/j.gastro.2005.06.017

17. Mitea C, Salentijn EMJ, Van Veelen P, Goryunova SV, Van der Meer IM, Van den Broeck HC, et al. *A universal approach to eliminate antigenic properties of alpha-gliadin peptides in celiac disease.* PLoS One. 2010; 5(12). http://dx.doi.org/10.1371/journal.pone.0015637

18. Xie Z, Wang C, Wang K, Wang S, Li X, Zhang Z, et al. *Molecular characterization of the celiac disease epitope domains in α-gliadin genes in* Aegilops tauschii *and hexaploid wheats* (Triticum aestivum L.). Theor Appl Gene. 2010; 121(7): 1239-51. http://dx.doi.org/10.1007/s00122-010-1384-8

19. Molberg Ø, Uhlen AK, Jensen T, Flæte NS, Fleckenstein B, Arentz-Hansen H, et al. *Mapping of gluten T-cell epitopes in the bread wheat ancestors: Implications for celiac disease.* Gastroenterology. 2005; 128(2): 393-401. http://dx.doi.org/10.1053/j.gastro.2004.11.003

20. Fire A, Xu S, Montgomery MK, Kostas SA, Driver SE, Mello CC. *Potent and specific genetic interference by double-stranded RNA in Caenorhabditis elegans.* Nature. 1998; 391(6669): 806-11. http://dx.doi.org/10.1038/35888

21. Mello CC, Conte D. *Revealing the world of RNA interference.* Nature. 2004; 431(7006): 338-42. http://dx.doi.org/10.1038/nature02872

22. Pistón F, Marín S, Hernando A, Barro F. *Analysis of the activity of a γ-gliadin promoter in transgenic wheat and characterization of gliadin synthesis in wheat by MALDI-TOF during grain development.* Mol Breed. 2009; 23(4):655-67. http://dx.doi.org/10.1007/s11032-009-9263-1

23. Pistón F, León E, Lazzeri PA, Barro F. *Isolation of two storage protein promoters from Hordeum chilense and characterization of their expression patterns in transgenic wheat.* Euphytica. 2008; 162(3): 371-9. ttp://dx.doi.org/10.1007/s10681-007-9530-3

24. Osorio C, Wen N, Gemini R, Zemetra R, Wettstein D von, Rustgi S. *Targeted modification of wheat grain protein to reduce the content of celiac causing epitopes.* Funct Integr Genomics. 2012; 12(3): 417-38. http://dx.doi.org/10.1007/s10142-012-0287-y

25. Gil-Humanes J, Pistón F, Hernando A, Alvarez JB, Shewry PR, Barro F. *Silencing of γ-gliadins by RNA interference (RNAi) in bread wheat.* J Cereal Sci. 2008; 48(3): 565-8. http://dx.doi.org/10.1016/j.jcs.2008.03.005

26. Pistón F, Gil-Humanes J, Rodríguez-Quijano M, Barro F. *Down-regulating γ-gliadins in bread wheat leads to non-specific increases in other gluten proteins and has no major effect on dough gluten strength.* PLoS ONE. 2011; 6(9): e24754. http://dx.doi.org/10.1371/journal.pone.0024754

27. Gil-Humanes J, Pistón F, Tollefsen S, Sollid LM, Barro F. *Effective shutdown in the expression of celiac disease-related wheat gliadin T-cell epitopes by RNA interference.* Proc Natl Acad Sci. USA. 2010; 107(39): 17023-28. http://dx.doi.org/10.1073/pnas.1007773107

28. Gil-Humanes J, Pistón F, Shewry PR, Tosi P, Barro F. *Suppression of gliadins results in altered protein body morphology in wheat.* J Exp Bot. 2011; 62(12): 4203-13. http://dx.doi.org/10.1093/jxb/err119

29. Camarca A, Anderson RP, Mamone G, Fierro O, Facchiano A, Costantini S, et al. *Intestinal T cell responses to gluten peptides are largely heterogeneous: implications for a peptide-based therapy in celiac disease.* J Immunol. 2009; 182(7): 4158-66. http://dx.doi.org/10.4049/jimmunol.0803181

30. Morita E, Matsuo H, Chinuki Y, Takahashi H, Dahlström J, Tanaka A. *Food-dependent exercise-induced anaphylaxis -importance of omega-5 gliadin and HMW-glutenin as causative antigens for wheat-dependent exercise-induced anaphylaxis-.* Allergol Int 2009; 58(4): 493-8. http://dx.doi.org/10.2332/allergolint.09-RAI-0125

31. Palosuo K, Alenius H, Varjonen E, Koivuluhta M, Mikkola J, Keskinen H, et al. *A novel wheat gliadin as a cause of exercise-induced anaphylaxis.* J Allergy Clin Immunol. 1999; 103(5): 912-7. http://dx.doi.org/10.1016/S0091-6749(99)70438-0

32. Sapone A, Lammers KM, Casolaro V, Cammarota M, Giuliano MT, Rosa MD, et al. *Divergence of gut permeability and mucosal immune gene expression in two gluten-associated conditions: celiac disease and gluten sensitivity.* BMC Medicine. 2011; 9(1): 23. http://dx.doi.org/10.1186/1741-7015-9-23

33. Carter BP, Morris CF, Anderson JA. *Optimizing the SDS sedimentation test for end-use quality selection in a soft white and club wheat breeding program.* Cereal Chem. 1999; 76(6): 907-11. http://dx.doi.org/10.1094/CCHEM.1999.76.6.907

Chapter 24

Intestinal Microbiota and Celiac Disease

Moisés Laparra, Marta Olivares, Yolanda Sanz

Microbial Ecology and Nutrition. Agrochemistry and Food Technology Institute. Scientific Investigation Board of Governors (IATA-CSIC). Valencia, Spain.

mlaparra@iata.csic.es, m.olivares@iata.csic.es, yolsanz@iata.csic.es

Doi: http://dx.doi.org/10.3926/oms.230

How to cite this chapter

Laparra M, Olivares M, Sanz Y. *Intestinal Microbiota and Celiac Disease.* In Rodrigo L and Peña AS, editors. *Celiac Disease and Non-Celiac Gluten Sensitivity.* Barcelona, Spain: OmniaScience; 2014. p. 477-494.

Abstract

Intestinal microbiota is considered to perform important metabolic and immunologic functions, which affect the host's health and disease risk. Evidence from epidemiologic studies suggests that environmental factors influencing the intestinal ecosystem, such breast-feeding practices and incidence of gastrointestinal infections, can also contribute to the risk of developing celiac disease (CD). Breast-feeding seems to exert a protective role against CD and it also favors bifidobacteria colonization in the infant's gut. Colonization of the newborn intestine is considered a critical stimulus for the adequate development of immune and intestinal barrier functions, modulating host protection mechanisms against allergens and pathogens. Observational studies indicate that gut colonization patterns of infants at genetic risk of developing CD differ from those of non-risk infants, which could also influence CD development. Imbalances in the gut microbiota of CD patients in comparison to healthy controls have also been reported in several observational studies. It is hypothesized that these alterations and specific bacteria isolated from patients could contribute to CD pathogenesis by activation of the pro-inflammatory Th$_1$-type response typical of the disease according to *in vitro* and animal studies. Therefore, dietary interventions based on the use of probiotics are being considered as potential adjuvants and preventive strategies to control the disease, as well as to improve quality of life of CD patients. These strategies could theoretically contribute to restoring the intestinal ecosystem, thereby ameliorating the severity of CD pathological manifestations and to developing a gluten-tolerant phenotype in subjects at risk via different mechanisms.

1. Introduction

Celiac disease (CD) is a chronic autoimmune enteropathy, caused by an intolerance to gluten proteins in cereals, including wheat, barley, rye and possibly oats, that causes severe functional and morphological alterations of the small intestinal mucosa. Typical cases of this disease usually occur in the first years of life, frequently manifested with gastrointestinal symptoms; however, extra-intestinal or atypical manifestations are increasingly more frequent, especially later in life. CD is also associated with other immune-based diseases such as dermatitis herpetiformis, IgA deficiency, diabetes mellitus type I, thyroiditis and autoimmune hepatitis.[1,2]

Genetic and environmental factors (mainly gluten) play a role in this pathology; however, other variables such as breastfeeding practices, incidence of gastrointestinal infections and intestinal microbiota composition could also be involved, as outlined in Figure 1.[3-5] Genetic susceptibility to CD is determined by the specific class II major histocompatibility complex (MHC) HLA-DQ encoding HLA-DQ2 or HLA-DQ8 heterodimers involved in antigen presentation. Most of celiac patients express HLA-DQ2/DQ8 molecules, indicating that it is a necessary factor for the disease development; however, these risk factors are also present in 30% of the general population and only a low percentage develops CD, indicating that their presence is not sufficient for the disease to become manifest. Studies on twins have also shown that in 25% of cases one twin does not develop CD,[6] indicating that other environmental factors besides genotype are also involved in the development of this disease.

In recent years imbalances in the intestinal microbiota composition of CD patients and in individuals at risk have been detected.[3,7,8] The colonization process in the early stages of life and the interaction between intestinal microbiota and the innate and adaptive immune systems in different stages of life could be crucial for the development of oral tolerance to gluten proteins and to determine the risk and severity of this pathology.

Currently, the only treatment for CD is a strict, lifelong gluten-free diet. Although symptoms usually resolve after following this dietary strategy, its maintenance is difficult due to the presence of gluten in most processed foods. In addition, a percentage (3-5 %) of patients have refractory CD and do not respond to this dietary pattern (reviewed by Mooney et al.[9]). This increases the need for developing additional preventive and therapeutic strategies to the gluten-free diet. Among these, we could include the use of proteolytic enzymes that hydrolyze the ingested gluten, intestinal permeability modulators and peptide-based vaccines with specificity for HLA-DQ2 molecules that facilitate desensitization to gluten as well as nutritional intervention based strategies, including food ingredients with immunomodulatory properties and a positive influence on the intestinal barrier function.[10]

2. Intestinal Microbiota, Breastfeeding and HLA-DQ Genotype

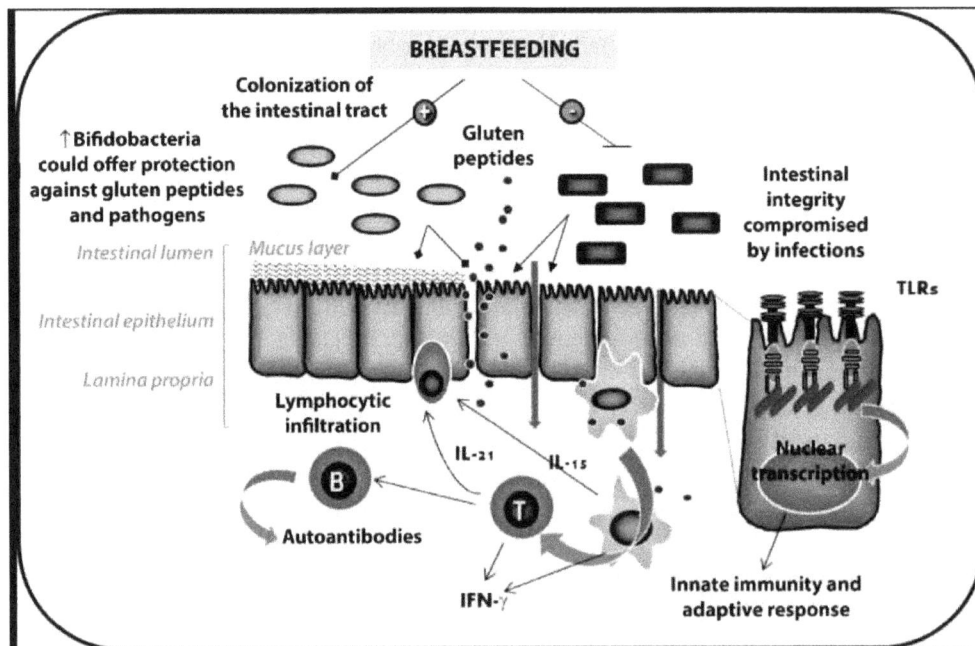

Figure 1. Influence of breastfeeding and intestinal microbiota on celiac disease pathogenesis.

Among the environmental factors related to CD etiology, besides gluten intake, we can include breastfeeding practices, timing of dietary gluten introduction, the incidence of infections and intestinal microbiota composition.[3,11,12] Epidemiological studies indicate that breastfeeding may have a protective effect against the development of CD.[13] Several studies have identified the presence of microorganisms and prebiotic oligosaccharides in breast milk and have described its effect on the composition of the infant gut microbiota and on the immune system modulation, which could also influence the risk for certain diseases (reviewed in Fernández et al.[14]). In breast-fed children, bifidobacteria dominate the intestinal microbiota, while artificial feeding promotes the colonization of a more heterogeneous microbiota which is similar to that of the adult population.[15,16] Furthermore, the comparative analysis of stool samples from twins, adults and children with different kinship degrees has led to the conclusion that genotype also affects the intestinal microbiota composition.[17-20] Toivanen et al.[21] pointed out that certain MCH genes might be involved in differences in fecal microbiota observed in mice with different genetic backgrounds.

In the context of CD, a prospective study of a cohort of new-borns with CD risk due to their family history using real-time PCR showed that both the type of breastfeeding as well as the HLA-DQ genotype influence the intestinal colonization process.[4,22] In children with a high risk disease, irrespective of breastfeeding practices, a reduction was observed in the number of *Bifidobacterium* spp. and in the species *B. longum*; however, breastfeeding attenuated the differences and favored colonization by species of this genus. An increase in the number of *Staphylococcus* spp. associated with increased genetic risk in infants fed with maternal and artificial formula was also observed. Furthermore, an increase was detected in the number of *B. fragilis* groups associated with genetic risk but only in children fed with formula.[4] In a subset of this cohort, colonization by species of the genus *Bacteroides* was also assessed using DGGE and showed that species diversity was higher in artificially fed infants than in breastfed infants.[22] Prevalence analysis, considering only the feeding type, showed that the intestinal microbiota of formula-fed infants was characterized by the presence of *B. intestinalis* and those who had been breast-fed by the presence of *B. uniformis*. Furthermore, analysis as a function of the genotype showed greater species diversity in low-risk infants than in the high-risk ones and increased prevalence of the *B. vulgatus* and *B. uniformis* in high and low risk infants, respectively. When considering the feeding type and genetic risk variables together, it was concluded that the prevalence of *B. uniformis* characterized the intestinal microbiota of children at low genetic risk and was favored by breastfeeding. Overall, it was observed that breastfeeding attenuated microbiota differences related to genotype, which could partly explain the protective effect that has been attributed to breastfeeding on the development of CD.

3. Infections and Celiac Disease

Some epidemiological studies have linked the incidence of infection of bacterial or viral origin, with the risk of CD. Several hypotheses have been proposed to explain the association between the incidence infections and CD, including the similarity between the bacterial or viral antigens and immunogenic gliadin peptides that could cause a similar reaction, and an over-stimulation of the immune system secondary to an infection with production of inflammatory cytokines such as TNF-α, INF-γ or IL-15 (reviewed in Jabri and Sollid[23]).

A study performed in Switzerland, which analyzed perinatal data from more than three thousand children who had developed CD showed that the main risk factor for its occurrence had been exposure to infections during the neonatal stage.[24] A subsequent study focused on establishing an association through serum level differences in antibodies to some infectious agents between healthy individuals and celiac patients. The results showed a lower IgG antibody prevalence in celiac patients, suggesting that infections by the three tested viruses (rubella, cytomegalovirus and Epstein-Barr virus) could exert a protective effect on the development of CD.[12]

Kagnoff et al.[25] proposed that the emergence of CD could be triggered by a type-12 adenovirus infection due to the similarity alpha-gliadin exhibits with this virus' E1d protein. The detection of an increase in IgG antibodies against the E1d protein in the sera of children with CD compared to the levels in the control group, seemed to support this hypothesis.[26] However, other studies have come to conflicting conclusions. Thus, Howdle et al.[27] found no difference in the serum levels of this protein between celiac patients and controls. Another infectious agent, which has been associated with CD in epidemiological studies, is hepatitis C. This association was based on the fact that the incidence of chronic liver diseases is 15 times higher in CD patients than in the non-celiac population[28], and in 5% of the cases, the onset of autoimmune liver diseases are accompanied by CD.[29] However, even though this virus is considered to be able to trigger secondary autoimmune processes, studies do not indicate an increase in CD in hepatitis C patients[30] and the association might simply be casual.[31] A prospective study of 1931 children with the CD risk genotype indicated that a higher rotavirus infection incidence (based on detection of positive serum antibodies against this pathogen), increased the risk of the disease. Similarly, studies associated CD with *Campylobacter jejuni*[32] and *Giardia lamblia*[33] infections in individual case studies. These observations seem to suggest the possible involvement of gastrointestinal infections in triggering CD, through increased intestinal permeability or amplification of the immune response to gluten peptides.

4. Intestinal Microbiota in Celiac Disease Patients

In recent years alterations in the intestinal microbiota composition of biopsies and feces from children and adults with CD have been detected compared to those of controls.[7,8,34] Microbiological analysis of duodenal biopsies by *in situ* hybridization techniques and flow cytometry showed that the ratio of Gram-positive to Gram-negative bacteria in CD patients, at the time of diagnosis and after treatment with a gluten-free diet for at least 2 years, was inferior than that detected in control individuals, as well as the ratio of potentially beneficial bacteria (*Bifidobacterium* + *Lactobacillus*) to potentially harmful ones (*E. coli* + *Bacteroides*).[7] Analyses by real-time PCR, have shown that the number of *Bacteroides* spp. in the duodenal and fecal microbiota of CD patients (treated or not with the gluten-free diet) was higher than those detected in control individuals.[34] The number of *E. coli* and *Staphylococcus* spp. was also higher in untreated patients compared to controls, but their concentrations were normalized after following a gluten-free diet. *Bifidobacterium* spp. and *B. longum* concentrations in CD patients' feces and biopsies were lower than in controls, although the differences between biopsies were statistically significant only between patients at the time of diagnosis and controls.[8]

Analysis of phylogenetic groups and gene prevalence associated with virulence factors in isolated enterobacteria from stools of CD patients and healthy children have also shown significant differences.[35] Analysis of phylogenetic groups (A, B, C and D) of *E. coli* clones showed that the control group had no differences in their proportion, while in the two groups of children with CD commensal isolates (A and B1) belonged mainly to phylogenetic group A. The virulent clone distribution represented by phylogenetic groups B2 and D, also exhibited differences between the two groups of children with CD; isolates of the group B2 were more abundant in patients with active CD and isolates of the group D were more abundant in CD patients treated with the gluten-free diet. Other authors also described an increased prevalence of virulent phylogenetic groups, especially the group B, in patients with Crohn's disease and ulcerative colitis.[36] In addition; *E. coli* clones belonging to virulent phylogenetic groups (B2 and D) from children with CD in active and non-active phases carried higher numbers of genes encoding virulence factors than those isolated from the control group. The prevalence of genes encoding for *P fimbriae*, K5 capsule and hemolysin was significantly higher in both CD patient groups than in healthy children. These results suggest that the enteric microbiota of CD patients have a higher pathogenic potential than in healthy subjects, which could favor the disease development or aggravate the disease symptoms.[35] Analysis of *Staphylococcus* isolates in a selective culture medium has also shown that children with CD, treated and untreated with a gluten-free diet, have greater *Staphylococcus epidermis* abundance with methicillin resistance genes, which is one of the main pathogens involved in nosocomial infections.[37] Finally, analysis of isolates from the genus *Bacteroides* has allowed detecting an increase in the species *B. fragilis*, which produces metalloproteases and is involved in opportunistic infections, in treated and untreated celiac patients compared with healthy subjects.[38]

Overall, these studies indicate that there are imbalances in the composition of the intestinal microbiota of CD patients compared with controls; the fact that these alterations are only partially restored after adherence to a gluten-free diet indicates that they are not only a secondary consequence the inflammatory process associated with active phase of the disease and it could play a greater role in its etiology and pathogenesis.

5. Pathogenic Mechanisms of gut microbiota

Oral tolerance to food components is a biologically complex process resulting from the interaction between environmental and individual genetic factors and that may depend on age, dose and postnatal antigen contact period, antigenic composition and structure, intestinal barrier integrity and degree of mucosal immune activation.[39,40] The mechanisms by which intestinal microbiota alterations could contribute to the etiology and pathogenesis of CD include (i) alterations of the microbiota interaction with epithelial and immunocompetent cells leading to activation of signaling mechanisms and inflammation mediators, (ii) alteration of the microbiota's ability to degrade or reduce the glycocalyx and secreted mucus that will influence the intestinal epithelium's barrier properties and (iii) the possible translocation of potentially pathogenic bacteria or derived molecules to the lamina propria.[41,42]

In situ studies of rat intestinal loops show that the presence of potentially pathogenic bacteria (*E. coli* CBL2) or real pathogens (*Shigella*) aggravates the intestinal permeability alterations caused by gliadins and facilitates their translocation to the lamina propria.[43] Under physiological conditions, the intestinal epithelium is a nearly impermeable barrier to macromolecules; however, CD is associated with an increased intestinal permeability[44], which facilitates access of gliadin-derived peptides to the lamina propria and their interaction with the components responsible for the immune response. Gliadins, as it is the case for some pathogens, cause alterations in intercellular tight-junction-related proteins and re-organization of different molecular components (zonulin, occludin, cadherin and claudins).[45] The re-organization of the tight-junction related proteins and the increased paracellular permeability occurs along with the inflammatory response characterized by the production of cytokines such as tumor necrosis factor α (TNF) and interleukin 1 β (IL-1β). They have an important function in further promoting increased intestinal permeability and lymphocyte infiltration[46,47] and activation of the nuclear factor kappa-B (NfkB) pathway.

The influence of the host genotype and the microbiota on the intestinal epithelium glycocalyx composition has also been considered to be a possible pathogenesis mechanism in the context of CD. The intestinal epithelium glycocalyx has an important role in preventing direct contact of ingested compounds and intestinal pathogens with epithelial cells.[43] Previous studies have demonstrated alterations in the rate and/or composition of glycoconjugates, which compose the glycocalyx and mucus layer in CD patients.[49] CD patients have a high proportion of D-galactose and α (1,2)-fucose residues, while these residues are not found in the mucosa of healthy individuals[49], who do have β-gal(1→3)galNAc residues.[50] Thus, it has been suggested that particular glycosylation patterns could promote the adhesion and colonization of a specific microbiota and pathogens. However, it has also been postulated that these changes in glycosylation patterns could be induced by alterations in the intestinal microbiota. Several studies have shown changes in the fucosylation and/or galactosylation patterns of different intestinal epithelium glycoconjugates in diverse animal models as a function of gut colonization.[51-53] However, there is a lack of studies concerning the particular role of host genotype and microbiota composition in glycosylation patterns and CD risk.

The mucus layer secreted into the luminal medium constitutes a physical barrier for dietary antigens and for intestinal commensal and pathogenic bacteria. This barrier depends largely on the mucus composition in different mucines.[41,42] Ex vivo studies have demonstrated higher expression levels (mRNA) of type 2 mucin (MUC2) in CD patient biopsies compared to biopsies from treated CD patients.[50] MUC2 biosynthesis and secretion is a process that has been associated with a possible bodily defense mechanism against infections by intestinal pathogens[54,55], which also limits the proportion of commensals being in contact with the epithelial mucosa.[55] However, the increased MUC2 expression in CD patients has also been associated with globet cell metaplasia[50] related intestinal mucosa atrophy and damage.[56] In rat intestinal loops it has been shown that gliadins reduce the number of mucus-producing cells and that this reduction is even more pronounced in the presence of intestinal pathogens (Shigella CBD8) and potential pathogens (E. coli CBL2).[43]

It has also been proposed that intestinal dysbiosis detected in individuals with CD may result from an alteration in the host's antimicrobial peptide production, such as defensins (HD5 and HD6).[50] However, another study conducted in adults with CD treated with a gluten-free diet demonstrated a lower HD1 expression in duodenal biopsies, while that of HD2, -3 and -4 did not show significant changes.[57] Defensin production is essential in host defense mechanisms and modulates the intestinal ecosystem composition.[58,59] These peptides are produced in response to bacterial antigens such as Gram-negative bacteria lipopolysaccharide (LPS) and Gram-positive peptidoglycan (muramyl dipeptide).[60] Although in CD patients fewer defensin-encoding gene copies have been detected, this is not always related to a reduction in the final production of active peptides.[61]

Toll like receptors (TLRs) have a crucial role during the development of the innate immune response to environmental antigens as well as in the discrimination between commensal bacteria and intestinal pathogens.[62] The stimulation of different TLRs activate signaling pathways and regulate the expression of various genes and inflammatory cytokines conferring them a critical role in the activation and severity of the innate immune response. The response to these stimuli appears to be associated with the interaction of histocompatibility molecules (MHC-II) contributing to the maturation of T "helper" lymphocytes.[63] Recent studies have suggested the involvement of TLRs in CD.[64-66] In these studies, an increased TLR2[64-66] and TLR9[65] expression is reported, while the effects on TLR4 expression are more controversial.[64-66] In no case significant alterations have been reported in expression of TLR3[65,66] (activated by viral RNA) and/or TLR5[65] (activated by bacterial flagellin). However, recent in vivo studies have demonstrated the critical role of IFN-α/β production in the activation and maturation of T CD4+ and CD8+ cells, in the initial stages of viral infections.[67] An increased TLR2 and TLR4 expression has also been detected on dendritic cells and monocytes of children with CD even after treatment with a gluten-free diet.[68] Several studies seem to suggest that molecular signaling through these receptors, mediated by interactions with bacterial components such as LPS from Gram-negative bacteria, may contribute to the activation and severity of the innate immune response in CD and to the enteropathy. Further, various components of the TLR family associated with the MyD88 molecular signaling pathway, are potent inducers of type I IFN production with subsequent activation of other inflammatory inducible genes in response to microbial and/or viral stimuli.[69] This interaction could contribute to the T cell-mediated immune response.[70] Besides, diverse pro-inflammatory cytokines such as IL-6, TNFα and IFN may promote the development of autoimmune processes.[71]

The possible influence of alterations in the intestinal microbiota composition on the inflammatory process typical of CD has been evaluated through *in vitro* studies.[72] In this study it was found that the fecal microbiota of CD patients induced an increased *in vitro* production of inflammatory cytokines in peripheral blood mononuclear cells (PBMCs) than that of healthy subject, which could contribute to the development of the Th1 type cytokine profile characteristic of CD. Subsequent studies confirmed that enterobacteria (*E. coli* CBL2 and *Shigella* CBD8), isolated from CD patient feces could trigger IL-12 and/or IFN-γ secretion associated with an increase in HLA-DR and CD40 molecule expression in PBMCs.[73] These results suggest that certain components of the altered microbiota of CD patients could contribute, together with gluten peptides, to the inflammatory process of CD. Using an intestinal loop animal model, co-inoculation of *E. coli* CBL2, gliadins and IFN-γ reduced the production of metalloproteinases inhibitor (TIMP-1) and an increased vascular endothelial growth factor secretion (VEGF).[73] In addition, recent *in vitro* studies suggest a potential role for different *Bacteroides fragilis* strains, which exhibit virulence factors that may favor epithelial permeability alteration and contribute to the production of potentially inflammatory peptides from gliadins, in CD.[38]

In general, existing scientific evidence suggests partial convergence of the pathogenic mechanism of action of gluten peptides and of potential pathogenic intestinal bacteria in CD, which could aggravate the inflammatory response and the intestinal permeability alteration.

6. Potential Probiotic Protection Mechanisms

Based on established associations between CD and intestinal dysbiosis, the possibility of using intervention strategies in the intestinal ecosystem, based on administration of probiotics[3,74] has been suggested for health restoration and for reducing the risk of disease in these patients. Probiotics are defined as live microorganisms which, when administered in adequate amounts, exert a beneficial effect on the host.[75] Among the probiotic mechanisms that could contribute to the acquisition of oral tolerance to dietary antigens, to reducing the severity of CD manifestation, and to health recovery in diagnosed patients, we can include the immunomodulatory effects and the ability to hydrolyze and reduce the toxicity of gliadin-derived peptides, to improve intestinal barrier function and restore intestinal microbiota composition.

Comparative studies of germ-free and conventional animals suggest that gut colonization by microbiota is necessary for the proper development of mucosal and systemic immune responses, such as the production of immunoglobulins and antigens.[76] Studies on some probiotic strains indicate that they have an important role in various processes that depend directly on mucosa-associated lymphoid tissue, such as oral tolerance to environmental antigens and to the commensal microbiota and the release of chemokines and cytokines that determines the balance of Th1/Th2 lymphocyte populations.[77] Besides, they can also participate in the innate response through their interaction with TLRs expressed by epithelial cells and antigen-presenting cells. Within the CD context, studies that evaluate the immunomodulatory capacity of probiotic strains or potentially beneficial bacteria are relatively scarce.[74,78-80] The transgenic mouse model expressing HLA-DQ8 molecules, sensitized with gliadin and adyuvant[74,78,79] that develops a characteristic Th1 cellular response although without intestinal mucosa damage, has been used to assess the effect of different *Lactobacillus* species (*L. paracasei, L. fermentum* and *L. casei*) and *Bifidobacterium lacti*s. These studies have shown that strains of these species have an activating rather than a suppressive effect on the innate and adaptive immune responses. It has been shown that these lactobacilli favor maturation of the immature bone marrow dendritic cells isolated from these animals *in vitro* and that some of the strains also favor TNF-α production upon gliadin stimulation in both *ex vivo* and *in vivo* experiments.[79] In addition, *L. casei* administration to sensitized animals potentiated the CD4+ T cell response against gliadins. In this context, it has been suggested that the strain *L. casei* ATCC 9595 could be used as a vaccine adjuvant for promoting cellular immune response.[78] In another study, the administration of the strain *Bifidobacterium longum* CECT 7347 to lactating rats sensitized with IFN-γ intraperitoneally and fed with gliadin,[80] led to partial enteropathy reproduction.[80,81] In this model, bifidobacteria administration resulted in a lower systemic proportion of CD4+ cells and CD4+Foxp3+ (regulatory T cells) and reduced the TNF-α production and increased IL-10 production in the small intestine compared to the disease model fed with placebo. IL-10 production plays a key role in modulating the cellular response triggered by gliadins, reducing IFN-γ production and antigen-specific cellular proliferation and inducing regulatory T cells.[82,83]

In this respect, *in vitro* studies also showed that different bifidobacterial strains (*B. longum* CECT 7347 and *B. bifidum* CECT 7365) have a positive effect favoring IL-10 production and inhibiting IFN-γ in PBMCs.[72] Subsequent *in vivo* studies with an animal intestinal loop model showed that *B. bifidum* CECT 7365 promotes the proliferation of globet mucus-producing cells, whose numbers are reduced by increased IFN-γ secretion in the context of CD.[43] In addition, bifidobacteria and IFN-γ co-administration caused no observable adverse effects regarding the zonulin-1 expression and increased chemotactic factors (MCP-1) and metalloproteinase (TIMP-1) inhibitors production, reducing the tissue damage caused by IFN-γ. On the other hand, *in vitro* studies have shown that the strain *B. longum* CECT 7347 is capable of increasing the gliadin digestion degree leading to the generation of peptide patterns with a lower inflammatory potential during gastrointestinal digestion.[84] Other studies have also shown that different species of the genus Rothia, mainly present in the oral cavity, have proteolytic activity on gliadins, but their possible *in vivo* effect is unknown.[85,86]

The immunomodulating potential of some probiotics has also been demonstrated in other inflammatory and autoimmune pathologies. In mice which reproduce an experimental colitis model it has been demonstrated that some probiotic strains, able to induce *in vitro* an increased IL-10 production and a reduced IL-12 production, exert an *in vivo* protective effect against colitis.[87] Likewise, the positive effects of the probiotic product VSL#3 on an autoimmune diabetic mouse model have been demostrated.[88] In humans, certain probiotics have also demonstrated their utility in pouchitis remission, although their efficacy is debatable in patients with ulcerative colitis and especially with Crohn's disease.[89]

In the context of CD, studies performed *in vitro* and in experimental animal models suggest that strains such as *B. longum* CECT 7347 could exert protective effects favoring anti-inflammatory and regulatory cytokine synthesis, reducing gliadin-mediated inflammatory and toxic response and microbiota alterations; however, human studies with an adequate experimental design are needed to assess the efficacy that the bacterium evaluated in pre-clinical tests may confer to the patients.

Acknowledgments

This study has been financed by the AGL2011-25169 project and Consolider Fun-C-Food CSD2007-00063 of the Spanish Economy and Competitivity Ministry. M. Laparra has a postdoctoral contract from CSIC y M. Olivares a postdoctoral scholarship from CSIC.

References

1. Setty M, Hormaza L, Guandalini S. *Celiac disease: risk assessment, diagnosis, and monitoring.* Mol Diagn Ther. 2008; 12(5): 289-98.
   http://dx.doi.org/10.1007/BF03256294

2. Schuppan D, Junker Y, Barisani D. *Celiac disease: from pathogenesis to novel therapies.* Gastroenterology. 2009; 137(6): 1912-33.
   http://dx.doi.org/10.1053/j.gastro.2009.09.008

3. Sanz Y, De Palma G, Laparra M. *Unraveling the ties between celiac disease and intestinal microbiota.* Int Rev Immunol. 2011; 30(4): 207-18.
   http://dx.doi.org/10.3109/08830185.2011.599084

4. De Palma G, Capilla A, Nova E, Castillejo G, Varea V, Pozo T et al. *Influence of milk-feeding type and genetic risk of developing coeliac disease on intestinal microbiota of infants: the PROFICEL study.* PLoS One. 2012; 7(2): e30791.
   http://dx.doi.org/10.1371/journal.pone.0030791

5. Pozo-Rubio T, Capilla A, Mujico JR, De Palma G, Marcos A, Sanz Y et al. *Influence of breastfeeding versus formula feeding on lymphocyte subsets in infants at risk of coeliac disease: the PROFICEL study.* Eur J Nutr. 2012; Doi: 10.1007/s00394-012-0367-8.
   http://dx.doi.org/10.1007/s00394-012-0367-8

6. Greco L, Romino R, Coto I, Di Cosmo N, Percopo S, Maglio M et al. *The first large population based twin study of coeliac disease.* Gut. 2002; 50: 624-8.
   http://dx.doi.org/10.1136/gut.50.5.624

7. Nadal I, Donat E, Ribes-Koninckx C, Calabuig M, Sanz Y. *Imbalance in the composition of the duodenal microbiota of children with coeliac disease.* J Med Microbiol. 2007; 56: 1669-74. http://dx.doi.org/10.1099/jmm.0.47410-0

8. Collado MC, Donat E, Ribes-Koninckx C, Calabuig M, Sanz Y. *Imbalances in faecal and duodenal* Bifidobacterium *species composition in active and non-active coeliac disease.* BMC Microbiol. 2008; 8: 232. http://dx.doi.org/10.1186/1471-2180-8-232

9. Mooney PD, Evans KE, Singh S, Sanders DS. *Treatment failure in coeliac disease: a practical guide to investigation and treatment of non-responsive and refractory coeliac disease.* J Gastrointest Liver Dis. 2012; 21(2): 197-203.

10. Sanz Y. *Novel perspectives in celiac disease therapy.* Mini-Rev Med Chem. 2009; 9(3): 359-67. http://dx.doi.org/10.2174/138955751090903035 9

11. Sollid LM. *Coeliac disease: dissecting a complex inflammatory disorder.* Nat Rev Immunol. 2002; 2(9): 647-55. http://dx.doi.org/10.1038/nri885

12. Plot L, Amital H, Barzilai O, Ram M, Nicola B, Shoenfeld Y. *Infections may have a protective role in the etiopathogenesis of celiac disease.* Ann N Y Acad Sci. 2009; 1173: 670-84. http://dx.doi.org/10.1111/j.1749-6632.2009.04814.x

13. Persson LA, Ivarsson A, Hernell O. *Breast-feeding protects against celiac disease in childhood epidemiological evidence.* Adv Exp Med Biol. 2002; 503: 115-23.
    http://dx.doi.org/10.1007/978-1-4615-0559-4_13

14. Fernández L, Langa S, Martín V, Maldonado A, Jiménez E, Martín R et al. *The human milk microbiota: Origin and potential roles in health and disease.* Pharmacol Res. 2012;
    http://dx.doi.org/10.1016/j.phrs.2012.09.001

15. Salminen S, Isolauri E. *Intestinal colonization, microbiota, and prebiotics.* J Pediatr. 2006; 149: S115-20. http://dx.doi.org/10.1016/j.jpeds.2006.06.062

16. Bezirtzoglou E, Tsiotsias A, Welling GW. *Microbiota profile in feces of breast- and formula-fed newborns by using fluorescence in situ hybridization (FISH).* Anaerobe. 2011; 17(6): 478-82. http://dx.doi.org/10.1016/j.anaerobe.2011.03.009

17. Van de Merwe JP, Stegeman JH, Hazenberg MP. *The resident faecal flora is determined by genetic characteristics of the host. Implications for Crohn's disease?* Antonie Van Leeuwenhoek. 1983; 49(2): 119-24. http://dx.doi.org/10.1007/BF00393669

18. Zoetendal EG, Akkermans ADL, Akkermans-van Vliet WM, de Visser JAGM, de Vos WM. *The Host Genotype Affects the Bacterial Community in the Human Gastrointestinal Tract.* Microb Ecol Health Dis. 2001; 13(3): 129-34.
http://dx.doi.org/10.1080/089106001750462669

19. Stewart JA, Chadwick VS, Murray A. *Investigations into the influence of host genetics on the predominant eubacteria in the faecal microflora of children.* J Med Microbiol. 2005; 54: 1239-42. http://dx.doi.org/10.1099/jmm.0.46189-0

20. Palmer C. Bik EM, DiGiulio DB, Relman DA, Brown PO. *Development of the Human Infant Intestinal Microbiota.* PLoS Biol. 2007; 5(7): e177.
http://dx.doi.org/10.1371/journal.pbio.0050177

21. Toivanen P, Vaahtovuo J, Eerola E. *Influence of major histocompatibility complex on bacterial composition of fecal flora.* Infect Immun. 2001; 69(4): 2372-7.
http://dx.doi.org/10.1128/IAI.69.4.2372-2377.2001

22. Sánchez E, De Palma G, Capilla A, Nova E, Pozo T, Castillejo G et al. *Influence of environmental and genetic factors linked to celiac disease risk on infant gut colonization b y Bacteroides species.* Appl Environ Microbiol. 2011; 77(15): 5316-23.
http://dx.doi.org/10.1128/AEM.00365-11

23. Jabri B, Sollid LM. *Tissue-mediated control of immunopathology in coeliac disease.* Nat Rev Immunol. 2009; 9(12): 858-70. http://dx.doi.org/10.1038/nri2670

24. Sandberg-Bennich S, Dahlquist G, Källén B. *Coeliac disease is associated with intrauterine growth and neonatal infections.* Acta Paediatr. 2002; 91(1): 30-3.
http://dx.doi.org/10.1111/j.1651-2227.2002.tb01635.x

25. Kagnoff MF, Paterson YJ, Kumar PJ, Kasarda DD, Carbone FR, Unsworth DJ et al. *Evidence for the role of a human intestinal adenovirus in the pathogenesis of coeliac disease.* Gut. 1987; 28(8): 995-1001. http://dx.doi.org/10.1136/gut.28.8.995

26. Lähdeaho ML, Lehtinen M, Rissa HR, Hyöty H, Reunala T, Mäki M. *Antipeptide antibodies to adenovirus E1b protein indicate enhanced risk of celiac disease and dermatitis herpetiformis.* Int Arch Allergy Immunol. 1993; 101(3): 272-86.
http://dx.doi.org/10.1159/000236457

27. Howdle PD, Blair Zajdel ME, Smart CJ, Trejdosiewicz LK, Blair GE, Losowky MS. *Lack of a serologic response to an E1B protein of adenovirus 12 in coeliac disease.* Scand J Gastroenterol. 1989; 24(3): 282-96. ttp://dx.doi.org/10.3109/00365528909093047

28. Lindgren S, Sjöberg K, Eriksson S. *Unsuspected coeliac disease in chronic "cryptogenic" liver disease.* Scand J Gastroenterol. 1994; 29(7): 661-74.
http://dx.doi.org/10.3109/00365529409092489

29. Volta U, De Franceschi L, Molinaro N, Cassani F, Muratori L, Lenzi M et al. *Frequency and significance of anti-gliadin and anti-endomysial antibodies in autoimmune hepatitis.* Dig Dis Sci. 1998; 43(10): 2190-5.
http://dx.doi.org/10.1023/A:1026650118759

30. Hernández L, Johnson TC, Naiyer AJ, Kryszak D, Ciaccio EJ, Min A et al. *Chronic hepatitis C virus and celiac disease, is there an association?* Dig Dis Sci. 2008; 53(1): 256-61. http://dx.doi.org/10.1007/s10620-007-9851-z

31. Garg A, Reddy C, Duseja A, Chawla Y, Dhiman RK. *Association between celiac disease and chronic hepatitis C virus infection.* J Clin Exp Hepatol. 2011; 1(1): 41-4. http://dx.doi.org/10.1016/S0973-6883(11)60116-3

32. Stene LC, Honeyman MC, Hoffenberg EJ, Haas JE, Sokol RJ, Emery L et al. *Rotavirus infection frequency and risk of celiac disease autoimmunity in early childhood: a longitudinal study.* Am J Gastroenterol. 2006; 101(10): 2333-40. http://dx.doi.org/10.1111/j.1572-0241.2006.00741.x

33. Verdú EF, Mauro M, Bourgeois J, Armstrong D. *Clinical onset of celiac disease after an episode of Campylobacter jejuni enteritis.* Can J Gastroenterol. 2007; 21(7): 453-5.

34. Collado MC, Donat E, Ribes-Koninckx C, Calabuig M, Sanz Y. *Specific duodenal and faecal bacterial groups associated with paediatric coeliac disease.* J Clin Pathol. 2009; 62(3): 264-9. http://dx.doi.org/10.1136/jcp.2008.061366

35. Sánchez E, Nadal I, Donat E, Ribes-Koninckx C, Calabuig M, Sanz Y. *Reduced diversity and increased virulence-gene carriage in intestinal enterobacteria of coeliac children.* BMC Gastroenterol. 2008; 8: 50. http://dx.doi.org/10.1186/1471-230X-8-50

36. Kotlowski R, Bernstein CN, Sepehri S, Krause DO. *High prevalence of Escherichia coli belonging to the B2+D phylogenetic group in inflammatory bowel disease.* Gut. 2007; 56(5): 669-75. http://dx.doi.org/10.1136/gut.2006.099796

37. Sánchez E, Ribes-Koninckx C, Calabuig M, Sanz Y. *Intestinal* Staphylococcus *spp. and virulent features associated with coeliac disease.* J Clin Pathol. 2012; 65(9): 830-4. http://dx.doi.org/10.1136/jclinpath-2012-200759

38. Sánchez E, Laparra JM, Sanz Y. *Discerning the role of Bacteroides fragilis in celiac disease pathogenesis.* Appl Environ Microbiol. 2012; 78(18): 6507-15. http://dx.doi.org/10.1128/AEM.00563-12

39. Brandtzaeg P. *History of oral tolerance and mucosal immunity.* Ann N Y Acad Sci. 1996; 778: 1-27. http://dx.doi.org/10.1111/j.1749-6632.1996.tb21110.x

40. Brandtzaeg P. *The gut as communicator between environment and host: immunological consequences.* Eur J Pharmacol. 2011; 668: S16-32. http://dx.doi.org/10.1016/j.ejphar.2011.07.006

41. Patsos G, Corfield A. *Management of the human mucosal defensive barrier: evidence for glycan legislation.* Biol Chem. 2009; 390(7): 581-90. http://dx.doi.org/10.1515/BC.2009.052

42. Koropatkin NM, Cameron EA, Martens EC. *How glycan metabolism shapes the human gut microbiota.* Nat Rev Microbiol. 2012; 10(5): 323-35. http://dx.doi.org/10.1038/nrmicro2746

43. Cinova J, De Palma G, Stepankova R, Kofronova O, Kverka M, Sanz Y et al. *Role of intestinal bacteria in gliadin-induced changes in intestinal mucosa: study in germ-free rats.* PLoS One. 2011; 6(1): e16169. http://dx.doi.org/10.1371/journal.pone.0016169

44. Sapone A, Lammers KM, Casolaro V, Cammarota M, Giuliano MT, De Rosa M et al. *Divergence of gut permeability and mucosal immune gene expression in two gluten-associated conditions: celiac disease and gluten sensitivity.* BMC Med. 2011; 9: 23. http://dx.doi.org/10.1186/1741-7015-9-23

45. Clemente MG, Virgiliis S, Kang JS, Macatagney R, Musu MP, Di Pierro MR et al. *Early effects of gliadin on enterocyte intracellular signalling involved in intestinal barrier function.* Gut. 2003; 52(2): 218-23. http://dx.doi.org/10.1136/gut.52.2.218

46. Ma D, Forsythe P, Bienenstock J. *Live* Lactobacillus reuteri i*s essential for the Inhibitory effect on tumor necrosis factor alpha-induced interleukin-8 expression.* Infect Immun 2004; 72(9): 5308-14. http://dx.doi.org/10.1128/IAI.72.9.5308-5314.2004

47. Victoni T, Coelho FR, Soares AL, de Freitas A, Secher T, Guabiraba R et al. *Local and remote tissue injury upon intestinal ischemia and reperfusion depends on the TLR/MyD88 signaling pathway.* Med Microbiol Immunol. 2010; 199(1): 35-42. http://dx.doi.org/10.1007/s00430-009-0134-5

48. Viatour P, Merville MP, Bours V, Chariot A. *Phosphorylation of NF-kappaB and IkappaB proteins: implications in cancer and inflammation.* Trends Biochem Sci. 2005; 30(1): 43-52. http://dx.doi.org/10.1016/j.tibs.2004.11.009

49. Vecchi M, Torgano G, Tronconi S, Agape D, Ronchi G. *Evidence of altered structural and secretory glycoconjugates in the jejunal mucosa of patients with gluten sensitive enteropathy and subtotal villous atrophy.* Gut. 1989; 30: 804-10. http://dx.doi.org/10.1136/gut.30.6.804

50. Forsberg G, Fahlgren A, Hörstedt P, Hammarström S, Hernell O, Hammarström ML. *Presenceof bacteria and innate immunity of intestinal epithelium in childhood CD.* Am J Gastroenterol. 2004; 95: 894-904. http://dx.doi.org/10.1111/j.1572-0241.2004.04157.x

51. Umesaki Y, Okada Y, Matsumoto S, Imaoka A, Setoyama H. *Segmented filamentous bacteria are indigenous intestinal bacteria that activate intraepithelial lymphocytes and induce MHC class II molecules and fucosyl asialo GM1 glycolipids on the small intestinal epithelial cells in the ex-germ free mouse.* Microbiol Immunol. 1995; 39: 555-62.

52. Bry L, Falk PG, Midtvedt T, Gordon JI. *A model of host-microbial interactions in an open mammalian ecosystem.* Science. 1996; 273: 1380-3. http://dx.doi.org/10.1126/science.273.5280.1380

53. Freitas M, Axelsson LG, Cayuela C, Midtvedt T, Trugnan G. *Microbial-host interactions specifically control the glycosylation pattern in intestinal mouse mucosa.* Histochem Cell Biol. 2002; 118: 149-61. http://dx.doi.org/10.1007/s00418-002-0432-0

54. Bergstrom KS, Kissoon-Singh V, Gibson DL, Ma C, Montero M, Sham HP et al. *Muc2 protects against lethal infectious colitis by disassociating pathogenic and commensal bacteria from the colonic mucosa.* PLoS Pathog. 2010; 6(5): e1000902. http://dx.doi.org/10.1371/journal.ppat.1000902

55. Johansson ME, Ambort D, Pelaseyed T, Schütte A, Gustafsson JK, Ermund A et al. *Composition and functional role of the mucus layers in the intestine.* Cell Mol Life Sci. 2011; 68(22): 3635-41. http://dx.doi.org/10.1007/s00018-011-0822-3

56. Rothey GA, Day DW. *Intestinal metaplasia in endoscopic biopsy specimens of gastric mocusa.* J Clin Pathol. 1985; 38: 613-21. http://dx.doi.org/10.1136/jcp.38.6.613

57. Intrieri M, Rinaldi A, Scudiero O, Autiero G, Castaldo G, Nardone G. *Low expression of human beta-defensin 1 in duodenum of celiac patients is partially restored by a gluten-free diet.* Clin Chem Lab Med. 2010; 48(4): 489-92. http://dx.doi.org/10.1515/cclm.2010.098

58. Salzman NH, Hung K, Haribhai D, Chu H, Karlsson-Sjöberg J, Amir E et al. *Enteric defensins are essential regulators of intestinal microbial ecology.* Nat Immunol. 2010; 11(1): 76-83. http://dx.doi.org/10.1038/ni.1825

59. Salzman NH. *Paneth cell defensins and the regulation of the microbiome: détente at mucosal surfaces.* Gut Microbes. 2010; 1(6): 401-6.
http://dx.doi.org/10.4161/gmic.1.6.14076

60. Vaishnava S, Behrendt CL, Ismail AS, Eckmann L, Hooper LV. *Paneth cells directly sense gut commensals and maintain homeostasis at the intestinal host-microbial interface.* Proc Natl Acad Sci USA. 2008; 105: 20858-63.
http://dx.doi.org/10.1073/pnas.0808723105

61. Fernández-Jimenez N, Castellanos-Rubio A, Plaza-Izurieta L, Gutierrez G, Castaño L, Vitoria JC et al. *Analysis of beta-defensin and Toll-like receptor gene copy number variation in celiac disease.* Hum Immunol. 2010; 71(8): 833-6.
http://dx.doi.org/10.1016/j.humimm.2010.05.012

62. Medzhitov R. *Toll-like receptors and innate immunity.* Nat Rev Immunol. 2001; 1: 135-45. http://dx.doi.org/10.1038/35100529

63. Frei R, Steinle J, Birchler T, Loeliger S, Roduit C, Steinhoff D et al. *MHC class II molecules enhance Toll-like receptor mediated innate immune responses.* PLoS One. 2010; 5(1): e8808. http://dx.doi.org/10.1371/journal.pone.0008808

64. Szebeni B, Veres G, Dezsofi A, Rusai K, Vannay A, Bokodi G et al. *Increased mucosal expression of Toll-like receptor (TLR)2 and TLR4 in coeliac disease.* J Pediatr Gastroenterol Nutr. 2007; 45(2): 187-93.
http://dx.doi.org/10.1097/MPG.0b013e318064514a

65. Kalliomäki M, Satokari R, Lähteenoja H, Vähämiko S, Grönlund J, Routi T et al. *Expression of microbiota, Toll-like receptors, and their regulators in the small intestinal mucosa in celiac disease.* J Pediatr Gastroenterol Nutr. 2012; 54(6): 727-32.
http://dx.doi.org/10.1097/MPG.0b013e318241cfa8

66. Eiró N, González-Reyes S, González L, González LO, Altadill A, Andicoechea A et al. *Duodenal expression of toll-like receptors and interleukins are increased in both children and adult celiac patients.* Dig Dis Sci. 2012; 57(9): 22778-85.
http://dx.doi.org/10.1007/s10620-012-2184-6

67. Huber JP, Farrar JD. *Regulation of effector and memory T-cell functions by type I interferon.* Immunology. 2011; 132(4): 466-74.
http://dx.doi.org/10.1111/j.1365-2567.2011.03412.x

68. Cseh Á, Vásárhelyi B, Szalay B, Molnár K, Nagy-Szakál D, Treszl A et al. *Immune phenotype of children with newly diagnosed and gluten-free diet-treated celiac disease.* Dig Dis Sci. 2011; 56(3): 792-8. http://dx.doi.org/10.1007/s10620-010-1363-6

69. Alexopoulou L, Holt AC, Medzhitov R, Flavell RA. *Recognition of double-stranded RNA and activation of NF-kappaB by Toll-lie receptor 3.* Nature. 2001; 413: 732-8.
http://dx.doi.org/10.1038/35099560

70. Schnare M, Barton GM, Holt AC, Takeda K, Akira S, Medzhitov R. *Toll-like receptor 3 control activation of adaptive immune responses.* Nat Immunol. 2001; 2: 947-50.
http://dx.doi.org/10.1038/ni712

71. Drakesmith H, Chain B, Beverley P. *How can dendritic cells cause autoimmune disease?* Immunol Today. 2000; 21: 214-7. http://dx.doi.org/10.1016/S0167-5699(00)01610-8

72. Medina M, De Palma G, Ribes-Koninckx C, Calabuig M, Sanz Y. Bifidobacterium *strains suppress* in vitro *the pro-inflammatory milieu triggered by the large intestinal microbiota of coeliac patients.* J Inflammation (London, U.K.). 2008; 5: 19.
http://dx.doi.org/10.1186/1476-9255-5-19

73. De Palma G, Cinova J, Stepankova R, Tuckova L, Sanz Y. *Pivotal advance: bifidobacteria and gram negative bacteria differentially influence immune responses in the proinflammatory milieu of celiac disease.* J Leukoc Biol. 2010; 87: 765-78. http://dx.doi.org/10.1189/jlb.0709471

74. D'Arienzo R, Stefanile R, Maurano F, Mazzarella G, Ricca E, Troncone R et al. *Immunomodulatory effects of Lactobacillus casei administration in a mouse model of gliadin-sensitive enteropathy.* Scand J Immunol. 2011; 74(4): 335-41. http://dx.doi.org/10.1111/j.1365-3083.2011.02582.x

75. FAO/WHO. *Guidelines for the Evaluation of Probiotics in Food. Report.* 2002. ftp://ftp.fao.org/es/esn/food/wgreport2.pdf

76. Tlaskalová-Hogenová H, Stepánková R, Hudcovic T, Tucková L, Cukrowska B, Lodinová-Zádníková R et al. *Commensal bacteria (normal microflora), mucosal immunity and chronic inflammatory and autoimmune diseases.* Immunol Lett. 2004; 93(2-3): 97-108. http://dx.doi.org/10.1016/j.imlet.2004.02.005

77. Isolauri E, Sütas Y, Kankaanpää P, Arvilommi H, Salminen S. *Probiotics: effects on immunity.* Am J Clin Nutr. 2001; 73: 444S-50S.

78. D'Arienzo R, Maurano F, Luongo D, Mazzarella G, Stefanile R et al. *Adjuvant effect of Lactobacillus casei in amouse model of gluten sensitivity.* Immunol Lett. 2008; 119: 78-83. http://dx.doi.org/10.1016/j.imlet.2008.04.006

79. D'Arienzo R, Maurano F, Lavermicocca P, Ricca E, Rossi M. *Modulation of the immune response by probiotic strains in a mouse model of gluten sensitivity.* Cytokine. 2009; 48: 254-9. http://dx.doi.org/10.1016/j.cyto.2009.08.003

80. Laparra JM, Olivares M, Gallina O, Sanz Y. Bifidobacterium longum *CECT 7347 modulates immune responses in a gliadin-induced enteropathy animal model.* PLoS One. 2012; 7(2): e30744. http://dx.doi.org/10.1371/journal.pone.0030744

81. Stepánková R, Kofronová O, Tucková L, Kozáková H, Cebra JJ, Tlaskalová-Hogenová H. *Experimentally induced gluten enteropathy and protective effect of epidermal growth factor in artificially fed neonatal rats.* J Pediatr Gastroenterol Nutr. 2003; 36: 96-104. http://dx.doi.org/10.1097/00005176-200301000-00018

82. Gianfrani C, Levings MK, SArtirana C, Mazzarella G, Barba G, Zanzi D et al. *Gliadin-specific type 1 regulatory T cells from the intestinal mucosa of treated celiac patients inhibit pathogenic T cells.* J Immunol. 2006; 177(6): 4178-86.

83. Salvati VM, Mazzarella G, Gianfrani C, Leving MK, Stefanile R, Giulio B et al. *Recombinant human interleukin 10 suppresses gliadin dependent T cell activation in ex vivo cultured coeliac intestinal mucosa.* Gut. 2005, 54(1): 46-63. http://dx.doi.org/10.1136/gut.2003.023150

84. Laparra JM, Sanz Y. *Bifidobacteria inhibit the inflammatory response induced by gliadins in intestinal epithelial cells via modifications of toxic peptide generation during digestion.* J Cell Biochem. 2010; 109(4); 801-7.

85. Helmerhorst EJ, Zamakhchari M, Schuppan D, Oppenheim FG. *Discovery of a novel and rich source of gluten-degrading microbial enzymes in the oral cavity.* PLoS One. 2010; 5(10): e13264. http://dx.doi.org/10.1371/journal.pone.0013264

86. Zamakhchari M, Wei G, Dewhirst F, Lee J, Schuppan D, Oppenheim FG et al. *Identification of Rothia bacteria as gluten-degrading natural colonizers of the upper gastro-intestinal tract.* PLoS One. 2011; 6(9): e24455. http://dx.doi.org/10.1371/journal.pone.0024455

87. Foligne B, Zoumpopoulou G, Dewul J, Younes BA, Charevre F, Sirard JC et al. *A key role of dendritc cells in probiotic functionality.* PLoS One. 2007; 2(3): e313. http://dx.doi.org/10.1371/journal.pone.0000313

88. Calcinaro F, Dionisi S, Marinaro M, Candeloro P, Bonato V, Marzotti S et al. *Oral probiotic administration induces interleukin-10 production and prevents spontaneous autoimmune diabetes in the non-obese diabetic mouse.* Diabetologia. 2005; 48(8): 1565-75. http://dx.doi.org/10.1007/s00125-005-1831-2

89. Veerappan GR, Betteridge J, Young PE. *Probiotics for the treatment of inflammatory bowel disease.* Curr Gastroenterol Rep. 2012; 14(4): 324-33. http://dx.doi.org/10.1007/s11894-012-0265-5

Chapter 25

Scientific Design of a Dairy Product aimed at Celiac Patients

Daniel Ramón

Biopolis SL; Scientific Park of University of Valencia; Valencia, Spain.

daniel.ramon@biopolis.es

Doi: http://dx.doi.org/10.3926/oms.222

How to cite this chapter

Ramón, D. *Scientific Design of a Dairy Product aimed at Celiac Patients*. In Rodrigo L and Peña AS, editors. *Celiac Disease and Non-Celiac Gluten Sensitivity*. Barcelona, Spain: OmniaScience; 2014. p. 495-504.

Abstract

After receiving a celiac disease diagnosis, patients need to follow a gluten-free diet. The technological bases of gluten-free products are focused on generating gliadin-free products, without providing any other nutritional benefits. Quite recently we have developed a milk supplement called *Proceliac* which aims to change this trend in the design of products for celiac patients. The basis of this product is a probiotic called ES1 that has shown strong anti-inflammatory effects in both experiments with human cell cultures and in preclinical animal experiments. The food safety of the ES1 probiotic has been evaluated following the World Health Organization guidelines. Moreover, its genome has been fully sequenced to ensure the absence of genes encoding conflicting proteins. Finally, two clinical trials on healthy adults and children with celiac disease at the beginning of gluten-free diet have been performed with excellent results that indicate this strain's ability to equilibrate the gut microbiota of celiac patients.

1. Introduction

1.1. Celiac Disease

Celiac disease (CD) is an autoimmune disease that occurs when genetically predisposed individuals ingest α-gliadin peptides from wheat or other cereals.[1,2] Clinical manifestations include intestinal inflammation symptoms and nutrient malabsorption, along with severe mucosal damage.[3] This inflammation occurs because, after consumption, α-gliadin is partially degraded by digestive proteases yielding proteolysis-resistant oligopeptides due to its high glutamine and proline content.[4,5] These peptides trigger the inflammatory immune response leading to the disease symptoms.[6-11] Along with these inflammatory effects, it should be noted that individuals with celiac disease suffer significant changes in intestinal microbiota, since it has a greater quantity of strains belonging to the *Bacteroides* and *Clostridium* genera, and a lower bifidobacteria proportion.[12-17]

CD incidence is estimated at 1% of the population, although it is estimated that, for every case diagnosed, there may be between 7 and 11 undiagnosed cases.[18] There is no therapeutic treatment for celiac disease. Therefore, the celiac individual must follow a lifelong gluten-free diet.[19] The global market for gluten-free food is widespread and grows beyond what was thought in market research early this decade. It is estimated that in 2012 in the U.S.A. alone sales of more than 4,200 million dollars were generated, and this figure is expected to rise to more than 6,500 million by the end of 2017. The 2012 annual compound growth rate stood at 28% and, more importantly, the number of consumers of such products increased from 15% to 18% in just two years.[20] Still, it must be remembered that the basis of this dietary offer is "no gluten" and that in no case products have been offered which, while lacking it, have additional nutritional or functional characteristics of interest for the celiac patients. So, a few years ago, the Asturian Milk Central, the Scientific Research Board of Governors (CSIC) and Biopolis SL, a biotechnological company, became interested in this problem and decided to tackle a research and development project that would yield a new product that would benefit the celiac patient's nutrition. It was a long-term wager, full of unknowns, but worthwhile (Figure 1). This product would be gluten-free and also have a nutritional profile that could help maintain the health of a celiac patient. The following pages describe the development of said product, called *Proceliac*.

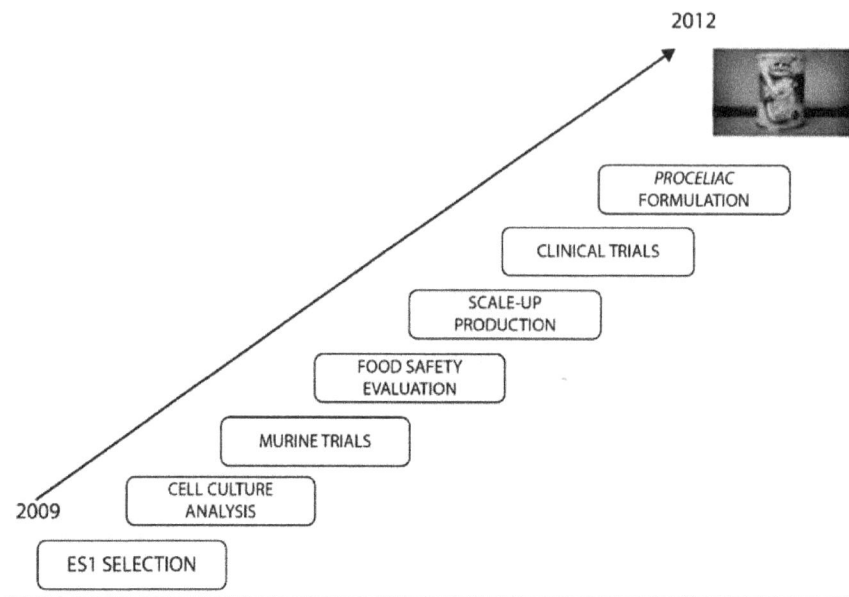

Figure 1. Proceliac development stages.

2. Selection of the ES1 Probiotic

Proceliac is based on a bacterium belonging to the genus *Bifidobacterium longum*. This bifidobacteria was isolated at the Institute of Agrochemistry and Food Technology, CSIC (IATA-CSIC) by Dr. Yolanda Sanz's group.[21] After screening hundreds of bifidobacteria isolates from the feces of children under three months of age, healthy and breastfed, they found a strain which they named ES1, which had the general properties of a probiotic. On one hand, this strain resisted extreme acidity values and high bile salt concentrations, on the other hand, it survived the passage through the digestive tract, as found in human volunteers that ingested it. It was also able to partially adhere to the surface of human intestinal cells. Besides, it also partially inhibited the growth of several bacterial pathogens found in excess in the intestinal microbiota of celiac patients.

All these properties were important since they conferred a probiotic character to the ES1 strain. Even more important was the fact that this strain partially degraded many of the gliadin peptides responsible for triggering celiac inflammation, as demonstrated in an experiment with suspension cultures of human intestinal epithelial Caco-2 cells to which gliadin samples were added which had been previously subjected to *in vitro* gastrointestinal digestion. The whole was co-incubated with the ES1 strain or other bifidobacteria and the resulting peptide mixtures for each case subjected to an RP-HPLC-ESI-MS/MS analysis. This helped determine the generated degraded peptides which were evaluated according to their toxicity. The results indicated that each bifidobacteria strain produced a distinct set of degraded gliadin peptides and that ES1 gliadin was the only one that did not produce α-β-gld (122-141) or α-β-gld (158-164), which cause inflammation by interacting with the CXCR3 receptor. Consequently, no cytotoxicity was detected only in the sample containing this probiotic strain.[22]

3. ES1 Strain Anti-inflammatory Capacity

In the IATA-CSIC laboratories it has been have shown that this strain is able to induce an anti-inflammatory response in three different cell models. The first study was conducted in collaboration with the University Hospitals La Fé and General and from the University of Valencia. Feces of celiac children, with symptoms and without symptoms, and of healthy children, were taken which were incubated with the ES1 probiotic or with a placebo. In turn, the whole was co-incubated with peripheral blood mononuclear cells from healthy adults. The results indicated that the feces of celiac children exposed to a placebo yielded a significant increase in the synthesis of the TNF-α inflammation-stimulating cytokine. In increase in CD86 production and decreased IL 10 anti-inflammatory interleukin synthesis and CD4 expression were also detected. In the case of feces from children with symptoms, a high IFN-γ expression indicative of an inflammation peak was detected. By contrast, feces incubated with the ES1 probiotic had no increased synthesis of all these inflammatory markers and, conversely, more IL-10 anti-inflammatory cytokine was synthesized.[23]

Subsequently, the IATA-CSIC group used another cellular model, Caco-2 human intestinal epithelial cells, which were treated with gliadin hydrolyzate in the presence or absence of the probiotic strain. Transcriptomics were used to quantify the expression of several encoding genes related to inflammatory response such as the CXCR3 receptor, NF-κβ and TNF-α, and the production of proinflammatory markers such as IL-1β, p50 was analyzed, as well as NF-κβ and TNF-α themselves. The results were very similar to those of the previous study, since epithelial cells co-incubated with the ES1 probiotic showed a decrease in the transcription of inflammation marker genes and, consequently, a decrease in the detection of the same.[22]

Finally, the effect of the addition of ES1 strain to human dendritic cell cocultures, Caco-2 human intestinal epithelial cells and gliadin hydrolyzate was studied. In this case, two enterobacteria isolated from the feces of celiac patients (CBL2 *Escherichia* coli and CBD8 *Shigella*) were used as controls. This work was performed within the framework of a collaboration between the IATA-CSIC and the Department of Immunology of the Czech Republic Academy of Sciences. The pathogenic microorganisms induced cytological changes in dendritic cells, such as podosoma dissolution, activation of adhesion and spreading, and also a peak in several inflammatory markers such as IFN-γ, IL-12 and TNF-α. These changes were not detected when adding the ES1 probiotic strain which also did not activate adhesion, reduced the CD40, CD86 and IFN-γ expression and increased anti- IL-10 inflammatory cytokine secretion.[24]

Finally, a proteomic study was performed in order to analyze the Caco-2 human intestinal epithelial cell secretome cultured with gliadin hydrolyzate in the presence of the ES1 probiotic or a placebo. Using 2DE and MALDI-TOF, a greater number of secreted proteins were detected in the case of the placebo than for ES1 strain. Most of these proteins were associated with cytoskeleton disorganization, inflammation and apoptosis. In the case of the group treated with the ES1 probiotic these proteins were not detected. On the contrary, the presence of proteins related to cell survival and function and calcium homeostasis was found. All these results were indicative of a gliadin toxicity decrease.[25]

4. Assays in Experimental Animals

Despite multiple efforts, unfortunately there is no animal model for celiac disease.[26] Following these tests in cell models, IATA-CSIC researchers decided to move to a study in newborn rats in which intestinal enteropathy was induced by treatment with IFN-γ. These rats were fed with gliadin and placebo or with the ES1 probiotic. After the test, the animals were sacrificed and a histological jejunum examination was performed, analyzing the expression of the gene encoding NFκβ and the production of various cytokines. The production of leukocyte populations and T-cells were also studied. Analysis of the results indicated that the group of rats that received the placebo showed changes in the structure of the intestinal epithelium, mainly a greater cellular infiltration, reduced villi width and enterocyte height reduction. By contrast, the group of rats that had ingested the ES1 probiotic had improved epithelial architecture. In addition, the rats that ate placebo had increased T CD4+, CD4+/Foxp3+ and CD8+ cells. In addition, it was found that ES1 probiotic intake reduced TNF production and increased the anti-inflammatory cytokines such as IL-10.[27] In a later study using the same animal model, an analysis was performed on the proteome of jejunal sections from animals sensitized with IFN-γ or not, which had been fed gliadin in the presence or absence of the ES1 probiotic, there being only significant differences in non-sensitized animals that had ingested ES1 compared with those who had not done so.[28]

5. Probiotic Strain ES1 Food Safety

All these encouraging results, determined the beginning of the ES1 strain food safety study which was undertaken at Biopolis SL, following the by FAO and the World Health Organization recommendations.[29] In the first stage the ES1 strain's production of toxic compounds such as biogenic amines or deconjugated bile salts was evaluated. The D and L-lactic acid productivity and their relationship where also quantified as well as the resistance levels to many antibiotics intended for hospital use. No problematic values were detected.

During the second phase, and in collaboration with the Pasteur Institute of Montevideo, an acute toxicity study was made using normal and immunosuppressed mice by means of pharmacological treatment. Both groups were fed a placebo or the ES1 probiotic. After a 9-day intake, no physiological problems were detected. After this time the animals were sacrificed and a pathological examination of all organs was performed; no abnormalities were detected. Finally, an analysis was made of the ES1 strain presence in all the isolated organs in order to detect their possible translocation. This search was unsuccessful, even in the case of immunosuppressed animals.[30]

Furthermore, the ES1 strain genome was sequenced at Biopolis SL using mass pyrosequencing technology, confirming the molecular absence of genes related to antibiotic resistance, virulence or pathogenicity factors. This study currently provides a complete annotation of the probiotic strain ES1 genome. Surely this fact will help understand the molecular basis of their anti-inflammatory behavior.

6. Clinical Trials

After the above, two ES1 probiotic clinical trials with human volunteers were conducted. Both were coordinated by the IATA-CSIC group. In the first, healthy adults were given probiotic or placebo pills for fifteen days. Subsequently, a two-week washout was performed and the groups were crossed. None of the trial participants expressed discomfort or intestinal problems or of any other type. Furthermore feces of these individuals were analyzed, determining the preponderance of the ES1 strain.

The second trial focused on celiac children who were beginning a gluten-free diet. They were given the probiotic or a placebo for three months. The study was conducted at the Sant Joan de Reus Hospital and the Sant Joan de Déu Hospital at Barcelona. The results indicated that some cell products involved in the inflammatory response are statistically reduced in a significant way in the group receiving the ES1 probiotic. Furthermore, the intestinal flora of the children receiving the probiotic had significant positive changes in relation to the group receiving the placebo, reducing *Bacteroides* and *Clostridium* counts and increasing bifidobacteria. At the time of this writing a scientific paper with all these results is being written.

7. Technological Development of *Proceliac*

Encouraged by these results, researchers from the R & D Department at the Asturian Milk Central developed *Proceliac*. To this end they combined the ES1 probiotic with a number of nutrients important for growth (calcium, iron and vitamins B1 and B5), or for the immune response (selenium, zinc, vitamins A, B6 and B12) in normal or celiac individuals.[31] It should be remarked that, regarding calcium, *Proceliac* provides 50% of the recommended daily dose while only 15% of the other nutrients (Table 1).

The product is a low-fat dehydrated milk that comes in two different formats: a family-sized can with a dispenser that offers 14 servings or a box containing 14 single-dose packages (Figure 2). Currently new product concepts are being developed which, based on these previous developments, improve the offer of these kind of products. For example, the development of this same kind of products, free of lactose and with added cocoa or vanilla is reaching its final stages.

The preceding pages allow us to conclude that *Proceliac* is a dairy product specifically aimed at and designed with celiac patients in mind. It is a new development in the gluten-free diet world by combining a probiotic and being backed by solid scientific experimentation that has produced scientific publications in prestigious journals. It should be noted that, by using it, an improvement in welfare of the celiac community is sought, but of course, this product is not intended to replace the gluten-free diet or to allow voluntary transgressions. Its role is different: to alleviate intestinal inflammation and restore the celiac patient's microbiota.

Important information	Contents of 30g/250 ml glass	% CDR
Energy value (Kcal/Kj)	105.9 / 449.6	
Protein (g)	8.2	
Carbohydrates (g)[1]	17.7	
Lactose (g)	< 0.01	
Glucose+ Galactose (g)	12.8	
Dextrose (g)	4.9	
Fats (g)[2]	0.25	
Of which saturated (g)	0.16	
Sodium (g)	0.13	
Calcium (mg)	400	50.0
Potassium (mg)	400	20.0
Iron (mg)	2.1	15.0
Zinc (mg)	1.5	15.0
Selenium (ug)	8.3	15.0
Vitamin A	120	15.0
Vitamin D	1.0	20.0
Vitamin E	1.8	15.0
Vitamin B1	0.17	15.0
Vitamin B5	0.9	15.0
Vitamin B6	0.21	15.0
Vitamin B12	0.38	15.0

Table 1. Proceliac Nutritional composition ([1] All sugars; [2] Saturated 0.16 g).

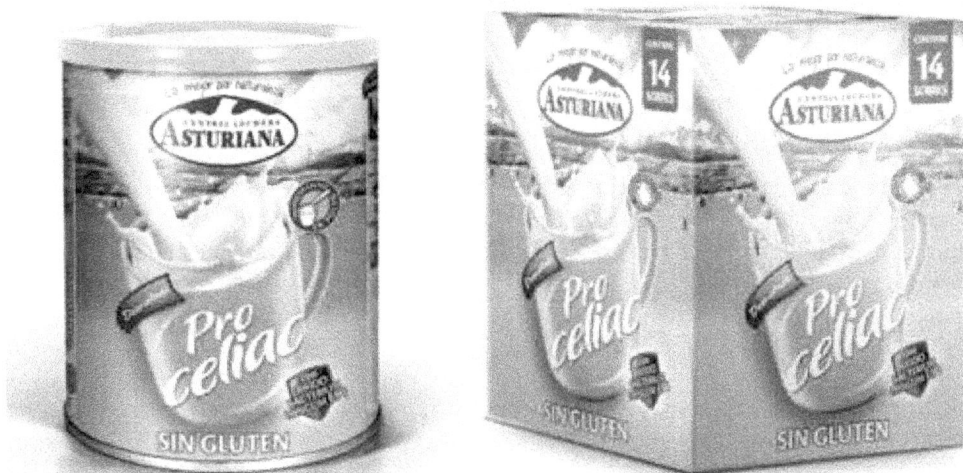

Figure 2. Proceliac formats.

References

1. Kagnoff MF. *Overview and pathogenesis of celiac disease.* Gastroenterology. 2005; 128: S10-8. http://dx.doi.org/10.1053/j.gastro.2005.02.008

2. Di Sabatino A, Corazza GR. *Coeliac disease.* Lancet. 2009; 373: 1480-93. http://dx.doi.org/10.1016/S0140-6736(09)60254-3

3. Wieser H, Koehler P. *The biochemical basis of celiac disease.* Cereal Chemistry. 2008; 85: 1-13. http://dx.doi.org/10.1094/CCHEM-85-1-0001

4. Wieser H. *Chemistry of gluten proteins.* Food Microbiology. 2007; 24: 115-9. http://dx.doi.org/10.1016/j.fm.2006.07.004

5. Shan L, Molberg O, Parrot I, Hausch F, Filiz F, Gray GM et al. *Structural basis for gluten intolerance in celiac sprue.* Science. 2002; 297: 2275-9. http://dx.doi.org/10.1126/science.1074129

6. Castellanos-Rubio A, Santin I, Irastorza I, Castano L, Carlos Vitoria J, Ramón Bilbao J. *TH17 (and TH1) signatures of intestinal biopsies of CD patients in response to gliadin.* Autoimmunity. 2009; 42: 69-73. http://dx.doi.org/10.1080/08916930802350789

7. Kleinschek MA, Boniface K, Sadekova S, Grein J, Murphy EE, Turner SP et al. *Circulating and gut-resident human Th17 cells express CD161 and promote intestinal inflammation.* Journal of Experimental Medicine. 2009; 206: 525-34. http://dx.doi.org/10.1084/jem.20081712

8. Skovbjerg H, Anthonsen D, Knudsen E, Sjöström H. *Deamidation of gliadin peptides in lamina propria: implications for celiac disease.* Digestive Diseases and Science. 2008; 53: 2917-24. http://dx.doi.org/10.1007/s10620-008-0450-4

9. Meresse B, Chen Z, Ciszewski C, Tretiakova M, Bhagat G, Krausz TN et al. *Coordinated induction by IL15 of a TCR-independent NKG2D signalling pathway converts CTL into lymphokine-activated killer cells in celiac disease.* Immunity. 2011; 21: 357-66. ttp://dx.doi.org/10.1016/j.immuni.2004.06.020

10. González S, Rodrigo L, López-Vázquez A, Fuentes D, Agudo-Ibáñez L, Rodríguez-Rodero S et al. *Association of MHC class I related gene B (MICB) to celiac disease.* American Journal of Gastroenterology. 2004; 99: 676-80. http://dx.doi.org/10.1111/j.1572-0241.2004.04109.x

11. Parrish-Novak J, Dillon SR, Nelson A, Hammond A, Sprecher C, Gross JA et al. *Interleukin 21 and its receptor are involved in NK cell expansion and regulation of lymphocyte function.* Nature. 2000; 408: 57-63. http://dx.doi.org/10.1038/35040504

12. Sanz Y, Sánchez E, Marzotto M, Calabuig M, Torriani S, Dellaglio F. *Differences in faecal bacterial communities in coeliac and healthy children as detected by PCR and denaturin gradient gel electrophoresis.* FEMS Immunology and Medical Microbiology. 2007; 51: 562-8. http://dx.doi.org/10.1111/j.1574-695X.2007.00337.x

13. Nadal I, Donat E, Ribes-Koninckx C, Calabuig M, Sanz Y. *Imbalance in the composition of the duodenal microbiota of children with coeliac disease.* Journal of Medical Microbiology. 2007; 56: 1669-74. http://dx.doi.org/10.1099/jmm.0.47410-0

14. Collado MC, Donat E, Ribes-Koninckx C, Calabuig M, Sanz Y. *Imbalances in faecal and duodenal Bifidobacterium species composition in active and non-active coeliac disease.* BMC Microbiology. 2008; 22: 232. http://dx.doi.org/10.1186/1471-2180-8-232

15. Collado MC, Donat E, Ribes-Koninckx C, Calabuig M, Sanz Y. *Specific duodenal and fecal bacteria are associated with pediatric celiac disease.* Journal of Clinical Pathology. 2009; 62: 264-9. http://dx.doi.org/10.1136/jcp.2008.061366

16. De Palma G, Nadal I, Collado MC, Sanz Y. *Effects of a gluten-free diet on gut microbiota and immune function in healthy adult human subjects.* British Journal of Nutrition. 2009; 102: 1154-60. http://dx.doi.org/10.1017/S0007114509371767

17. Pozo-Rubio T, Olivares M, Nova E, De Palma G, Mujico JR, Ferrer MD et al. *Immune development and intestinal microbiota in celiac disease.* Clinical and Developmental Immunology. 2012; ID 654143. http://dx.doi.org/10.1155/2012/654143

18. Schuppan D, Junker Y, Barisani D. *Celiac disease: from pathogenesis to novel therapies.* Gastroenterology. 2009; 137: 1912-33. http://dx.doi.org/10.1053/j.gastro.2009.09.008

19. Stoven S, Murray JA, Marietta E. *Celiac disease: advances in treatment via gluten modification.* Clinical Gastroenterology Hepatology. 2012; 10: 859-62. http://dx.doi.org/10.1016/j.cgh.2012.06.005

20. Celiac.com. http://www.celiac.com/articles/23103/1/Gluten-free-Market-to-Top-66-Billion-by-2017/Page1.html

21. Sanz Y, Sánchez E, Medina M, De Palma G, Nadal I. *Microorganisms for improving the health of individuals with disorders related to gluten ingestion.* 2009; WO 2009/080862 A1.

22. Laparra JM, Sanz Y. *Bifidobacteria inhibit the inflammatory response induced by gliadins in intestinal epithelial cells via modifications of toxic peptide generation during digestion.* Journal of Cell Biochemistry. 2010; 109: 801-7.

23. Medina M, de Palma G, Ribes-Koninckx C, Calabuig M, Sanz Y. Bifidobacterium *strains suppress* in vitro *the pro-inflammatory milieu triggered by the large intestinal microbiota of coeliac patients.* Journal of Inflammation. 2008; 3: 5-19. http://dx.doi.org/10.1186/1476-9255-5-19

24. De Palma G, Kamanova J, Cinova J, Olivares M, Drasarova H, Tuckova L et al. *Modulation of phenotypic and functional maturation of dendritic cells by intestinal bacteria and gliadin: relevance for celiac disease.* Journal of Leukocyte Biology. 2012; 92: 1043-52. http://dx.doi.org/10.1189/jlb.1111581

25. Olivares M, Laparra M, Sanz Y. *Influence of* Bifidobacterium longum *CECT 7347 and gliadin peptides on intestinal epithelial cell proteome.* Journal of Agricultural and Food Chemistry. 2011; 59: 7666-71. http://dx.doi.org/10.1021/jf201212m

26. D'Arienzo R, Maurano F, Lavermicocca P, Ricca E, Rossi M. *Modulation of the immune response by probiotic strains in a mouse model of gluten sensitivity.* Cytokine. 2009; 48: 254-9. http://dx.doi.org/10.1016/j.cyto.2009.08.003

27. Laparra JM, Olivares M, Gallina O, Sanz Y. Bifidobacterium longum *CECT7347 modulates immune responses in a gliadin-induced enteropathy animal model.* PLoS ONE 7. 2012; e30744 http://dx.doi.org/10.1371/journal.pone.0030744

28. Olivares M, Laparra M, Sanz Y. *Oral administration of* Bifidobacterium longum *CECT7347 modulates jejunal proteome in an* in vivo *gliadin-induced enteropathy animal model.* Journal of Proteomics. 2012; 77: 310-20. http://dx.doi.org/10.1016/j.jprot.2012.09.005

29. FAO/WHO. *Guidelines for the evaluation of probiotis in foods.* Joint FAO/WHO Working Group Report. 2002.

30. Chenoll E, Codoñer FM, Silva A, Martínez-Blanch JF, Bollati-Fogolín M, Crispo M et al. *Genomic sequence and safety assessment of* Bifidobacterium longum *CECT 7347, a probiotic able to reduce* in vitro *and* in vivo *toxicity and inflammatory potential of gliadin-derived peptides.* Enviado para su publicación.

31. Malterre T. *Digestive and nutritional considerations in celiac disease: could supplementation help?* Alternative Medicine Review. 2009; 14: 247-57.

www.ingramcontent.com/pod-product-compliance
Lightning Source LLC
Chambersburg PA
CBHW080120220326
41598CB00032B/4901